Foundations of
# HEALTH
# INFORMATION
# MANAGEMENT

SIXTH EDITION

# Foundations of
# HEALTH INFORMATION MANAGEMENT

**NADINIA DAVIS,** MBA, FAHIMA
Instructor (retired)
Delaware Technical Community College
Wilmington, Delaware

ELSEVIER

Elsevier
3251 Riverport Lane
St. Louis, Missouri 63043

FOUNDATIONS OF HEALTH INFORMATION MANAGEMENT, SIXTH EDITION

ISBN: 978-0-323-88218-7

Previous editions copyrighted 2020, 2017, 2014, 2007, and 2002.

*Senior Content Strategist:* Luke Held
*Director, Content Development:* Laurie Gower
*Content Development Specialist:* John Tomedi
*Marketing Manager:* Joshua Capras
*Publishing Services Manager:* Deepthi Unni
*Senior Project Manager:* Manchu Mohan
*Senior Book Designer:* Renee Duenow

Printed in India.

Last digit is the print number: 9 8 7 6 5 4 3 2 1

*Thank you to the many editorial and production
staff who worked with us for your support, encouragement,
and fabulous work.*

*Many thanks to all of the contributors to previous editions,
on whose work we have continued to build.*

*Thank you to our students: past, present, and future.
We wrote this for you.*

**Nadinia Davis**

# About the Author

**Nadinia Davis, MBA, FAHIMA**

Nadinia Davis has more than 20 years of teaching experience, encompassing associate, baccalaureate, and master's level curricula. She has held program director-level positions in two associate programs, both of which she successfully led to timely accreditation. She holds a bachelor's degree in political science from Villanova University in Pennsylvania and an MBA with a concentration in accounting from Fairleigh Dickinson University in New Jersey. Nadinia worked for 12 years in the financial services industry before returning to school to obtain her postbaccalaureate certificate in health information management (HIM) from Kean University in New Jersey. She has worked in a variety of capacities, including consultant coding, HIM department management, and revenue cycle director. Before her retirement, she held RHIA, CHDA, and CCS certifications.

Nadinia has volunteered extensively for the American Health Information Management Association (AHIMA), including a term on the board of directors. Her state-level volunteer work includes the presidency of both the New Jersey Health Information Management Association (NJHIMA) and, more recently, the Delaware Health Information Management Association (DHIMA). In 1999 she received the NJHIMA Distinguished Member Award; in 2004 she was granted Fellowship in the AHIMA; and in 2007 she was inducted into the Honor Society of Phi Kappa Phi, Kean University Chapter. In recognition of her contribution to HIM education, DHIMA named an HIM scholarship for her.

# Contributors

**Lisa R. Reilly, MSHCA, RHIA, CCS**
Health Information Management Director
College/University Adjunct Instructor

Lisa R. Reilly has more than 23 years of experience in the health information industry. She started her HIM career as a Medicare biller for a small community hospital in Alaska before moving back to the east coast to take a position as an Inpatient Coder, progressing to Clinical Documentation Specialist, HIM management, and ultimately HIM Director in both the acute and physical rehabilitation settings. Lisa also serves as an adjunct HIM instructor. She holds a BS in HIM from Stephens College and an MS in Health Care Administration from Valparaiso University. She is a member of Pinnacle Non-Traditional Honor Society. Lisa's HIM volunteer activities include various positions on the Delaware Health Information Management Association Board of Directors, including president.

**Tina M. Cartwright, RHIT, CCS**
Senior Medical Coder
OptumInsight
UnitedHealth Group
Minneapolis, Minnesota

HIM Technician
Health Information Management
PAM Rehabilitation Hospital
Dover, Delaware

Tina M. Cartwright has more than 23 years of experience in health insurance. She started as a claims processor before transferring to IT as a developer working on benefits, contracts, and membership. Upon moving to the provider side of health care, she worked in the HIM Department at Post-Acute Medical Rehabilitation Hospital and is currently employed as an HCC risk adjustment coder for OptumInsight. Tina has a bachelor's degree in agriculture from the University of Delaware and an associate degree in health information management from the Delaware Technical Community College. Tina has been a member of the American Health Information Management Association and the Delaware Health Information Management Association since 2018.

# Previous Edition Reviewers

**Patricia S. DeVoy, EdS, LPN, RHIT, CPC, CPPM**
Assistant Professor
University of Detroit Mercy
Detroit, MI
United States

**Mara E. McAuley, RHIA, CHDA, CHTS-IS**
Interim Program Director, Health Information Technology
Brookdale Community College
Lincroft, NJ
United States

**Cheryl A. Miller, MBA/HCM**
Program Director/Assistant Professor
Westmoreland County Community College
Youngwood, PA
United States

**Susan F. Slajus, MBA, RHIA**
HIT Program Director
Kirtland Community College
Roscommon, MI
United States

**Romel Celanese Smith, BS, MIS**
School Director
Urban Training Center
Dallas, TX
United States

**Janine Vance, MBA, RHIA**
Adjunct Faculty
University of Central Florida
Orlando, FL
United States

**Yolanda Maria Zesati, BS,**
Healthcare Administration, CPAR
National Louis University
Chicago, IL
United States

# Preface

The purpose of this text is to introduce the reader to health information management (HIM) both as a work-based, task-oriented function and as a contributing discipline to health care organizations, patients, and the health care industry. The sixth edition of *Foundations of Health Information Management* has been revised, updated, and expanded to reflect the most recent changes in HIM practice and the health care industry.

Ever since physicians and other caregivers began documenting their care of patients, they have had individuals working with them to help, at a minimum, store and retrieve that documentation. In the late 19th century and early 20th century, the individuals who performed that function, most notably in hospitals, were the medical record librarians. (We like to imagine these people in the basement with cobwebs and dust mites, scurrying around trying to file and retrieve charts.) With each wave of change, HIM professionals have stepped up and embraced new challenges and opportunities: computerization, reimbursement, privacy and security, electronic health records, and the current transition to health information exchanges.

The HIM profession has grown over the last 90 years as a result of HIM professionals, both individually and collectively, assuming increasing responsibilities as health care delivery has become a more complex industry. The field of HIM embraces an increasing variety of individual functions and professional competencies, and a number of national and international professional organizations reflect the diversity of the profession in general.

Since the second edition of this title, the continued implementation of technology in this field has brought about major changes in the HIM landscape and the work performed by HIM professionals. This book introduces the way the health care industry records, maintains, and shares patient health data, taking into account the evolving role of the Registered Health Information Technician (RHIT) from that of record filer and keeper to that of health care analyst, who turns data into useful, high-quality information for a wide variety of purposes, including management decision-making, strategic planning, and research.

The field of HIM today is so broad that its elements and the knowledge that individuals must acquire in order to successfully practice cannot be contained in one volume. This book is designed to meet the needs of students at the beginning of their course of study. It can easily fit into a one-quarter or one-semester course as an introduction to HIM, both in degree programs and in certificate courses such as coding and tumor registry. It can also be used by individuals who wish to acquire some basic knowledge of HIM and how it fits into the health care arena. To that end, we have endeavored to keep this text as current and comprehensive as it is user friendly, written in a style that is clear and concise, with concrete examples of the way the HIM profession works.

## Organization of the Text

This book opens with a highly relatable vision of modern health care delivery. The foundation is then laid with basic concepts of data collection and electronic health records. Building on this foundation, we construct the components of the core competencies of health information in logical sequence: what's in a record, what happens to a patient record after treatment, how reimbursement for services is accomplished, what happens in settings other than acute care, how data is analyzed and managed, and what data quality means. We complete the structure with a discussion of general management topics.

We have stressed accessibility and comprehension in every edition of this text. Each chapter begins with a list of learning objectives, vocabulary terms, and a chapter outline. A boxed feature at the chapter opener lists the exact 2018 HIM Associate Degree Curriculum competencies satisfied in the text. Although these competencies originate at AHIMA, we have labeled them CAHIIM Competencies to reflect their importance in students achieving standards set forth by the Commission on Accreditation of Health Informatics and Information Management programs. Features within each chapter include exercises to reinforce the material, summary tables and figures, screen shots, and sample forms. End-of-chapter features include a bibliography, chapter summary, a Professional Profile highlighting a key HIM professional related to the topics discussed, and a Career Tip instructing the reader on a course of study and work experience required for the position. We have also retained the correlating Patient Care Perspective, which ties the HIM professional's role to tangible customer/patient care scenarios. Finally, the text checks for student comprehension with tailored competency assessments, ethics challenges, and critical thinking questions. While ethics is covered explicitly in two chapters, it is inherent in virtually all aspects of HIM practice. Look for an Ethics Challenge at the end of every chapter.

## New to This Edition

This edition presents a realistic, practical view of the technology and trends at work, right now, in the contemporary health care environment. To that end, we brought in industry professionals to review and revise chapters in their areas of expertise. You will also see some additional critical thinking questions and a revised and updated mock RHIT exam.

One thing in particular that has not changed is the tone of the narrative. Our students have told us repeatedly that this is a very easy book to read and understand. As that was our original goal, we are pleased to maintain that aspect of the text.

For whatever reason you are reading this book, remember that it is the beginning of the journey. You will not have achieved understanding of HIM by the end of Chapter 10. You will need to obtain additional skills. You must acquire more knowledge from other sources to be a successful practicing professional in this field. Also, the industry and the profession are changing constantly. We have no doubt that some elements in this book will be outdated the moment it goes to press. However, that is the challenge of a dynamic profession and illustrates the need for lifelong learning.

We believe that HIM is an exciting and rewarding career choice for students, and we have tried our best to infuse the narrative with that enthusiasm. We hope you enjoy using this text and would welcome any comments that you may have to improve it for our next edition.

## Student Resources on Evolve

The Evolve companion website offers additional resources to students using the text. Sample paper forms are available on Evolve, enabling students to print blank copies of each form for practice.

## Instructor Resources on Evolve

The TEACH Instructor's Resource Manual provides detailed lesson plans, PowerPoint slides, and a comprehensive and customizable test bank. The lesson plans allow instructors to quickly familiarize themselves with the material in each chapter. PowerPoints are tailored to each lesson, highlighting the most important concepts from the text. The test bank includes more than 1000 questions. Each question is tied to a specific learning objective. A mock RHIT exam is tied to the 2018 Curriculum.

Instructors using this textbook also have access to a full suite of course management tools on Evolve. The Evolve website may be used to publish the class syllabus, outlines, and lecture notes. Instructors can set up email communication and "virtual office hours" and engage the class using discussion boards and chat rooms. An online class calendar is available to share important dates and other information.

**Nadinia Davis**

# Contents

## Unit I: The Environment of Health Care, 1

1  **The Health Care Industry, 1**
   *Tina Cartwright*

2  **Collecting and Storing Health Care Data, 29**
   *Lisa Reilly*

## UNIT II: Content, Structure, and Processing of Health Information, 64

3  **Sources of Data, 64**
   *Tina Cartwright*

4  **Data Quality and Management, 118**
   *Lisa Reilly*

## UNIT III: Use and Analysis of Data, 155

5  **Coded Data, 155**
   *Tina Cartwright*

6  **Financial Management, 192**
   *Lisa Reilly*

7  **Statistics and Data Analytics, 235**
   *Nadinia Davis*

## UNIT IV: Administration and Operations, 288

8  **Confidentiality and Compliance, 288**
   *Lisa Reilly*

9  **Management and Leadership, 325**
   *Lisa Reilly*

10  **Performance Improvement and Project Management, 379**
    *Tina Cartwright*

Appendix A  **Paper Health Records, 413**

Appendix B  **Electronic Documentation, 459**

Appendix C  **Using Microsoft Excel to Perform Calculations, 469**

**Glossary, 476**
**Index, 485**
**Abbreviations, 498**

1

# The Health Care Industry

TINA CARTWRIGHT

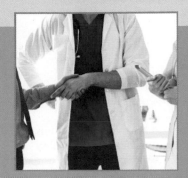

## CHAPTER OUTLINE

**Health Care Professionals**
Physicians
Nurses
Physician Assistants
Allied Health Professionals
Health Information Management
Credentials and Continuing Education
Professional Associations
Interdisciplinary Collaboration

**Providers**
Inpatient Providers
Outpatient Providers
Patient Population
Services
Facility Size
Continuity of Care
Ownership
Tax Status
Evolving Organizational Models

**Payers**
Insurance Companies
Employers
Federal and State Government

**Patients**
Customer Satisfaction
Healthy People 2030

**Manufacturing and Distribution**
**External Forces**
Federal Government
State Government
Local Government
Accreditation
Professional Standards
Independent Organizations

**Chapter Summary**
**Competency Milestone**
**Ethics Challenge**
**Critical Thinking Questions**
**The Role of Health Information Management Professionals
in the Workplace**
Professional Profile—Physician Office Liaison
Patient Care Perspective
**Works cited**
**Further Reading**

## CHAPTER OBJECTIVES

*By the end of this chapter, the student should be able to:*

1. Describe the roles of clinicians and allied health profession-als, including health information management profes-sionals, and their interrelationships across the health care delivery system;
2. Summarize the structure of the health care system, includ-ing types of providers and their patients, third-party payers and the role of the employer, pharmaceutical companies

and device manufacturers, and the interrelationships working to provide continuity of care; and
3. Discuss the external forces that guide policy-making and health care delivery, including the impact of various levels of government, accreditation agencies, and professional organizations.

## VOCABULARY

accreditation
activities of daily living (ADLs)
acute care facility
admission
allied health professionals
ambulatory care facility
American Health Information Management Association (AHIMA)
bed count
Centers for Medicare and Medicaid Services (CMS)
Commission on Accreditation for Health Informatics and Information Management (CAHIIM)
Conditions of Participation (COP)
continuing education (CE)
continuity of care
continuum of care
credentials
deemed status
Department of Health and Human Services (DHHS)
discharge
dual governance
entitlement program
ethics
health information management (HIM)
health information technology (HIT)
health record

Health Insurance Portability and Accountability Act (HIPAA)
hospital
inpatient
integrated delivery system (IDS)
licensed beds
licensure
Medicaid
Medicare
National Integrated Accreditation for Healthcare Organizations (NIAHO)
nurse
occupancy
outpatient
palliative care
patient care plan
payer
physician
physician assistant
physician's orders
primary care provider (PCP)
privileges
profession
reimbursement
resident
The Joint Commission (TJC)

### CAHIIM COMPETENCY DOMAINS

V.4. Identify the impact of policy on health care. (3)
VI.7. Assess ethical standards of practice. (5)

Welcome to the world of health information management (HIM)! We are excited that you have chosen to learn about this profession. To help you understand the HIM profession, we must begin by explaining the basic structure and terminology of the health care industry. The health care industry is an increasingly complex environment that is affected by many forces both within the industry itself, such as the rules and guidelines of health care professionals, and external forces, such as regulations and laws. As you read this chapter, keep in mind that the topics in Chapter 1 will establish the foundation for discussions in subsequent chapters as we explain the tenets of HIM.

Most people have experienced the need for health care at some time, either at birth or for treatment of a particular illness or an injury. Some people know a lot about certain types of health care because of their own illness or the illness of a family member or friend. While reading this chapter, you may find it helpful to try to recall such personal experiences to link what is presented here to your previous experiences and understanding of the health care industry. HIM professionals must be able to distinguish among

providers and organizations in the health care industry. As you read, pay particular attention to how health care facilities differ from each other, which types of professionals are employed in those facilities, and how those organizations and professionals interact with each other. The setting and type of provider will impact the rules and requirements for the documentation in the health records of the patients who receive care in that facility.

## Health Care Professionals

A **profession** is characterized by specific training in a body of knowledge that is supported by an explicit code of ethics and continuing education (CE). A professional is a member of a profession. As we discuss the various professions and their practitioners, note the variations in training, body of knowledge, and CE that contribute to health care.

Health care professionals vary from physicians and nurses to therapists and technicians to administrative and financial personnel. Each of these professionals plays a vital role in the delivery of health care. Nurses and therapists often work on teams with physicians, helping to make decisions and carry out the recommended treatments. Technical and administrative personnel support the teams by administering and evaluating tests, organizing data, and evaluating processes and procedures.

## Physicians

Most people are familiar with the health care professional called a physician, also known as a *doctor*. **Physicians** identify and treat illnesses; they make decisions about the patient's condition and advise treatment. They can also help prevent illnesses through patient education and various types of inoculations. Physicians are vital to the health care team, because typically, they are the individuals who direct the treatment plan, through **physician's orders**. A physician's order is a verbal or written direction regarding the patient's care. Nurses and professionals in other health-related disciplines help physicians prevent, identify, and treat illnesses. Identification of the illness is the *diagnosis*. A *procedure* is performed to help in the identification (diagnostic) and treatment (therapeutic) processes.

| Diagnosis | Procedure | |
| --- | --- | --- |
| | Diagnostic | Therapeutic |
| A disease or abnormal condition | The evaluation or investigative steps taken to develop the diagnosis or monitor a disease or condition | The steps taken to alleviate or eliminate the cause or symptoms of a disease or condition |
| **Examples** | | |
| Appendicitis | Physical examination | Appendectomy |
| | Blood test | |
| Cerebrovascular accident (stroke) | Physical examination | Medication |
| | Neurologic examination | Physical therapy |
| | Computed tomography scan | Occupational therapy |
| | | Speech therapy |
| | | Psychological counseling |
| Myocardial infarction (heart attack) | Physical examination | Medication |
| | Blood test | Coronary artery bypass graft |
| | Electrocardiogram | |

A physician is licensed to practice medicine. The practice of medicine is regulated by the individual state that issues the license and the requirements for licensure vary by state. Generally, to become licensed, a candidate attends college and medical school, earning a college degree as a Doctor of Medicine (MD) or a Doctor of Osteopathy (DO) (Box 1.1). He or she then serves a residency in his or her specialty. A **resident** performs professional duties under the supervision of a fully qualified physician. Residency can last from 4 to 8 years, depending on the specialty. The medical

The schools that train MDs and DOs focus on different philosophies of medical treatment and diagnosis. Historically, DOs relied on physical manipulation of the patient, particularly the spine, to alleviate symptoms of disease. MDs, on the other hand, used drugs and surgery, also called *conventional medicine*, to treat patients. The term *allopathic* is sometimes used in reference to the conventional approach. In the United States, DOs take a whole-body approach and are likely to use both manipulation (osteopathic manipulative treatment) and conventional methods. However, in other countries, the historical differences may remain. All states in the United States license both MDs and DOs (American Osteopathic Association, 2021).

Physicians are categorized by their medical specialty. They can treat patients according to the area of the body, according to specific diseases, or by assisting with diagnosis. For example, an oncologist is a physician who diagnoses and treats cancers. A gastroenterologist specializes in diseases of the digestive system. A physician who does not specialize in any particular body system or specific disease process is a "general practitioner." Physicians in general practice see patients for a wide variety of illnesses and of all ages. They consult with specialists as needed. Treatments by a physician range from ordering diet and exercise to prescribing oral medications to performing procedures, such as surgical removal of diseased tissue. Some specialties may focus more narrowly on the patient's age group; a pediatric oncologist deals with children's cancers, for example. Table 1.1 lists some common medical specialties.

licensing examination can be taken after the first year of residency. States may administer their own exam or, more commonly, accept an exam from a relevant agency. MDs take the United States Medical Licensing Examination, which is developed and administered by the Federation of State Medical Boards in collaboration with the National Board of Medical Examiners. The USMLE is a three-step examination process that tests both the knowledge and the ability of the candidate to apply that knowledge in the clinical setting (United States Medical Licensing Examination, 2022). DOs may take the USMLE or the Comprehensive Osteopathic Medical Licensing Examination (COMLEX), which is developed and administered by the National Board of Osteopathic Medical Examiners. The COMLEX is also a multistep examination process (National Board of Osteopathic Medical Examiners, 2021). Examination results are provided to the individual state medical boards for licensing purposes. Examples of differences in state licensure requirements include the years of residency and the time limits for completing the USMLE and COMLEX (Federation of State Medical Boards, 2021).

Several of the tasks that physicians perform are considered specialties, even though many physicians may perform those tasks to a certain extent. For instance, a radiologist is a specialist who interprets radiographs and images from other types of examinations of internal organs. A gastroenterologist knows how to read a radiograph, but it is not his or her specialty. A growing practice is physicians who specialize

---

◆ **NOTE**

### Medical Terminology is a Supporting Body of Knowledge for Health Information Management

If you have not yet studied medical terminology, here is a brief lesson. Medical terms consist of root words/combining forms, prefixes, and suffixes. These parts are assembled to form words that can easily be deciphered when you know the definitions of the parts. For example, we just used the word *oncologist*. This word is assembled from the following parts:

*onc/o*=combining form for cancer
*-logy*=suffix meaning process of study
*-ist*=suffix meaning one who specializes

*Therefore an* oncologist is one who specializes in the study of cancer. The following are the word parts of some of the other specialties we mentioned:

*gastr/o*=stomach
*enter/o*=intestine
*ped/i*=children
*iatr/o*=treatment
*-ic*=pertaining to
*oste/o*=bone
*-pathy*=process of disease

Can you decipher the words in Table 1.1 now that you know the meaning of the parts?

---

in treating hospitalized patients. So, although many physicians admit patients into hospitals and care for them there, **hospitalists** care only for patients in that environment.

Beyond licensing and completing the residency, physicians pursue additional training and take an examination to become board certified. Board certification is developed and administered by the specialty board that sets standards of education for the physician's specialty. The American Board of Medical Specialties is an umbrella group representing the 24 medical specialty boards (American Board of Medical Specialties, 2021). Among the 24 medical specialties, there are additional subspecialties. For example, geriatrics is a subspecialty of family medicine. A board-certified family practitioner is referred to as a *Diplomate of the American Board of Family Medicine*. See Box 1.2 for a list of medical specialty boards.

Most individuals have a relationship with a family practitioner. This physician is trained to identify and treat a wide variety of conditions. However, the family practitioner also seeks guidance from other specialists as needed. For example, the family practitioner may identify a suspicious skin problem and send the patient to a dermatologist for evaluation and treatment. The process of sending a patient to another physician in this manner is called a *referral*. The family practitioner may ask the dermatologist to evaluate the patient's condition and confirm the family practitioner's ideas or give recommendations for treating the patient. The process of a specialist reviewing and reporting their opinion regarding a patient's condition at the request of another physician is called a *consultation*.

Physicians may be in practice alone or in groups (see Chapter 3). They may practice as employees of a health care facility or have **privileges** at a health care facility. Physician privileges are determined by the facility, based on

| TABLE 1.1 | Common Medical Specialties and Subspecialties |
| --- | --- |

| Physician Specialty | Description |
| --- | --- |
| Allergist | Diagnoses and treats patients who have strong reactions to pollen, insect bites, food, medication, and other irritants |
| Anesthesiologist | Administers substances that cause loss of sensation, particularly during surgery |
| Cardiologist | Diagnoses and treats patients with diseases of the heart and blood vessels |
| Dermatologist | Diagnoses and treats patients with diseases of the skin |
| Family practitioner | Delivers primary health care for patients of all ages |
| Gastroenterologist | Diagnoses and treats patients with diseases of the digestive system |
| Gynecologist | Diagnoses and treats disorders of, and provides well care related to, the female reproductive system |
| Hospitalist | Employed by a hospital; medical practice focuses on patient care situations specific to acute care settings |
| Neonatologist | Diagnoses and treats diseases and abnormal conditions of newborns |
| Obstetrician | Cares for women before, during, and after delivery |
| Oncologist | Diagnoses and treats patients with cancer |
| Ophthalmologist | Diagnoses and treats patients with diseases of the eye |
| Orthopedist | Diagnoses and treats patients with diseases of the muscles and bones |
| Pathologist | Studies changes in cells, tissue, and organs to diagnose diseases and/or to determine possible treatments |
| Pediatrician | Delivers health care to children |
| Psychiatrist | Diagnoses and treats patients with disorders of the mind |
| Radiologist | Uses radiography and other tools to diagnose and treat a variety of diseases |

experience, education, and specialty, through the credentialing process. Privileges define what a physician is permitted to do at the facility: admit patients, consult, or perform surgery, for example. Whether an employee or a nonemployee with privileges, all physicians must satisfy the facility's credentialing process, which is discussed further in Chapter 8.

## • BOX 1.2  Medical Specialty Boards: American Board of Medical Specialties Member Boards

American Board of Allergy and Immunology
American Board of Anesthesiology
American Board of Colon and Rectal Surgery
American Board of Dermatology
American Board of Emergency Medicine
American Board of Family Medicine
American Board of Internal Medicine
American Board of Medical Genetics and Genomics
American Board of Neurological Surgery
American Board of Nuclear Medicine
American Board of Obstetrics and Gynecology
American Board of Ophthalmology
American Board of Orthopaedic Surgery
American Board of Otolaryngology-Head and Neck Surgery
American Board of Pathology
American Board of Pediatrics
American Board of Physical Medicine and Rehabilitation
American Board of Plastic Surgery
American Board of Preventive Medicine
American Board of Psychiatry and Neurology
American Board of Radiology
American Board of Surgery
American Board of Thoracic Surgery
American Board of Urology

A physician who coordinates the care of a patient, through referrals and consultations, is called a **primary care provider (PCP)**. A family practitioner is most often the PCP for his or her patients. However, not all PCPs are family practitioners. For example, some women choose to use their gynecologist as their PCP. A pediatrician is frequently the PCP for a child. Although the PCP is typically a physician, a nurse practitioner or **physician assistant (PA)** may also serve in this capacity, depending on state law.

## Nurses

A **nurse** is a clinical professional who has received postsecondary school training in caring for patients in a variety of health care settings. There are several levels of nursing education, each qualifying the nurse for different health care positions. Historically, most nurses graduated from a hospital-based certificate program. Another large percentage received their training through associate degree programs. A growing number of nurses have a bachelor's or Master of Science degree in nursing, and today, almost all nurses are college educated at some level. Nurses, like doctors, take licensing examinations. Table 1.2 lists the various levels of nursing and their educational requirements.

A licensed practical nurse (LPN), sometimes referred to as a *vocational nurse*, receives training at a hospital-based, technical, or vocational school. The training consists of learning to care for patients' personal needs and other types of routine care. LPNs work under the direction of physicians or registered nurses (RNs), or both. The extent of their practice depends on the rules of the state in which they are

## TABLE 1.2  Levels of Nursing Practice

| Title | Credentials | General Description and Requirements |
|---|---|---|
| Licensed Vocational Nurse; Licensed Practical Nurse | LVN, LPN | High school graduate or equivalent; graduation from a 1- to 2-year state-approved Health Occupations Education practical/vocational nurse program; pass NCLEX-PN examination. Licensed by state of employment or by the National Federation of Licensed Practical Nurses. |
| Registered Nurse | RN | Programs leading to registration are offered at the diploma, associate's, bachelor's, and master's degree levels. Pass NCLEX-RN; licensure in state of practice. May be eligible to practice in other states participating in the Enhanced Nurse Licensure Compact (eNLC). |
| Advanced Practice Registered Nurse | APRN (may vary in some states) | Registered nurse; completion of an accredited course in nurse practitioner training. Licensure and scope of practice vary. The National Council of State Boards of Nursing has initiated programs to encourage consensus and a multistate license compact. |
| Advanced Practice Nursing examples: | (BC=Board Certified) | |
| Adult Gerontology Clinical Nurse Specialist | AGCNS-BC | Completion of practice requirements and examinations offered by the American Nurses Credentialing Center, a subsidiary of the American Nursing Association. |
| Family Nurse Practitioner | FNP-BC | |
| Pediatric Primary Care Nurse Practitioner | PPCNP-BC | |

From American Nurses Credentialing Center: https://www.nursingworld.org/our-certifications/; National Council of State Boards of Nursing, 2021. https://www.ncsbn.org/compacts.htm. Accessed September 13, 2021.

licensed. LPNs take vital signs, monitor patient condition, care for wounds and dressings, administer certain medications, document patient status and care, and report changes to RNs or other professionals.

In addition to caring for patients' personal needs, an RN administers all types of medication and renders other care at the order of a physician. RNs particularly focus on assessing and meeting patients' needs for education regarding their illness. RNs may specialize in caring for different types of patients. For example, a nurse may assist in the operating room or care for children or older adults, each of which requires special skills and training. RNs who want to move into management-level or teaching positions generally pursue a master's degree, a doctoral degree, a specialty certification, or some combination of these qualifications. Although RNs are licensed by the states in which they practice, under the Enhanced Nurse Licensure Compact, a nurse who is licensed in a participating state and meets 11 uniform licensure requirements is eligible to practice in any member state (National Council of State Boards of Nursing, 2021a).

In response to physician shortages and nurses' desire for greater independence, several advanced degrees in nursing practice have developed under the general title *advanced practice registered nurse* (APRN) who have a minimum of a master's degree and additional training and certification beyond the RN. Although the scope of practice varies by state, an APRN usually diagnoses and treats patients and provides care under the supervision of a physician, who is ultimately responsible for the care of the patient. Some APRNs pursue specialties, such as nurse midwives and nurse anesthetists. A *nurse midwife* focuses on the care of women during the period surrounding childbirth: pregnancy, labor, delivery, and after delivery. A *nurse anesthetist* is trained to administer anesthesia and to care for patients during the delivery of anesthesia and recovery from the process.

A hospital may grant privileges to a nurse practitioner, if permitted by state law but may also require a formal relationship with a physician to do so. For example, a nurse midwife may be entirely responsible for the care of the pregnant patient up through and including delivery, but the hospital may require that documentation by the midwife be reviewed by the related physician.

The National Council of State Boards of Nursing is involved in two initiatives regarding APRNs. The APRN Compact will allow APRNs licensed in a participating state to practice in other participating states. As of September 2021 five additional state approvals were required in order to implement the Compact (National Council of State Boards of Nursing, 2021b). An APRN Campaign for Consensus, which advocates consistency in licensure standards, is also ongoing (National Council of State Boards of Nursing, 2021c).

The American Nurses Credentialing Center, a subsidiary of the American Nursing Association (ANA), offers a variety of nurse practitioner certifications in subspecialties such as forensic nursing and pediatrics (American Nurses Credentialing Center, 2021).

## Physician Assistants

Physician assistants (PAs) grew out of the need for more PCPs during the mid-1960s. Like APRNs, PAs are not physicians but fulfill some or all of the roles of a physician in certain settings. They are responsible for diagnosing and treating patients, along with patient education and the documentation of treatment. They prescribe medication, and although their scope of practice varies according to state and care setting, most PAs work independently from a physician, instead of maintaining an agreement with a supervising physician.

A PA will have earned a master's degree from an accredited school in either Physician Assistant Studies (MPAS), Health Science (MHS), or Medical Science (MMSc) and must pass the Physician Assistant National Certifying Examination administered by the National Commission on Certification of Physician Assistants. Licensure is regulated by the medical boards of the individual states (NCCPA, n.d.).

## Allied Health Professionals

Allied health professionals can include both clinical and nonclinical professionals who provide a variety of services to patients. A clinical professional is one who provides health care services to a patient, generally pursuant to orders from a physician or APRN. Clinical professionals include radiology technicians and a variety of therapists. Nonclinical professionals support the clinical staff and provide other types of services to a patient. Nonclinical allied health staff includes HIM professionals. Table 1.3 provides examples of clinical allied health professions, their principal work environments, and their basic educational requirements.

## Health Information Management

Health information management (HIM) encompasses all the tasks, jobs, titles, and organizations involved in the administration of health information, including collection, storage, retrieval, securing/protecting, and reporting of that information. Traditionally, HIM professionals have worked in departments within providers and other health care–related organizations in roles that support these activities. Over time, HIM professionals have frequently expanded their practice to related activities, including the financial and technical operations of a health care practitioner or organization. For example, HIM professionals may assist in the development and implementation of electronic health records (EHRs), oversee the maintenance of those databases, provide support services such as patient registration, retrieve data for reporting and continuing patient care, and participate in the billing process.

HIM professionals have been partners in improving the quality of health care data for almost 100 years. In 1927 the American College of Surgeons (ACS) sought assistance in the implementation of its Medical Record Improvement program. They found that assistance in what was then the

| TABLE 1.3 | Examples of Clinical Health-Related Professions | |
|---|---|---|
| **Title** | **Description** | **Requirements** |
| Occupational Therapist | Focuses on returning patient to maximal functioning in activities of daily living (ADLs). Primarily employed in rehabilitation facilities but may work in virtually any health care environment. | Master's degree; licensure required in all states; certification (registration) can be obtained from the American Occupational Therapy Association. |
| Phlebotomist | Draws blood for donation and testing. Primarily employed in health care facilities and community blood banks. | High school graduate or equivalent. Completion of 10- to 20-hour certification program in a hospital, physician's office, or laboratory. Completion of a vocational education program as a phlebotomist. |
| Physical Therapist | Focuses on strength, gait, and range-of-motion training to treat movement dysfunctions and injuries. Often works in a private office, clinic, or hospital but may be employed in many different settings. | Doctor of Physical Therapy (DPT) degree; licensure by state of practice. Currently, the doctoral degree is a requirement for certification. |
| Registered Dietitian | Manages food services; evaluates nutritional needs, including planning menus and special diets and educating patients and family. Primarily employed in health care facilities. | Bachelor's degree; registration can be obtained from American Dietetic Association; licensure, certification, or registration required in many states. |
| Respiratory Therapist | Delivers therapies related to breathing. Employed primarily in health care facilities. | Associate's or bachelor's degree; licensure or certification required in most states; registration can be obtained from the National Board for Respiratory Care. |

Medical Librarians. As the librarians embraced the challenge and expanded their formal organization, they also developed academic and credential standards. In the 1960s they accepted the challenge to abstract data from the paper records and code clinical data for input into computers. In the early 1980s, with the implementation of coded diagnosis-related groups as a reimbursement mechanism, the role of HIM professionals rose to greater prominence. Ultimately, the renaming of AMRA in 1993 to the American Health Information Management Association (AHIMA) reflected the profession's acceptance of the increasing focus on the data and information as opposed to the paper records. HIM professionals continue to expand their role and presence in health care as the demand for their skills increases.

While many of the traditional roles continue to exist, they have been transformed by the increased use of technology in both applications and communication. Virtual offices and telecommuting are increasingly viable options for many HIM professionals, leading to the description *HIM Without Walls*. This is never more dramatically illustrated than when walking a group of students through an HIM department in a hospital, during which someone typically asks, "Where are the people?" The file clerks are now scanning and indexing; the coders are working from home, and patients can download a lot of their own data from a patient portal. Another illustration of the evolution of the profession is the migration from focusing on the paper to focusing on the data that is collected. Chapters 2 and 3 talk about that data and the computerization that supports its collection and use. Chapters 4–6 discuss some of the traditional professional roles within an HIM department and in a variety of settings.

Literally, hundreds of different jobs with many different titles are performed by HIM professionals throughout the world. This text presents specific job descriptions and job titles that can assist in planning a career in HIM (Table 1.4).

HIM professionals work in every area of the health care delivery system virtually, from physician offices and hospitals to insurance companies and government agencies. They are also employed by suppliers, such as computer software vendors, and educational institutions as well as consulting firms. Throughout this text are discussions of the historical roles, emerging roles, and future of the HIM profession. As you review the opportunities available to HIM professionals, it would be useful to check industry publications and websites for information about those specific jobs in your geographic area and around the world.

## Credentials and Continuing Education

One of the standards of professional practice that can improve health care is mandatory vocational education, both formal education and CE. Formal education in the discipline supports consistency of education, research, and growth of the knowledge base of the profession. For example, physician candidates must attend medical school, and physical therapists require a doctorate. The formal

**TABLE 1.4    Examples of Health Information Management Professionals**

| Job Title/Certifications | Description | Requirements for Certification |
| --- | --- | --- |
| **Medical Coder**<br>Certified Coding Specialist (CCS) or Certified Coding Specialist/Physician-based (CCS-P) or Certified Coding Associate (CCA)/AHIMA<br>Certified Professional Coder/AAPC | Assigns, collects, and reports codes representing clinical data. Primarily employed in health care facilities, insurance companies, and consulting firms. | Certification by examination. Prerequisites vary but may include experience, technical training, or an existing credential. |
| **Release of Information Specialist**<br>Privacy Officer<br>Certified in Healthcare Privacy and Security (CHPS)/AHIMA | Specializes in privacy and security aspects of HIM practice. Typically employed in hospitals and other provider settings. | A combination of education or credentials and health care data experience, ranging from a high school graduate or equivalent and 6 years of experience to a master's degree and 1 year of experience. |
| **Data Analyst**<br>Certified Health Data Analyst (CHDA) | Analyzes health care data. Employment can be any health care or related setting. | An RHIT or RHIA certification or a bachelor's degree or higher. |
| **Clinical Documentation Improvement (CDI) Professional**<br>Clinical Documentation Improvement Professional (CDIP)<br>Certified Clinical Documentation Specialist (CCDS)/ACDIS | Supports the collection of clinical documentation. Originally working in acute care hospitals, specialists are needed in many different settings. | An RHIA, RHIT, CCS, CCS-P, RN, MD, or DO and 2 years of experience in clinical documentation improvement, or an associate degree or higher and 3 years of experience in the clinical documentation setting. |
| **Health Unit Coordinator**<br>Certified Health Unit Coordinator (CHUC)/National Association of Health Unit Coordinators | Transcribes physician's orders, prepares and compiles records during patient hospitalization. Primarily employed in acute care facilities, LTC facilities, and clinics. | High school graduate or equivalent; community college; hospital training program; completion of a vocational education program as a ward clerk, unit secretary, or health unit coordinator. |
| **Registered Health Information Technician (RHIT)/CCHIIM** | Provides administrative support targeting the collection, retention, and reporting of health information. Employed primarily in health care facilities but may work in a variety of settings, including insurance, consulting, and pharmaceutical companies. | Associate degree from accredited Health Information Technology program; registration by examination. |
| **Registered Health Information Administrator (RHIA)** | Provides administrative support targeting the collection, retention, and reporting of health information, including strategic planning, research, and systems analysis and acquisition. Employed primarily in health care facilities but may work in a variety of settings, including insurance, consulting, and pharmaceutical companies. | Bachelor's degree from accredited Health Information Administration program; registration by examination. |

*DO*, Doctor of Osteopathy; *HIM*, health information management; *LTC*, long-term care; *MD*, Doctor of Medicine; *RN*, registered nurse.

education process is often a requirement to sit for an examination that is designed to measure the competence of the individual. The specific level of competence varies from entry-level (basic) competence to advanced or specialty practice. Nursing education, for example, starts at an entry-level certificate or diploma and progresses through increasing levels of education and competencies. Satisfaction of the profession's requirements for education evidence of competence (by examination) entitles the individual to certain **credentials**. Nurses, for example, can progress from LPN to RN to APRN and can earn specialty credentials as well. Maintenance of a professional credential generally requires **continuing education (CE)**. CE for nurses is regulated by the states. Professions with a national credential and no licensing requirement, such as HIM professions, rely on their certifying bodies to establish CE requirements. Continuing professional education supports the currency of professional knowledge among practitioners.

## Professional Associations

Increasing demand for health care workers and the special emphasis on particular groups of patients have led to a proliferation of professional associations and credentials. One of the primary roles of a professional association is to improve the practice of the profession. Therefore professional associations play a critical role in the development of professional standards and improvement in health care delivery. Professional standards also have an impact on the documentation of patient care in health care records.

Professional associations are typically national (or international) and membership primarily consists of the professionals who are represented by the association. Physicians are served by the American Medical Association (AMA), nurses by the ANA, and physical therapists by the American Physical Therapy Association. Most professional associations are not-for-profit (you can tell by the .org in the website address). Professional associations are generally supported by a body of volunteers.

Some associations, such as the AMA, support the profession; however, the credentialing is housed elsewhere. Other associations, such as the **American Health Information Management Association (AHIMA)**, both support the profession and are affiliated with the credentialing body—in this case, the Commission on Certification of Health Informatics and Information Management Professionals.

HIM is an example of a category of allied health professionals with multiple related professional associations and a variety of credentials. AHIMA supports the HIM by promoting high-quality information standards through a variety of activities, including, but not limited to, CE, professional development and educational publications, and legislative and regulatory advocacy. Another organization, the American Academy of Professional Coders (AAPC), promotes the accuracy of coding and billing in all health care settings, but particularly outpatient. AAPC offers multiple credentials in coding, auditing, and training. Coding is discussed in Chapters 4–6 as it is an important HIM function. The Healthcare Financial Management Association offers professional support and credentials for health care billing functions (see Chapter 6). The Association of Clinical Documentation Improvement Specialists supports clinical documentation improvement and offers a related credential similar to that of AHIMA (see Chapter 5). Thus HIM professionals have a wide range of opportunities for both professional development and career growth.

## Interdisciplinary Collaboration

Clinical professionals work together to care for the patient. Developing a diagnosis is generally the responsibility of the physician who directs the care of the patient. The physician nurse practitioner, or PA, will also prescribe any medication or therapies. However, the care of the patient involves many different individuals, including the patient. The **patient care plan** is the formal set of directions for the treatment of the patient. It may be as simple as instructions to "take two aspirin and drink plenty of fluids," or it may be a multiple-page document with delegation of responsibilities to many different types of health care professionals. Suppose a patient has been diagnosed with Type I diabetes mellitus, a disease characterized by chronic high blood glucose that

> ◆ **NOTE**
>
> **Alphabet Soup**
> The decoding of professional credentials is simplified by familiarity with a few guidelines:
> **R**—generally stands for Registered. Individuals who are registered have complied with the standards of the registering organization. Standards may include passing an examination, completing academic requirements, and demonstrating experience in the field. Examples: RHIA—Registered Health Information Administrator, RHIT—Registered Health Information Technician.
> **C**—means the individual is Certified. This term is synonymous with Registered. Examples: Certified Coding Associate, the entry-level credential for coding; Certified Coding Specialist (CCS), the mastery credential for coding; and Certified Coding Specialist/Physician-based (CCS-P).
> **F**—signifies a Fellow. A Fellow has generally demonstrated a significant long-term contribution to his or her discipline or a specific high level of competence. Fellowship is granted in a professional organization. For physicians, board certification is expressed as a fellowship. Example: FAHIMA (Fellow of the AHIMA).
> **L**—refers to a License. Separate from other designations, licensure denotes compliance with state regulations. Individuals may be licensed. Facilities may also be licensed. In some disciplines, licensure is a prerequisite to practice. Example: LPN.
> These guidelines refer to the acronyms of the credential. Some credentials imply dual meanings. For example, RNs are so designated when they are licensed to practice.

can be controlled only with medication (i.e., insulin). The clinical professionals involved in developing the patient care plan might have the following roles:

- A nurse or medical assistant may be responsible for educating the patient about medication regimens.
- A psychologist can help the patient deal with the stress of chronic illness.
- An HIM professional can provide the patient with documentation of the diagnosis and treatment for continuing patient care.
- A social worker may help the patient's family learn about the disease and what to do in a crisis.
  If the patient is older and lives alone:
- A home health care worker may be brought in to check the patient's blood glucose level at home.
- A registered dietician may provide the patient with education about proper diet.
- A physical therapist may provide the patient with training for safe conditioning exercises.

The patient, of course, must be involved every step of the way. All the information about the illness or health problem, the treatments provided, and the directions for self-care are documented in the patient's **health record**. Clinical and allied health professionals use the health record to communicate with one another and monitor the patient's health. HIM professionals are responsible for making sure the health record is complete and accessible each time the person visits a clinical professional. A well-documented patient care plan helps all members of the interdisciplinary care team work together to deliver the best possible care to the patient.

## Providers

Think about all the different places where people receive health care services. Hospitals and physicians' offices, pharmacies and imaging centers, laboratories, physical therapists, chiropractors, nursing care homes, and many others work to help diagnose and treat patients. Perhaps, at first, the differences among these providers seem obvious—they each offer different services—but in truth many of these settings have similar capacities. For example, a women's clinic, urgent care center, and a pharmacy might all administer flu shots and other immunizations, treat insect bites, and perform pregnancy tests, and it is their operational variations that give each setting a place in the health care landscape.

Some chiropractors have X-ray machines, but the patient in a bicycle accident probably would not want to be rushed to the chiropractic clinic. A patient suffering from a persistent cold would not walk into a nursing home for treatment, even though the nursing home certainly has the staff and resources to treat it. Each type of provider has some overlap in the services offered and the patient populations it treats. Furthermore, many facilities offer a variety of services, making it difficult to describe the facility as one type. Because no single characteristic separates one provider from another, the comparison of facilities requires consideration of their many characteristics to obtain a real understanding of the differences, discussed in Chapter 3. This section outlines the primary distinction among providers, namely, the length of time during which the patient is treated, which determines whether the facility treats on an *inpatient* or *outpatient* basis. Other defining characteristics are the scope of services provided, tax status, and types of ownership.

---

 **COMPETENCY CHECK-IN 1.1**

### Health Care Professionals

#### Competency Assessment

*Match the activity on the left with the name of the specialty on the right.*

| | |
|---|---|
| _____ 1. Administers substances that cause loss of sensation | A. Allergist |
| _____ 2. Cares for patients with cancer | B. Anesthesiologist |
| _____ 3. Provides care related to the female reproductive system | C. Cardiologist |
| _____ 4. Cares for women before, during, and after delivery | D. Dermatologist |
| _____ 5. Delivers primary health care for children | E. Family practitioner |
| _____ 6. Delivers primary health care for patients of all ages | F. Gastroenterologist |
| _____ 7. Treats diseases and abnormal conditions of newborns | G. Gynecologist |
| _____ 8. Treats diseases of the digestive system | H. Neonatologist |
| _____ 9. Treats diseases of the heart and blood vessels | I. Obstetrician |
| _____ 10. Treats diseases of the muscles and bones | J. Oncologist |
| _____ 11. Treats diseases of the skin | K. Ophthalmologist |
| _____ 12. Deals with disorders of the mind | L. Orthopedist |
| _____ 13. Provides care related to eye diseases | M. Pathologist |
| _____ 14. Treats patients who have strong reactions to pollen and insect bites | N. Pediatrician |
| _____ 15. Studies changes in cells, tissue, and organs | O. Psychiatrist |

16. Table 1.1 lists common medical specialties, but there are many others. List as many other medical specialties as you can find and describe what they do.
17. Physicians diagnose diseases and perform certain procedures, both diagnostic and therapeutic. Distinguish between *diagnosis* and *procedure*. Give examples of both.
18. List three different levels of nursing education and the duty or role each is qualified to perform.
19. Much of the care for patients is performed by various allied health professionals. List as many allied health professionals as you can remember and describe what they do. Refer to Table 1.3 to see how well you did.
20. List the HIM professional credentials and what they represent.
21. What is a patient care plan?

## Inpatient Providers

We can separate providers broadly into two kinds: *inpatient* facilities and *outpatient* facilities. Before we define an inpatient, we need to understand the concept of admission. **Admission** is the process that occurs when a patient is registered for evaluation or treatment by a provider on the order of a physician. The physician has determined that the patient's health status requires the resources of a facility which can monitor and care for the patient for a longer length of time, at least overnight. To admit the patient, the physician writes an order to admit. Sometimes, the order will state, "admit to inpatient status." Therefore the term *inpatient* is an administrative status within a facility. In most facilities, the admission process involves a variety of data collection activities, which we will discuss in Chapter 3.

The admission date is defined as the actual calendar day that the order to admit was written. Whether the patient arrives at 1:05 a.m. or 11:59 p.m. on January 5, the admission date is the same: January 5.

**Discharge** is the process that occurs when the patient leaves the facility. Discharge implies that the patient has already been admitted to the facility. The day of discharge is defined as the actual calendar day that the patient leaves the facility. Note that a physician's order for a patient to leave the facility is required for a normal discharge. However, a patient may die, leave against medical advice (AMA), or be transferred to another facility. All these events are discharges as of the calendar day on which they occur.

An **inpatient** is a patient who typically remains in the facility at least overnight and whose evaluation and treatment therefore result in admission to and discharge from the facility on different days. Exceptions can occur, such

---

**NOTE**

For this discussion, we will use the term *provider* to include both organizations as well as individuals in solo practice.

---

as if a patient dies or is transferred on the day of admission. However, these patients are still considered inpatients because the physician's orders to admit the patient reveal the intention of the physician to keep the patient at least overnight. A hospital is one type of inpatient provider. Other types of inpatient facilities include inpatient rehabilitation and inpatient behavioral health.

A **hospital** is a facility that offers 24-hour, around-the-clock nursing, beds for patients who stay overnight, and an organized medical staff that directs the diagnosis and treatment of the patients.

Hospitals are governed by a board of directors or a board of trustees, which is ultimately responsible for the facility and its activities. The board oversees strategic (long-term financial and operational) planning and approves administrative policies and procedures, budgets, and physician staff appointments. Hospitals typically have shared or dual governance. **Dual governance** means that from the governing board run two separate lines of authority: administration and medical staff. The administration, headed by the chief executive officer (CEO), is responsible for the day-to-day operations of the facility, such as ensuring adequate resources for patient care. The medical staff, which includes physicians and other practitioners, is responsible for the clinical care rendered in the hospital. Fig. 1.1 shows an example of the organization of the upper management of a hospital and some of the departments that might report to those administrators.

An **acute care facility** (or short stay facility) is a type of hospital. The word *acute* means sudden or severe. Applied to illnesses, it refers to a problem that generally arises swiftly or severely. An acute care facility treats patients who require a level of care that can be provided only in the acute care setting, such as serious injuries or illnesses and surgical procedures that require significant postoperative care. The typical patient in an acute care facility either is acutely ill or has some problem that requires the types of evaluations and treatment procedures that are available in the facility. In recent literature, the term *short stay facility* is being used synonymously with *acute care facility*. However, because the term *short stay* can also refer to the length of time a patient is in a facility and is occasionally used to describe facilities that are not also acute care, this text will continue to use the term *acute care*. Typically, an acute care facility is distinguished by the presence of an emergency department (ED) and surgical (operating) facilities.

In state licensure standards, the average time that patients stay in an acute care facility is less than 30 days. Exceptions can and do occur; greater lengths of stay are not uncommon but do not have an impact on the facility's acute care designation. The average number of days that a patient spends in each acute care facility depends on what types of patients are treated in the facility. Many acute care facilities have an average patient stay between 3 and 6 days, significantly less than 30 days. Unlike acute care hospitals, inpatient rehabilitation and behavioral health facilities are not particularly characterized by the length of stay of the patients, as we will see in later sections.

## Outpatient Providers

An **outpatient** is any patient who is not an inpatient. In an outpatient or **ambulatory care facility**, patients usually receive the services on the same day on which they present. Physicians' offices, diagnostic laboratories, and imaging centers are classified as ambulatory care facilities that treat outpatients. Many therapies can also be rendered as outpatient, such as dialysis or chemotherapy, as well as some types of surgeries. Ambulatory surgery centers, also called same-day surgery centers, routinely perform eye surgeries, colonoscopies, excisions, and many types of orthopedic surgeries on an outpatient basis, wherein the patient returns home after the procedure is performed.

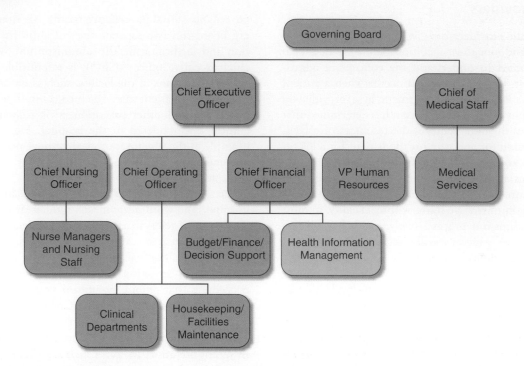

• **Fig. 1.1** Hospital organization chart. This is a very simple example of the possible organization of a hospital. There are many more possible departments than those depicted here and many different organizational structures. For example, an HIM department may report to any of the administrative chiefs, even the Chief Nursing Officer. *HIM,* Health information management.

The concepts of admission and discharge have little relevance in an ambulatory care facility because both processes typically are intended to take place on the same day. An ambulatory care admission, then, is referred to as a *visit* or an *encounter*. In general, outpatient services are rendered in a matter of minutes or hours and the patient returns home quickly. However, some hospital-based outpatient services blur the lines between outpatient and inpatient, either in duration or appearance. Two examples are emergency and observation visits.

Though most often located in part of a hospital, an ED is another example of an ambulatory care service. An ED patient is always an outpatient, even if the visit extends from one calendar day to the next, as is often the case late at night. A patient who is experiencing excessive nausea and vomiting may remain in the hospital overnight; however, the visit is still classified as outpatient. If, after evaluation, the physician determines that the patient needs inpatient care, the order to admit results in an inpatient admission. See Chapter 6 for a discussion of the billing issues related to this change in status. Sleep studies and ambulatory surgery are other examples of outpatient services that occasionally extend from one calendar day to the next.

From an administrative and billing standpoint, a patient in *observation* status is also an outpatient. These patients are experiencing signs or symptoms that may indicate a serious condition; however, the definitive etiology has not been determined. Chest pain, for example, may be acid reflux or it might signal an impending myocardial infarction. Shortness of breath, abdominal pain, and syncope (fainting) are other symptoms that may take considerable time to evaluate. For

these patients, a period of observation may be appropriate. Patients in observation status may remain in the hospital for 24–48 hours, during which time they are considered outpatients—regardless of their actual location in the hospital or what specific bed they occupy. The purpose of observation status is to give the physician an extended period in which to decide whether to admit the patient for inpatient treatment or to discharge the patient.

## Patient Population

While acute care facilities treat inpatients for a few days, there are other inpatient facilities where the focus is on patients who require longer or very different kinds of care than is routinely provided in such a short stay. Typically, these facilities are characterized by the populations of patients rather than their length of stay. In fact, some of these facilities offer both inpatient and outpatient services.

Many facilities specialize in treating only certain types of diseases. For example, the Deborah Heart and Lung Center in New Jersey specializes in treating cardiac and respiratory problems. It would not accept a patient whose only problem is a broken leg. Another common type of specialty hospital is a *children's hospital*. The medical treatment of children requires smaller equipment as well as specialized training. A children's hospital would not normally accept a 35-year-old patient.

Some types of patients are best served in a *long-term care* (*LTC*) facility, which treats a wide variety of patients who need more care than they would be able to get at home but who do not need the intensity of care provided by an acute care facility. Historically referred to as nursing homes, LTC facilities cared primarily for older patients who were ill or whose families could no longer care for them at home. Patients often moved into a nursing home and lived there until they died. Today, the philosophy of these facilities has changed so that the focus is less on making a home for the patient and more on maintaining the patient's health and preparing him or her to go home, if possible. In LTC, patients are termed *residents*. By definition, an LTC facility has an *average length of stay (ALOS)* in excess of 30 days. This is an important difference between acute care and LTC.

Another type of specialized hospital is an inpatient behavioral health facility. Patients in a *behavioral health facility* either have or are being evaluated for psychiatric illnesses. Such a facility may also be referred to as a *mental health facility* or *psychiatric facility*. Facilities that treat substance abuse and addiction are classified as behavioral health facilities. These facilities can be inpatient, outpatient, or both. Large behavioral health facilities may be administered by the state or county government. In addition, there are many small, private facilities. There is no standard in terms of ALOS. Outpatient services may be provided in stand-alone clinics or as part of an inpatient facility.

A *rehabilitation facility* treats patients who have suffered a debilitating illness or trauma or who are recovering from a certain type of surgery. One typical patient may have survived a car accident but has suffered head trauma and other injuries that require extensive therapy. Another patient may have had knee replacement surgery and needs therapy to learn to function with the prosthetic joint. The focus is to return the patient to the maximal possible level of function in terms of **activities of daily living (ADLs)**. ADLs include self-care functions such as bathing and toileting as well as practical concerns such as ironing and cooking. This type of rehabilitation is referred to as *physical medicine and rehabilitation*. These facilities may be inpatient, outpatient, or both.

A *hospice* provides palliative care for the terminally ill. **Palliative care** involves making the patient comfortable by easing his or her pain and other discomforts. Hospice care can be delivered to the patient in an inpatient residential setting or in the home. A hospice also provides support groups and counseling for both the patient and his or her family and friends. Hospice services may provide follow-up services to the survivors for up to a year after the patient's death.

As the name implies, *home health care* involves a variety of services provided to patients in the home. Services range from assistance with ADLs to physical therapy and intravenous drug therapy. Personnel providing these services also vary, from aides to therapists, nurses, and doctors.

## Services

Depending on the types of patients that they treat, facilities offer a variety of services. These services are often organized into departments. For example, an acute care facility has an ED and a surgery department. It also offers radiology, laboratory, and pathology services. If an acute care facility offers physical therapy, the physical therapy department may be small. Often, therapy is provided at the patient's bedside. Some hospitals offer acute inpatient behavioral health care, and others have no behavioral health services at all. Some hospitals have a neonatal intensive care unit to specialize in the care of premature newborns, and other small hospitals lack even a maternity ward.

A rehabilitation facility does not have an ED, but it may have a room set aside for the performance of minor surgical procedures. It may have radiology and laboratory services, but it probably does not have a pathology department. Because physical therapy is a major component of rehabilitation, the physical therapy department is large. A large amount of space is available for treatment, including a variety of specialized equipment.

## Facility Size

Another way of distinguishing one facility from another is by size. Frequently, not only is a facility described as being *acute care* or *LTC* or *ambulatory care* or *rehabilitation*, but also it is differentiated by number of beds or number of discharges. The size of an ambulatory care facility is defined by the number of encounters or the number of visits. These concepts are detailed in the following sections.

### Number of Beds

In an inpatient facility, beds are set up for patients to occupy. There are two basic ways to view beds: licensed beds and bed count. **Licensed beds** are the number of beds that the state has approved for the hospital. One can think of licensed beds as the maximum number of beds allowed to the facility under normal circumstances.

Facilities do not always use all of their licensed beds. For example, a facility may not have enough patients to fill all beds. It is very expensive to maintain the equipment and staff members for an empty room. If the number of occupied beds is low over a long period, then administrators may decide to close some of the beds. For economy, a facility may equip and staff only as many beds as it needs for the foreseeable future. A hospital may choose to offer private rooms as a courtesy or a marketing strategy, thereby reducing the number of available beds. This number of available beds, which can be less than the number of licensed beds but not more, is called the *bed count*. **Bed count** is the number of beds that the facility has set up, equipped, and staffed, that is, the beds that are ready to treat patients.

### Discharges

Another measure of the size of a facility is the number of discharges in a period, usually expressed monthly or annually. Number of discharges is a measure of activity, as opposed to a measure of physical size. Although two acute care facilities may each have 250 beds, one of them may discharge 15,000 patients per year while the other discharges 25,000 patients per year. Higher numbers of discharges require larger numbers of administrative and other support staff.

Occupancy, the percentage of available beds that have been used over a certain period, is one explanation for the difference in the number of discharges. To calculate occupancy, divide the number of days patients used hospital beds by the number of beds available. For example, if there are 100 licensed beds in the facility and there are 75 patients currently in those beds, then the day's occupancy is 75% (Fig. 1.2). The number of beds available can be based on either bed count or licensed beds. A facility may use bed count internally to monitor the rate at which available beds are being used, but it may use licensed beds to compare use over time because licensed beds are less likely to change.

The length of stay is another explanation for different discharge numbers. The longer a patient stays in the hospital, the fewer individual patients can be treated in the bed being used by the patient. Therefore, if a hospital has an ALOS of 6 days, it can treat half as many patients as a hospital of the same size with an ALOS of 3 days (Fig. 1.3).

For example, to calculate the capacity of a 200-bed hospital in the month of June, multiply 200 beds by 30 days in June to equal 6000 "beds" or "days" available to treat patients. If the ALOS is 6 days, then the hospital can treat an estimated 1000 patients for 6 days (6000 divided by 6 equals 1000). If the ALOS is 3 days, then the hospital can treat an estimated 2000 patients—twice as many as the hospital with an ALOS of 6 days (Fig. 1.4). That means twice as many admissions, twice as many discharges, and twice as much work for many of the administrative support staff who process these activities.

## Continuity of Care

With so many different caregivers working in such a variety of facilities, communication among them is essential. The coordination among caregivers to treat a patient is called the continuity of care or continuum of care. Continuity of care is a concept with two separate but related elements. First, it refers to communication among all the patient's care providers in a facility from his or her admission to discharge. As a patient moves from place to place in a facility, communication among all his or her caregivers ideally should be as smooth and coordinated as possible. This means that each individual rendering care should be aware of and responsive to all known relevant data about the patient. For example:

- The nurses need to know about the orders: What has been completed, what is outstanding, and what critical results must be communicated to the physician.
- The radiology staff needs to know whether the patient has any drug allergies if they are doing a test that requires contrast dye.
- The physician needs to be aware of the results and whether the nursing staff has reported any issues since the previous visit.

All of this is accomplished when health care professionals document the patient's data in the health record. A nurse or medical assistant collects the patient's history, including any allergies; the physician examines the patient and orders diagnostic imaging, entering this data into the health record; the radiographer reads the patient's health record for instructions, noting any allergies; the radiologist views the images and records his analysis of the imaging in the record; the physician or provider reads the radiologist's

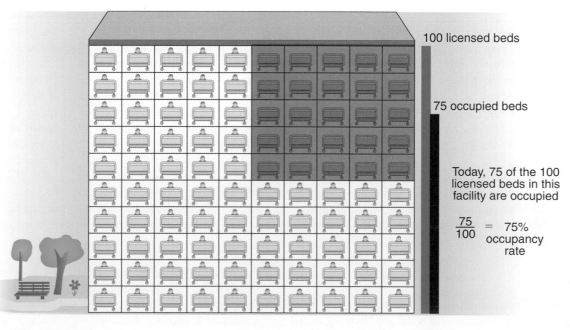

100 licensed beds

75 occupied beds

Today, 75 of the 100 licensed beds in this facility are occupied

$$\frac{75}{100} = 75\% \text{ occupancy rate}$$

• **Fig. 1.2** Calculating occupancy.

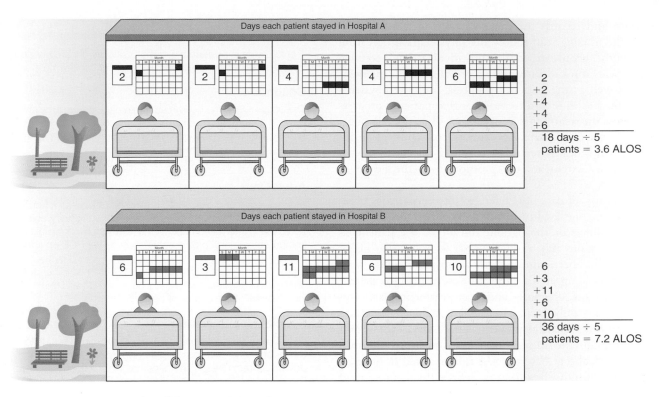

• **Fig. 1.3** The calculation of ALOS. *ALOS*, Average length of stay.

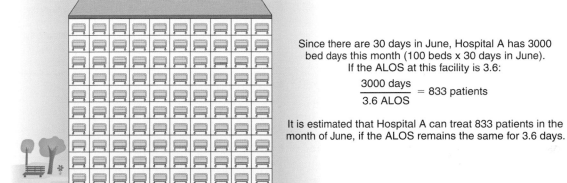

Hospital A has 100 licensed beds

Since there are 30 days in June, Hospital A has 3000 bed days this month (100 beds x 30 days in June). If the ALOS at this facility is 3.6:

$$\frac{3000 \text{ days}}{3.6 \text{ ALOS}} = 833 \text{ patients}$$

It is estimated that Hospital A can treat 833 patients in the month of June, if the ALOS remains the same for 3.6 days.

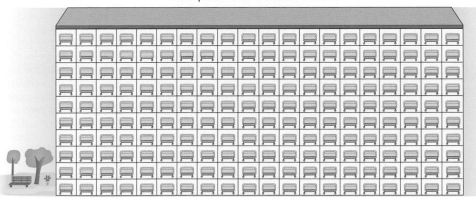

Hospital B has 200 licensed beds

Hospital B has twice as many licensed beds and therefore twice as many bed days in June:

200 beds x 30 days in June = 6000 days

But since Hospital B's patients average a stay that is twice as long, an ALOS of 7.2 days, it is estimated that it will treat the same amount of patients in June (833). Maybe Hospital B's patients were more severely ill or maybe Hospital A is just more efficient.

Because Hospital A has a shorter ALOS it can treat about the same amount of patients in June as Hospital B, even though Hospital B is twice the size.

$$\frac{6000 \text{ days}}{7.2 \text{ ALOS}} = 833 \text{ patients}$$

• **Fig. 1.4** The comparison of ALOS in two facilities. *ALOS*, Average length of stay.

findings, and records the diagnosis and orders for treatment; the nursing staff follow the physician's orders from the health record to administer medications, perform patient teaching and care, and record all of their interventions as well as the patient's progress; and the physician checks the health record to monitor that patient's progress and adjust the treatments as necessary. Thus the complete, comprehensive, accurate, and timely collection of health data into the health record is required for continuity of care and, by extension, the promotion of the health of the patient.

Continuity of care also refers to all the patient's experiences from one facility to another, either throughout a particular illness or throughout the life of the patient, as illustrated in Box 1.3. A PCP needs to know that his or her patient has been admitted to the hospital so that he or she can follow up at discharge to ensure that the patient understands the diagnosis and the treatment plan. This follow-up not only helps the patient manage the illness effectively but also helps prevent unnecessary readmissions to the hospital. The seamless continuity of care as described here is an ideal that has yet to be fully realized in practice. The World Health Organization defines this continuity of care as *integrated care*: a concept bringing together inputs, delivery, management, and organization of services related to diagnosis, treatment, care, rehabilitation, and health promotion. Integration is a means to improve services in relation to access, quality, user satisfaction, and efficiency (O Gröne, 2021).

## Ownership

Health care facilities may exist under many different types of ownership. Some facilities, such as physician group practices and radiology centers, are owned by individuals or groups of individuals. Facilities may also be owned by corporations, government entities, or religious groups. Hospital Corporation of America (HCA) is a corporation that owns many facilities. The Veterans Administration facilities are examples of government-owned facilities. The Catholic Church operates many hospitals throughout the country. Frequently, the ownership of the organization has an impact on both the operations and the services provided by the facility. For example, a facility owned by a religious organization may not allow abortions to be performed by their physicians. A government-owned facility may require supplies to be purchased from government-approved vendors.

## Tax Status

Another way to distinguish institutions from one another is by their tax status: for-profit or not-for-profit. A for-profit, or proprietary, organization has owners. It can have few or many owners (or shareholders). HCA is an example of a for-profit organization with many shareholders. A not-for-profit institution operates solely for the good of the community and is considered to be owned by the community. It has

---

### • BOX 1.3   Continuity of Care Across the Life span

The following is an example of the continuity of care needed to treat a particular female patient throughout her lifetime.

#### Childhood

The patient, Emily, is born in an acute care facility. As a child, Emily is treated by a pediatrician. The pediatrician is her PCP. She receives extensive well-child care: preventive vaccinations, checkups, and developmental assessments. Each visit is documented in Emily's health care record.

#### Adult Care

As Emily ages and grows into adulthood, she visits a family practitioner as her new PCP. The family practitioner would benefit from having information about all of Emily's childhood diseases, immunizations, and problems. Emily sees her PCP on a regular basis. As she becomes an adult, she also visits a gynecologist for regular examinations. Emily moves several times in her adult life, changing physicians each time. The new PCP and gynecologist would benefit from copies of her prior records.

#### Special Health Issues

When Emily becomes pregnant, she is examined and followed by her obstetrician throughout the pregnancy and cesarean delivery. Later in life, as she becomes older, other illnesses arise. For example, in her late 30s, Emily develops diabetes. Her PCP refers her to an endocrinologist for treatment of the diabetes. After Emily discovers a lump in her breast, she undergoes mammography and is referred to a surgeon for a diagnosis. Then she enters an acute care facility to have a lumpectomy. Note that at this point, Emily has had at least three admissions to an acute care facility and has visited at least three specialists in addition to her PCP. When she is seeing specialists concurrently, it is important for Emily to ask them to communicate with one another about her care. To do so, each specialist will need to share the documentation they added to Emily's health care record. This communication helps avoid unnecessary duplication of tests and conflicting plans of care.

#### Elder Care

Maturing past menopause, Emily falls and breaks her hip. She needs to have a hip replacement and is treated by an orthopedic surgeon in an acute care facility for hip replacement surgery, after which she is transferred to a rehabilitation facility for a couple of weeks of rehabilitation to enable her to resume her ADLs. Eventually, Emily becomes incapacitated and is unable to take care of herself. She is diagnosed with Alzheimer's disease and is seen by a neurologist and a psychiatrist. Ultimately, she is admitted to a nursing home for 24-hour monitored nursing care.

Throughout these encounters with various facilities and specialists, the history of Emily's care should follow her smoothly. The orthopedic surgeon will want to know her experiences under anesthesia when she had breast surgery and her reaction to anesthesia when her baby was born. This information should be available to subsequent surgeons. Emily can maintain a personal health record (PHR): copies of important documents such as operative reports, discharge summaries, immunizations, and test results. Her PHR can be a folder with the paper documents or an electronic file. There are also websites on which Emily can maintain her data. Increasingly, physicians and some hospitals are providing patient access to certain elements of the patient's records for this purpose. As the technology evolves, the communication among caregivers, and hence the continuity of care, is facilitated.

no shareholders who have a vested interest in the economic viability of the organization. Not-for-profit institutions enjoy certain tax benefits, including exemption from property and certain corporate income taxes. Most community hospitals are not-for-profit.

Although for-profit institutions are often criticized, the tax status of an organization should have little or no impact on the day-to-day operations of the organization. The fundamental impact is on the distribution of net income. Net income is the excess of revenue (mostly income from patient services) over expenses (the resources used to provide the services) over a specified period. In a not-for-profit organization, net income (called *surplus*) must be used for charitable purposes. In a for-profit organization, net income belongs to the shareholders and may, at the discretion of the board of directors, be distributed in whole or in part to these owners of the organization. Because board members are elected by the shareholders, the board is answerable to them.

## Evolving Organizational Models

Hospital mergers have increased in recent years. Many health care organizations are consolidating along the continuum of care. In other words, they are not just buying multiple acute care facilities; they are buying physician's office practices, rehabilitation facilities, and LTC facilities as well as acute care facilities. Thus they can provide patients with seamless coordination of care along this continuum. Such enterprises are referred to as **integrated delivery systems (IDSs)**. Many see this approach as an efficient delivery of health care throughout a patient's lifetime. As these new health care organizations evolve, they are coordinating the exchange of health information among the various health care providers. Sometimes the organizations that join will share the same EHR system; in other situations, they may use a health information exchange to share information on their patients. We will discuss these scenarios further in Chapter 2. Evolving relationships among PCPs and other providers, as well as the emphasis on alternatives to expensive inpatient care, have led to the development of *Accountable Care Organizations (ACOs)* and the *Medical Home model.*

The *Medical Home model* has its foundation in the concept that the PCP is the gatekeeper for services to patients and the coordinator of those services. In this model, the PCP does not just refer patients to specialists but also coordinates the follow-up and any subsequent required care. In this model, the PCP is the patient's "home" for all medical care, regardless of the actual provider rendering the service. Transitioning from one setting to another is a key component of the Medical Home model.

Normally, all providers are paid separately for care that is rendered to patients. Physicians who care for patients in acute care facilities are entitled to payment separate from the hospital's facility charges. Because inpatient care is expensive, one way to incentivize hospitals and physicians to work together toward efficient and effective inpatient care is through *ACOs*, in which payment for inpatient services flows through the hospital and out to other providers. In this manner, the hospital and the physicians have a vested interest in working together to ensure the necessity and efficiency of services rendered. We will discuss ACOs in more detail in Chapter 6.

## ❖ COMPETENCY CHECK-IN 1.2

### Providers

#### Competency Assessment

1. What are the characteristics of a hospital?
2. The fundamental difference between ambulatory care and acute care is the patient's length of stay. Ambulatory patients are called *outpatients*, and acute care patients are called *inpatients*. In your own words, describe the differences between the two. What problems arise in an acute care facility in distinguishing between an outpatient and an inpatient? What are some other differences between ambulatory care and acute care?
3. Define admission and discharge.
4. If a patient is admitted as an inpatient on Monday at 10 a.m. but dies on Monday at 3 p.m., is that patient still considered an inpatient?
5. A hospital with an average length of stay of less than 30 days, an ED, operating suite, and clinical departments to handle a broad range of diagnoses and treatments is most likely a(n) _____.
6. A specialty inpatient facility that focuses on the treatment of individuals with psychiatric disorders is a(n) _____.
7. Care for the terminally ill is the focus of _____ care.
8. The Community Care Center has 200 beds. It has an average length of stay of 2 years. Most of the patients are older, but there are some younger patients with serious chronic illnesses. Community Care Center is most likely a(n) _____.
9. _____ focuses on treating patients where they reside.
10. What is the difference between a facility's bed count and its number of licensed beds?
11. Chapone Health Care is an organization that owns a number of different health care facilities: three acute care hospitals, two LTC facilities, and a number of physician offices. Chapone also owns a rehabilitation hospital and an assisted living facility, which also delivers home care. This organization delivers care to patients at every point along the continuum of care. Chapone Health Care can be described as a(n) _____ _____.
12. The coordination among caregivers to provide services to a patient within a facility or among different providers is referred to as _____.

## Payers

When providers render a service, they expect to be compensated. The payment to a health care provider is called a **reimbursement**. The individual or organization responsible for compensating the provider is called the **payer**. The payer may be the patient, government entity, or it may be an insurance company, for example. In Chapter 6, we will discuss insurance and the financial relationships among these parties.

## Insurance Companies

Insurance companies have existed for centuries. Notably, Lloyd's of London insured cargoes on merchant ships, which were frequently subject to loss from piracy, inclement weather, and other catastrophes. The beginnings of insurance in health care date only to the mid-19th century, when companies insured railroad and paddleboat employees in the event of catastrophic injury or death. A lump sum was paid to an employee or employee's family after such an event.

The origins of modern health care insurance, as we know it today in the United States, began during the Great Depression in the 1930s. A decline in health care industry income prompted the development of hospital-based insurance plans. For a payment of a small sum, a hospital guaranteed a specific number of days of hospital care at no additional charge. The most successful of these plans was developed at Baylor University by Justin Ford Kimball (Sultz and Young, 2006; Blue Cross, 2021)—Baylor's plan eventually became the model for what we know today as the Blue Cross plans.

To obtain insurance, an individual pays a fixed amount of money each month, called a *premium*. In exchange for the monthly premium, the health insurer pays for all or part of the individual's medical bills in the event he or she needs care. Often, the insurer requires the individual to share the cost of care through *deductibles*, *copays*, and *coinsurance*, commonly called "out-of-pocket" costs. We will explore these concepts in detail in Chapter 6. Table 6.1 contains definitions of several terms that are useful during any discussion of health insurance.

In the early days of the industry, health care insurance was paid for by the recipient of the coverage, sometimes through the employer, union, or other organizations. In the original Baylor University scheme, teachers paid $0.50 a month, which entitled them to 21 days of hospital care should they need it (Sultz and Young, 2006). The insurance company became what is called a *third-party payer* in the relationship between the provider and patient.

## Employers

Some people today purchase their health insurance privately from an insurance company, but most people have health insurance through their employer. During World War II, some companies started offering health insurance as an employee benefit. Soon employers around the country began to offer paid health insurance to attract employees. Employer-sponsored health coverage grew in popularity in the years that followed. In 2019 49.6% of Americans aged 18–65 received their health insurance coverage through their employer (Kaiser Family Foundation, 2021). You can think of the employer as the fourth party in the physician–patient–payer–employer relationship.

Because of their position as a payer, employers have a very large role in the structure of the health care system. As the cost of health care rises, so do insurance premiums. Employers routinely shop the alternatives as they attempt to control their insurance costs. Such negotiations affect the coverage available to employees. To lower premiums, employers may choose an insurance plan that does not cover some services. The employer may also decide to lower its premiums by pushing more of the cost of services to employees in the form of higher deductibles or copays. Employees may also be incentivized to seek less expensive treatment options, such as using a particular laboratory for testing and a mail-order pharmacy service as opposed to local laboratories and pharmacies. For employees, annual changes in plans because of price sensitivity can lead to a decrease in insurance choices. These are just some examples of how employers have an impact on the health care industry in general.

## Federal and State Government

At the same time, rates of employer-sponsored coverage grew in the 1950s and 1960s, and expensive new technologies promised life-saving treatments. The cost of hospital care skyrocketed, and the cost of health insurance rose along with it. Policymakers soon realized that the problem with relying on employers to pay health care costs is that those who do not work have less access to health insurance. The country's most vulnerable populations—the elderly, the unemployed, and the very poor—were unable to purchase affordable insurance coverage. In 1965 Title XVIII and Title XIX of the Social Security Act initiated **Medicare** to pay for health care for the elderly and **Medicaid** to help pay for the health care of the poor. The federal government became the payer for millions of Americans. Medicare and Medicaid are called **entitlement programs** because their benefits are guaranteed to anyone who meets certain requirements, like age, employment status, or other circumstances. A federal agency called the **Centers for Medicare and Medicaid Services (CMS)** oversees both programs, although individual states administer Medicaid based on their needs. Today, CMS covers most of the cost of health care for over 120 million people and is the largest payer in the United States.

## Patients

Historically, patients played little role in their own care other than to devise ways to pay for it. In recent decades, though, partly in response to rising out-of-pocket costs and partly because of increased availability of medical information, patients have played an increasing role in the direction of their own care. Hence, the industry trends toward patient-centered care.

## Customer Satisfaction

One driver of the focus on patients is their increasing importance in measuring the quality of care. We will discuss this in greater detail in Chapter 10, but for now, think of customer satisfaction as an important measure of quality. If patients at hospital A report that the care areas are noisy, unfriendly, or unclean, then hospital A will get a poorer rating for these factors than hospital B, the patients' report of which is quiet, friendly, and clean. This is not merely a social media observation, a blog, or a comment on the provider's website. There are multiple, professional, and in some cases regulatory surveys that are used to formally collect this type of feedback, which is then published on websites.

## Healthy People 2030

The US government has an interest in monitoring and improving the health and well-being of the public. Healthy People is a national program that gathers and compiles data on the indicators of health, reflecting major health threats in the United States. These health indicators include data on individual behaviors, like tobacco use, substance abuse, and nutrition; environmental factors like air and water quality; social factors like sexual health and violence; mental health; oral health; maternal, infant, and child health; as well as the ability of people to access health care and preventive services. Combined, these indicators are designed to grant policymakers insight into the overall health of the population, as well as the health of population subsets. Within these topic areas, policymakers create measurable objectives to address the causes of poor health. These topic areas and objectives, currently up to 355, are updated every 10 years to promote the health of all Americans. The Department of Health and Human Services (DHHS), Office of Disease Prevention and Health Promotion, works in collaboration with other agencies and communities across the country to achieve the objectives of each plan. Information on the current Healthy People plan can be found on the website healthypeople.gov.

## Manufacturing and Distribution

The cost of health care is not all about the providers and insurers. The manufacture and distribution of supplies, medical devices, and pharmaceuticals, for example, also contribute to the cost of care. Everything from bandages to cardiac pacemakers to aspirin must be developed, manufactured, marketed, sold, and delivered to the end user.

Pharmaceutical companies often cite research and development costs as a main cause of high drug prices. Similarly, computer-based operating tools require years of trials and intense hours of training before they can be used on patients. Genetics-based cancer treatments designed specifically for the individual patient also require long development periods. These technological advances have vastly improved patient outcomes and life spans but have also made the cost of care more and more expensive.

Once developed, products need to be manufactured. The availability of materials and appropriately skilled labor as well as the cost of all components of the process will drive where and how the manufacturing will take place. Outsourcing manufacture to contractors around the world is not uncommon. The supply shortages experienced during the COVID-19 pandemic illustrated some of the difficulties that arise in a global marketplace. Masks, pharmaceuticals, and semiconductors are just a few examples of supply shortages that resulted from sudden, increased demand combined with slowdowns in manufacturing and shipping.

An increasingly common phenomenon is the marketing of products not just to the providers who will use or recommend them but also directly to patients. Patients in turn are urged to speak to their provider about whether the product is right for them. Providers can experience pressure from patients to prescribe a new drug or other product, even though a less expensive, well-known alternative is available.

## External Forces

Various facilities have different ways of operating, but the mandate under which activities are performed often arises from legislation, regulation, and accreditation requirements.

Federal, state, and local governments all have an impact in varying degrees on health care institutions and delivery. For example, patients have guaranteed rights at the federal level as well as at the state level through court actions, laws, and regulations, depending on the state. The legal and regulatory environment is discussed in greater detail in Unit IV, but the following discussion is a general overview of how government affects health care. Table 1.5 summarizes the agencies of the federal government that impact health care.

### Federal Government

The federal government has a major impact on health care through policy and regulatory activity. The federal legislature enacts laws, which the executive branch must then enforce. For example, a patient's right to privacy is mandated at the federal level by the privacy provisions of the Health Insurance Portability and Accountability Act (HIPAA). Hospital EDs are required to evaluate patients regardless of their ability to pay, per the Emergency Medical Treatment and Active Labor Act. Another important area of

| Department | Agency | Health-Related Functions |
|---|---|---|
| Department of Health and Human Services | Food and Drug Administration | Ensures safety of foods, cosmetics, pharmaceuticals, biological products, and medical devices |
| | Centers for Medicare and Medicaid Services | Oversees Medicare and the federal portion of Medicaid |
| | National Institutes of Health | Supports biomedical research |
| | Centers for Disease Control and Prevention | Provides a system of health surveillance to monitor and prevent outbreak of diseases |
| | Health Resources and Services Administration | Helps provide health resources for medically underserved populations |
| | Indian Health Service | Supports a network of health care facilities and providers to American Indians and Alaska Natives |
| | Office for Civil Rights | Protects patients from discrimination in health care |
| Department of Defense | Military Health Services System | Maintains a network of health care providers and facilities for service personnel and their dependents |
| Department of Veterans Affairs | Veterans Affairs facilities | Maintains a network of facilities and services for armed services veterans and sometimes their dependents |
| Department of Labor | Occupational Safety and Health Administration | Regulates workplace health and safety |

**TABLE 1.5  Federal Agencies Involved in Health Care**

different agencies including the following that play key roles related to health care delivery in the United States:

- **Centers for Medicare and Medicaid Services (CMS)**: This agency administers Medicare and part of Medicaid.
- **Agency for Healthcare Research and Quality**: This agency supports quality health care by providing research in a meaningful way so that it can be used by health care providers and policymakers.
- **Office of the National Coordinator for Health Information Technology**: This office coordinates efforts for the use of health information technology (HIT) and electronic exchange of health information (Office of the National Coordinator for Health Information Technology, 2021).
- **Centers for Disease Control and Prevention**: This agency protects the people of the United States from various health threats by providing a system of health surveillance to monitor and prevent outbreaks of diseases.
- **Office of Inspector General**: This agency monitors compliance with Medicare and Medicaid rules/regulations.
- **National Institutes of Health**: This agency provides leadership, coordination, and funding for medical research in the United States and around the world.
- **Food and Drug Administration**: This agency monitors the nation's food supply as well as the safety and effectiveness of drugs and medical devices.
- **Health Resources and Services Administration**: This agency administers programs to improve access to health care services for people who are geographically isolated or medically vulnerable. It also oversees organ, bone marrow, and cord blood donation.
- **Indian Health Service**: This agency provides health services to American Indians and Alaska Natives.
- **Substance Abuse and Mental Health Services Administration**: This agency engages in public health efforts to reduce the impact of mental illness and substance abuse.

As we have seen, Medicare is an entitlement to health care benefits for persons of advanced age (older than 65 years) or those with certain chronic illnesses (e.g., end-stage renal disease). Health care facilities are not automatically eligible for full reimbursement from Medicare simply based on treating a Medicare patient. To be eligible for full reimbursement from Medicare, a health care facility must comply with Medicare's **Conditions of Participation (COP)**. COP standards include the quality of providers, certain policies and procedures, and financial issues; these are updated in the *Code of Federal Regulations* and published in the *Federal Register*.

## State Government

Aside from the administration of Medicaid and Children's Health Insurance Program, the impact of state government on health care organizations varies from state to state and consists primarily of licensure and reporting.

federal regulation concerns the release of information pertaining to patients with drug and alcohol diagnoses.

Enforcement arises from the delegation of executive responsibilities to various agencies. In terms of health care, the critical regulatory agency is the **Department of Health and Human Services (DHHS)**, which includes many

## Licensure

For operation of any health care facility, a license must be obtained from the state in which the facility will operate. The process of **licensure** varies among states. Often, the state's legislature passes a hospital licensing act or a similar law that requires hospitals to be licensed and delegates the authority to regulate that process to a state agency, possibly the state's Department of Health. The delegated agency then develops and administers the detailed regulations, which are part of the state's administrative code. The licensure regulations contain a great deal of useful information pertaining to the operations of a health care facility, including the minimum requirements for maintaining patient records. Some states' regulations are very detailed and specific as to the organization and structure of a facility, including such items as services to be provided, medical staff requirements, nursing requirements, committees, and sanitation. Licensure is specific to the type of health care facility being operated. The regulations governing acute care facilities differ somewhat from those for LTC facilities, which are in turn different from those for rehabilitation facilities.

It is fundamentally the responsibility of the board of directors or board of trustees of a facility to ensure compliance with each of the requirements of the license. The board delegates the day-to-day operations of the facility to management, through the CEO or administrator of the hospital.

> **NOTE**
>
> **Abbreviations and Acronyms**
> You may have noticed that many of the terms and phrases used in health care frequently are shortened to a few recognizable letters. An abbreviation made from the initial letters or parts of a term is called an *acronym*. Acronyms and other abbreviations shorten writing time and save space. However, acronyms can also cause confusion. AMA, for example, means "against medical advice." It is also the abbreviation for the American Medical Association and the American Management Association. There are also interdisciplinary issues with abbreviations. "Dr." means doctor to a health care professional. To an accountant, it means debit. Therefore abbreviations should be used carefully. Health care facilities must define acceptable abbreviations and should restrict the use of abbreviations to only those that have been approved. CMS maintains an acronyms and abbreviations lookup tool at https://www.cms.gov/acronyms.

Many state agencies visit hospitals regularly and review the hospital operations and the documentation for compliance with the license of the facility. Of note are LTC facilities, which tend to be scrutinized very closely. State surveyors may visit a facility as part of a general audit plan or in response to patient complaints. CMS may also delegate to state surveyors the task of conducting COP reviews.

## Reporting

A tremendous amount of reporting occurs among health care facilities and state agencies. Typically, reporting includes information about general patient data, cancer, trauma, birth defects, and infectious disease. Additional reporting may result from health care workers' observation of inappropriate activities, such as child abuse; health care workers have an obligation to report certain types of suspected abuses to the authorities.

One of the key reporting relationships between health care facilities and the state is the reporting of service activity. States typically require the transmission of specific data about patients, which is discussed in Chapter 2. For example, the New Jersey Department of Health and Senior Services requires acute care facilities to upload all acute, ambulatory surgical, and ED discharges electronically to the New Jersey Discharge Data Collection System. States use this activity data to study the patterns of use of health care facilities and allocate resources for underserved populations, for example. The federally required component of the data collected is then forwarded to the federal government (See Data Sets, Chapter 2).

## Local Government

Local government may also become involved in health care organizations, particularly in the aspect of zoning regulations. For example, a health care organization is a business, and zoning regulations may require that businesses be located only in certain areas of a town. If a health care organization is not-for-profit, it is likely exempt from property taxes. A facility that is not taxable is an economic burden to the local government. Therefore health care organizations often become deeply intertwined with the interests of the communities in which they are located. Current Internal Revenue Service regulations require not-for-profit organizations, including hospitals, to measure and report the benefit that they provide to their communities.

## Accreditation

Another issue that has a visible impact on the operation of a health care facility is voluntary accreditation. Whereas licensure is mandatory to operate a health care facility within a given state, accreditation is voluntary.

**Accreditation** begins with voluntary compliance with a set of standards that are developed by an independent organization. That organization then audits the facility to ensure compliance. Examples of accreditation standards include the existence and enforcement of policies and procedures regarding activities surrounding medical staff, environment of care, information management, and provision of care. Numerous accrediting bodies exist for different industries. Table 1.6 lists some health care accrediting bodies and the subjects of their activities.

### The Joint Commission

Within the health care industry, the most important accrediting body is **The Joint Commission** (TJC). TJC is an organization located in Chicago that sets standards for acute

| TABLE 1.6 | Accrediting Organizations in Health Care |
| --- | --- |
| **Accrediting Organization** | **Facilities/Organizations Accredited** |
| Accreditation Association for Ambulatory Health Care (AAAHC) | Ambulatory care facilities |
| American Osteopathic Association (AOA) | Osteopathic hospitals |
| The Joint Commission (TJC) | Acute care, ambulatory care, behavioral health LTC, and rehabilitation facilities |
| DNV GL's National Integrated Accreditation for Healthcare Organizations (NIAHO) | Acute care facilities |
| Commission on Accreditation of Rehabilitation Facilities (CARF) | Rehabilitation facilities |
| National Committee for Quality Assurance (NCQA) | Managed care organizations |
| Healthcare Facilities Accreditation Program (HFAP) | Acute care, ambulatory care, behavioral health LTC, and rehabilitation facilities |
| Community Health Accreditation Program (CHAP) (National League for Nursing) | Home- and community-based health care organizations |
| Accreditation Council for Occupational Therapy Education (ACOTE) | Occupational therapist and occupational therapy assistant programs |
| American Physical Therapy Association (APTA) | Physical therapist and physical therapist assistant programs |
| Committee on the Accreditation of Allied Health Education Programs | Education programs for multiple allied health specialties, including anesthesiologist assistant, cardiovascular technologist, blood bank technologist, medical assistant, exercise science, and respiratory therapist |
| Commission on Accreditation of Health Informatics and Information Management Education (CAHIIM) | Health information and informatics programs |
| Accreditation Council for Education in Nutrition and Dietetics (ACEND) | Dietitian/nutritionist and dietetic technician programs |
| Liaison Committee of the Association of American Medical Colleges and the American Medical Association (LCME) | Medical schools |
| National League for Nursing Accrediting Commission (NLNAC) | Nursing schools |

*LTC*, Long-term care.

care facilities, ambulatory care networks, LTC facilities, and rehabilitation facilities as well as certain specialty facilities, such as hospice and home care agencies.

The standards set by TJC reflect best practices and in many ways define how a health care facility should operate in terms of patient care, the clinical flow of data, and documentation standards. Much of TJC's activity stems from the original 1913 ACS medical documentation standardization project. For many years after that project, ACS not only maintained the development of the standards of documentation for hospitals but also conducted the approval proceedings. In 1951 the ACS, along with the American Hospital Association, the American Medical Association, and the Canadian Medical Association, formed the Joint Commission on Accreditation of Hospitals, which took over that accrediting function. In 1987 the organization changed its name (Joint Commission on Accreditation of Healthcare Organizations) to reflect the variety of organizations that were seeking accreditation. In 2009 the current name, The Joint Commission, was adopted.

TJC has a tremendous impact on health care facilities for several reasons. First, on-site accrediting surveys take place on a scheduled 3-year (maximum) cycle. Therefore, at least every 3 years, the facility is subject to an intensive on-site review. The accreditation standards change to differing degrees annually, with interim changes as needed. Thus, within the 3-year cycle of review, facilities are required to stay abreast of the changes and implement procedures to comply.

Second, whether a facility attains favorable accreditation status has an impact on its relationship with government entities. As previously discussed, the CMS, through Medicare, allows reimbursement from Medicare to those facilities that comply with Medicare's COP. This ordinarily entails a survey to ensure that the facility complies with COP. However, a facility that is accredited by TJC is typically not subjected to the COP review; this situation is called **deemed status** because the facility is deemed to have complied with the COP because of its TJC accreditation. In addition, in some states TJC accreditation reduces the incidence of state licensure surveys. So, in some cases, the voluntary accreditation by TJC can alleviate two additional surveys: for the state department of health and for Medicare COP. Many health insurance companies also require TJC or other accreditation before they reimburse the organization.

Finally, accreditation is also desirable as a symbol of quality for marketing purposes.

### National Integrated Accreditation for Healthcare Organizations

Until 2008 TJC was the only accreditation option for general acute care facilities that wanted to achieve deemed status. In 2008 CMS approved accreditation by Det Norske Veritas (DNV), a Norwegian global firm that specializes in risk management. DNV serves a wide range of business sectors, including maritime, energy, food and beverage, and health care industries.

DNV's **National Integrated Accreditation for Healthcare Organizations (NIAHO)** program integrates International Standards Organization (ISO) 9001 quality compliance and the CMS COP. Surveys are conducted annually and are focused on education and performance improvement. As of August 2021 over 600 US hospitals had achieved NIAHO accreditation.

### Commission on Accreditation of Rehabilitation Facilities

Another important accrediting body is the Commission on Accreditation of Rehabilitation Facilities (CARF), also known as the Rehabilitation Accreditation Commission, which focuses on facilities that provide physical, mental, and occupational rehabilitation services. Accreditation of adult day care, assisted living, and employment and community services is also available. TJC also accredits rehabilitation facilities, but it has slightly different requirements and standards, adapting acute care and ambulatory care requirements. In fact, many rehabilitation facilities may be accredited by both TJC and CARF. The focus of the two reviews is slightly different, and rehabilitation facilities that are accredited by TJC find themselves in something of a dilemma in complying with both sets of requirements. CARF requirements tend to be more prescriptive, and surveyors focus beyond physician/nurse documentation to emphasize documentation of occupational, physical, and other therapies. In recent years, TJC and CARF have collaborated to offer joint survey options to facilities. In this way, the surveys can be simultaneous and partially coordinated to reduce duplication of effort.

Many organizations accredit health care facilities and health care professional education programs. A partial list of these organizations and the facilities and institutions that they accredit is provided in Table 1.6.

### Commission on Accreditation for Health Informatics and Information Management

If you are studying HIM in a college that has an accredited HIM program, your program is accredited by the **Commission on Accreditation for Health Informatics and Information Management (CAHIIM)**. CAHIIM serves the public interest by establishing quality standards for the educational preparation of future HIM professionals. When a program is accredited by CAHIIM, it has voluntarily undergone a rigorous review process and has been determined to meet or exceed the standards set by CAHIIM. CAHIIM is an independent affiliate of the AHIMA. CAHIIM accreditation is a way to recognize and publicize best practices for HIM Education Programs (Commission on Accreditation for Health Informatics and Information Management Education, 2021).

## Professional Standards

In addition to licensure and accreditation requirements, yet another level of requirements must be followed in a health care organization: professional standards. On the one hand, licensure and accrediting bodies take a general overview of the facility and tend not to specifically address the day-to-day activities of individual practitioners. On the other hand, professional standards are developed by the professional organizations that represent the individuals performing health-related tasks. So, the American Medical Association promulgates professional standards for doctors, the American Nurses Association for nurses, and the AHIMA for HIM professionals. Often, it is the professional standards of the individual practitioner that dictate the type and extent of documentation required in the performance of any type of therapy or evaluation of patients.

Medical professions have a code of **ethics** that governs the conduct of their members. For example, nurses are bound by the Code of Ethics for Nurses set forth by the American Nurses Association. HIM professional standards tend to revolve around the issues of ethics and best practices. They also tend to target data quality, confidentiality, and access to health information. It is important HIM professionals know and adhere to these professional standards. Professional standards in HIM are developed by the AAPC and AHIMA. They take the form of an ethics statement as well as practice briefs and position papers. AHIMAs are routinely published in the *Journal of the American Health Information Management Association*. Box 1.4 shows the AHIMA Code of Ethics.

Ethical Principles: The following ethical principles are based on the core values of the American Health Information Management Association and apply to all AHIMA members.

A health information management professional shall:

1. advocate, uphold, and defend the consumer's right to privacy and the doctrine of confidentiality in the use and disclosure of information;
2. put service and the health and welfare of persons before self-interest and conduct oneself in the practice of the profession so as to bring honor to oneself, their peers, and to the health information management profession;
3. preserve, protect, and secure personal health information in any form or medium and hold in the highest regard health information and other information of a confidential nature obtained in an official capacity, taking into account the applicable statutes and regulations;
4. refuse to participate in or conceal unethical practices or procedures and report such practices;
5. use technology, data, and information resources in the way they are intended to be used;
6. advocate for appropriate uses of information resources across the health care ecosystem;
7. recruit and mentor students, peers, and colleagues to develop and strengthen professional workforce;
8. represent the profession to the public in a positive manner;
9. advance health information management knowledge and practice through continuing education, research, publications, and presentations;
10. perform honorably health information management association responsibilities, either appointed or elected, and preserve the confidentiality of any privileged information made known in any official capacity;
11. state truthfully and accurately one's credentials, professional education, and experiences;
12. facilitate interdisciplinary collaboration in situations supporting ethical health information principles; and
13. respect the inherent dignity and worth of every person.

Reprinted with permission from the American Health Information Management Association. Copyright 2022 by the American Health Information Management Association. All rights reserved. No part of this may be reproduced, reprinted, stored in a retrieval system, or transmitted, in any form or by any means, electronic, photocopying, recording, or otherwise, without the prior written permission of the association. Adapted with permission from the Code of Ethics of the National Association of Social Workers.
Revised and adopted by AHIMA House of Delegates, April 29, 2019.

## Independent Organizations

Because health care is an industry that affects everyone, it is not surprising that a variety of independent organizations have arisen, the purpose of which is to monitor and report on health care activities, research best practices, or both. We will revisit this topic in Chapter 8, but here are some examples.

The National Academy of Medicine (NAM), formerly the Institute of Medicine, is one of three academies that make up the National Academies of Sciences, Engineering, and Medicine (the National Academies) in the United States. The National Academies are private, nonprofit institutions that work outside of government to provide objective advice on matters of science, technology, and health. NAM defines itself as:

- an independent, evidence-based scientific advisor;
- a national academy with global scope;
- committed to catalyzing action and achieving impact;
- collaborative and interdisciplinary; and
- an honorific society for exceptional leaders.

As the Institute of Medicine, this organization published *To Err is Human: Building a Safer Healthcare System*, a critical report on medical errors that was the catalyst for many quality efforts in health care.

The Leapfrog Group is another independent organization focused on health care improvement. Leapfrog started as a collaboration among industry and watchdog groups. It describes itself as an important and influential voice for health care purchasers. Leapfrog collects, analyzes, and disseminates hospital data to promote transparency. Its programs include a voluntary hospital survey on safety, quality, and resource use; a hospital grading system; a value-based purchasing program; and an ambulatory surgery center survey (The Leapfrog Group, n.d.).

The Institute for Healthcare Improvement (IHI) is an independent not-for-profit organization based in Boston, Massachusetts. It promotes innovation through collaborative activities, focusing on four key areas:

- Pursuing Safe and High-Quality Care
- Improving the Health of Populations
- Building the Capability to Improve
- Innovating and Sparking Action

The IHI offers many educational tools focusing on quality improvement, including free downloadable case studies (Institute for Healthcare Improvement, 2023).

The Patient-Centered Outcomes Research Institute (PCORI) funds research that helps patients and their caregivers make informed choices about their treatment options. Unlike the other organizations highlighted in this section, PCORI's focus is on providing specific, useful information directly to patients and those who treat and care for them. Their primary activity is funding research into the outcomes of specific treatments so that data can be compared among alternatives (Patient-Centered Outcomes Research Institute, 2021).

**COMPETENCY CHECK-IN 1.3**

**Interrelationships**

**Competency Assessment**

1. An insurance company is a type of third-party payer. Who are the first two parties?
2. How do employers affect the delivery of health care in the United States?
3. _____ is an entitlement program created in 1965 to provide health care to the poor.
4. List three reasons the cost of health care is rising from a manufacturing perspective.
5. List and describe the purposes of the agencies within the Department of Health and Human Services.
6. How does the government, as a payer, ensure providers are offering quality care to patients?
7. Medicare waives compliance audits for appropriately accredited facilities by granting them _____.
8. Voluntary compliance with a set of standards developed by an independent agency is part of the _____ process.
9. Health care facilities must be licensed to conduct business. However, they often choose to be accredited as well. What is licensure? What is accreditation? What is the difference between licensure and accreditation?
10. How do accreditation agencies like The Joint Commission know that facilities are adhering to the standards they establish?
11. Who sets professional standards and how can they affect the delivery of health care?

## Chapter Summary

Health care is provided by a variety of different practitioners, including physicians, nurses, and therapists. Each time the patient receives health care, documentation of that care is entered into the patient's health care record. Practitioners in multiple disciplines work together to care for the patient; to do so, they must exchange health information about the patient. Physicians may maintain their own offices as solo practitioners or work with other physicians in group practices. Physicians' offices are a type of ambulatory care facility. Other types of facilities are acute care, LTC, and a variety of specialty facilities, including rehabilitation facilities, mental health facilities, and children's hospitals. Facilities also can be classified by length of stay, inpatient versus outpatient services, ownership, and financial status (i.e., for-profit or not-for-profit).

Government plays a role in the health care industry. Federal and state governments enact laws and enforce them through regulations. Health care facilities are licensed

through the state, and there are a number of very specific reporting requirements. Another aspect of facility organization is accreditation status. Accreditation is very important to ensure quality and efficient reimbursement. Last, professional standards play a role in determining the activities of a facility because each profession has its own standards of both care and documentation as well as education and certification.

As we mentioned at the beginning of this chapter, to understand the HIM profession, you must understand the basic structure and terminology of the health care industry. After reading this chapter, you are beginning to see that the health care industry has become a complex environment and that it is affected by the rules and guidelines of health care professionals, insurance companies, federal regulations, state laws and licensing, and accreditation standards. As you read the remaining chapters of this text you will use the knowledge learned here to understand the tenets of HIM.

## Competency Milestone

**CAHIIM Competency**

*V.4. Identify the impact of policy on health care. (3)*

**Rationale**

The structure of the US health care system is a complex interrelationship of providers of care, patients, payers, and regulating bodies. Working in HIM requires an understanding of the interests of all parties and the relationship between them and health policy.

**Competency Assessment**

1. A hallmark of being a professional is promoting the public good. Looking at the job descriptions of HIM professionals, how do you think members of this occupation serve society?
2. How does the health record promote quality patient care?
3. How does the health record facilitate continuity of care?
4. Select three health care facilities in your state. Prepare a table to compare the facilities in terms of size, ownership, tax status, patient population, and services. Do these facilities compete? Do they have any affiliation(s)?

5. How does the government, as a payer, ensure providers are offering quality care to patients?
6. What indicators does Health People monitor? What do policymakers do with this information?
7. How do the independent organizations discussed in this chapter contribute to health care policy?
8. Why is government involved in the delivery of health care?
9. If the Department of Health and Human Services were dissolved tomorrow, what impact would that have on the health care industry? Why?

## Ethics Challenge

### CAHIIM Competency

*VI.7. Assess ethical standards of practice (5)*

### Competency Assessment

1. Vanessa is the supervisor of HIM at Community Hospital. She is a member of AHIMA and is studying to become a registered health information technician. Community Hospital has a new chief operating officer, Brad, who is new to the hospital and comes from another state. Brad is concerned that too many physicians are not completing their paperwork when patients are discharged. He would like Vanessa and her staff to send the paperwork out of the hospital to the physicians' offices for completion because he thinks that the physicians would be more likely to do the work if it were on their desks. Vanessa knows that the state licensure regulations prohibit the removal of the paperwork from the hospital under normal circumstances. Should Vanessa comply with Brad's request? Is compliance with Brad's request a violation of the AHIMA Code of Ethics?
2. Sandra has just graduated from an associate degree program, achieving a perfect 4.0 GPA. She is sure that she will pass the RHIT exam and has scheduled to sit for it next month. Sandra inserts the credential RHIT after her name in her resume that she is sending out to potential employers. Is this ethical or not?
3. Mike is an RHIT and has been working for Diamonte Community Hospital for the past 6 months. Mike is not happy with his salary and thinks he should be making more than noncredentialed employees. His instructor from the HIM program has asked him to participate on a panel to talk about the profession to new HIM students. Mike participates in the panel and is very vocal and candid about his dissatisfaction with his job and the HIM profession in general. Is this ethical or not?

## Critical Thinking Questions

1. What are the licensure requirements for physicians in your state?
2. Log on to the AHIMA website (http://www.ahima.org). Explore the site. What does AHIMA say about careers in HIM? How many schools offer degrees in HIM? What courses are included in these programs?
3. What HIM certifications are offered by Commission on Certification for Health Informatics and Information Management?
4. If you were just diagnosed with diabetes, how would you go about finding a physician to care for you?
5. The lines between inpatients and outpatients may become blurred under certain circumstances. An ED patient who is treated and released is clearly an outpatient. However, if the patient entered the ED at 11 p.m. and left at 4 a.m., the patient clearly arrived on one day and left on the next. Is this patient an inpatient or an outpatient? Why?
6. Some patients are kept in the hospital for observation. This is a special category of patients, neither outpatients nor inpatients, who may stay in the hospital for as many as 24–48 hours without being admitted as inpatients. What problems does this present for hospitals?
7. Several organizations have recently announced their intention to enter the health care arena in a variety of ways, including merging drug store chains with insurers and non–health care corporations collaborating to control health care costs. Search the Internet to find at least two examples of this phenomenon. Discuss the implications for consumers.
8. Find two drugs or other products that are advertised to the public. Identify what alternatives are available. What are the pros/cons of each? Is pharmaceutical marketing a good idea? Should drug ads include pricing?
9. This chapter mentioned the groundbreaking report 1999 entitled *To Err is Human: Building a Safer Health System* from NAM, formerly the Institute of Medicine. This report is available in full at https://www.ncbi.nlm.nih.gov/books/NBK225182/. Review the report. How do you think it has influenced health care?
10. Differentiate among these organizations: Leapfrog Group, NAM, IHI, and PCORI.
11. Essay: What are the components of the US health care system and how do they interact with each other?
12. What behaviors are required of HIM professionals by the AHIMA code of ethics, but not by law?

# The Role of Health Information Management Professionals in the Workplace

### Professional Profile—Physician Office Liaison

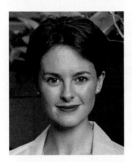

My name is Melanie, and I am a physician office liaison in the Medical Staff Office at Diamonte Hospital. I am responsible for helping the hospital maintain good relationships with the physicians and our staff. We are a small community hospital with 250 licensed beds. Our physicians are not employees of the hospital; they have privileges. This means that the hospital allows the physicians to admit their patients for treatment at the hospital.

These physicians have private practices with their own offices and staff. It is my job to know them, to help with any problems they may have communicating with the hospital, and to coordinate the filing of their professional documentation.

To be able to help a physician's office staff member, I have to know the various professionals who might work in an office and what they might do. It really helps that I know the difference between a medical assistant and a nurse practitioner. It is important that I know how a group practice works so that I can help the hospital keep track of which physicians can cover for one another.

The hospital collects statistics on physicians: How many patients they admit, what diagnoses they are treating, what procedures they are performing, and other information. I collaborate with other hospital departments to collect these reports and help present them at medical staff meetings. To do this, I have to know all the departments in the hospital and how they are related. I also need to understand the reports.

One of my most important tasks is credentialing. When a physician applies for privileges, I do a background check, collect the licensing documentation, and prepare a presentation for the credentialing committee. Because privileges are not permanent, I remind the physicians when they need to reapply and help gather the updated documentation. In addition to assisting physicians seeking privileges, I also check on physicians who write orders for services provided in the hospital. I research the physician to ensure they are licensed in the state and that they are not prohibited from participation in Medicare, Medicaid, or state-funded services. For all of these credentialing activities, I need to understand the differences among the medical specialties and what board certification means, and how to research authoritative websites.

Finally, I coordinate CE sessions for physicians and their office staff. My next project is to develop a newsletter of hospital and physician activities that I can email to the physicians' offices.

How did I get this job? I'm a registered health information technician. I have an associate degree in health information technology (HIT) from my local community college. In the HIT program, I learned about physicians, hospitals, and other health-related professions. The hospital administrators were very happy to find a candidate for the job who already understood the system.

### Career Tip

For a career in physician relations or a medical staff office, an associate degree in HIM is a good start. Consider a bachelor's degree in HIM or hospital administration. In your academic plan, be sure to include written and oral communications as well as information technology courses. You should have good organizational skills and be outgoing and comfortable meeting and working with new people.

### Patient Care Perspective

### Maria, Mother of Two

When my husband and I moved to town, we needed to find a pediatrician right away. We contacted Diamonte Hospital because they had a physician referral service. I had some follow-up questions, so I called the hospital and spoke with Melanie in the Medical Staff office to help me understand how the referral service worked. We were able to interview several physicians and establish a great relationship with the pediatrician we chose.

## Works Cited

American Board of Medical Specialties: *Member boards: specialty and subspecialty certificates*, 2021. https://www.abms.org/member-boards/specialty-subspecialty-certificates/. Accessed September 5, 2021.

American Nurses Credentialing Center: *Certified Nursing Excellence*, 2021. https://www.nursingworld.org/our-certifications/. Accessed September 5, 2021.

American Osteopathic Association (AOA): *History of the AOA*, 2021. https://osteopathic.org/about/. Accessed September 5, 2021.

Blue Cross: An Industry Pioneer: *Blue Cross: origins*, 2023. https://www.bcbs.com/about-us/industry-pioneer/. Accessed January 6, 2023.

Commission on Accreditation for Health Informatics and Information Management Education (CAHIIM): 2021. https://www.cahiim.org/. Accessed September 20, 2021.

Federation of State Medical Boards: *State-specific requirements for initial medical licensure*, 2021. https://www.fsmb.org/step-3/state-licensurehttps://www.fsmb.org/step-3/state-specific/. Accessed September 5, 2021.

Institute for Healthcare Improvement: *About Us*, 2023. http://www.ihi.org/about/Pages/default.aspx. Accessed January 6, 2023.

Kaiser Family Foundation: *Health insurance coverage of the total population*. KFF (Kaiser Family Foundation), 2019. https://www.kff.org/other/state-indicator/total-population/. Accessed September 19, 2021.

National Board of Osteopathic Medical Examiners: *COMLEX-USA*, 2021. https://www.nbome.org/assessments/comlex-usa/https://www.nbome.org/exams-assessments/comlex-usa/. Accessed September 5, 2021.

National Commission on Certification of Physician Assistants: *About NCCPA*, n.d. https://www.nccpa.net/about-nccpa/. Accessed September 13, 2021.

National Council of State Boards of Nursing: *Licensure compacts*, 2021a. https://www.ncsbn.org/compacts.htm. Accessed September 5, 2021.

National Council of State Boards of Nursing: *APRN compact*, 2021b. https://www.ncsbn.org/aprn-compact.htm. Accessed September 5, 2021.

National Council of State Boards of Nursing: *APRN campaign for consensus: moving toward uniformity in state laws*, 2021c. https://www.ncsbn.org/campaign-for-consensus.htm. Accessed September 13, 2021.

O Gröne, M Garcia-Barbero: Integrated care, *Int J Integr Care* 1(2), 2001. http://doi.org/10.5334/ijic.28. Accessed 19 September 2021.

Office of the National Coordinator for Health Information Technology: 2021 https://www.healthit.gov/topic/about-onc. Accessed September 25, 2021.

Patient-Centered Outcomes Research Institute: *Our story*, 2014. https://www.pcori.org/about-us/our-story. Accessed September 25, 2021.

Sultz H, Young K: *Health care USA: understanding its organization and delivery*. ed 5, Sudbury, MA, 2006, Jones & Bartlett.

The Leapfrog Group: *Who we are and our mission*, n.d. http://www.leapfroggroup.org/about. Accessed September 25, 2021.

United States Medical Licensing Examination: *Bulletin. USMLE Bulletin of Information: 2022 Bulletin*, 2022. https://www.usmle.org/bulletin/. Accessed January 6, 2023.

## Further Reading

American Health Information Management Association (AHIMA): *AHIMA Code of Ethics*, 2021. https://library.ahima.org/doc?oid=105098#.YU9tYuySlaQ. Accessed September 25, 2021.

American Health Information Management Association: *Certifications & careers*, 2021. https://www.ahima.org/certification-careers/certification-exams/. Accessed September 13, 2021.

American Nurses Association: *ANA Standards for Excellence®*, n.d. https://www.nursingworld.org/ana/about-ana/standards/. Accessed September 13, 2021.

Bureau of Labor Statistics, U.S. Department of Labor: *Occupational outlook handbook*, 2021. https://www.bls.gov/ooh/. Accessed January 5, Labor 2023.

Institute of Medicine (US) Committee on Quality of Health Care in America Kohn LT, Corrigan JM, et al: *To err is human: building a safer health system*. Washington, DC: National Academy Press; 2000. 10.17226/9728.

National Association of Health Unit Coordinators, Inc.: *NAHUC Certification and Recertification*. n.d. https://nahuc.org/532-2/certification-2/. Accessed September 25, 2021.

The National Academies of Sciences, Engineering, and medicine. *Who we are*, 2021. https://www.nationalacademies.org/about. Accessed September 25, 2021.

# 2

## Collecting and Storing Health Care Data

### LISA REILLY

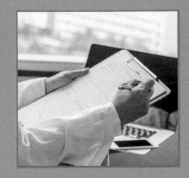

## CHAPTER OUTLINE

**Basic Concepts**
    Health
    Data
    Information
    Health Data
    Health Information

**Data Architecture**
    Data Quality
    Building a Database
    Master Patient Index
    Data Sets

**Data Collection and Storage**
    Forms
    Electronic Health Record
    Storing Health Care Data

**Planning for Electronic Health Record Migration and Implementation**
    Selection

    Design
    Implementation
    Evaluation
    Support

**Chapter Summary**

**Competency Milestones**

**Ethics Challenge**

**Critical Thinking Questions**

**The Role of Health Information Management Professionals in the Workplace**
    Professional Profile—Health Information Management Implementation Specialist
    Patient Care Perspective

**Works Cited**

**Further Reading**

## CHAPTER OBJECTIVES

*By the end of this chapter, the student should be able to*

1. Distinguish health data and health information.
2. Explain the purpose and contents of a data dictionary.
3. Describe the structure of a relational database.
4. Define the data sets used in health care and compare their applications and purposes.
5. Describe the importance of forms and their application to data collection.
6. Compare and contrast an electronic health record (EHR) with a hybrid EHR.
7. Discuss the importance of interoperability and the longitudinal use of the EHR.
8. Explain the use of the data repository, data warehouse, and data mapping in the storage of health data.
9. Explain the system acquisition and evaluation process.

## VOCABULARY

aggregate data
algorithm
authentication
character

clinical decision-making system (CDS)
compliance
computerized physician order entry (CPOE)
countersigned

data analytics
data collection device
data dictionary
data repository
data set
data warehouse
data
database
Digital Imaging and Communications in Medicine (DICOM)
document imaging
electronic data interchange (EDI)
electronic document management system (EDMS)
electronic health record (EHR)
epidemiology
evidence-based medicine (EBM)
field
file
health data
health information exchange (HIE)
health information
Health Level 7 (HL7)
health record
hybrid record
information
infrastructure

interface
interoperability
master forms file
master patient index (MPI)
medical record number (MRN)
Minimum Data Set (MDS 3.0)
morbidity
mortality
Nationwide Health Information Network (NHIN)
Outcome and Assessment Information Set (OASIS)
patient account number
patient portal
personal health record (PHR)
picture archiving and communication system (PACS)
point-of-care documentation
record
relational database
request for proposal (RFP)
stakeholder
superuser
system development life cycle (SDLC)
Uniform Bill (UB-04)
Uniform Hospital Discharge Data Set (UHDDS)
vital statistics

## CAHIIM COMPETENCY DOMAINS

I.3.   Identify policies and strategies to achieve data integrity (3)

III.7.  Summarize standards for the exchange of health information (2)

III.7.  **DM** Identify standards for the exchange of health information (3)

Chapter 1 contains a discussion of various health care professionals and the settings in which they work. While caring for patients, these health care workers listen to patients and make observations. They record those observations, including their evaluation of the patient's condition and plans for further assessment and treatment. All of the assessment and treatment activities are documented as they occur along with the outcomes of these activities. This chapter begins with a discussion of the ways that health care workers record (document) what they observe and what they do. We will cover some of the organizational issues pertaining to the capture and quality assurance of that documentation. This chapter is a foundation for subsequent discussions in the text about the content of patient health records and the management of the data that go into the record as well as the information that is derived from those data.

Although the technology for electronic documentation certainly exists and is used in most settings to some extent, its universal implementation has not arrived. In fact, even

with an "all-electronic" documentation system, there will likely always be the need to capture and save documentation that originates in paper form. Although both paper and electronic documentation currently coexist, we will focus our attention on the electronic form. We have archived the discussion of paper documentation, workflow, and storage issues into an appendix accessible on the Evolve website.

## Basic Concepts

Some basic terminology will assist your understanding of the material in this chapter, as well as the rest of the text. Although these terms may have other meanings, it is important to understand them in the context of health care.

### Health

A person who is healthy is free of disease and is also free of outside physical, social, and other problems that could lead to a disease condition. To achieve and maintain health, individuals need to access the health care system at various points in their lives. Lack of access or the inability to pay for health care, therefore, is a concern—not just for the individual but also for society in general. And, it is not just our genetics and exposure to diseases that affect our well-being. There are also social factors influencing our health (called *social determinants of health*), including the conditions in which we live, work, and play. Our knowledge about health comes from our analysis of a wide variety of data, including health care data (Centers for Disease Control and Prevention, 2022).

## Data

**Data** are items, observations, or raw facts. We have to understand the context in which the data are collected to use them. For example, say we are told that there are 100 patients in Community Hospital today. What does that mean? Is the hospital full? How many patients are usually there? The number of patients in the hospital is not meaningful without understanding the context of the data collection. When data are presented in context, we have *information*.

## Information

To analyze data—to make sense of the facts and use them—the data must be organized. The goal of organizing the data is to provide **information**. The terms *data* and *information* are often used synonymously, but they are not the same. "Get me the data" usually really means "get me useful information." Data are the units of observation, and information is data that have been organized to make them useful. In Fig. 2.1A, we see that Community Hospital has had around 100 patients every day for the past month. Although the isolated observation about the number of patients on a particular day was not useful to us, we can see that putting that observation in context, by collecting that same observation over a period of time and organizing it into this table, gives us useful information. This information enables us to answer the previous questions:

*Is the hospital full?* No—the hospital can hold more.

How many patients are usually there? About 100.

Fig. 2.1B provides an organized report of the 100 patients that gives the user information about the patients who are currently in the hospital. Comparison of those patients' details over time can give us an understanding of our patient population and how it might be changing. Thus we might

**The daily volume of inpatients in the month of August. Community Hospital: Inpatient Volume, August 20XX**

| Date | Number of Inpatients |
|---|---|
| 8/1 | 103 |
| 8/2 | 98 |
| 8/3 | 102 |
| 8/4 | 99 |
| 8/5 | 108 |
| 8/6 | 95 |
| 8/7 | 94 |
| 8/8 | 109 |
| 8/9 | 108 |
| 8/10 | 101 |
| 8/11 | 109 |
| 8/12 | 97 |
| 8/13 | 110 |
| 8/14 | 104 |
| 8/15 | 97 |
| 8/16 | 104 |
| 8/17 | 108 |
| 8/18 | 97 |
| 8/19 | 93 |
| 8/20 | 100 |
| 8/21 | 103 |
| 8/22 | 96 |
| 8/23 | 96 |
| 8/24 | 104 |
| 8/25 | 101 |
| 8/26 | 98 |
| 8/27 | 109 |
| 8/28 | 97 |
| 8/29 | 93 |
| 8/30 | 94 |
| 8/31 | 98 |

A

**Detailed explanation of the 100 patients in the facility on August 20, 20XX**

| | | |
|---|---|---|
| Total Inpatients | | 100 |
| | | |
| Service | | |
| | Medical | 42 |
| | Surgical | 23 |
| | Obstetrical | 7 |
| | Psychiatric | 24 |
| | Nursery | 4 |
| | | |
| Length of Stay | | |
| | 1 day | 23 |
| | 2 days | 22 |
| | 3 days | 29 |
| | 4 days | 14 |
| | 5 days | 7 |
| | 6 days | 3 |
| | 7 or more days | 2 |

B

• **Fig. 2.1** Patient volume report two different ways. (A) is the volume of patients each day of August. (B) is an example of a detailed volume report for a single day.

normally have a lot of medical and surgical patients, but over time, perhaps there will be a shift toward maternity patients if we make an effort to grow that service.

Here is another example of data versus information. On the left in Fig. 2.2 is a list of data pertaining to Maria Gomez. The user cannot tell what the data on the left signify until it is determined that they are her oral temperatures taken at 1-hour intervals. Only then do the data become useful and therefore information. The temperatures are listed in chronological order. Based on these few observations, it is easy to see that Maria's temperature was highest (spiked) at 2 p.m. and has been going down since then. The example in Fig. 2.2 is just a small number of observations or data points. If a nurse took Maria's temperature every hour for 5 days, there would be 120 data points. With that much data, even listing the data points in order would not be helpful because there would be too many numbers to process visually. Therefore the most useful information is often data organized into a picture, such as the graph shown in Fig. 2.3, which shows 24 observations. Here, we can see that Maria's temperature was high in the morning but that it returned to normal later in the evening and stayed there. The figure shows that the usefulness of data—turning them into information—depends on how we organize and present them. As we will discuss later, a patient's temperature would be observed and recorded as an entry into the patient's record. In an electronic health record (EHR) the user could choose to display those observations in a graph. In a paper record the recorder would need to write the temperature *and* place a mark on a graph to see such a display.

## Health Data

**Health data** are facts or observations in reference to an individual patient or a group of patients. The series of temperatures collected and reported by Maria Gomez in Fig. 2.2 is an example of specific health data from one patient. We can also list all of the diseases that a patient has (e.g., for continuing patient care) or all of the patients who have a certain disease (e.g., to see what types of diseases the hospital is treating).

Similarly, one can obtain vast quantities of data on individual patients or groups of patients. Imagine a list of 10,000 patients and their diseases. Is this list useful? What could be done with this data? Unless one is prepared to organize it, the list is not very informative. However, a list of the top 10 most common diseases of 10,000 residents in a particular location would be quite useful. This type of information is published frequently. For example, Fig. 2.4 shows the top 10 causes of death in the United States in 1900 and 2015.

 **NOTE**

Is *data* a plural word or a singular word? *Datum* is the singular form of the Latin word, and it represents a single item, observation, or fact. However, we rarely refer to one item of knowledge. Generally, we discuss a group of similar items, such as the temperatures listed in Fig. 2.2, and we call the group *data*. In this book the plural form is used to refer to items of related data ("the data are significant").

---

**Data versus Information**

| DATA | INFORMATION |
|---|---|
| Definition: Individual units of knowledge | Definition: Data with a frame of reference |
| Example: Maria Gomez | Example: Maria Gomez Temperature (oral) March 15, 20XX |

| | |
|---|---|
| 104 | |
| 105 | |
| 104 | 1 p.m.    104° |
| 103 | 2 p.m.    105° |
| 102 | 3 p.m.    104° |
| 101 | 4 p.m.    103° |
| 100 | 5 p.m.    102° |
| 99 | 6 p.m.    101° |
| | 7 p.m.    100° |
| | 8 p.m.     99° |

On the left, the data about Maria Gomez are not useful, because we do not have a frame of reference. Those same data, within the frame of reference of date and time, tell a story that is clinically significant.

• **Fig. 2.2** A list of data with a frame of reference becomes information.

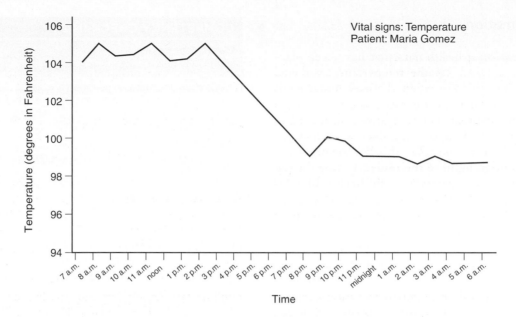

• **Fig. 2.3**  The data presentation graph displays a large amount of data.

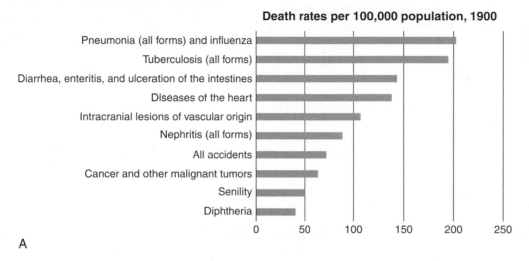

A

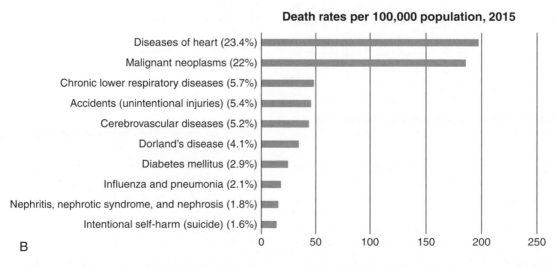

B

• **Fig. 2.4**  The top 10 causes of death in the United States. (A) Death rates per 100,000 people, 1900. (B) Death rates per 100,000 people, 2015. ((A) From Linder FE, Grove RD: *Vital statistics rates of the United States, 1900-1940*, Washington, DC, 1947, U.S. Department of Commerce, Bureau of the Census, U.S. Government Printing Office. (B) From Murphy SL, Xu, J, Kochanek KD, Curtin S, Arias E, Division of Vital Statistics: *Deaths: final data for 2015. National Vital Statistics Reports 66, No. 6*, November 27, 2017. https://www.cdc.gov/nchs/data/nvsr/nvsr66/nvsr66_06. pdf. Accessed November 25, 2018.)

## Health Information

**Health information** is health data that have been organized. In Figs. 2.2 and 2.3 the temperatures gathered become health information when the user understands that those temperatures are for one patient at certain times of the day. Expand that to health data related to 10,000 city residents. A large data collection such as this becomes health information when the data are organized in a way that is meaningful to the reader. Listing the top 10 diseases of a city's residents is useful health information. This is information that hospital administrators, public health officials, and physicians can use to make decisions. In Fig. 2.4, for example, tuberculosis and diarrhea/enteritis are no longer on the list of the top 10 causes of death (mortality) in the United States. **Mortality** data are a **vital statistic** captured through the death certificate filing process, discussed in detail in Chapter 7. Births and marriages are also vital statistics. **Morbidity**, or disease, data are captured through the reporting of patient-specific data from various types of facilities. Upon study, one finds that the development of antibiotics and vaccines and improvements in sanitation have significantly reduced the number of deaths caused by tuberculosis and diarrhea/enteritis. The graphs in Fig. 2.4 present interesting information that helps us ask questions that lead to more information. The study of these types of health trends or patterns is called **epidemiology**. Epidemiology is important to public health officials and others who are interested in the spread of disease and the treatment/prevention of disease.

Health information is a broad category. It may refer to the organized data that have been collected about an individual patient, or it can be the summary of information about that patient's entire experience with his or her physician. Health information can also be **aggregate data** or summary information about all the patients that a physician has seen. A table showing the top five diagnoses of patients seen by the physician during the year is an example of aggregate data. Furthermore, health information management (HIM) professionals can take all the available information about patients in a particular geographical area and make broad statements on the basis of this array of information (public health information). The process of examining the data and exploring them to create information is called **data analytics**.

Health information therefore encompasses the organization of a limitless array of possible data items and combinations of data items. It can range from data about the care of an individual patient to information about the health trends of an entire nation. HIM professionals are important and active participants in health information, through the analysis of existing data and the management of the quality of data at the facility level.

❖ **COMPETENCY CHECK-IN 2.1**
**Basic Concepts**

1. Give two examples in your personal life of data and two examples of information. Think of two examples of ways that health data differ from health information.
2. How do data become information?
3. What is health information?

## Data Architecture

Data are collected for a reason and stored for later use. The process is a little like grocery shopping. One buys food that is needed both now and later and stores it in the proper place for current and future use. Similarly, health care providers collect the data that are needed both now and later and store these data in the proper places for both current and future use.

Historically, the data collected by health care providers have been recorded on paper forms, which are bound and filed by patient. The development and implementation of appropriate computer systems for the capture, storage, and transmission of clinical data into *EHRs* have taken decades. Currently, there are versions of EHRs in a wide variety of health care settings in the United States and many other countries. As we discuss the foundations of electronic records, keep in mind that the principles related to the basic data collection (documentation) are similar, whether working in a paper or electronic format. Further, there is still a significant volume of paper data collection, so that format cannot be ignored.

Health data must be collected and organized in such a way that it can be found quickly when it is needed. Data collected electronically are organized into a **database**. The first step in creating a database is determining what data elements are needed. The specific elements that are collected will vary depending on the health care provider, the patient population, the needs of the facility, and the requirements of other users such as the payer.

## Data Quality

If data are wrong when being recorded, they are not useful to anyone, hence the expression: "garbage in, garbage out." In other words, if the data entered into the EHR are wrong, then the data extracted from the EHR will be wrong. Those responsible for entering data must exercise extreme care to ensure that the data are correct. The same rule applies to data collected on paper. If the data on the paper record are incorrectly recorded, then users will be presented with incorrect data upon review. High-quality data collection starts with an understanding of the data needs of the users:

both those who document (collect the data) and those who utilize the data after it is documented. Data collection devices (e.g., forms, interactive screens, and scanners) must be designed to capture data with an emphasis on the integrity of the data, or data quality.

## Building a Database

To take the analogy of grocery shopping further: Just as food comes in appropriate containers, data also come in packages. Data are collected piece by piece in logical segments. The logical segments are called *characters, fields, records,* and *files.*

### Characters

This chapter focuses on the way data are collected electronically; however, the concepts also pertain to paper data collection with a few modifications. Regarding computers, the smallest segment of data is referred to as a *bit*. A bit is the computer's electronic differentiation between two choices: on and off. Small strings of bits in specific combinations of on/off patterns make bytes, which are represented on the computer screen as characters. A character is the smallest segment of written data.

A character is a letter, a single-digit number, or a symbol. "A" is a character, as are "3" and "&." A character is the smallest unit of data that is collected. Characters are the building blocks of data. Characters are strung together to make words, larger numbers, and other types of written communication.

### Fields

The individual who is recording the data needs to know what characters to combine to make the words that are the patient's name, for example. Placing the characters in the correct order is important so that the data collected are accurate (correct). For example: If a patient's name is Gomez, recording the name as Goemz is not accurate.

A field is a series of related characters that have a specific relationship to one another. They express a data element, such as name, gender, or birth date. Usually, a field is a word, a group of related words, or a specific type of number. For example, a patient's address in the United States contains a postal service zip code. The zip code for Linden, New Jersey, is 07036. Therefore the field "zip code" contains five characters: 0, 7, 0, 3, and 6.

Fields are defined by the type of data that they contain. A field containing only letters would be an alphabetic field, abbreviated as *alpha*. For example, the address field for the name of the city is an alphabetic field. A field containing only numbers is a numeric field. A field for dollars is an example of a numeric field. A field can also be a combination of alphabetic and numeric characters; this is called an *alphanumeric field*. A field for street address is an alphanumeric field. The designation of a field as alphanumeric means that it is acceptable to have both numeric and alphabetic characters, not that they are required.

When creating fields in a database, you may find it useful to designate that a series of numerical characters is not to be treated as a number. For example, zip codes are made up of numeric characters. If a zip code field is labeled numeric, any leading zero would not be recognized. Zip code 07036 then becomes 7036 both on the screen and when printed out. This is not desirable if you are printing labels for mailing envelopes. Mail addressed this way would most certainly be delayed. Social Security numbers are another tricky field to define. Since the first character in a Social Security number can be a zero, a field containing a Social Security number should be defined as alphanumeric or text to preserve the zeros. Some software allows the user to preserve leading zeros, while other programs do not.

Fields are generally given logical names to identify them. Fig. 2.5 illustrates data fields and definitions. The listing of fields is one component of creating a data dictionary. A data dictionary is a listing of all fields to be collected: their size, name, and description. Some fields, such as the month of the year, have a limited number of possible contents or values. The data dictionary describes the specific contents or values that can be contained in each field. For example, in the specific contents of the field for the month of the patient's admission, the whole numbers 1 through 12 are the only acceptable (or *valid*) values. Whether the data are collected on paper or in a computer, the size of the field must be considered to ensure uniformity in recording and retrieving the data (standardization). The data dictionary also describes how the data are collected, who is allowed to amend it, and where these will be stored.

| Name | Definition | Size | Type | Example |
| --- | --- | --- | --- | --- |
| FNAME | Patient's first name | 15 Characters | Alphabetic | Jane |
| LNAME | Patient's last name | 15 Characters | Alphabetic | Jones |
| TELE | Patient's phone number | 12 Characters | Alphanumeric | 973-555-3331 |
| TEMP | Patient's temperature | 5 Characters | Numeric | 98.6 |

• **Fig. 2.5** Common fields of data, including definitions.

To illustrate how a data dictionary might be constructed, consider a patient's first name:

Field: Patient First Name

Field Name: ptfname

Size: 15 characters

Description: The patient's given name, as it appears on identification presented at registration. Should match the patient's insurance card, if applicable, or other identification such as driver's license or passport.

Type: alphanumeric

Valid: none

Origination: patient registration

Amendment: patient registration

Location: Master Patient Index

Imagine what would happen if the designers of the data collection did not specifically define these elements. Users may not see or even be aware of this underlying documentation; however, it is the foundation for efficient and accurate data collection and communication among different parts of the system. Ideally, the patient's first name is collected and recorded once at registration. Although it may be used many times throughout the patient's care, the different programs, displays, and reports always use that initial data collection as the source of truth about the patient's name.

### Records

In the same way, that characters combine to make fields, fields combine to make **records**. A very simple example of fields that combine to make a record is an entry in a contact list in an electronic device such as a smart phone. First name, last name, street address, city, state, zip code, and multiple telephone numbers are listed. Similarly, a physician keeps track of patients using groups of fields that combine to make a record of the patient's contact data. An example of how fields combine to make a record is shown in Fig. 2.6.

### Files

The physician collects numerous records of different types of data, and this group of related records is called a **file**. In Fig. 2.7 the entire contact list is a file made up of individual records. Files can be large or small, depending on the number of records that they contain. A patient's entire health history can be contained in one file. An EHR is developed by linking the data records collected for each patient. In common usage the terms *file* and *record* are often used interchangeably, even though they have different technical meanings.

## Master Patient Index

If we were drawing a picture of a database, we would make tables to represent the records and show how they link together. These tables or entities contain a set of fields or elements that define the entity. Each field is a row on the table and the tables link together by common fields. This structure is called a **relational database** because the data items are organized into tables of related data. One table can link to any number of other tables through the identification of a key field. The picture of these linked tables is called an entity relationship diagram. This advantage of a relational database means that fields can be accessed directly

| Name | Definition | Size | Type | Example |
|---|---|---|---|---|
| FNAME | Patient's first name | 15 Characters | Alphabetic | Marion |
| LNAME | Patient's last name | 15 Characters | Alphabetic | Smith |
| ADDRESS | Patient's home street address | 25 Characters | Alphanumeric | 23 Pine St |
| CITY | City associated with ADDRESS | 15 Characters | Alphabetic | Anywhere |
| STATE | State associated with ADDRESS | 14 Characters | Alphabetic | IOWA |
| ZIP | Postal zip code associated with ADDRESS | 10 Characters | Alphanumeric | 31898-0578 |
| TELE | Patient's primary contact number | 14 Characters | Alphanumeric | (319) 555-1234 |

FNAME: Marion

LNAME: Smith

ADDRESS: 23 Pine St.

CITY: Anywhere

STATE: Iowa

ZIP: 31898-0578

TELE: (319) 555-1234

Marion    Smith

23 Pine Street

Anywhere    Iowa    31898-0578

(319) 555-1234

Each field in the record above is blocked to illustrate the number of characters allowed, compared to the number this record required.

• **Fig. 2.6** An example of how fields combine to make a record in a contact list.

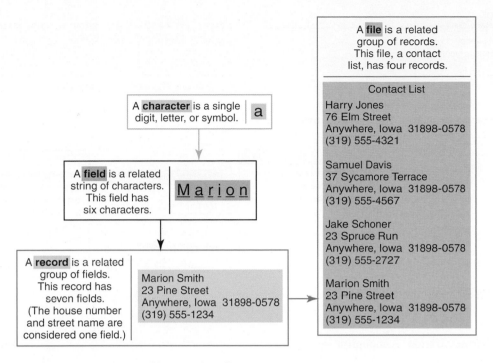

• **Fig. 2.7** Contact list example of how records combine to make a file.

for both data collection and data reporting. The human/database interaction is accomplished through a Structured Query Language. One critical example of how relational databases are constructed is the Master Patient Index (MPI).

The first time a patient visits a provider, a unique **medical record number (MRN)** is assigned. On subsequent visits, the registrar will use the MRN that already exists. For accounting purposes, each visit is also assigned a unique number, frequently called the **patient account number**, *patient number,* or *billing number.* The account number is linked to the MRN so that all visits can be identified and tracked. The MRN uniquely identifies the patient and each visit is linked to that MRN through the patient account number. The patient account number uniquely identifies the visit so that data collection can be associated with that visit.

The number of health records (or files) generated by a provider quickly becomes unmanageable without a way to reference them. The **master patient index (MPI)** is the key to identifying patients and locating their records. The data contained in the MPI are, at a minimum, the patient contact data collected during the patient registration process. These data are used to identify each patient within that health care facility and to locate the data in the patient's health record.

In a paper-based environment the MPI is primarily a look-up for finding patients and their visits. However, more powerfully, this numbering and linking of patient identity to visits and the health data are the foundation for the database that becomes the EHR. In the entity relationship diagram, Fig. 2.8 example, note the basic MPI record contains the patient's unique identification number (MRN), which links to the patient's contact record, financial record, and patient account index. The patient account index further links to the radiology visit record. Thus a query could be written to

display any configuration of data available in the records. For example, the user can look up the patient's MRN using the patient's last name, first name, and date of birth. A display of all the associated patient account numbers is often presented, which the system obtains by searching for the records in the patient account index that match the MRN being searched. Those patient account numbers will link to records associated with the individual visits and so forth. This small example contains a tiny fraction of the possible tables or entities needed to represent a complete patient health record.

## Data Sets

Throughout the course of the patient's care, data are collected by many health care professionals. The elements of data collected are used for different purposes. Physicians use the data to improve the quality of their services and help treat individual patients. Health care consumers may use the data to select a physician or a treatment. Insurance companies and government agencies require health data to pay patients' bills or track health trends. Without a specific requirement, facilities might not collect data elements that are helpful to users who wish to perform an analysis.

For this reason, many of these users, such as the Centers for Medicare and Medicaid Services (CMS), are very particular in their data needs and give health care providers specifications for the data they require, called a *data set.*

A **data set** is a defined group of fields that are required for a specified purpose. One common example of a data set is a mailing address. To mail a letter through the US Postal Service, the data set is defined as the following:

- addressee
- street address

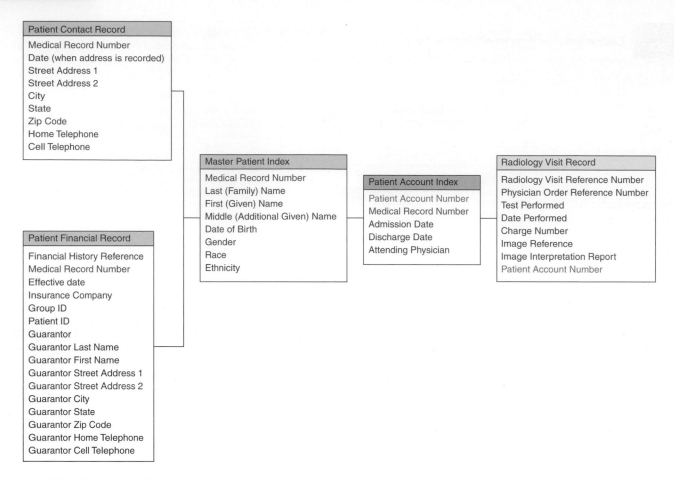

• **Fig. 2.8** Using the master patient index table as the key point of reference, the user can look up the medical record number, which links to the patient's contact, financial, and clinical data.

- apartment or unit number (if applicable)
- city
- state
- zip code

Each of these elements is part of the required data set to mail a letter. Online shoppers are familiar with the dual data sets of "billing address" and "shipping address," as well as the "payment" data set, which includes the credit card, name on the card, card number, expiration date, and security code. As we will see, the users of health information specify their own data sets telling HIM professionals what data to collect and how to report it.

### Defined Data Sets

A data set requires a standard method for reporting data elements so that they can be compared with similar data collected either in a different time or from a different facility. To compare data, everyone must collect the data in the same manner that can be readily converted into the same format. For example, certain data are collected on all patients regardless of the health care services needed-name, address, phone number, gender, and date of birth. This data set is for the patient's personal identification. It allows the facility to distinguish one patient among other patients and to distinguish between men and women, mothers and babies, and

seniors and pediatric patients. The patient's living arrangements, on the other hand, are not a required field in all settings.

The collection and reporting of defined data sets enable users to compare activities, volumes, patient care, and some outcomes among the reporting facilities. The detailed data can be aggregated and analyzed to make public health decisions and to study the spread of disease. Proper and complete comparison is only possible when facilities know what data to collect and how to report it.

Even for a required field, however, there are no specific rules governing the way in which the data are captured. Thus, even when the patient's gender is identified and recorded, facilities may choose to capture those data in the way that is most convenient or useful. For example, without a specific rule to follow, the field that captures the patient's gender could read F, 1, or A for female; M, 2, or B for male; and O, U, 3, or C for *nonbinary* patients, or those patients who do not identify as male or female. Table 2.1 illustrates data collection of gender as a numeric value that is converted to an alphabetic character on reporting. The decision as to how to store data elements may depend on system capacity and data quality issues. For example, a Social Security number may be stored as a single, nine-character alphanumeric field (i.e., 123456789) but can be displayed for ease of reading in

| TABLE 2.1 | Collection and Report of Gender Data | |
|---|---|---|
| | Collected Numerical | Reported Alpha |
| Female | 1 | F |
| Male | 2 | M |
| Nonbinary | 3 | O |

the recognizable 3-2-4 pattern (123-45-6789), since there is no need to store two dashes every time.

If each health care facility determined its own method for collecting the patient's gender data and reported it that way, users would have to interpret each facility's method for classifying this information as they attempt to analyze the data. In fact, facilities may collect the data in any format that is useful to the facility as long as it complies or can be converted to comply with regulatory and accreditation reporting requirements. For example, a hospital may decide to store patient admission and discharge dates as Microsoft Excel dates (January 1, 1900 = day "1"; October 3, 2014 = day "41915") to facilitate manipulation of downloaded data. But to report that data, the hospital must convert those dates into the format required by the user.

Here are two examples of data sets that we will be exploring in detail in subsequent chapters: billing data and patient visit data.

The standard billing form for institutional providers (such as hospitals) is the Health Insurance Portability and Accountability Act 837I data set, which is represented on the **Uniform Bill (UB-04)**. The UB-04 tells providers exactly what data to collect and report to bill payers for their services. The data set of the UB-04 was developed by the National Uniform Billing Committee (NUBC), which consists of the users of this billing data. Current member organizations of the NUBC are the American Hospital Association, industry associations, insurance companies, and government agencies such as CMS (National Uniform Billing Committee, n.d.).

For most types of health care delivery, a minimum set of data must be collected and reported for each patient. Acute care hospitals, for example, report the **Uniform Hospital Discharge Data Set (UHDDS)**, which includes demographic, clinical, and financial data about individual patient visits. Health care entities provide UHDDS data to states through a defined reporting system. Within a specified time frame after discharge, the institution must report all of the elements to the state Department of Health or other designated agency, along with any additional data elements required by the state. A summary of these elements is shown in Box 2.1. Skilled nursing facilities use their **Minimum Data Set (MDS 3.0)** and home health organizations report, the **Outcome and Assessment Information Set (OASIS)**. These setting-specific data sets are prescribed by CMS.

Other data sets, such as those collected for disease-specific registries, are discussed in subsequent chapters in relation to the appropriate discussion of the health care setting or topic. Table 2.2 contains a summary of the data sets discussed in this chapter for use in various health care settings.

When various providers report the same data in the same way, the data can be compared among different providers. Trends in patient care can be identified, as well as opportunities for improvement. For example, the defined data set of the UHDDS allows government entities to analyze patients, the health care provider, and services. The analysis is possible because each data element is being reported the same way for every inpatient receiving acute care in the United States.

The standardization of this reporting allows analysts to compare health care services received by Medicare patients regardless of where they receive those services. CMS

| • BOX 2.1 | Uniform Hospital Discharge Data Set (UHDDS) Summary of Data Elements |
|---|---|

Personal/unique identifier medical record number (MRN)
Date of birth
Gender
Race and ethnicity
Residence
Health care facility identification number
Admission date
Type of admission
Discharge date
Attending physician's identification number
Surgeon's identification number
Principal diagnosis
Other diagnoses
Qualifier for other diagnoses
External cause of injury
Birth weight of neonate
Significant procedures and dates of procedures
Disposition of the patient at discharge
Expected source of payment
Total charges

| TABLE 2.2 | Summary of Minimum Data Sets | |
|---|---|---|
| **Data Set** | | **Setting** |
| Uniform Hospital Discharge Data Set (UHDDS) | | Acute care |
| Uniform Ambulatory Care Data Set (UACDS) | | Ambulatory care |
| Minimum Data Set (MDS) | | Long-term care |
| Outcome and Assessment Information Set (OASIS) | | Home health care |
| Data Elements for Emergency Department Systems (DEEDS) | | Emergency departments |

provides a definition for each data element specifying what should be captured for that data element. For example, the *principal diagnosis* is defined in the UHDDS as "that condition established after study to be chiefly responsible for occasioning the admission of the patient to the hospital for care" (Centers for Medicare and Medicaid Services [CMS], 2022).

## Data Collection and Storage

All of the data that have been collected about an individual patient are called a **health record** or medical record. A health record may refer to the patient's record that is kept by a particular health care provider or to the patient's lifelong medical history. For the sake of clarity, we refer to a patient's information as the health record, whether it refers to a single visit or the patient's collective experience.

Data collection is rarely the collection of a single data field but is more often a record of several data fields collected repeatedly over time. We do not just collect one patient's contact data; we collect all patients' contact data. We collect these data in the same way every time within a particular organization. The data collected in various health care settings vary somewhat depending on the needs of the users in that setting and the type of care being rendered. So, the methods of data collection, recording, and storage of data vary as well.

The primary difference between the data compiled in a physician's office record and the data collected in a hospital lies in the volume of data collected about a patient

and the way the data are organized in a record. In the physician's office, there are a limited number of individuals recording data in the record. The receptionist, a nurse, a medical assistant, and a doctor might contribute to collecting and recording data. The categories of data are the same (see Chapter 3) when a patient is receiving care in a facility, such as a hospital; however, the volume of data collected in a hospital is much greater than that collected in a physician's office. While the patient is in the hospital, an entire team of clinical personnel is collecting and recording data about everything that happens to the patient. Even a patient with multiple complications who visits a physician's office has a brief record until he or she has visited many times. In a hospital, however, sometimes even the smallest procedures generate enormous volumes of data. Paper forms and computer hardware are the primary data collection devices for health data. We use the term **data collection device** to refer to any tool that facilitates the collection and recording of data, including paper forms and computerized data entry screens.

## Forms

In a paper-based record, most of the data are collected in a standard format that is devised by the individual facility. With some exceptions, notably the forms for newborns and women delivering babies, the forms in one hospital do not look exactly the same as those in another hospital. Although most facilities are well on their way to having entirely EHRs, note that the foundation for the development of the computer screens that guide the capture of data is the original paper forms and is guided by similar purposes. In the context of a computer program, forms improve the data collection. On a paper-based form the patient's name and MRN are added manually. Someone has to write it in, stamp it in, or affix a label in the corner of every page. In an EHR the patient's name is entered once, at the point of registration, and associated with the MRN. Subsequent users who are recording data in that patient's record may select the patient from a directory of existing patients. Thus the patient name and MRN are entered once and used many times. Further, EHRs need backup if there is a system failure and data cannot be captured electronically. Forms have certain benefits, whether electronic or paper, such as

- reminding the user of which data must be collected,
- providing a structure for capturing that data so that the reader knows where to look for the desired data, and
- ensuring that complete data are collected according to the clinical guidelines of the facility and profession and according to regulation.

Paper forms are designed to meet documentation standards specific to the clinical discipline, the facility, facility guidelines, and regulatory considerations. They are frequently created by committees of the people who use them. Forms related to *medication administration*, for example, would be created by the nursing department in collaboration with the pharmacy and probably with physician input. Some facilities have an oversight committee, simply called the *forms committee* or *documentation committee*. This committee may be charged with ensuring that forms are created only when necessary, that duplicate forms are not created, and that the forms conform to facility and regulatory guidelines. The most important consideration in the development of a form is the needs of the users of the form. Those needs include regulatory compliance, clear communication, ease of data entry, and ease of data retrieval.

Even facilities that collect the clinical data on paper tend to have computerized patient registration data. The patient's contact information and billing data collected during the patient registration process can usually be printed out on one paper form, called the *admission record*, although several computer screens may be necessary to capture these data. In a paper record the admission record would typically be the first page in the patient's record. In an electronic record the patient's record typically opens on a home page that may contain summary or recent care data and generally has tabs or a menu to access specific types of data.

## Form Content

Many considerations go into the development of a health data form. Consider the development of a physician's order form in the following example. The physician directs the care of the patient. The form for a physician's order has the very important function of communicating the physician's plan for the patient's care to all members of the health care team. All lab tests, for example, must start with the physician's order. The form must satisfy every user's needs, not just the physician's.

If a physician wants to administer penicillin to a patient, the nurse and the pharmacy need to know the following information:

- to which patient the medication is being dispensed,
- the exact medication, including whether a brand name or generic drug is required
- the exact dosage, including precise measurements,
- the specific route of administration (e.g., oral or intravenous [via a needle into the bloodstream]),
- the ordered frequency of administration,
- when the order was given (time and date),
- who gave the order (author of the order and authorized signature).

Thus the order form must be flexible enough to record the hundreds of different medications, therapies, and instructions that a physician might give and to communicate accurately the instructions needed by the recipient of the order, such as the radiology department.

Generally, the patient's name, MRN, and other identifying data are recorded in the top right-hand corner of every page of every form or computer screen. Patient identification data must be on every page so that the data can be matched to the correct patient. The patient data usually go in the right-hand corner of a paper record page because most records, particularly when the patient is still in the hospital, are kept in three-ring binders and it's easy to see the patient identification in the top right corner as you flip through the pages. It is equally important that the patient be identified at the top of every computer screen in an EHR, to minimize the potential for errors that could occur by working in the wrong patient's record.

In addition to identifying the patient on the form or screen, some information identifying the form is needed. Typically included on a paper form are the name of the facility, the title of the form, and any special instructions about the form. The top left-hand corner of the page is a convenient place to put the name of the hospital and possibly its location (which is useful if the hospital has many facilities), along with the title of the form. In an electronic record the name of the page or type of data collection generally appears prominently on the page or the menu tab.

### Formatting the Form

How many physician orders can be put on one page of a paper record? Should there be separate blocks for each order, or should the form be designed to have a lot of lines on which the physician may write as much as he or she desires for each order? The answers to these questions are a matter of facility preference. Forms with the orders in blocks, with each block containing only one set of orders, and forms that consist of a page of blank lines on which the physician may write free-form are both common. Some facilities may create separate forms for every type of order. Thus orders pertaining to newborns would be on one type of form; order forms for surgical patients would be different; orders for the general patient population would be on a third form.

A major consideration in constructing a form is the size of the fields that will be included. In the previous discussion about data dictionaries the size of a field was illustrated. On a paper form, the size of the field in characters must be accommodated, as well as the space needed to handwrite the data. The size of the printing on the page is a consideration. How close to the edge of the page can the form be printed? Will holes be punched in the form? If so, where will they be and how much space should be allowed? Fig. 2.9 shows a form design template. Table 2.3 summarizes paper form design issues.

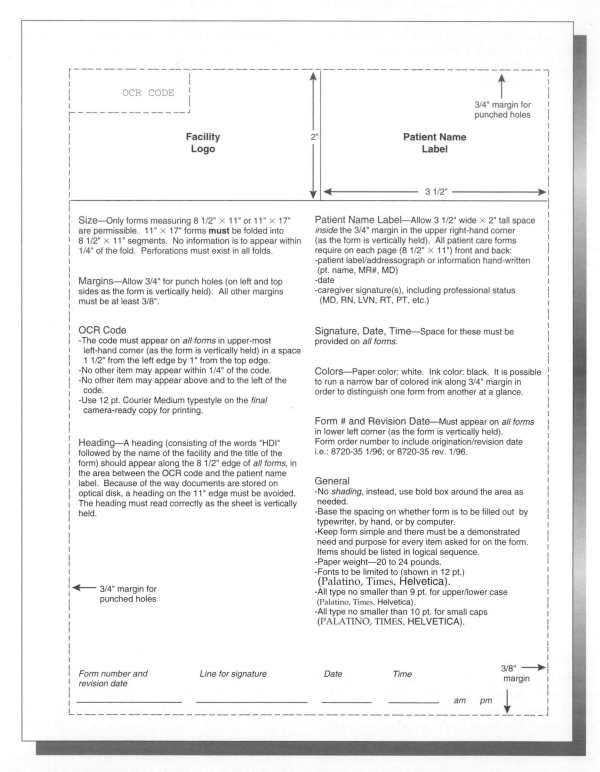

• **Fig. 2.9** Forms design template. (From Abdelhak M, Grostick S, Hanken MA, Jacobs E: *Health information: management of a strategic resource*, ed 4, Philadelphia, 2012, Saunders, p 122.)

| | |
|---|---|
| **TABLE 2.3** | **Data Collection Device Design Issues** |

| Issue | Considerations |
|---|---|
| Identification of user needs | Not limited to the collectors of the data; also necessary to consider subsequent users of both the device and the data it contains |
| Purpose of the data collection device | Necessary to ensure both data collection and controls for quality |
| Selection of the appropriate data items and sequencing of data collection activities | Should fulfill the purpose of the device, without unnecessary fields; important to consider the order in which data are collected |
| Understanding the technology used | Not just paper versus computer (e.g., How is the paper used? How is the computer used? What input devices are available and how will they be used?) |
| Use of standard terminology and abbreviations and development of a standard format | Communication among users improved by consistency in language and format |
| Appropriate instructions | Consistency improved by instructions on the form |
| Simplicity | The simpler the device, the easier to use |

On a computer screen, there are additional considerations. For example, if there is a lot of data to be collected at one time, how many screens will be needed and in what order should the data be collected? Should the software require the user to complete each screen before moving to the next or will the user be able to go back and make changes? In a computer-based record, it is not necessary to "allow room" for variable handwriting; exactly enough room is allowed for the particular data field because the size of the field is defined in the data dictionary. Electronic data collection also benefits from validity checks, radio buttons, and drop-down menus. A validity check could issue a warning to a user who attempts to enter a number higher than 12 to represent the month. A drop-down menu could be accessed to enter the patient's gender, race, and ethnicity according to the valid choices. In the vital signs entry screen shown in Fig. 2.10 the user selects from drop-down menus to enter the patient's pulse, blood pressure, and oxygen saturation were measured. Among the choices of sites from which the patient's pulse was measured, this medical assistant has selected "radial," meaning that the patient's pulse at was taken at her wrist. In the illustration the patient's oxygen delivery is entered using radio buttons.

Another example of improvement in data collection that results from EHR implementation is the **computerized physician order entry (CPOE)**. When ordering medication, instead of typing or writing out the name of the drug, the dosage, and the route of administration, the provider

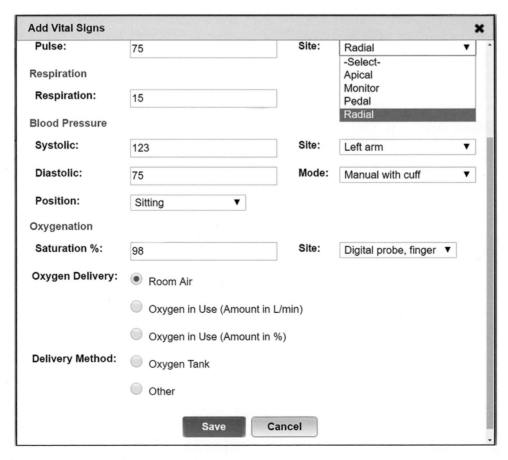

• **Fig. 2.10** Use of drop down menus and radio buttons on a vital signs entry screen.

selects this information from drop-down menus and radio buttons. CPOE greatly reduces errors due to poor handwriting or incorrectly input data. In addition, the provider can only order items that are on the facility's approved drug list because they are the only options on the menu. In this instance the use of a menu-driven computer-based data collection system significantly reduces the chance that a physician orders a nonapproved drug. Such a mistake might very well happen if the physician has privileges at a variety of different hospitals because approved drug lists in various hospitals are not necessarily identical. Moreover, CPOE can be linked to the pharmacy, which might generate the medication request without nursing intermediation. In addition, the CPOE can be linked to health data that have already been collected about the patient, such as sex, height, weight, age, and diagnosis. Then, if a physician ordered a drug at a dosage that exceeds the maximal amount that is considered safe for a newborn, for instance, the software could automatically generate a warning that the drug dosage was inappropriate, thereby alerting the physician of his or her error before any harm was done.

## Compliance

**Compliance** with licensure and accreditation standards is another consideration. Whether forms are maintained on paper or in an electronic medium, documentation standards for the record remain the same. The Joint Commission, for example, requires that a physician's orders must be authenticated: signed, dated, and timed. Therefore the order form should facilitate compliance with these requirements by having a labeled space for the signature, date, and time. Occasionally, a clinician may write an order but forget to sign it, meaning that the order is not *authenticated*. The "signature" is in ink on the paper form, but on the electronic form, it will be a notation generated by the physician's acceptance of the order (Fig. 2.11).

Two concepts are necessary to understand "signed." The first concept is authorship: the author of an order is the person who wrote or entered it. The second concept is **authentication**: the author's mark or signature. The distinction between author and authentication is important for compliance with rules regarding signing of clinical and other documentation. For example, a first-year resident may be the author and signer of an order or progress note; however, that order or note will likely be **countersigned** by a supervising, licensed physician. The potential need for this

> ### ◆ NOTE
>
> Patient gender is recorded, however, patients identify regardless of their sex at birth. Gender categories can become problematic when software is programmed to identify gender/diagnosis mismatches, such as a prostate disease in a female patient. HIM professionals are aware of these issues and must be sensitive in determining whether there was a registration error or perhaps the patient had a gender-reassignment or made a gender identity declaration.

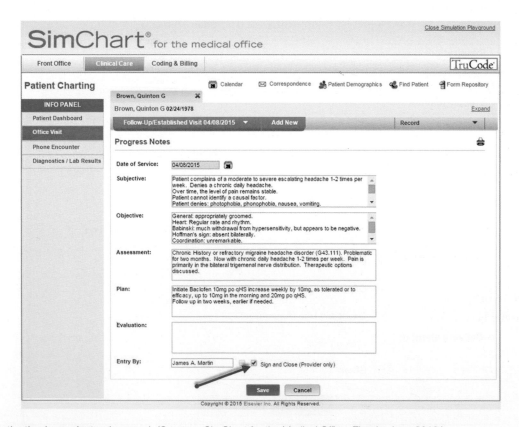

• **Fig. 2.11** Authentication in an electronic record. (Courtesy SimChart for the Medical Office, Elsevier, Inc., 2018.)

second authentication must be taken into consideration in the design of forms. Another example of an authentication without authorship is the discharge instruction form. Discharge instructions are often prepared by nursing staff and then completed and authenticated by the discharging physician.

On a paper record, that mark or signature takes the form of the author's formal signature or his or her initials. Consequently, in the design of the form, places are provided for the author's authentication and a note of the date and time of the orders. This detail is important from a clinical perspective because the time between the writing of the order and the execution of the order is a compliance issue. In an electronic record, since there is no signature line, there must be a prompt or space for the clinician to enter a code or accept the documentation.

Next, the designers must consider what other information will be necessary on the form. The physician's orders are written to communicate instructions to other health care providers. In a paper record the physician's orders are maintained in the nursing unit near the patient. The orders are not directly accessible to the radiology department, laboratory department, pharmacy, and so on. Someone has to communicate the orders to the correct party. Members of the nursing staff are usually charged with that responsibility. Therefore the form must contain an area for these staff members to indicate that they have read and executed the order. In the case of medication the nurse may send the order to the pharmacy, verify the drug when it is received, and document the administration of the drug which it is given to the patient. In an electronic record the order may be communicated directly to the pharmacy for dispensing. However, the verification and medication administration documentation is still required.

Another compliance issue revolves around the nature of the form. As we will explore in subsequent chapters, there are certain forms that are required for legal reasons. In your own experience, you may have had to sign such forms at the hospital or physician's office. With the advent of EHRs, many facilities print these forms when they are needed (on demand) rather than have stacks of blank forms that require patient-identifying data to be added. So, after the patient's registration data are collected, the software is able to generate the form with the appropriate patient data already included. The patient can then sign the form, which is then scanned back into the patient's record, or sign a signature pad, which the software affixes to the form in the patient's record.

## Other Considerations

So far, the focus has been on the data that must be recorded on the form. In a paper record a number of other issues must be considered:

- How heavy should the paper be? Should it be heavy card stock or copy machine weight?
- Should the form be one part, two parts, or more?
- If it is a multipart form, should each part be a different color?
- On what color paper should the form be printed? White is best for photocopying, but would another color help the users of the form?

These are considerations that the forms committee reviews to ensure that the form conforms to the institution's guidelines. Designing forms was once a difficult and time-consuming process because they had to be developed with a pencil and paper, given to a printer, created, and then returned to the organization for editing-frequently multiple times. Today, it is relatively simple to create a form in a word-processing document for review and editing.

Another consideration is how to keep track of the existing, approved forms. In a paper-based system, forms are used selectively depending on the type of patient record and the department using them. Someone in the hospital, frequently the director of the HIM department, must keep track of all approved forms to ensure that documentation standards are met. In reality, forms get passed around, photocopied, and shuffled from department to department. If a form is not used frequently, it can become lost. When the form is needed but not readily available, the users may create a new form even though the old form still exists. Therefore a **master forms file** should be created and maintained by the director of the HIM department. The master forms file contains every form used by the hospital and can be organized in any way that the hospital finds useful.

One very efficient way to save a master forms file is to keep forms in categories corresponding to the departments that use them and then alphabetically by department name. Another way to maintain a master forms file is to give each form a numerical assignment and then save the forms in numerical order. In either case, the creation of an index and table of contents for the master forms file is necessary. The index is at the front of the file, and the title of each form and its individual number are listed in the table of contents. The responsibility for ensuring that forms are not duplicated and that each form conforms to the institution's needs usually lies with the forms committee, as previously mentioned.

The forms committee is an institution-wide committee that has the responsibility of reviewing and approving all forms on a regular basis. Therefore representatives of all the major clinical services must be included. The committee should include a representative from nursing, physician staff (probably several representatives if the facility offers numerous services), laboratory, and radiology. Because HIM personnel are frequently in charge of the master forms file, a representative from the HIM department should be included in the forms committee.

In a computer-based environment, the forms are created and displayed on computer screens. The development of or addition of forms/data to a computer system should be under the direction of a systems development team. However, only the clinicians and other health practitioners are truly aware of the data that must be collected and how the data should be organized. The data dictionary then becomes critical in the development process. The data fields that are collected, the staff members who have access to them, and whether those with access can print, change, or view the data become increasingly important considerations. Existing institutional committees become involved in the development of computer-based forms according to institution policies. In any event, HIM personnel should be directly involved in this process.

## Electronic Health Record

The health care industry relies on computer technology to deliver quality patient care. The terminology of computerization is often confusing. The terms *electronic*, *computerized*, *computer-assisted*, and *computer-based* are sometimes used interchangeably. At the time of this writing, the generally accepted term for a computerized patient record is the **electronic health record (EHR)**. An EHR is a digital version of the patient's paper health record that collects and maintains data about the patient. Unlike a paper health record that can only be accessed by having the physical file, the data in the EHR can be collected, viewed, and updated from any location. Patient data are quickly retrieved and available to multiple health care professionals at the same time. When a paper record is used, the record is accessible wherever the patient is being treated because it goes where the patient goes. Therefore only one health care provider at a time is usually able to see the record. The EHR allows the record to be viewed by several caregivers at the same time, regardless of the location of the patient or the caregivers. In the HIM department the EHR allows several staff members to use the record at the same time to support the many functions that occur. Having the ability to accomplish these tasks simultaneously leads to greater efficiency.

Additionally, the EHR does more than simply store and maintain health data. Modern EHR systems are highly sophisticated and take advantage of the ability to send and receive information instantly. For example, EHR technology allows providers to order tests and send prescriptions directly to pharmacies. The EHR also suggests treatment plans and reports data to authorities. Table 2.4 lists the key characteristics of a comprehensive EHR.

### The Hybrid Record

For organizations that have not transitioned to a full EHR, an interim step is the **hybrid record**: part paper, part electronic. There are various degrees of computerization in the hybrid record. In a hybrid record, some departments of the hospital use computer information systems to document patient care, but other departments continue to use paper documentation. Recording of clinical data at the time treatment is delivered to the patient is called **point-of-care documentation**. Some clinical point-of-care documentation may be captured electronically through the system, making data collection into the patient's health record immediate.

| TABLE 2.4 | Functions of the Electronic Health Record |
|---|---|
| **Topic** | **Function** |
| Health information and data | Allows providers to have immediate access to key information such as allergies, medications, and lab test results |
| Result management | Allows providers to quickly access new and past test results, increasing patient safety and effectiveness of care |
| Computerized physician order entry (CPOE) | Allows providers to enter and store orders for prescriptions, tests, or services in a computer-based system that improves legibility, reduces duplication, and increases the speed of executing the orders |
| Clinical decision-making support (CDS) | Allows the use of reminders, alerts, and prompts that suggest treatment plans, improve compliance with best clinical practices, and ensure regular screening |
| Electronic communication and connectivity | Allows for efficient, secure, and readily accessible communication among providers and patients that will improve the continuity of care, enhance the timeliness of diagnoses and treatments, and reduce the frequency of adverse occurrences |
| Patient support | Provides tools that give patients access to their own health records, provides internet education, and assists them in carrying out home monitoring and self-teaching, which can help improve chronic conditions |
| Administrative processes | Allow for administrative tools such as scheduling, which would improve efficiency and provide more timely service |
| Reporting | Allows electronic data storage using uniform data standards that will enable organizations to respond to third-party regulatory agencies |

Modified from Institute of Medicine (US) Committee on Data Standards for Patient Safety: *Key capabilities of an electronic health record system: letter report*, Washington (DC), 2003, National Academies Press (US). https://www.ncbi.nlm.nih.gov/books/NBK221802/. Accessed November 20, 2018. doi:10.17226/10781.

Physicians and other health care professionals may capture patient information directly into the health record using several different documentation systems, which are detailed throughout this text. The hybrid record represents a midpoint between the traditional paper record and the fully functional EHR, in which all the documentation surrounding patient care is captured and maintained electronically. In fact, even when all point-of-care documentation is electronic, there may be some documentation, such as externally prepared reports, that arrive in paper form. There will always be paper that must be reconciled, for example, due to system downtime or records from other organizations, often resulting in scanning or other electronic storage. It can be anticipated that health records will always be in some form of hybrid. Therefore EHRs typically facilitate the scanning of paper documentation into the record.

Some facilities transfer or scan the paper-based portion into a digital format using a **document imaging** system, creating an electronic copy of that information. In document imaging a scanner converts the paper document into a digital image, which is then stored on a document server, optical disk, or other storage media. An example is illustrated in Fig. 2.12. An **electronic document management system (EDMS)**, such as the one pictured, may be used as a storage and retrieval mechanism and allows for additional documents to be added to an electronic record. For example, an EDMS may be used to scan records transferred from another facility to the EHR. Document imaging can be performed after discharge or at the point-of-care.

Even facilities that rely on paper documentation for their clinical data tend to use computer systems for the MPI. Once this database is created, it can be used by other systems within the organization via **interface**: the process by which two independent systems are configured to communicate with each other. The hospital EHR system can interface with the billing system and the ancillary systems, enabling data to be shared in both directions. Because information can be shared, communication among departments is faster, less redundant, and more accurate. Since the MPI is the key to referencing the data to the correct patient, the MPI database must be present to develop an electronic record. Because part of the patient registration process is the collection of data related to the method of payment, financial data are also collected and stored electronically.

Clinical data, consisting of, for example, physician, nursing, and diagnostic testing data, make up the bulk of a traditional health record. Clinical data can be collected and stored electronically or collected on paper and scanned into the system.

Ancillary departments, such as laboratory, radiology, and pharmacy, may also use information systems to collect data and generate reports. Their data may be held in a separate database or interfaced with the HIM and/or financial systems. Collectively, these ancillary systems make up a great portion of the health record. Having this information available electronically to multiple users is a great advantage for providers, resulting in better quality of care. However, although many ancillary departments adopted electronic systems long ago, they did not necessarily interface with the hospital systems for access by providers. This resulted in the need to print and distribute large quantities of paper reports that would have to be delivered to the patient care area and ultimately filed in the patient record. In a certified EHR the ancillary systems interact with the EHR, eliminating this costly and cumbersome step.

The challenges associated with managing a hybrid record are substantial. Because portions of the record may be saved as scanned images, locating a specific data element in a document may be difficult. Controlling the various versions of the record is also important to ensure that the most up-to-date version of the record and documentation is stored in all parts of the patient's record. For example, if a patient changes his or her address and it is updated in the MPI, that change should be reflected in every system, including anything that has been scanned. The need to scan large volumes of patient care documentation diminishes as EHRs are fully implemented; however, as mentioned earlier, scanning will likely never be eliminated.

The goal is always to have a reliable and accessible patient record, in whichever way that record may be organized or stored. Many facilities have utilized hybrid records as a sensible, affordable solution to make progress toward an EHR.

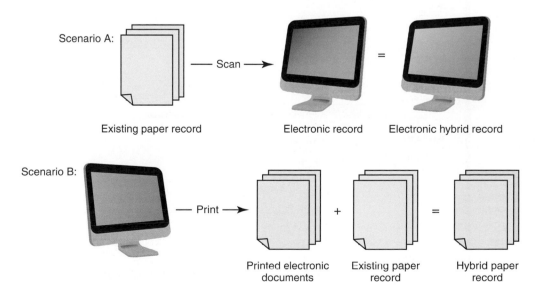

• **Fig. 2.12** Two kinds of hybrid records.

## *Features of the Electronic Health Record*

An EHR results from computer-based data collection. Physicians and other clinicians capture data at the point-of-care, with the ability to retrieve the data later for reporting and use in research or administrative decision-making. Health care workers document care via input ports on the various clinical units, using laptops, handheld tablets, and bedside terminals. Very few, if any, paper reports are generated. The EHR allows all departments (e.g., nursing) to document care electronically using these templates. A fully functional EHR incorporates the patient history, demographics, patient problem lists, list of current medications, and patient's allergies, in addition to physician clinical notes, which include patients' medical history and follow-up notes. The laboratory and radiology tests are ordered and viewed electronically, with the results being incorporated into the EHR. Further, the out-of-range values for the laboratory tests are highlighted as they are included within the EHR.

Order entry is the beginning of the process in which instructions from the physician are communicated. Physicians' orders were historically handwritten. The traditional method of handwriting prescriptions and orders can be difficult, tedious, or even dangerous. The electronic entry of physicians' instructions for the treatment of the patients may reduce medical errors. For this reason, the EHR has CPOE allowing a physician to enter orders for medications, tests, treatments, or procedures directly into a system (Fig. 2.13). As stated above, the CPOE system provides the physician with a list of medications that can be used for the specific treatment of the patient's diagnosis. From a menu, the provider selects the drug, dosage, and frequency of administration (e.g., as needed, three times per day). User interfaces through software on laptops, handheld electronic devices, and mobile computing terminals in hospitals have made order entry at point-of-care convenient for physicians. The CPOE system also provides alerts to the physician based on the patient's drug list, allergies, interactions, or other potential contraindications. It can provide certain prompts or alerts specific to the physician's orders and provide drug–drug and drug–allergy interaction checks. As shown in Fig. 2.14, the EHR prompts the possibility of a moderate drug interaction between the previously prescribed drug, lisinopril, and the newly prescribed drug, glyburide. The CPOE does not stand alone. Ideally, it is interfaced with the pharmacy and ancillary department systems, as well as the billing system and nursing's medication administration record. In this way, the provider's order is sent electronically to the pharmacy of the patient's choice. This communication among systems or modules allows the order to initiate the cascade of events that result in a completion of the order's instructions. Thus an unfulfilled order creates a flag in the system that helps prevent orders from being missed.

Many EHR software technologies also have a **clinical decision-making system (CDS)**. The CDS suggests appropriate patient care strategies to the physician through an **algorithm**, a set of step-by-step instructions for solving

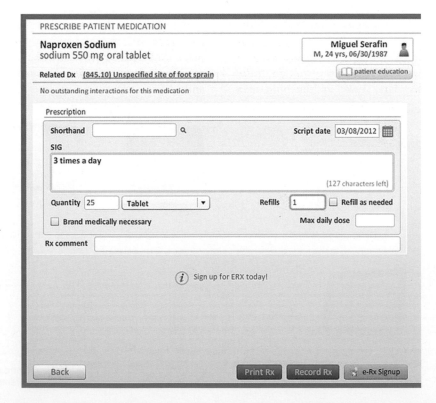

• **Fig. 2.13** A computerized physician order entry (CPOE) e-prescribing screen. (Courtesy Practice Fusion, Inc., San Francisco, CA.)

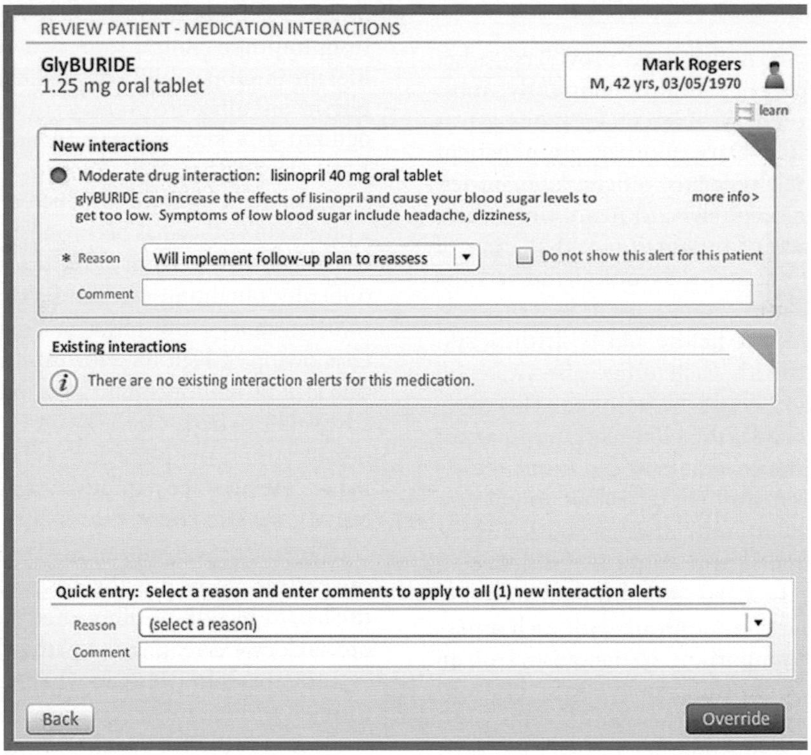

REVIEW PATIENT - MEDICATION INTERACTIONS

**GlyBURIDE**
1.25 mg oral tablet

**Mark Rogers**
M, 42 yrs, 03/05/1970

learn

**New interactions**

Moderate drug interaction: lisinopril 40 mg oral tablet
glyBURIDE can increase the effects of lisinopril and cause your blood sugar levels to
get too low. Symptoms of low blood sugar include headache, dizziness,

more info >

* Reason    Will implement follow-up plan to reassess        □ Do not show this alert for this patient

Comment

**Existing interactions**

ⓘ There are no existing interaction alerts for this medication.

**Quick entry: Select a reason and enter comments to apply to all (1) new interaction alerts**

Reason    (select a reason)

Comment

Back                                                                                    Override

• **Fig. 2.14** Drug interaction prompt. (Courtesy Practice Fusion, Inc., San Francisco, CA.)

a problem. Once the patient's information is entered into the EHR, the CDS guides the physician by recommending certain diagnostic tests, treatments, and monitoring strategies. In this way, the EHR integrates into the physician's workflow a wealth of **evidence-based medicine (EBM)**, a decision-making approach based on the idea that the best care results from the conscientious, explicit, and judicious use of current best evidence. Ideally, the CDS is linked to the CPOE so the physician can create orders based on the recommendations from the CDS.

Other important features included in the EHRs are to send reminders to patients for patient preference or preventive follow-up care, to print out the diagnosis summary and current medication list, and to provide patients with timely electronic access to their health information. Reference material may be available for electronic use when specific diagnoses are documented. Lastly, most EHR systems help connect patients to their providers. Some EHRs allow patients to actively participate in their records. Through the Web, portions of an EHR may be made available to the patient to view or print. Patients are given a unique ID and password that grant them access to their own records. The patient logs onto a website, often referred to as a **patient portal**. On the patient portal, users can send messages to the clinical staff and physicians. They may also view their lab results and track and monitor information regarding their personal health. For example, they can add information such as allergies or new over-the-counter medications they are taking. Administratively, the patient can schedule appointments,

edit billing information, and request their health records be sent to a specific provider. Table 2.4 summarizes the functions of the EHR.

The health care industry has undergone dramatic changes as a result of the greater use of EHRs. In 2011 CMS established the Medicare and Medicaid EHR Incentive Program (now known as the Promoting Interoperability Program) to encourage eligible providers, eligible hospitals, and Critical Access Hospitals (CAHs) to adopt, implement, upgrade, and demonstrate meaningful use of certified electronic health technology (CEHERT). The US federal government, through the CMS, provided financial incentives to the health care providers who use certified EHRs in a "meaningful" way, called *meaningful use*, to hasten the widespread use of the EHRs. Initially, the federal government paid providers more for using EHRs with specific features. Later in the program, providers were financially penalized if they did not use functional EHRs. This compelled providers to use technology in the right way to save time and money, improve patient care, and facilitate patient participation in their own care. Concurrent with the development and implementation of the meaningful-use program were multiple quality-based initiatives focusing on patient outcomes and quality reporting. These two strategic efforts appear to have converged into the Merit Based Incentive Payment Program (MIPS), which is part of the Medicare Access and CHIP Reauthorization Act of 2015 (MACRA) (Office of the National Coordinator for Health Information Technology [ONC], 2022a). We will discuss quality initiatives in Chapter 10.

## Interoperability

During a patient's lifetime, health care providers gather information about the patient's health. Currently, most clinical information is stored in different locations across the health care community. Data about a given patient may be held in systems in physicians' offices, laboratories, imaging systems, or other hospitals, and many times these systems do not "talk." Lack of integration and sharing of clinical information that is stored electronically affects the quality of care across the United States, just as lack of access to paper records hampered care before EHRs. If these systems could communicate with each other effectively, all of the patient's information could be accessed, effectively creating a **longitudinal record**, the compilation of patient health data from all providers over a period of time, ideally from birth to death. The longitudinal record would provide a more complete picture of an individual's medical history. Theoretically, a longitudinal record could be compiled in paper form, but realistically a true longitudinal record is more likely with EHRs that communicate with each other.

Thus one of the most important characteristics of an EHR while storing the clinical information is its **interoperability** with other systems. In other words, the EHR systems should operate with one another to share information. If information systems within the same hospital cannot communicate or interact with each other, then sharing patient information is not possible. To achieve the objective to exchange clinical information, a secure, interoperable EHR is required that can share the information with other EHRs. Because data may be acquired about a patient from multiple clinical sources over the course of his or her life, the interoperability of provider data, from hospitals and physicians' offices to grocery store pharmacies, has been recognized as a key objective in utilizing the potential of an EHR (Fig. 2.15).

Consider a scenario in which a patient who usually visits a physician's office has been transported to a nearby hospital because of an emergency. The attending physician may have difficulty obtaining the patient's complete information. In some instances, the physician may have to repeat certain tests owing to lack of prior information about the patient. The lack of interoperability can be an enormous obstacle to advancing patient care. The interoperability between these organizations, the physician's office and the hospital, would reduce the need for redundant tests and would save the associated time and cost.

Moreover, without interoperable systems, the treatment the patient received at the hospital may not become part of the health record, possibly affecting the treatment decisions of the doctor directing the patient's care in the future.

Interoperable EHRs must standardize the health record formats and language used within the various information systems in order for systems to integrate data. This interoperability among the systems is critical in order for users to gain maximum use of and efficiency from the EHR. When information is collected in different formats, it cannot be shared or exchanged with another organization without intervention by a user. For example, the data element Date

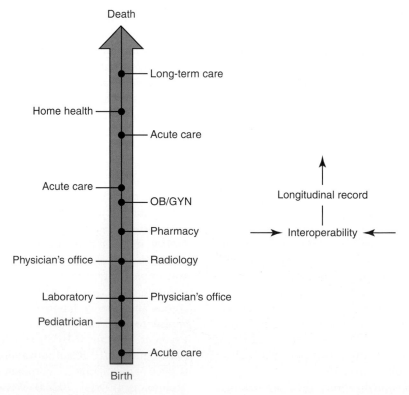

• **Fig. 2.15** Interoperable systems creating a longitudinal record.

of Birth can be collected in numerous ways. Some systems may collect it in the format of 2-digit date, 2-digit month, 4-digit year. Other systems may collect month first, then date, then year. Alternatively, some may collect the month as alphabetical characters (Oct instead of 10):

System 1: 09/10/1975
System 2: 10/09/1975
System 3: Oct/09/1975

Attempting to exchange or share information among these three systems will be difficult because of the lack of standardization in the Date of Birth field. Critical errors may result when systems cannot share information, such as misinterpreting treatment plans, medication strengths, or diagnoses.

The Institute of Electrical and Electronics Engineers (IEEE, 1990) defines *interoperability* as the "ability of two or more components to exchange information and to use the information that has been exchanged." In simple terms, interoperability exists between two systems when both the systems can send and receive information and perform the necessary tasks in an appropriate manner without any intervention. Interoperability can be classified into three categories as follows (Garde et al., 2007):

*Syntactic interoperability*—The two systems should be capable of exchanging *data*. In other words, the data should be accessible and in a machine-readable format. "Syntax" is the description of the rules by which the structure and the meaning are clearly defined.

*Structural interoperability/semantic interpretability*—The meaning of the information should be clear and understood by all users. An example of semantic interpretability is discrete code sets, such as in the International Classification of Diseases, 10th Revision-Clinical Modification (ICD-10-CM).

*Semantic interoperability*—The two or more systems that exchange information should be able to interpret the meaning of the information exchanged without any ambiguity. Semantic interoperability creates coherence among systems that do not speak the same language. To achieve semantic interoperability, the systems exchanging information should refer to a common information exchange reference model, such as Health Level 7 (HL7).

To illustrate the impact of interoperability, consider the impact of electronic data capture and storage on medical imaging (radiography). Advances in medical imaging have ushered in a new era of noninvasive diagnostic tools in health care, but the way these images are captured and shared has evolved as well. Digital imaging has made the use of film increasingly rare in radiography, and it has also changed the way these data are stored. Rather than developing, filing, and retrieving film jackets, modern medical imaging requires the storage and transmittal of very large digital pictures.

The technology that allows the effective use of these images is called a **picture archiving and communication system (PACS)**. A PACS allows many different kinds of diagnostic images (e.g., x-rays, magnetic images, ultrasound scans, computed tomography scans) obtained by many different kinds of machines to be archived and accessed from any computer terminal in the network and even implemented into a patient's EHR (Fig. 2.16).

Just as the data contained in an EHR require certain standards to be interoperable, images must follow a certain standard. Furthermore, some types of digital images generate so much data that their use is impractical without compression. The **Digital Imaging and Communications in Medicine (DICOM)** standard enables the management of these images—with regard to both storage and transmission over networks. Specifically, DICOM dictates the formats, protocols, means of compression, and even printing of images, making their exchange among physicians and other providers possible.

### Health Information Exchange

One means of achieving interoperability is participation in a **health information exchange (HIE)**. HIEs serve as a communication link among systems, allowing health care providers to request and receive patients' records from other providers. For example, the HIEs facilitate sharing of electronic information that is requested by a physician at facility A for a patient from facility B (Fig. 2.17). The rationale behind the establishment of HIEs and the way they are

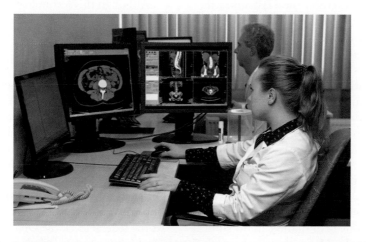

• **Fig. 2.16** A radiologist interprets diagnostic images on a picture archiving and communication system (PACS) capable of transmitting very large files. (Copyright Medvedkov/iStockphoto.com.)

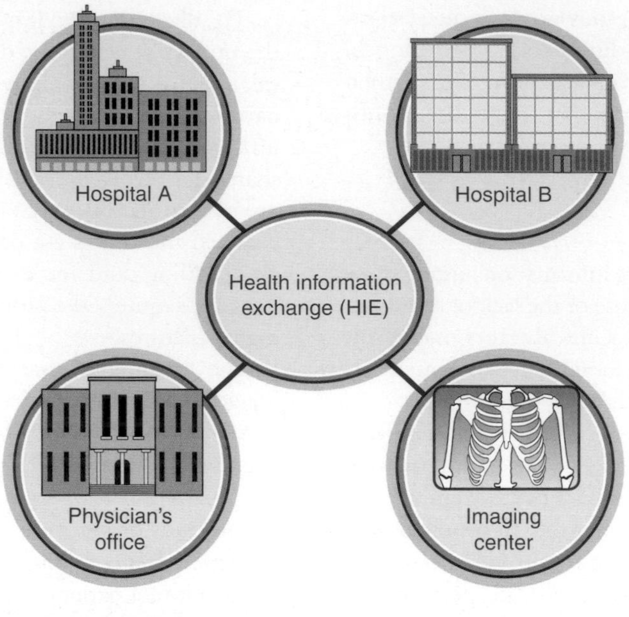

• **Fig. 2.17** Components of a sample health information exchange.

managed varies, as some are established by the state government and others by private organizations. Most HIEs were formed to share and gather electronic information among health care providers in geographic areas such as state, county, region, or nation. The HIEs benefit the health care providers by reducing costs through the elimination of duplication of tests and increased staff efficiencies. Other benefits include

- easy access to a health record,
- better continuity of care for patients,
- decreased medical errors with the ability to reconcile medications,
- improved patient outcomes and quality of care,
- potential for a longitudinal record, and
- support reduction in prescription drug abuse.

Although HIEs have existed for many years, their financial sustainability has been problematic. Theoretically, the provider pushes either patient index data or patient records to the HIE. In a distributed structure, the HIE stores the index and facilitates data requests from other providers—passing the request from the provider to the originator and passing the information back to the requester. In a centralized structure, the HIE receives both the index and the actual records from the originator and requestors access the data in the HIE. The mechanics of such sharing are hampered by variations in the technology and the ability of the providers to share data electronically—a hurdle being overcome thanks to provisions of meaningful use that require electronic exchange of data.

But the mechanics are not the biggest hurdles. The most difficult aspect of developing and implementing HIEs has to do with competitors achieving a level of trust sufficient to allow sharing of that precious commodity: information. Thus it is easy to understand why HIEs in general are relatively slow to develop.

In spite of the numerous benefits of HIEs, they face challenges in their long-term sustainability as they try to connect hundreds to thousands of participants in their networks. Each HIE usually receives seed grant money to establish itself, but as the money from the grant dries up, it becomes difficult for the HIE to sustain itself financially. Seed grant money may come from federal or state government projects or a combination of both. Private grant funding may also be available for certain aspects of development. Once the HIE is developed, it needs to be maintained, which requires facilities and staffing. Since grant funding is generally finite, the HIE must find other sources of revenue. Revenue may come from the organizations that provide the data, from the users of the data, or from a combination of both. The Delaware Health Information Network (DHIN) is an example of a self-sustaining HIE. The DHIN is a public/private partnership that connects providers with over 1.6 million unique patients (DHIN, 2022).

Although this technology promises improved health care delivery by making it easier to access patient data, obstacles such as the cost of implementation, agreement on technology standards, and concerns about privacy have limited the adoption of fully functional, interoperable EHRs. Both private consumer groups and government agencies have been working to speed up EHR implementation. These groups and agencies are working toward the goal of standardizing the technologies and content associated with EHRs to ensure confidentiality, accuracy, comprehensiveness, and the ability to share information among systems.

### Office of the National Coordinator for Health Information Technology

At the federal level, the *Office of the National Coordinator for Health Information Technology (ONC)* guides the nationwide implementation of an interoperable EHR in both the public and private sectors. One of the initiatives taken by the ONC to move the entire nation from paper records to EHRs was to establish the **Nationwide Health Information Network (NHIN)**. The NHIN's goal is to provide an interoperable HIE among providers, consumers, and others involved in supporting health and health care that is secure and capable of sharing information nationwide over the internet. Initial efforts were geared toward articulating applicable standards. The aim was to set common computer language requirements and secure messaging to allow regional and state-based networks of HIEs, laboratories, pharmacies, physicians' offices, and other entities involved in health care delivery to share information in a safe, efficient manner (ONC, 2022c).

The ONC has also worked to address the problem of health care organizations and EHR vendors who are reluctant to share their data. It has recently published the Trusted Exchange Framework and Common Agreement, a common set of nonbinding foundational principles to promote exchange among HINs (Box 2.2). The ONC hopes that industry alignment with these principles will help various stakeholders "enter into effective contractual relationships for the secure electronic flow of digital health information where and when it is needed" (ONC, 2022c). (Many of these goals were realized with eHealth Exchange.) eHealth Exchange promotes interoperability among regional HIEs. At the time of this writing, 75% of US hospitals through 61 regional and state HIEs and 5 federal agencies exchange patient data within eHealth Exchange along with 70,000 medical groups, 5800 dialysis centers, and 8300 pharmacies (eHealth Exchange, 2022).

A primary goal of the ONC is to allow authorized users to have access to medical information wherever and whenever it is needed, whether in a physician's office, acute care facility, or home health agency. Rural facilities will be able to access the records from urban facilities where the specialists practice. Consumers will have personal health records (PHRs) that they can share with the caregivers at any facility.

One of the key advantages of a functional EHR linked to the eHealth Exchange is the accessibility of the patient's information by the providers regardless of the location of the patient. For example, consider a patient who enters a health care facility through the emergency department because of shortness of breath. The physician can retrieve the patient's previous encounters, including test results and treatments that the patient received in the past from any facility. A surgery consultation is ordered for the patient. The surgeon is just finishing another patient's procedure and receives notice of the consultation. While in the surgery unit, he can access the patient's previous and current records and have some knowledge of the patient's health status before assessing the patient during this treatment encounter. The patient undergoes surgery during which an organ is removed. The organ is sent to the pathology laboratory for review. The pathologist may access the patient's record to review the clinical history and surgical findings before performing the pathologic examination of the organ. The patient is discharged and has a follow-up appointment with the surgeon. The surgeon wants to review the pathology report again before discussing the findings with the patient. He can access the pathology report from his office rather than going to the HIM department to view the paper record.

Many other initiatives have been sponsored by the ONC, which is a valuable resource for organizations seeking guidance and knowledge regarding Health IT (Office of the National Coordinator for Health Information Technology, 2022b).

Markle Foundation was founded in 1927 by a husband and wife initially to encourage the progression of knowledge and the general good of mankind. One of its goals was to eliminate barriers to the implementation of the EHR. Two of these barriers are lack of interoperability (the ability to exchange information) among computer systems and privacy issues. The Markle Foundation fostered collaboration in both private and public sectors through an initiative called Connecting for Health, which seeks to improve patient care by promoting standards for electronic medical information. In addition, the Markle Foundation provided information and promoted meaningful use and the development of HIEs. Although the Markle Foundation has shifted its focus in recent years to workforce initiatives, its impact on health information has been significant with respect to technology innovation and health care policy (http://www.markle.org).

**• BOX 2.2   The Trusted Exchange Framework (TEF): Principles for Trusted Exchange**

Principle 1—Standardization: HINs should prioritize federally recognized and industry-recognized technical standards, policies, best practices, and procedures.
Principle 2—Openness and Transparency: HINs should conduct activities openly and transparently, wherever possible.
Principle 3—Cooperation and NonDiscrimination: HINs should collaborate with stakeholders across the continuum of care to electronically exchange digital health information, even when a stakeholder may be a business competitor.
Principle 4—Privacy, Security, and Safety: HINs should exchange digital health information in a manner that supports privacy; ensures data confidentiality, integrity, and availability; and promotes patient safety.
Principle 5—Access: HINs should ensure that Individuals and their authorized caregivers have easy access to their digital health information and understand how it has been used or disclosed and HINs should comply with civil rights obligations on accessibility.
Principle 6—Equity: HINs should consider the impacts of interoperability on different populations and throughout the life cycle of the activity.
Principle 7—Public Health: HINs should support public health authorities and population-level use cases to enable the development of a learning health system that improves the health of the population and lowers the cost of care.

## Health Level 7

Because standardization is a critical element in achieving a seamless exchange of information, numerous standards have been issued, resulting in a need for coordination of these standards into one set. Health Level 7 (HL7), a nonprofit group composed of providers, vendors, payers, consultants, government groups, and others, is working to develop standards that will aid the interoperability of the exchange of electronic data in and among health care organizations. HL7 has established standards specifically for the EHR and how it should be designed and formatted, as well as the functions it should be capable of and the content it should contain. The standards are divided into three categories: *direct care*, *supportive*, and *information infrastructure* standards. Direct care standards relate to which EHR functions would relate to providing care to patients. The supportive standards section involves financial and administrative functions in a health care organization. Finally, the information infrastructure category is a more technical set of functions including security, user identification, and approved terminologies. For each standard, conformance criteria are listed that indicate how that standard is applied to the EHR system. HL7 has released various functional models describing these standards and how they should be incorporated into an EHR so that interoperability is ensured (Health Level 7, 2004).

This group is one of many standards-developing organizations that are producing standards for particular health care domains, such as pharmacy and radiology. Separate businesses or organizations can use the same standard to exchange information in an electronic data interchange (EDI). While EDIs are used in many industries to transmit documents such as invoices, in health care, an EDI can send patient information. HL7 standards allow messaging for clinical and administrative domains. In its current version (2.5.1), the HL7 standard uses 85 different types of messages to send information about events in the facility, specifically the exchange, management, and integration of data supporting clinical patient care and the evaluation of health services. For example, one type of HL7 message sends information about a patient admission; another type sends an order to a pharmacy; other types of HL7 messages transmit patient financial information, lab results, charges, and confirmations that a message was received. These specifications ensure that data from one system or organization can be accepted and interpreted by HIE systems. An HL7 "patient admit" message is shown in Fig. 2.18, as indicated by the message code ADT^A01. The message shows the patient's contact information, physician, and payer information. Each field in the HL7 message is separated by the pipe character (|).

## Certification Commission for Health Information Technology

Originally, the Certification Commission for Health Information Technology (CCHIT), a nonprofit organization, took a leadership role in the advancement of HIT by creating industry-approved certifications for EHRs. Although health care professionals agreed in general that it was essential to move from paper-based records to an electronic format, there was little consensus on what components would constitute an EHR and how these systems would securely share data. The problem was made more complex by the large number of EHR products available and the knowledge that many EHR implementations do not succeed.

CCHIT took on the task of defining the key functional components of an EHR, how it should communicate with other systems, and how it should protect patient information. The CCHIT criteria consisted of a list of detailed product

```
MSH|^~\&|AcmeHIS|StJohn|ADT|StJohn|20050518073622||ADT^A01|MSGID
20050518073622|P|2.3

EVN|A01
```

| | |
|---|---|
| PID\|\|\|12001\|\|Jones^John^^^Mr.\|\|19670822\|M\|\|\|123 West St.^^Denver^CO^80020^USA\|\|(850)555-0809\|\|\|\|\|99345\|460-99-2928 | PID – Patient Info |
| PV1\|\|I\|Main^802^1\|\|\|\|^Quacker^John\|\|\|IP\|\|\|\|\|\|\|\|\|\|1\|\|\|\|\|\|\|\|\|\|\|\|\|\|\|\|\|\|\|\|\|\|20050518073622 | PV1 – Visit Info |
| IN1\|1\|EPO\|80\|AETNA US HEALTHCARE\|PO BOX 981114^""^EL PASO^TX^79998^""\|\|\|\|1500004000001\|AETNA SERVICES INC\|19\|AETNA US HEALTHCARE\|""\|""\|\|2\|SOUTAR^RENEE^D\|3\|19700722\|13324 WHITE CEMETERY RD^""^HANNIBAL^NY^130740000^""\|\|\|\|\|\|\|\|\|\|\|\|\|\|\|\|\|\|\|124705454\|\|\|\|\|1\| F\|225 GREENFIELD PARKWAY^^LIVERPOOL^NY^13088\|185428 IN2\|1\|\|124705454\|\|461-1200\|\|\|\|\|\| | IN1 & IN2 Insurance Info |

• **Fig. 2.18** An Health Level 7 (HL7) "patient admit" (ADT) message. The rows of an HL7 message are called segments. The fields contained in each segment are separated by a pipe character (|). (Courtesy Corepoint Health, Frisco, Texas. https://corepointhealth.com/resource-center/hl7-resources/hl7-adt/.)

capabilities against which EHRs were evaluated. CCHIT developed and maintained a certification process for EHRs but ceased its certification activities at the end of 2014 due to economic pressures from uncertain revenue streams as a result of the delay in enforcement of the second stage of meaningful use. The current ONC Health IT Certification Program is a collaboration among various agencies, as well as industry. Current ONC-accredited certification organizations include ICSA Labs, Drummond Group, and SLI Compliance (Office of the National Coordinator for Health Information Technology [ONC], 2022c).

### Patient Access to Records

As mentioned earlier, access to a patient portal is an important feature of an EHR. But to make it possible, good information governance requires an examination of the impact of allowing access, including not only the mechanics of access (e.g., passwords and user names) but also the type of access. Since health data are captured by clinicians and are displayed for the use of clinicians, it is not necessarily layperson friendly. So right away we know that we have to have a different format for patients. Also, we do not necessarily want patients having access to our entire system—just the information itself. So, we need to create a patient-friendly space in which key information can be displayed without allowing full access to the system.

Many organizations have had patient portals for years. Cleveland Clinic has *My Chart* (https://mychart.cleve-landclinic.org/), for example, and Mayo Clinic Health Services has its *Patient Online Services* portal (http://mayo-clinichealthsystem.org/online-services). A patient portal can contain as little as your recent lab results or it can contain dictated reports, clinical notes, authoritative articles and videos for patient education, and secure email. Patients may even have the ability to upload and store documentation or to enter additional data to support their **personal health record (PHR)**, an individual's record of his or her own health information, which may be needed in making health decisions. In the PHR the individual owns and manages the health information and decides who has access to it. It can be paper-based, computer-based, Web-based, or some kind of composite thereof. In recent years, personal fitness trackers and other patient-controlled devices and applications are being discussed as possible additions to PHRs and even EHRs. A small device that links with a cell phone to generate an EKG is available online (AliveCor.com). In a study published in Cell Reports Medicine, Mayer et al. (2022) looked at how wearable a wearable tracking device could monitor the progress of COVID-19 symptoms from onset through infection periods. How that data are communicated, stored, and potentially shared with providers are some of the issues that arise in that discussion. Kaiser Health News reports that the profusion of data generated by wearables can cause anxiety and confusion on the part of patients and increased workload to the provider as so much

data are not necessarily helpful in diagnosing and treating patients (Tahir, 2022).

Patient portals can be accessible from mobile devices, such as smartphones and tablets, making it easier and more convenient for patients but problematic for providers from an information security perspective. Providers have no way to ensure that patients are using password-protected devices, so applications should have time-outs to help prevent unauthorized individuals from accessing the patient's account if they obtain access to the device.

Another way that patient portals could be used is for outreach and patient navigation. If the portal has secure messaging, then providers can push information to the patient, such as reminders about medications and appointments, as well as patient education and safety. In addition, the portal could contain information about care coordination or the messaging could facilitate patient navigation. Care coordination/patient navigation are activities in which the patient is guided through multiple levels of care, such as primary care to acute care to rehabilitation to home care. Typically, the primary care provider would lead the coordination effort. Although the Patient Centered Medical Home model is based in part on this coordination concept, it is increasingly important for all providers to participate in ensuring smooth transition of care to support the best patient outcomes and even to optimize reimbursement.

## Storing Health Care Data

So far, we have been talking about how data are collected and stored in an EHR. EHRs are designed to collect, display, and report data about patient care. As you can imagine, the volume of data collected quickly becomes unmanageable without the ability to store the data in an accessible way.

### Data Repository

Since the data in a patient's health record can come from many different facilities or sources, in many systems, a **data repository** is used. The data repository stores data from unrelated software programs that may be created by different vendors and have different applications. A data repository can store the data from these different systems and make them usable through an interface without the need to run reports from each system. Consider a patient who has diabetes: the data repository would store data from the pharmacy software program extracted from the medication administration report indicating the amount of insulin the patient receives. The laboratory software program submits its findings, storing the patient's glucose levels, and the nursing notes would contain the glucose monitoring results obtained from the nursing flow sheets.

While a data repository is useful in that it consolidates data into a single source, it is simply a storage medium.

Users can view the repository to obtain data about a patient. However, they generally do not facilitate analytics, such as reviewing a patient's history over time. For a fully functional database that provides useful analytics, we need a data warehouse.

## Data Warehouse

A **data warehouse** collects information from different databases and organizes it for use in creating reports and for analytical research. Data warehousing facilitates the use of the data in the health records of many individuals by making all this information available for analysis. Data warehousing is used to make a variety of vital decisions in health care. Stakeholders in the health care industry use this information for many reasons, including

- analyzing revenue, such as calculating the cost of treating a patient with specific conditions;
- clinical management, such as determining the average amount of insulin needed by a patient with diabetes in a specific age group;
- operational applications, such as the staffing pattern for patients on a diabetic nursing unit; and
- outcome management, such as estimating the percentage of patients who showed improvement after treatment.

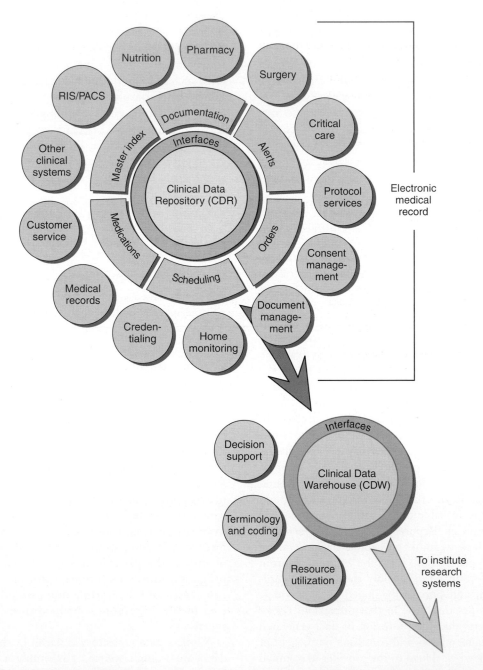

• **Fig. 2.19** Data repository/warehouse. *PACS*, Picture archiving and communication system; *RIS*, radiology information system.

In a true EHR, data are collected, used, and shared with authorized hospital departments and users, as shown in Fig. 2.19. The traditional HIM department functions can be performed electronically, either while the patient is still receiving treatment (concurrently) or after discharge (Foran et al., 2017).

### Data Mapping

Data mapping is the matching of a data element in one system or database to the same element in another system or database. One of the key principles of EHRs is that the data should be able to be shared electronically. Sharing can be the downloading and transmission of specific data via telecommunication, such as email. It can also be the direct transmission of data from one system to another. As we discussed earlier in the chapter, data may be collected differently in one system than another. To facilitate that sharing, we need to identify what data in the source system matches the same data element in the target system. This is the purpose of HL7. There is a great deal of work going on at the facility and vendor levels in creating interfaces between systems. There is also work going on at stakeholder organizations, such as the CDC, to identify and catalog vocabulary that is useful for general-use data mapping (Centers for Disease Control and Prevention, 2018).

## Planning for Electronic Health Record Migration and Implementation

Federal mandates, driven by the need for improved patient care and the long-term reduction in health care costs, have meant that facilities across the United States accelerated their implementation of EHRs. Today's HIM department managers are important members of the team in an organization that is implementing an EHR for the first time, replacing an existing system, or merging with another organization that has a different system in place.

There are many things that must be considered to successfully implement an EHR in a health care facility. Health care organizations and HIM professionals can use the **system development life cycle (SDLC)** for the large-scale design and implementation of information systems. Box 2.3 shows the phases of the SDLC.

---

**• BOX 2.3   Phases of Information System Development Life Cycle**

1. Selection
2. Design
3. Implementation
4. Evaluation
5. Support

---

❖ **COMPETENCY CHECK-IN 2.3**

**Data Collection and Storage**

**Competency Assessment**

1. Compare and contrast the considerations in the development of paper-based versus computer-based data collection devices.
2. The nursing department in your facility has submitted a form to the forms committee for approval. The form is printed on dark gold paper so that it will stand out in the chart. You recommend a light yellow paper instead because it photocopies better than dark gold. This is an example of taking which of the following into consideration:
   a. The purpose of the data collection device.
   b. The needs of all users of the device.
   c. An understanding of the technology used.
   d. Simplicity.
3. What is the purpose of instructions on a data collection device?
   a. To ensure that the correct form is used.
   b. To help users with complicated data collection.
   c. To ensure the consistency of data collection.
   d. To organize the data in the correct sequence.
4. What is the most important consideration in developing data collection forms and screens?
5. What consideration is important in screen development that is less important in forms development?
6. Explain the difference between the hybrid medical record and the EHR.
7. List the features of an EHR. Explain how these features are advantages for health care.
8. How are data in an EHR stored?
9. Recording of clinical data at the time treatment is delivered is called _____.
10. A _____ system is an application that allows a physician to enter orders for medications, tests, treatments, or procedures into a system.
11. Explain how an algorithm can improve the quality of care.
12. The database of a network of health care providers allowing access to patient records within the network from approved points-of-care is called a _____.
13. Information systems that provide clinical best knowledge practices to make decisions about patient care are called _____.
14. How does a data warehouse differ from a data repository?
15. How has the federal government encouraged providers to adopt EHR technology?

## Selection

Selection of an EHR product is a major project for the health care organization. It requires involvement from those employees who will use and maintain the system. These employees are often called stakeholders. Corporate facilities often choose one product to use in all of their facilities; while in independent health care facilities, the product may be chosen/dictated by the CEO, governing board, or partner organizations. Health care facilities start by identifying their needs or system requirements. The needs are incorporated into a list that will serve as the rubric or method for evaluating each proposed EHR product.

With the list of system requirements, a facility can formulate a request for proposal (RFP). The RFP is used to explain to EHR vendors what the health care organization intends to accomplish and requires of an EHR product. EHR vendors who are interested in doing business with the health care organization will review the RFP and submit a proposal explaining how their product can fulfill the needs of the health care facility/organization.

The RFP is a document created by the health care facility to explain its expectation for a particular service or product to potential vendors, for example, EHR software or an outsource service contract. The RFP describes the health care facility and also explains what the facility requires in the software product it wishes to purchase. A vendor who is interested in being chosen to provide the system or service for the health care organization reviews the RFP and submits a proposal explaining how his or her product or company can fulfill the needs listed in the RFP.

One of the biggest challenges in adopting, implementing, or changing an EHR is cost. Estimating the cost of an EHR is difficult because of the complex and varied infrastructures of health care organizations. Infrastructure can be defined as the standard operating nomenclature, specifications, or protocols of a system. Modern health care delivery systems are diverse, and their structures and needs vary greatly from simple to complex. Logically, a more complex health system would require a more expensive EHR with greater functionality. Despite the variances in structure, a large portion of the costs relate to the acquisition of both hardware and software. Organizations must also consider planning, design, reliable IT support, effective training, appropriate licenses, and maintenance fees. All of these issues will be considerations in a well-prepared RFP.

Once proposals are received, then a committee of stakeholders reviews the proposals to determine the vendor that best meets their needs, keeping in mind costs and the vendor's ability to provide support. Once a vendor is chosen, the stakeholders can move to the next SDLC phase: design.

## Design

During the design process, the stakeholders work to ensure that the product performs to meet the needs of the health care organization (as they requested in the RFP). The EHR vendor will help the organization establish a time line for the implementation. Some vendors have products that are easy to implement but allow very little flexibility in custom design. Other vendors allow the organization options to customize the product so that it meets their specific needs. Generally speaking, without compromising quality, a facility will work within time and budget constraints to ensure that the new technology matches its current or anticipated workflow needs.

In addition, this is the point at which the facility will ensure that the product can work with other information systems or software products being used in the facility. This is often called *integration*, making sure that the data from one system can be integrated into another system for optimal use. Integration can require additional cost and time to make sure all of the data are shared accurately in a way that functions correctly.

## Implementation

As the organization transitions from the design to the implementation phase, there is a period when the stakeholders and the vendor create a "test" environment so that they can determine whether the product works as it was designed. Once testing is complete, the facility is ready to implement the system in the "live" environment. There are several ways to accomplish this. One way is to implement it in pilot stages, by which it is used only partially in small areas until the stakeholders are sure that the product functions correctly. Another method is to run the new system parallel (at the same time) with the old system, and still another way is to switch over, to simply stop using the old system on a particular date and start using the new system. There are pros and cons to each system, so the implementation method should suit the size and capability of the new system and the method for implementation is chosen by the stakeholders or implementation team.

A pilot phase implementation could work well when a system such as CPOE is being implemented. The implementation could begin on a particular patient care unit in the health care facility. Prior to implementation, the training would be focused and specific to the needs of the group of physicians and nurses who work on the unit. The implementation date would be chosen, and the progress of the implementation would be localized to one unit and group of stakeholders. Then, as the comfort level and function of the new system become stable, a new unit would be chosen for the next phase of implementation to include training and so on.

When systems are implemented in a parallel situation, the health care facility chooses to keep the old system operational while training and beginning to use the new system. This may happen when a health care facility begins to scan health care records into a document imaging system. This method requires double processing of health care records. Training would begin with the HIM scanning technicians learning the new process to prepare records for scanning into the document imaging system. The double processing would occur once the paper pages of the record were scanned; the HIM technicians would still assemble the record in the paper method (organizing them and attaching them to a file folder labeled accordingly) for maintenance and record completion. The parallel systems would continue for a time to allow comfort with the new system and to ensure that the new system facilitated the accurate storage, retrieval, and record completion requirements of the HIM department. At some point, the old method of assembly and paper record identification and storage would stop, and the document imaging system would be the primary method of record processing.

The switchover implementation method is simple: The health care facility simply stops using the old method and from that date forward only uses the new system. It is best to prepare for this method of implementation by performing a significant amount of testing prior to the go-live date—the day the new equipment is put into service. The employees who will use the new system need to be trained and comfortable with the new system. It is also a good idea to have a number of support tools available to employees when they begin using the system: for instance, a team of superusers well trained and able to monitor the implementation from all areas and help desk contact numbers and/or specific employees in their unit to report problems and ask questions and easily accessible training modules/policy (online knowledge base) to access online if they forget a procedure.

Regardless of the method used for implementation, it is important to manage this stage closely and to prepare/plan ahead of time for the transition period. Implementation is exciting and daunting. Proper planning is required. Training is essential. Support tools and problem-reporting methods provide mechanisms to keep the implementation on track.

Training users involves coordination among IT, HIM, all employees, and physicians. Even though computers are a part of our daily lives, many health care workers may not feel as comfortable managing electronic records rather than paper records. Initially, productivity is expected to decrease as employees adjust to the new information management system. Good leadership practices should be utilized during the transition to help the organization meet established goals for the transition. Employees should be encouraged to learn the system properly, and managers should be patient during the transition phase. If delays are expected that would affect internal or external users, proper explanation and communication of the reason for the delay should be offered.

Training will cost an organization in development, time, personnel, and resources. Training methodology will vary according to the type, size, and complexity of the organization. Some organizations choose to train users in an electronic or online model with simulations in which users can learn at their own pace. Other organizations use a traditional approach whereby users learn on site with hands-on practice. Organizations may customize training according to their users' comfort with technology.

However an organization chooses to train users, it is critical that training be carefully planned and executed. Training is essential to the success of any HIT implementation. Failure to train or poor training can have catastrophic effects on the success of the EHR. The EHR is only as good as the individuals who use it. Identifying a superuser and making sure it is accessible to staff is one method of ensuring that users have adequate support during the migration and transition.

A **superuser** is an individual who has been trained in all aspects of the system and can serve as an on-site help desk for users who may experience difficulties with the system. The superuser can also be the main contact for the facility and may communicate technology issues with the software vendor. Many facilities train numerous superusers to meet the needs of their staff.

## Evaluation

Once the system is implemented in the real work environment, it is evaluated to ensure that it is working the way it was designed. This is different from testing because the system is being evaluated in the real or live situation it is serving. The evaluation process can include feedback from users, surveys of satisfaction, and monitoring of reported problems where the system does not perform correctly. These indicators help pinpoint places where modifications can be made in the system to ensure that it functions as intended.

## Support

As with any information system, there must be a way for users to report problems associated with the function or access to the system. The support is typically called a *help desk* or *technical support hotline*. In some organizations, there may be one phone number to report these problems, although more advanced systems also have an email, live chat feature, or online knowledge base so that users have access to technical support 24 hours a day, 7 days a week. Reporting a problem with the system usually results in a ticket, or record of the reported problem, so that the problem can be tracked through the process until it is resolved. This allows technical support to keep a record of frequent problems, have answers ready when a similar problem arises, and work on ways to correct the problem permanently, improving overall efficiency.

**COMPETENCY CHECK-IN 2.4**

### Planning for EHR Migration and Implementation

#### Competency Assessment

1. The process of planning, designing, implementation, and evaluation used in updating and improving or implementing a new health information system is called the _____.
2. An individual who is trained on all aspects of a computer system and who can help others on-site who are having difficulty is called a(n) _____.
3. What is the foundation for the RFP?
4. What is the purpose of an RFP?
5. Compare and contrast EHR implementation strategies.
6. The framework that enables interoperability by using standard operating nomenclature, specifications, or protocols is called _____.

## Chapter Summary

Data are collected about patients' health. Then those data are organized to provide information. HIM professionals are concerned with the collection, storage, retrieval, and documentation of health information.

Within the health record, data are organized into databases that are built from characters, fields, records, and files. The data dictionary describes the specific contents or values that can be contained in each field. The records and files are linked through the MPI in an EHR.

A data set is a defined group of fields that are required for a specified purpose. Many different data sets are collected about patients, including UHDDS and OASIS. The collection and reporting of defined data sets enable users to compare activities, volumes, patient care, and outcomes among the reporting facilities. The detailed data can be aggregated and analyzed to make public health decisions and to study the spread of disease. Researchers and government entities are examples of users of these data.

Data are collected on forms and screens. The general structure of a paper form is useful in designing electronic data capture screens. Using CPOE, the provider selects choices from menus which greatly reduces errors related to handwriting.

Many health care organizations are using either hybrid health record or EHRs. An EHR is a digital version of the patient's health record that collects health data at the point-of-care and makes the data available instantly. Health care organizations will standardize their EHR systems to enable interoperability, which is necessary for the creation and maintenance of records across the continuum of care. Widespread use of the interoperable EHR would make health information more accessible to users and thereby improve the quality of health care. The federal government has provided incentives and penalties to promote the use of EHRs.

Health data are stored in data warehouses, clinical data repositories, and other large databases at the institutional, local, state, regional, and national levels. Researchers can use the data warehouse to analyze health information and make health policy and financial decisions.

The SDLC—selection, design, implementation, evaluation, and support—is the process by which providers choose an EHR vendor and product. During this process, the RFP is used to explain to EHR vendors what the health care organization intends to accomplish and requires of an EHR product.

## Competency Milestones

### CAHIIM Competency

*I.3. Identify policies and strategies to achieve data integrity. (3)*

### Rationale

The integrity of the data being collected and stored is essential to support the many uses of that data that we will be exploring in subsequent chapters.

### Competency Assessment

1. Define data integrity.
2. List and describe three ways that data integrity is supported within the facility.
3. What does a database manager have to consider when deciding how to store data?
4. Explain how a relational database supports data integrity.
5. What challenges does patient self-collection of data (e.g., personal health monitors, at-home blood pressure, and blood glucose testing) present in terms of data integrity?

### CAHIIM Competency

*III.7. Summarize standards for the exchange of health information. (2)*

### Rationale

The use of standards enables consistent data collection and interoperability.

### Competency Assessment

1. Explain the benefits of interoperable systems and the importance of a longitudinal record.
2. The term interoperability describes two independent systems configured to communicate with each other. Give an example of this concept.
3. Explain the impact of HL7.
4. Why is standardization important for the widespread use of the EHR?

CAHIIM Competency

*III.7. **DM** Identify standards for the exchange of health information. (3)*

### Rationale
The use of standards enables consistent data collection and interoperability.

### Competency Assessment
1. Explain interoperability.
2. What is an HIE? How does it facilitate interoperability?

### Case Study
*PART 1. Prepare a data dictionary entry for the collection of a patient's race, using the categories from the United States 2010 Census (see Part 2 before responding).*
*PART 2. Construct a database table to store the valid values for the field Patient Race.*
*PART 3. Construct a map from the 2010 Census race field to the UHDDS. Alternatively, map from your state's race data collection value set to the UHDDS.*
*PART 4. Review the Value Set Concepts on the CDC web page: Public Health Information Network Vocabulary Access and Distribution System (PHIN VADS). https://www.cdc.gov/phin/tools/PHINvads/index.html.*
1. What is the purpose of PHIN VADS?
2. Access PHIN VADS: http://phinvads.cdc.gov/. Click on the link for CDC Race Category and Ethnicity Group. Select Race Category Value Set. In the Value Set Description, there is a statement that is not accommodated by UHDDS reporting. Why is this statement important?
*PART 5. Go back to PART 2 and reconfigure the table using the PHIN VADS value set ID.*

## Ethics Challenge

*VI.7. Assess ethical standards of practice. (5)*

1. You are the Practice Manager for a group of Family Medicine physicians. The physicians have decided to change EHRs because they find the current one cumbersome to use. You are given the task of investigating and recommending the best of three systems that they have heard about from their colleagues. Upon investigation, it seems that all three systems are an improvement over the current one, but during the process, you discover that the sales representative for one of the systems, Lynchpin Inc., is your cousin's wife. Your family learns about this and is pressuring you to select that system for your work. To keep the peace, you recommend Lynchpin's system to your physician group. Ethical or not?
2. You are the coding supervisor at the Diamonte Community Hospital. In the course of training for the implementation of a new computer system, you discover that one of your staff has not attended the training. When asked, he states that his previous employer used the new system, so he does not feel that he needs the training and asks you to please mark him as trained. Because he seems sincere, you mark him as trained. Ethical or not?

## Critical Thinking Questions

1. In Fig. 2.4, we illustrated the shift in causes of death between 1900 and 2015. Look at the Provisional Mortality Data for the United States, 2021 on the CDC website: https://www.cdc.gov/mmwr/volumes/71/wr/mm7117e1.htm#. Click on the link to Figure 2 and see the provisional number of leading causes of death. What is different? Why is 2021 so different from 2015?
2. You are a health information professional working for Dr. Heath in his private practice. Dr. Heath has a large practice with several ancillary services attached. He and his partner see 50 patients a day in the practice, many of whom receive on-site diagnostic procedures. The diagnostic areas that Dr. Heath has are radiology, electrocardiography, and laboratory. He is concerned because a number of patients have complained that in each area of care, the health personnel seems to ask the same questions. The redundancy is annoying. He is considering computerizing his data collection to streamline the data collection process. Before he does, he wants to make sure that he understands the clinical flow of data in the facility. Dr. Heath seeks your advice and assistance in resolving his problem. What do you recommend? How would you go about implementing your recommendations?
3. Think about a disease with which you are familiar, and create a list of all the data elements that you think a physician and allied health personnel in a physician's office would generate for this disease. You can make up the data but make the list as

complete as you can. This exercise will give you an idea of how complex health information is, even at the physician's office level.

4. Go to the ONC and HL7 Web sites and prepare a brief report on the current activities of these organizations relating to the implementation of the EHR. Prepare this report as if you were presenting it to the next monthly HIM department meeting at your hospital.

5. The health care facility is implementing a new patient portal for access to the patient health record, appointments, prescription refills, and bill pay. Prepare a pamphlet or online tutorial to provide information to patients about this new portal.

6. Go to Healthit.gov and locate the page for the Trusted Exchange Framework and Common Agreement. Download the pdf files and review the documents.

   a. Beginning on page 4 of the Common Agreement, review the contract vocabulary. Identify language that is new to you. Why do you think this Agreement is needed?

   b. What is the purpose of the Trusted Exchange Framework? What issues does this document attempt to resolve?

# The Role of Health Information Management Professionals in the Workplace

### Professional Profile—Health Information Management Implementation Specialist

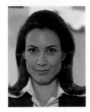

My name is Ann, and I am an HIM Implementation Specialist in a 250-bed facility, Diamonte Hospital. This facility provides acute care, emergency services, and ambulatory services and has a cancer center and two offsite rehabilitation centers. Our hospital is one of four hospitals in the city owned by the same corporation. We have approximately 500 physicians on the medical staff.

The four hospitals share a medical record database, working in a fully implemented EHR. Each hospital has an HIM implementation specialist who works on different HIM applications in the electronic record. I am an RHIT and was promoted from clerical supervisor to implementation specialist when I finished my bachelor's degree in health information management. This is a very exciting position. It has given me an opportunity to learn about and work with the information systems throughout the facility and I network with employees throughout all the hospitals in our network.

I am a member of the implementation team at our facility and provide input on HIM functions, forms, and communication. I work with a joint forms committee with representatives from all four hospitals to revise the record forms to an electronic format. I also work closely with the vendor and IT department to develop the workflow for the electronic record. I spend many hours testing the HIM functions for my assigned applications as they are developed and provide feedback on the results of the application testing to the vendor and implementation committee. Currently, we are working on a new scanning and indexing application, and I am developing training materials for the HIM employees at all four hospitals.

This position allows me to use my computer skills, work with a team, and use my knowledge of HIM workflow and processes. Being part of the team developing the foundation for the EHR is very rewarding.

### Career Tip

An associate's or bachelor's degree in HIM or a clinical field is important for this position, because an intimate knowledge of the components of the health record, as well as legal, regulatory, and professional standards, is necessary. A certificate or degree in informatics will open more doors.

### Patient Care Perspective

### Dr. Lewis's partner, Dr. Boonton

One thing we are trying very hard to accomplish is electronic communication between our practice and the hospitals at which we have privileges. Diamonte Hospital has negotiated a relationship with a software vendor who creates a connection among hospitals, physician offices, and patients. I send quite a few patients to Diamonte, although I do not admit them myself; the hospitalists care for them. So if one of my patients is admitted to Diamonte, key data elements flow automatically from the hospital to my office system. I am aware of the admission on a timely basis and can contact the hospitalist if necessary. For example, Maria's mother, Isabel, was admitted to Diamonte last week after a fall. I saw the notification the following morning, and the hospitalist called me to confirm her medications and discuss her condition and discharge plan. The day after she was discharged, we set up an appointment for follow-up.

## Works Cited

DHIN: *DHIN funding*, 2022. The Delaware Health Information Network. http://www.dhin.org/about/dhin-funding. Accessed April 29, 2022.

eHealth Exchange. *Home page* (website). ehealthexchange.org. Accessed April 30, 2022.

Foran DJ, Chen W, Chu H, et al: Roadmap to a comprehensive clinical data warehouse for precision medicine applications in oncology, *Cancer Inf* 16:1176935117694349, 2017. https://doi.org/10.1177/1176935117694349

Garde S, Knaup P, Hovenga EJS, Heard S: Towards semantic interoperability for electronic health records, *Methods Inf Med* 46:332–343, 2007.

Health Level 7: *HL7 EHR system functional model: a major development towards consensus on electronic health record system functionality*, 2004. https://www.hl7.org/documentcenter/public_temp_F1AA40BB-1C23-BA17-0CE5FC5FE22D8769/wg/ehr/ehr-swhitepaper.pdf. Accessed November 25, 2018.

Institute of Electrical and Electronics Engineers (IEEE): *IEEE standard computer dictionary: a compilation of IEEE standard computer glossaries*, 1990. New York, IEEE.

Mayer C, et al: Consumer-grade wearables identify changes in multiple physiological systems during COVID-19 disease progression, *Cell Rep Med* 3(4):100601, 2022. https://doi.org/10.1016/j.xcrm.2022.100601. https://www.cell.com/cell-reports-medicine/fulltext/S2666-3791%2822%2900118-5?utm_source=newsletter&utm_medium=email&utm_campaign=newsletter_axiosvitals&stream=top. Accessed April 29, 2022.

National Uniform Billing Committee: *About the NUBC*, n.d. National Uniform Billing Committee. http://www.nubc.org/about-NUBC. Retrieved April 28, 2022.

Tahir D: Heartbeat-Tracking Technology Raises Patients' and Doctors' Worries, *Kaiser Health News*, April 20, 2022. https://khn.org/news/article/heartbeat-technology-wearables-afib-google-apple-doctor-worries/?utm_source=newsletter&utm_medium=email&utm_campaign=newsletter_axiosvitals&stream=top. Accessed April 29, 2022.

## Further Reading

AHIMA e-HIM Personal Health Record Work Group: The role of the personal health record in the EHR, *J AHIMA* 76:64A–64D, 2005.

Arzt NH: Standards: NHIN and NHIN Direct Specifications—The Impact on HIEs, *HIMSS News,* 2010, April 1. https://www.himss.org/news/standards-nhin-and-nhin-direct-specifications-impact-hies. Retrieved November 25, 2018.

Center for Medicare and Medicaid Services. *ICD-10-CM Official Coding Guidelines. Section II. Selection of principal diagnosis*, 2022. p 101. https://www.cms.gov/files/document/fy-2022-icd-10-cm-coding-guidelines-updated-02012022.pdf. Accessed April 28, 2022. Updated April 1, 2022.

Centers for Disease Control and Prevention: *PHIN VADS hot topics*, December 5, 2018, Public Health Information Network Vocabulary Access and Distribution System (PHIN VADS). https://phinvads.cdc.gov/vads/SearchVocab.action. Retrieved April 29, 2022.

Centers for Disease Control and Prevention: *Social determinants of health: know what affects health*, December 8, 2022, Centers for Disease Control and Prevention. https://www.cdc.gov/socialdeterminants/. Retrieved April 19, 2023.

Centers for Medicare and Medicaid Services: *Promoting interoperability (PI)*. Centers for Medicare and Medicaid Services. April 12, 2023. https://www.cms.gov/EHRIncentivePrograms/30_Meaningful_Use.asp Accessed April 19, 2023.

HealthIT.gov: *Certification bodies and testing laboratories*, 2014, HealthIT.gov. http://www.healthit.gov/policy-researchers-implementers/certification-bodies-testing-laboratories. Accessed November 26, 2018.

Devine E, Totten AM, Gorman P, et al: Health information exchange use (1990–2015): a systematic review, *EGEMS (Wash DC)* 5(1):27, 2017. https://doi.org/10.5334/egems.249

Healthcare Information and Management Systems Society (HIMSS): *Electronic health records*, 2018, Healthcare Information and Management Systems Society (HIMSS) Resource Library. https://www.himss.org/library/ehr. Retrieved November 25, 2018.

Institute of Medicine (US) Committee on Data Standards for Patient Safety: *Key capabilities of an electronic health record system: letter report*, 2003. Washington, DC, National Academies Press (US). https://www.ncbi.nlm.nih.gov/books/NBK221802/ doi: 10.17226/10781. Accessed November 20, 2018.

Moja L, Kwag KH, Lytras T, et al: Effectiveness of computerized decision support systems linked to electronic health records: a systematic review and meta-analysis. *Am J Public Health* 104(12):e12–e22, 2014. https://doi.org/10.2105/ajph.2014.302164

Office of the National Coordinator for Health Information Technology (ONC): *Promoting interoperability*, 2022a, HealthIT.gov. https://www.healthit.gov/topic/meaningful-use-and-macra/meaningful-use-and-macra. Retrieved April 29, 2022.

Office of the National Coordinator for Health Information Technology (ONC): *At a glance: the certification process*, 2022b, HealthIT.gov: Official Website of the Office of the National Coordinator for Health Information Technology (ONC). https://www.healthit.gov/topic/certification-ehrs/certification-health-it. Retrieved April 29, 2022.

Office of the National Coordinator for Health Information Technology: *Trusted Exchange Framework and Common Agreement (TEFCA)*, 2022c, HealthIT.gov. https://www.healthit.gov/topic/interoperability/trusted-exchange-framework-and-common-agreement-tefca. Retrieved April 30, 2022.

Sackett DL, Rosenberg WM, Gray JA, et al: Evidence based medicine: what it is and what it isn't, *BMJ* 312:71–72, 1996.

# 3

# Sources of Data

TINA CARTWRIGHT

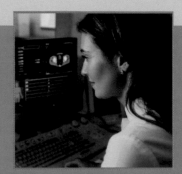

## CHAPTER OUTLINE

**Health Records Defined**
  Key Data Categories
**Clinical Flow of Data**
  The Order to Admit
  Medical Decision-Making
**Clinical Documentation**
  Physicians
  Nurses
  Laboratory Data
  Radiology Data
  Special Records
  Clinical Oversight
**Discharge Data Set**
**Documentation in Nonacute Care Providers**
  Physicians' Offices
  Emergency Department
  Radiology and Laboratory Services
  Ambulatory Surgery

  Long-Term Care
  Behavioral Health Facilities
  Rehabilitation Facilities
  Hospice
  Other Specialty Care
  Home Health Care
  Telehealth
**Chapter Summary**
**Competency Milestone**
**Ethics Challenge**
**Critical Thinking Questions**
**The Role of Health Information Management Professionals in the Workplace**
  Professional Profile—Records Manager
  Professional Profile—Patient Registration Specialist
  Patient Care Perspective
**Works Cited**
**Further Reading**

## CHAPTER OBJECTIVES

*By the end of this chapter, the student should be able to:*

1. Define the health record and understand the types of data it contains.
2. Describe the flow of clinical data through an acute care facility.
3. Differentiate the various providers and disciplines who contribute to clinical documentation.
4. Examine the elements of the Uniform Hospital Discharge Data Set.
5. Assess patient records to ensure compliance with organizational policy and procedures, and with regulatory and accreditation requirements.

6. Discuss the services, care providers, data collection, data sets, licensure, and accreditation of ambulatory care settings,
7. Discuss the services, care providers, data collection, data sets, licensure, and accreditation of long-term care, behavioral health, rehabilitation, hospice care, home health, and other settings.

# VOCABULARY

activities of daily living (ADLs)
administrative data
admission consent form
admission denial
admission record
admitting diagnosis
admitting physician
advance directive
against medical advice (AMA)
ambulatory care
ambulatory surgery
anesthesia report
assessment
assisted living
attending physician
authenticate
bar code
board-certified social worker (BCSW)
behavioral health facility
case management
chief complaint
clinic
clinical data
clinical pathway
cognitive remediation
Commission on Accreditation of Rehabilitation
    Facilities (CARF)
Community Health Accreditation Program (CHAP)
consultant
consultation
continued stay denial
countersigned
Data Elements for Emergency Department Systems (DEEDS)
demographic data
diagnosis
Diagnostic and Statistical Manual of Mental Disorders,
    5th Edition (DSM-5)
dialysis center
differential diagnosis
direct admission
discharge disposition
discharge planning
discharge summary
encounter
evidence-based medicine
financial data
group practice
guarantor
health record
history and physical (H&P)
history
hospice
hospitalist
intensity of service (IS)
laboratory
longitudinal record

long-term care (LTC) facility
medical record number (MRN)
medication administration
Minimum data sets
Medicare Severity diagnosis-related group (MS-DRG)
National Committee for Quality Assurance (NCQA)
nosocomial infection
nursing assessment
nursing progress notes
objective
observation
operative report
order set (protocol)
Outcome and Assessment Information Set (OASIS)
outcome
outpatient
palliative care
patient care plan
physiatrist
physical examination
physician's office
plan of care (treatment)
point-of-care documentation
primary care provider (PCP)
primary caregiver
procedure
progress notes
protocol (order set)
radiology
remote patient monitoring (RPM)
Resident Assessment Instrument (RAI)
Resident Assessment Protocol (RAP)
respite care
retail care
rule out
same-day surgery
severity of illness (SI)
skilled nursing facility (SNF)
soap
socioeconomic data
store-and-forward
subjective
Substance Abuse and Mental Health Services
    Administration (SAMHSA)
symptom
telemedicine
treatment
triage
Uniform Ambulatory Care Data Set (UACDS)
Uniform Hospital Discharge Data Set (UHDDS)
Urgent Care Association (UCA)
urgent care center
utilization review (UR)
visit
vital signs
working DRG

In Chapter 2 we discussed data and you learned about the Uniform Hospital Discharge Data Set (UHDDS) for inpatient records. In this chapter we continue the discussion of data collection, building the data set for a given patient receiving care in various settings. Each type of facility (acute care, long-term care [LTC], ambulatory, medical office) has a specific data set that must be considered in the planning of data-collection strategies, inclusive of the discharge data set required for the US Department of Health and Human Services (DHHS). In the previous chapter, we discussed the structure of data collection on forms and computer screens, as well as how it is stored and shared electronically. In this chapter, we focus on the nature of the data and how it is collected.

## Health Records Defined

The primary purpose of recording data is communication, which is necessary for a variety of reasons. Clinical professionals record data about the patient's health status, treatments, and procedures so that they or others can review it later to see what has been done and whether the patient is improving. For example, a medical assistant may take a patient's vital signs and record them for the physician's reference. Physicians record their observations so that they can measure the patient's progress at a later date. Thus recording health data is an important way for health care professionals to communicate and facilitate patient care.

Beyond patient care, there are many other uses for health data. Hospital administrators use health data to make decisions about what services to offer and how best to serve the communities in which they are located. Lawyers use health data to defend the actions of providers or demonstrate the extent of injuries suffered by a client. Payers, such as insurance companies and Medicare, use health data to determine reimbursement to providers. Government entities use health data for a variety of purposes, such as monitoring diseases.

These uses of health data will be discussed throughout this text. Chapter 6 discusses the use of health data for reimbursement. Chapter 7 discusses examples of the statistical analysis and administrative uses of health data.

All data collected about an individual patient are called a health record or medical record. Although there is literature to support that there is a difference between a health record and a medical record, the difference is primarily in the scope of the record. A medical record might be the documentation of a single visit in a hospital or a record in a physician's office. The health record would be a more comprehensive compilation of data, such as all of the records of all of the practitioners who treated the patient. An interesting blog post at healthit.gov discusses this issue (Garrett and Seidman, 2011). If the compilation consists of data over a significant period of time and incorporates all of the settings in which the patient received care, it is also called a longitudinal record.

The specific content of a patient's record will be unique to the patient; however, patients with similar conditions, diseases, or treatments will tend to have similar data in their records. Thus maternity records will all contain specific data about labor and delivery, and patients undergoing hip replacement may have different reasons for the surgery but will all have data about the operation and recovery from the same. We will discuss data collection later in this chapter. For now, we will turn our attention to the types of data that are collected.

## Key Data Categories

Health data that are collected in a consistent, systematic process are most easily organized into information. Therefore the health data collected about individual patients is collected in a systematic process in which the required data are clearly defined and both the data collection and the data storage are uniform.

There are four broad categories into which health data are collected: demographic, socioeconomic, financial, and clinical.

### Demographic Data

Demographic data identifies the patient. Name, address, age, and gender are examples of demographic data. The physician needs the patient's name and address to send the patient correspondence, follow-up notices, or a bill. Other necessary data include the home phone number, place of employment, work telephone number, race, ethnicity, and Social Security number. The physician needs these data both to contact the patient and to distinguish one patient from another. These data also help the physician answer questions such as How old are my patients? Where do my patients live? Fig. 3.1 shows demographic data collected for a patient.

Demographic data comprise the admission, discharge, and transfer (ADT) data that systems use to communicate with each other in order to match up a patient with the data associated with that patient. In Chapter 2 we described the master patient index (MPI) table, which is the location in the facility database in which the patient-identifying data are stored. Depending on how the database is structured, an ADT transmission would contain identifying data from the MPI and visit data from the visit/encounter table, if applicable.

### Socioeconomic Data

Another type of data about a patient that a health care professional collects is socioeconomic data. These personal data include the patient's marital status, sexual orientation, education, religion, and personal habits. An example

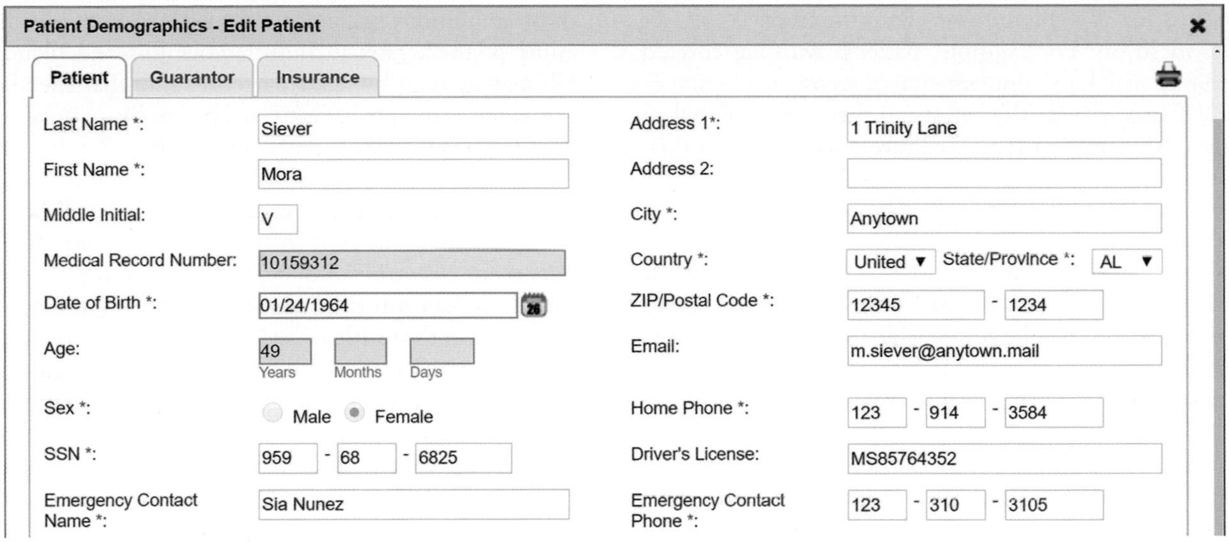

• **Fig. 3.1** Demographic data: data that help the user contact the patient or to distinguish one patient from another. (Courtesy SimChart for the Medical Office, Elsevier, Inc., 2023.)

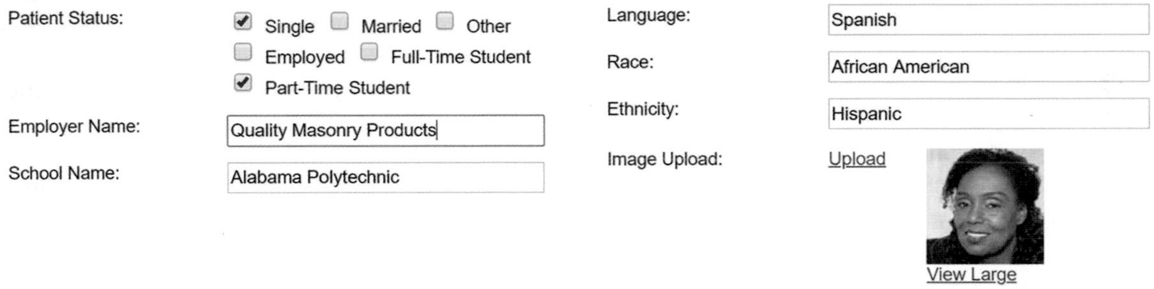

• **Fig. 3.2** Socioeconomic data are personal data that give the user clues about potential problems and assistance in planning care. (Courtesy SimChart for the Medical Office, Elsevier, Inc., 2023.)

of socioeconomic data is presented in Fig. 3.2. One of the reasons that such data are important is that the diagnosis of many illnesses, and sometimes their treatment, depends on the doctor's understanding of the patient's personal situation.

A patient with asthma who smokes will likely be advised by his or her physician to quit smoking. This is an example of a personal habit that directly affects a disease condition. In addition, the socioeconomic situation or personal life of a patient sometimes dictates whether the patient will follow a medication regimen or even whether he or she is able to obtain treatment. For example, if an older patient has just undergone a hip replacement, sending that patient home to a third-story walk-up apartment might be a problem. It will be very difficult for the patient to get in and out of the apartment and certainly very difficult for the patient to leave the apartment for therapy, particularly if there is no caregiver at home. Treatment at home might be needed, as well as assistance with routine activities such as grocery shopping. In some cases, the patient may need residential placement in an assisted living facility.

Sometimes, the knowledge that a patient travels widely can lead a physician to suspect an illness that he or she would not consider if the patient never traveled. Travel in certain areas of the world could have caused exposure to diseases that are uncommon in the patient's native area. Thus a patient's complaint of abdominal pain could lead the physician to suspect a parasite (an organism that may have been swallowed and is living in the intestines), whereas ordinarily the physician would consider only bacterial or viral causes. Therefore understanding a patient's personal life and living situation is important to the planning of how to care for the patient.

## Financial Data

When requesting services from any health care provider, one expects at some point that payment of some sort will be required. The provider asks the patient who will be responsible for paying the bill. **Financial data** relate to the development of the bill for services rendered. The data collected at registration comprise the basic data about the patient's financial relationship with the provider.

The party (person or organization) from whom the provider is expecting payment for services rendered is called the payer. The payer is frequently an insurance company. It may also be a government agency, such as Medicare or Medicaid.

Many patients have more than one payer. The primary payer is billed first for payment. A secondary payer is approached for any amount that the primary payer did not remit, and so on. For example, patients who are covered by Medicare may have supplemental or secondary insurance with a different payer. The physician first sends the bill to Medicare. Any amount that Medicare does not pay is then billed to the secondary payer. The patient may also have some responsibility for part of the payment.

The patient is typically financially responsible for payment of the bill for services that he or she has received. If the patient is a dependent, the patient's guardian or an other authorized person may be responsible for the bill. The person who is ultimately responsible for paying the bill is called the **guarantor**. For example, if a child goes to the physician's office for treatment, the child, as a dependent, cannot be held responsible for the invoice. Therefore the parent or legal guardian is responsible for payment and is the guarantor. In some cases, such as a child personally eligible for Medicaid, the child may be technically responsible for payment; however, collection from the child is unlikely. Fig. 3.3 shows financial data required by a health care provider.

Payer data are typically collected at registration, and charges incurred for services rendered are collected during the patient's encounter. In Chapter 2, we discussed the UHDDS and the UB-04, the standard billing form. The hospital has already collected all the necessary data for billing, so the UB-04 compiles a variety of fields, including demographic data and summarized charge data, as well as diagnoses, procedures, and physician identification, from the database tables in which they are stored. Fig. 3.4 shows the location of UHDDS data elements on the form locator (FL) fields of the UB-04. Patients receiving hospital treatment will often receive two bills, however. A physician or other provider who has privileges at the hospital bills the patient separately. The form for the provider bill is the CMS-1500. It requires similar data, although the charges tend to be less voluminous than the facility charges on the UB-04. Payer data and charges are discussed in greater detail in Chapter 6.

### Clinical Data

Clinical data are probably the easiest to understand and relate to the health care field. **Clinical data** comprise all of the data that have been recorded about the patient's health, including:

- the **assessment**, the provider's evaluation of the patient;
- the **diagnosis**, the physician's conclusion about the patient's condition; and
- the recommended **treatment**, a procedure, medication, or other measure designed to cure or alleviate the symptoms of disease.

Say the patient presents in the physician's office for pain in the abdomen. The physician knows that pain in the abdomen can be caused by a variety of conditions. The pain is merely a **symptom**, a description of what the patient feels or is experiencing. Other symptoms may include nausea, dizziness, and headache. The physician orders tests and performs a physical examination to determine which of

those conditions is responsible for the abdominal pain. Some of these tests include radiographs and blood tests. Ultimately, the physician may conclude that the abdominal pain is caused by an inflamed appendix, or appendicitis. Appendicitis is the diagnosis, and the blood test and physical examination are the **procedures**. The physician records both the findings of the examination and the evaluation of the results of the tests in the patient's record. The blood tests themselves are conducted in a laboratory. The reporting of results from the laboratory to the clinician is a part of the patient's health record. The laboratory typically has its own computer system that receives patient demographic data and the physician order from the main hospital system and returns the test results. As discussed in Chapter 2, the laboratory's computer system is independent of that in the physician's office, but the two systems are interoperable. Radiology systems work similarly, as do pharmacy systems that are not a part of the main hospital system.

Clinical data constitute the bulk of any patient's record. All of the previous data that have been discussed—demographic, socioeconomic, and financial—can usually be printed out onto one or two pages or displayed on one or two summary screens. The rest of the record is the clinical data. Box 3.1 lists examples of clinical data.

### Administrative Data

In addition to the data that are collected from and about the patient, a provider will assign administrative data to a patient for identification and tracking purposes. One type of administrative data is the **medical record number** (MRN), a unique number assigned to each patient in a health care system; this code is used for the rest of the patient's encounters with that specific health system.

**Administrative data** enable the facility to distinguish one patient from another and to identify specific episodes of care for a particular patient or group of patients. Thus the provider can list all patients who were discharged on a certain day or all episodes of care for a particular patient.

Other examples of administrative data include patient account number, admission/discharge dates for the episode of care, room number, and identification of clinical staff providing services. Typically, the identification of the physician who is ordering the admission of the patient to the facility or who wrote the order for outpatient treatment is entered by registration personnel. The patient registration clerk selects the name of the physician from a drop-down menu of physicians. Although the name of the physician typically appears on screens and forms, it is the physician's identification number that is stored in the system. Maintenance of the physician identification database in a facility is typically the responsibility of the Medical Staff Office. The Medical Staff Office serves as a liaison between facility staff and the medical staff. Credentialing of providers (the verification of credentials, education, and experience) and routine compliance checks (such as ensuring that a provider is not sanctioned by the Centers for Medicare and Medicaid Services [CMS]) are generally the responsibilities of Medical Staff Office.

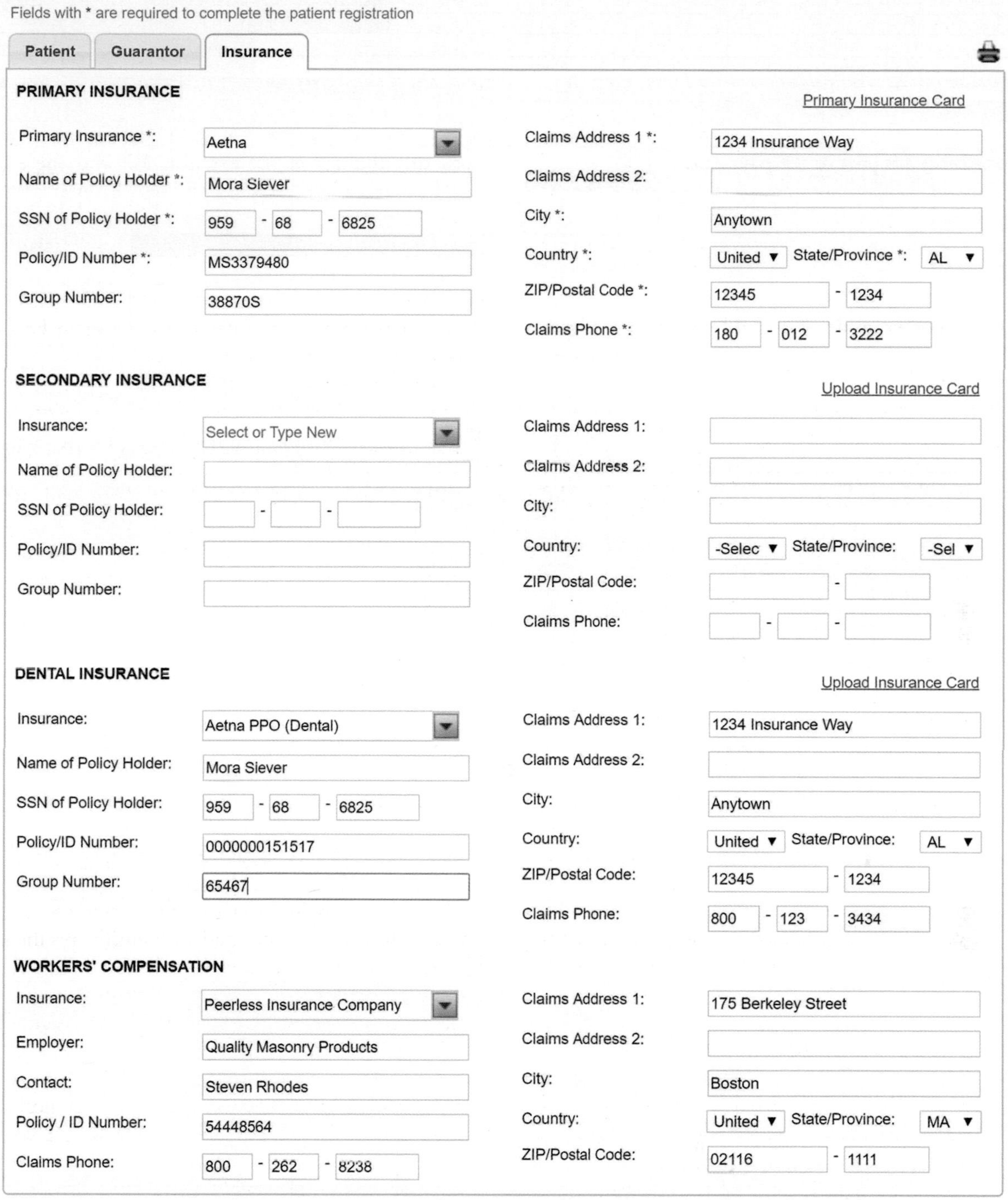

Fields with * are required to complete the patient registration

| Patient | Guarantor | **Insurance** |

## PRIMARY INSURANCE

Primary Insurance Card

| Primary Insurance *: | Aetna ▼ | Claims Address 1 *: | 1234 Insurance Way |
| Name of Policy Holder *: | Mora Siever | Claims Address 2: | |
| SSN of Policy Holder *: | 959 - 68 - 6825 | City *: | Anytown |
| Policy/ID Number *: | MS3379480 | Country *: | United ▼  State/Province *: AL ▼ |
| Group Number: | 38870S | ZIP/Postal Code *: | 12345 - 1234 |
| | | Claims Phone *: | 180 - 012 - 3222 |

## SECONDARY INSURANCE

Upload Insurance Card

| Insurance: | Select or Type New ▼ | Claims Address 1: | |
| Name of Policy Holder: | | Claims Address 2: | |
| SSN of Policy Holder: | - - | City: | |
| Policy/ID Number: | | Country: | -Selec ▼  State/Province: -Sel ▼ |
| Group Number: | | ZIP/Postal Code: | - |
| | | Claims Phone: | - - |

## DENTAL INSURANCE

Upload Insurance Card

| Insurance: | Aetna PPO (Dental) ▼ | Claims Address 1: | 1234 Insurance Way |
| Name of Policy Holder: | Mora Siever | Claims Address 2: | |
| SSN of Policy Holder: | 959 - 68 - 6825 | City: | Anytown |
| Policy/ID Number: | 0000000151517 | Country: | United ▼  State/Province: AL ▼ |
| Group Number: | 65467 | ZIP/Postal Code: | 12345 - 1234 |
| | | Claims Phone: | 800 - 123 - 3434 |

## WORKERS' COMPENSATION

| Insurance: | Peerless Insurance Company ▼ | Claims Address 1: | 175 Berkeley Street |
| Employer: | Quality Masonry Products | Claims Address 2: | |
| Contact: | Steven Rhodes | City: | Boston |
| Policy / ID Number: | 54448564 | Country: | United ▼  State/Province: MA ▼ |
| Claims Phone: | 800 - 262 - 8238 | ZIP/Postal Code: | 02116 - 1111 |

• **Fig. 3.3** Financial data include the identities of the parties responsible for paying the invoice. (Courtesy SimChart for the Medical Office, Elsevier, Inc., 2023.)

The patient status is also recorded, classifying each patient in the hospital as an outpatient, inpatient, or observation patient (Box 3.2). The patient's status is important for billing purposes because reimbursement varies according to patient status. The patient's room number is important because registration needs to know what beds are occupied and by whom in order to place an incoming patient in a bed. Furthermore, the patient's bed during a specific stay may be important if it becomes necessary to identify what nursing and other health care workers attended the patient. Clinical staff who provide services, such as physicians and therapists, are associated with a patient's visit via identification numbers. This association enables the hospital to track patients by physician and to review physician activity, for example. The amount of administrative data assigned to a patient encounter depends on the needs of the provider.

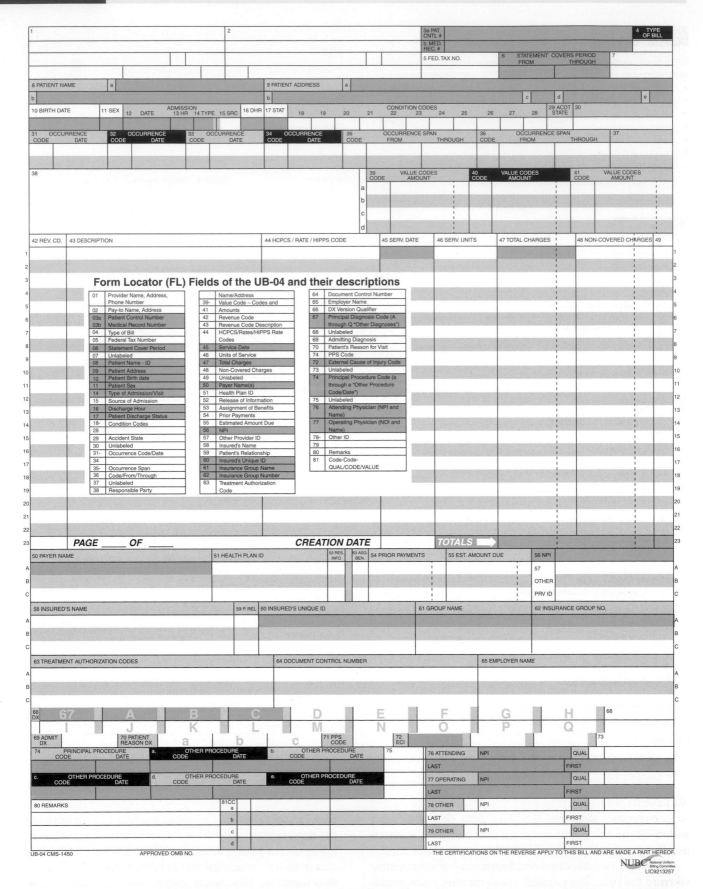

• **Fig. 3.4** UHDDS data elements on the UB-04. In this illustration, the fields highlighted in green represent data items required by the UHDDS that are also found here on the Universal Bill. *UHDDS*, Uniform Hospital Discharge Data Set.

Clinical data are specific to the patient's diagnosis and treatment; examples are as follows:
- diagnosis
- body temperature
- blood pressure
- laboratory reports
- radiographs and other types of imaging
- medications
- surgical procedures

**• BOX 3.2    Patient Status**

**Outpatient:** a patient whose health care services are intended to be delivered within 1 calendar day or, in some cases, a 24-hour period.
**Inpatient:** a patient admitted to the hospital by order of a physician with the intention of staying overnight for at least 1 night.
**Observation:** a patient not admitted to the hospital but monitored in the facility for a period of not more than 48 hours.

**❖ COMPETENCY CHECK-IN 3.1**

**Health Records Defined**

1. How does the health record facilitate communication among health care professionals?
2. List and describe the five key data categories. For each category of data, give four examples of data elements that would be contained in that category.

## Clinical Flow of Data

In any health care delivery encounter, there is a pattern of activity and data collection that is characteristic of the facility and the type of care being rendered. Although there are unique differences, most encounters have some basic points in common: patient registration, clinical data collection and evaluation, assessment, and treatment. This section specifically addresses data in an acute care setting. Following that is a discussion of the unique data requirements in nonacute care settings.

## The Order to Admit

All patients who seek treatment in any health care setting (e.g., emergency department [ED], clinic, inpatient unit) within a hospital must be registered. Inpatient admissions usually correspond to one of the following four scenarios:

*Emergency*—Unexpected, in which case the patient is taken to the ED and admitted as an emergency admission. These patients have life-threatening conditions that require immediate medical care, such as myocardial infarction (heart attack).

*Urgent*—The patient may be admitted because of an exacerbation of a medical condition. The physician or someone from the physician's office calls in advance in much the same way that a patient calls a physician's office and makes an appointment. This type of admission is referred to as a **direct admission**. Other patients may be admitted directly as transfer patients from other hospitals or skilled nursing facilities (SNFs).

*Elective*—The patient's visit is planned, in which case the patient has an appointment (i.e., the patient's physician or someone in the physician's office arranges for, or schedules, the admission). For example, a woman may be coming in to give birth by elective Cesarean section.

*Other*—Newborns are considered admitted at the time of birth and are registered soon thereafter.

In most of the situations listed above, the inpatient admission is initiated by a physician's order. The physician who issues the order to admit the patient is termed the **admitting physician**. The physician who directs the care given to the patient while hospitalized is termed the **attending physician**. The admitting physician can be different from the attending physician. For example, an on-call or staff physician may admit a patient with chest pain. The patient's cardiologist may then take over the case and become the attending physician. While nurses and physician assistants may have certain privileges within a facility and may write certain orders, only a physician can be listed as the attending physician. The admission order must come from a practitioner who has admission privileges at the facility. According to Medicare:

*Qualifications of the ordering/admitting practitioner: the order must be furnished by a physician or other practitioner ("ordering practitioner") who is: (a) licensed by the state to admit inpatients to hospitals, (b) granted privileges by the hospital to admit inpatients to that specific facility, and (c) knowledgeable about the patient's hospital course, medical plan of care, and current condition at the time of admission. The ordering practitioner makes the determination of medical necessity for inpatient care and renders the admission decision (Department of Health and Human Services, Centers for Medicare and Medicaid Services, 2014).*

If the patient is to be an inpatient, the physician order should state "admit to inpatient status." In a computerized physician order entry (CPOE), the patient status may be a required field with a short menu of options. The status of the patient is very important because the billing and coding are different for inpatients and outpatients.

Sometimes, a patient has a suspected condition that the physician would like to monitor, but the situation does not appear to need inpatient admission. In that case, the physician would write an order to place the patient in observation or outpatient status. If the patient is to remain in the hospital for observation, the physician's order is to keep the patient on outpatient status so that the patient can be monitored by the clinical staff. Typically, chest pain and syncope (fainting) are symptoms that might require close monitoring while laboratory tests and radiologic examinations are performed and their findings reviewed. CMS considers 48 hours to be the maximum amount of time that a patient would reasonably be held in observation status, at which point a decision to admit or to discharge should have been made. In exceptional circumstances, a patient might be held longer; however, the documentation should be very specific as to why the patient was held in observation for longer than 48 hours.

In recent years, whether a patient is admitted as an inpatient or given outpatient observation status has become a problematic issue for hospitals. The reimbursement for outpatient observation is minimal in comparison with that for inpatient admission. Short-stay inpatient admissions (length of stay [LOS] 1 or 2 days) are targets of CMS auditors, who may deny the admission for lack of medical necessity.

To change the patient status from outpatient observation to inpatient admission, the physician writes a new order to admit to inpatient status. However, if a patient is admitted to inpatient status first and is later (during the admission) changed to outpatient observation status, a specific order must be written and the UB-04 must contain a condition code 44 to reflect this action. This condition code is placed in a field (also known as an FL) on the UB-04 that communicates to the payer-specific details of the patient's stay. Many hospitals post **case management** personnel in the ED or patient registration department to coordinate the patient's care and services. They help to facilitate the placement of patients in the correct status and to work with physicians in the event of uncertainty about the nature of a physician's order. This coordination activity is part of utilization review (UR), which is discussed later in this chapter.

In 2013 CMS implemented a rule clarifying the requirements for an inpatient admission. In essence, CMS assumes, absent documentation to the contrary, that an inpatient will require 2 days of hospitalization. Called the "two-midnight" rule, this underlying assumption is an effort to focus providers and facilities on selecting the appropriate setting for the care of a patient.

## The Patient Registration Department

Hospitals often have an entire department, the function of which is similar to that of the registration or reception area of a physician's office. The patient registration department is responsible for ensuring the timely and accurate registration of patients. Employees who perform the clerical function of completing the paperwork may be called *patient registration clerks* or *registrars*. In a small hospital, the admissions department may consist of only one person; however, in a larger facility, dozens of health care professionals may be trained to register patients. Like other departments in the hospital, the name of the patient registration department may vary from facility to facility, as shown in Box 3.3.

The registration function is said to be *centralized* if there is one place in the hospital where all registration activities are performed. In some facilities, the registration function may be decentralized; to that is, registrars are placed in locations

---

**• BOX 3.3    What is in a Name?**

Department names, job titles, and other administrative details vary among organizations. Here are a few common variations:

| | |
|---|---|
| Patient Registration Department | Patient Access Admissions |
| Patient Registration Clerk | Patient Access Clerk Admitting Clerk Registrar |
| Health Information Management Department | Health Records Services Medical Records Department |

---

throughout the facility. For example, dedicated registration areas may be located in the ED, clinics, and ambulatory (same-day) surgery area. However registration is organized, it is a function that must be staffed around the clock, every day of the week.

### Precertification

The patient registration staff must determine whether the patient has health insurance and whether the insurance covers the care that the physician has requested. The attending physician must provide an **admitting diagnosis** to explain the reason for admission and a list of any planned procedures as part of the preapproval process (Fig. 3.5). This preapproval, or precertification/insurance verification, process is extremely important to the hospital. Without the authorization that the insurance company will pay for the patient's stay, the hospital is exposed to the risk of financial loss if the patient is unable to pay for his or her treatment. When the patient's hospitalization is planned, the patient completes the initial registration process and possibly some preadmission testing (e.g., laboratory tests and radiology procedures) before the actual hospitalization. This process gives the patient registration department time to obtain the necessary information.

The registration process can be complicated because the registrars must be able to handle all admission scenarios and must understand a variety of insurance rules. Because the patient registration clerk is often the first hospital staff member that patients and their families meet, providing excellent customer service is important for this professional. Many facilities prefer patient registration clerks to speak at least two languages, depending on the patient population served. In addition, facilities may subscribe to translation services or maintain a call list of employees who speak multiple languages. Many registration departments are staffed and managed by health information professionals. Patient registration clerks have a professional association, the National Association of Healthcare Access Management (http://www.naham.org). The American Association of Healthcare Administrative Managers and the Healthcare Financial Management Association also serve patient registration constituents.

**Tri-State Medical Group**

**FAX Request Form for Precertification Review**

To:_____  Date:_____

(Area Code) Fax:_____

(Area Code) Phone:_____

Attn:_____

From:_____  Fax:_____

Number of Pages (Including Cover Sheet):_____
If there is problem with the receipt of this fax, please call _____.Thank you.

Recipient/Patient Name:_____
Complete Recipient
Address _____

_____

ID Number:_____  CAMA  ☐ Yes     ☐ No

Requested Admit Date:_____  Diagnosis Code(s):_____

Procedure Date(s): _____

Days Requested: _____  Procedure Code(s):_____

New Admit? ( )  Transfer ( )

Recertification Review? Y( )  If So, Par/Reference #_____

Setting:              ☐ Inpatient                    ☐ Physician Office
                      ☐ Outpatient                   ☐ Out of State

Admit Type:           ☐ Non-urgent/Emergent          ☐ Urgent/Emergent

Physician Name:_____  Phone:_____
                                              Fax:_____

Facility:_____  Phone:_____
                                              Fax:_____

Clinical Information:_____
_____
_____
_____
_____

This message is intended for the use of the individual entity to which it is transmitted and may contain information that is privileged, confidential and exempt from disclosure under applicable laws.  If the reader of this communication is not the intended recipient, you are hereby notified that any dissemination, distribution or copying of this communication is strictly prohibited.  If you have received this communication in error, please notify us immediately by telephone and return the original communication to us at the address below via U.S. Postal Service.  We will reimburse you for the mailing costs.
Thank you.
400 North 4th Street, Anytown, Iowa 50622
Phone: 319-555-5734  Fax: 319-555-5758

• **Fig. 3.5** A generic precertification form. (From Beik J: *Health insurance today: a practical approach*, 2021, ed 7, St. Louis, MO, Elsevier, pp. 167.)

## Registration Process

After the patient arrives at the patient registration reception area, the registration clerk asks the patient for proof of identity and insurance, as well as demographic data, certain socioeconomic data, and financial data. These data are used to populate (or update) the MPI. Collectively, the data recorded and stored at registration can be printed together on a form known as an **admission record** (Table 3.1).

If the hospital uses a bar code system for scanning any paper documents, labels with the patient's identification data may be provided by the registrar. **Bar codes** represent data in a way that is easily readable by a machine. Some systems allow the printing of forms with the patient's identification data and bar code preprinted on them, which facilitates postdischarge scanning of the paper documents (Fig. 3.6).

In addition to beginning the data-collection process for the health record and the labeling of documents (if required), the registrar must properly label the patients themselves. Typically, facilities use wristbands to identify each patient. These bands might include the patient's name, birth date, admission date, MRN, patient account number, account number, the bar code from admission, and the attending physician's name (Fig. 3.7). Recent technology has enabled a picture of the patient to be included on the wristband as well. Once the wristband is placed, it is difficult to remove, so the patient can always be identified from it during the

| TABLE 3.1 | Sample Data Included in a Patient Registration[a] | |
|---|---|---|
| **Data Element** | **Explanation or Common Choices** | |
| Patient's identification number | Number assigned by the facility to this patient | |
| Patient's billing number | Number assigned by the facility to this visit | |
| Admission date | Calendar day: month, day, and year | |
| Discharge date | Calendar day: month, day, and year (entered at discharge) | |
| Patient's name | Full name, including any titles (MD, PhD) | |
| Patient's address | Address of usual residence | |
| Gender | Male, female, other | |
| Marital status | Married, single, divorced, separated | |
| Race and ethnicity | Must choose from choices given on the admissions form | |
| Religion | Optional | |
| Occupation | General occupation (e.g., teacher, lawyer) | |
| Current employment | Specific job (e.g., professor, district attorney) | |
| Employer | Company name | |
| Insurance | Insurance company name and address | |
| Insurance identification numbers | Insurance company group and individual identification numbers | |
| Additional insurance | Some patients are insured by multiple companies; all information must be collected | |
| Guarantor | Individual or organization responsible for paying the bill if the insurance company declines payment | |
| Attending physician | Usually physician identification number, which is linked to the physician database in the organization's system | |
| Admitting diagnosis | Reason the patient is being admitted | |

[a]These are typical items that are included in an admission record.

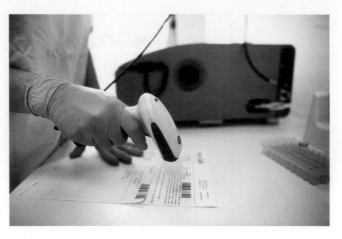

• **Fig. 3.6** The laboratory technician scans forms that have been printed with the patient's bar code. (Copyright zeljkosantrac/iStockphoto.com.)

Occasionally, the facility requires that patients be photographed for identification. If photographs are taken, care must be taken to comply with all applicable Health Insurance Portability and Accountability Act (HIPAA) privacy standards to ensure patient privacy.

Additional data collected at this point include whether the patient has an **advance directive** (a written document that specifies a patient's wishes for his or her care) and the name of the patient's primary care provider (PCP). The patient is also asked to sign an **admission consent form**, with the patient's signature witnessed by the registration clerk. If the patient or the patient's representative is unable to sign this form, the registrar must make a note of this fact and follow up with an attempt to obtain a signature during the hospitalization. In some cases, if the patient is unconscious or not of legal age, an alternative signature is obtained from a parent, guardian, or spouse. The general consent form also contains the following key permissions that the patient grants to the facility:

- permission for caregivers in the hospital to provide general diagnostic and therapeutic care, such as laboratory tests, radiology examinations, most medications, and intravenous fluids and
- permission to release patient information to the patient's designated third-party payer, if applicable, to obtain payment for the services rendered and to appeal denials of payment.

Consent for invasive procedures, such as surgical procedures, requires additional consent, as discussed later in this chapter. The general consent form also contains acknowledgments that the patient has received certain notifications, such as the notice of patients' rights. In recent years, the acknowledgment of the patient's receipt of the notice of patients' rights is typically a separate document.

Depending on the patient population that the hospital serves, admission consent forms may be printed in various languages, such as Spanish, Polish, Chinese, and Arabic, as well as English. Great care must be taken when translating

hospitalization or encounter. Physicians and all hospital staff must check each patient's wristband before administering any treatments to confirm that they are performing the appropriate treatment on the right patient.

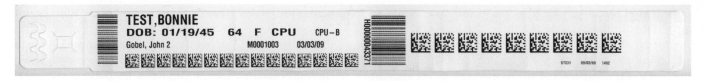

• **Fig. 3.7** The bar code on the patient's wristband contains the patient's medical record number, which links the patient to the patient's medical record. (Courtesy Zebra Technologies Corporation, Lincolnshire, IL.)

a form from English to other languages because this form becomes part of the legal patient record. Hospitals often send their forms to companies that specialize in such translations. See Chapters 6 and 9 for a discussion of some additional documents that patients might sign at registration.

## Medical Decision-Making

After being formally admitted, the patient is taken to the appropriate treatment area. This area may be a patient unit, or sometimes it is the preoperative area, where the patient is prepared immediately for surgery. Patient units are generally designed to accommodate patients who need a specific level of nursing care. Medical/surgical, telemetry, intensive care, labor and delivery, and neonatal intensive care are examples of some unique patient units. In the treatment area, the patient is assessed by nursing staff to determine the patient's needs during care and obtain vital signs and is assessed by the physician to start the diagnostic and treatment process.

One of the key elements of clinical data is the physician's documentation of how they diagnosed the patient and what they decided to do about it. A logical thought process supports the medical evaluation process or development of a medical diagnosis. That thought process is called *medical decision-making*. Ideally, the medical decision-making process is documented in a uniform pattern. In a common format for documenting clinical data, this pattern consists of data collected in four specific categories: the patient's *subjective* view, the physician's *objective* view, the physician's opinion or *assessment*, and the care *plan*. This pattern of recording the observations or clinical evaluations that comprise medical decision-making is called the SOAP format: subjective, objective, assessment, and plan. Although physicians may not always follow this format exactly, they record their thoughts in this general manner. Table 3.2 lists the elements of a medical evaluation.

In conducting the evaluation, the physician collects data sufficient to develop a medical diagnosis. Initially, the data may support several different diagnoses. The physician continues to collect and analyze data until a specific diagnosis can be determined. For example, chest pain and shortness of breath can be the symptoms of many conditions, including myocardial infarction (heart attack), congestive heart failure (a heart-pumping problem that causes a buildup of fluid), and pneumonia (inflammation of the lungs). The possible diagnoses are called the **differential diagnosis**. The physician examines the patient and orders enough tests to conclude which diagnosis (or diagnoses) applies in each case.

| TABLE 3.2 | Elements of Medical Evaluation (SOAP) |
|---|---|
| **Data Element** | **Explanation** |
| **S**ubjective | The patient's report of symptoms or problems |
| **O**bjective | The physician's observations, including evaluation of diagnostic test results |
| **A**ssessment | The physician's opinion as to the diagnosis or possible diagnoses |
| **P**lan | Treatment or further diagnostic evaluation |

### Subjective

The physician begins the medical evaluation process by asking the patient about the medical problem and the symptoms that he or she is experiencing. The patient's description of the problem, in his or her own words, is the subjective, or history, portion of the evaluation process. For example, the patient may have stomach pain. The patient may describe this as "abdominal pain," "pain in the belly," or "pain in the stomach." The physician's task is to narrow the patient's description through questioning. For instance, the patient can be assisted to identify the pain as a sharp, stabbing pain in the lower right portion of the abdomen. The physician also asks when the pain began, whether it is continuous or intermittent, and whether there are any other symptoms, such as nausea and vomiting. The physician will record the patient's description in the patient's own words.

### Objective

Once the physician has obtained and recorded the patient's subjective impressions about the medical problem, the physician must look at the patient objectively. The physician conducts a physical examination, exploring the places where the stomach pain may be located. The patient says his or her stomach hurts, but the physician records that the patient has "tenderness on palpation in the right lower quadrant." Tenderness on palpation in the right lower quadrant is a classic indication of appendicitis. Other possible differential diagnoses are ovarian cyst and a variety of intestinal disorders, such as diverticulitis (inflammation of the intestines). The physician's objective notation is the specific anatomic location of the pain, vital signs, and the results of any laboratory tests that the physician ordered. The physician orders tests to confirm a likely diagnosis or to **rule out** (eliminate) a possible diagnosis. In this example, the physician is looking for an elevation of the white blood cell (WBC) count, which indicates the presence of an infection. The physician may rule out a differential diagnosis such as appendicitis if the WBC count is normal. Additional tests, such as an abdominal ultrasound, might be ordered if the blood test results are negative or inconclusive.

### Assessment

Once the physician has obtained the patient's subjective view and has conducted an objective medical evaluation, he or she develops an *assessment*. The assessment is a description of what the physician thinks is wrong with the patient: the diagnosis or possible (provisional) diagnoses. If there are multiple possible diagnoses, the physician would record "possible appendicitis versus ovarian cyst" or "rule out appendicitis, rule out ovarian cyst." The phrase "rule out" means that the diagnosis is still under investigation. "Ruled out" means that the diagnosis has been eliminated as a possibility. Alternatively, the physician might make a list of the differential diagnoses and label them as such: "differential diagnoses: appendicitis, ovarian cyst." In this abdominal pain example, if the physician has eliminated the possibility of an ovarian cyst and has concluded that the patient has appendicitis, the documentation would read, "appendicitis, ovarian cyst ruled out."

### Plan

Once the physician has assessed what is potentially wrong with the patient, he or she writes a **plan of care**. The plan may be for treatment or further evaluation, particularly if the assessment includes several possible diagnoses. So, for a patient with sharp pain in the right lower abdomen, the plan of care might be diagnostic and include a blood test to check for infection and an ultrasound to differentiate between possible diagnoses of appendicitis or an ovarian cyst. The plan is executed, and then the physician reviews the objective results, assesses those results, and makes a new plan. Say the blood test comes back with increased white cell count, indicating infection, and the ultrasound shows no ovarian cyst. The new plan might include surgery to remove the appendix.

Because the plan of care may involve many medical specialties, each patient is often assigned to a patient care team that consists of various health care professionals in addition to physicians. The initial plan may consist of tests and other diagnostic procedures. All procedures, whether diagnostic or therapeutic, are undertaken only on the direct order of the physician. Orders may also specify whether the patient has bathroom privileges, may ambulate independently, requires a special diet, or can have visitors.

Other disciplines involved in the care of the patient include, but are not limited to, nurses, case managers, social workers, psychologists, nutritionists, physical and occupational therapists (PTs and OTs, respectively), and respiratory therapists (RTs). In the acute care setting, these allied health professionals are directed by the physician. In other words, they collaborate in developing and implementing the plan of care but cannot independently direct patient care. Some clinical personnel, such as physician assistants, nurse midwives, and advanced practice registered nurses, may be licensed as independent practitioners. These providers may be approved to direct specific, limited types of patient care independent of a physician through the hospital's credentialing process. In other cases, they may be dependent practitioners, directing patient care under the supervision of a particular physician.

Although physicians direct patient care and are responsible for the overall plan, they are not always present with the patient during the entire inpatient stay. They may have office hours elsewhere or admit patients to multiple facilities. An exception to this situation is the **hospitalist**, a type of physician employed by the hospital whose practice is primarily focused on patient care situations unique to the acute care setting. Other physicians who spend most of their time on the hospital premises are intensivists, who focus their efforts on patients in critical care units.

Fig. 3.8 illustrates the pattern of data collection in progress notes in the SOAP format, and the resulting orders from those progress notes. Other clinical personnel also record their observations but not necessarily in the SOAP format. Nursing practice has evolved standards of practice, and nurses are diligent in documenting patient care and the events surrounding care. Because nurses spend far more time with a patient than the attending physician, nurse feedback is important to the physician's medical decision-making.

### Outcome

Once the patient has been diagnosed and treated, the patient is discharged. The patient may leave the facility to return home or may transfer to another facility for additional treatment. For example, an appendectomy patient may return home, but a hip-replacement patient may transfer to a rehabilitation facility. The destination of the patient after discharge is a data element called **discharge disposition**, typically recorded by designated clinical personnel, stored in the patient's visit/encounter table, and included on the UB-04. As with admission, a discharge is typically preceded by a physician order. Patients who choose to leave the facility before clearance from the physician may be considered to have left **against medical advice (AMA)**.

Discharge disposition is entered in the form of one of the codes listed in Table 3.3.

An increasingly important component of the medical decision-making process is the **outcome**: the result of the plan or series of plans. In other words, did the plan clarify and effectively treat the diagnosis? Insurance companies may use the history and trending of outcomes to determine which health care providers will be included in their networks.

| Physician's Progress Note | Physician's Order | What Happened |
|---|---|---|
| S Patient complains of abdominal pain<br>O Pain on palpation, right lower quadrant<br>A Rule out appendicitis versus ovarian cyst<br>P CBC with differential<br><br>*Frank Blondeau MD 07/02/2019 1700* | CBC with differential<br>NPO<br><br>*Frank Blondeau MD 07/02/2019 1715* | The doctor isn't sure whether the patient has appendicitis or an ovarian cyst, so he orders a blood test and directs that the patient have no food or drink in case they have to operate |
| S Patient states abdominal pain slightly improved. Diarrhea, but no nausea or vomiting<br>O Pain on palpation, right lower quadrant<br>A CBC normal, appendicitis ruled out. Rule out ovarian cyst versus gastroenteritis versus diverticulosis<br>P CT scan today<br><br>*Frank Blondeau MD 07/03/2019 1830* | CT scan abdomen, with contrast<br>Liquid diet<br><br>*Frank Blondeau MD 07/03/2019 1845* | The blood test showed no elevated white blood count, so the doctor is expanding the rule outs to include gastroenteritis and diverticulosis. He has ordered a CT scan and is allowing the patient to have liquids |
| S Patient states abdominal pain improved and no diarrhea since noon<br>O Minimal pain on palpation; CT scan negative<br>A Diagnosis: gastroenteritis; cannot rule out diverticulosis<br>P Discharge and follow up for outpatient colonoscopy to rule out diverticulosis<br><br>*Frank Blondeau MD 07/03/2019 1715* | Discharge to home<br>Follow up for outpatient colonoscopy<br><br>*Frank Blondeau MD 07/03/2019 1730* | The patient's symptoms are abating and the CT scan came back negative. The patient does not need to be an inpatient for additional follow-up for possible diverticulosis. |

• **Fig. 3.8** The link between physician's progress notes (taken in SOAP format) and physician's orders.

**TABLE 3.3 Partial List of Discharge Disposition Codes**

| Code | Discharge Status |
|---|---|
| 01 | Discharged to home or self-care |
| 02 | Discharged/transferred to another short-term general hospital for inpatient care |
| 03 | Discharged/transferred to a skilled nursing facility (SNF) with Medicare certification in anticipation of covered skilled care |
| 04 | Discharged/transferred to an intermediate care facility |
| 05 | Discharged/transferred to a designated cancer center or children's hospital |
| 06 | Discharged/transferred to home under care of organized home health service organization in anticipation of covered skilled care |
| 21 | Discharged/transferred to court/law enforcement |
| 43 | Discharged/transferred to a federal health care facility |
| 51 | Discharged/transferred to hospice-medical facility (inpatient only) |
| 61 | Discharged/transferred within this institution to a hospital-based Medicare-approved swing bed |
| 62 | Discharged/transferred to an inpatient rehabilitation facility, including distinct part units of a hospital |
| 63 | Discharged/transferred to a long-term care hospital (LTCH) |
| 64 | Discharged/transferred to a nursing facility certified under Medicaid but not certified under Medicare |
| 65 | Discharged/transferred to a psychiatric hospital or psychiatric distinct part unit of a hospital |
| 66 | Discharged/transferred to a critical access hospital (CAH) |
| 70 | Discharged/transferred to another type of health care institution not defined elsewhere in the code list |

A swing bed hospital is a hospital or critical access hospital (CAH) participating in Medicare that has CMS approval to provide post-hospital SNF care and meets certain requirements. A swing bed is an acute bed used by such a hospital to provide this service. http://www.cms.gov/Medicare/Medicare-Fee-for-Service-Payment/SNFPPS/SwingBed.html. A long-term care hospital (LTCH) is defined by Medicare as a hospital having an average length of stay of over 25 days. https://www.cms.gov/Outreach-and-Education/Medicare-Learning-Network-MLN/MLNProducts/html/medicare-payment-systems.html#LongTerm. A CAH is a special designation to hospitals that provide necessary care in remote locations. http://www.cms.gov/Outreach-and-Education/Medicare-Learning-Network-MLN/MLNProducts/downloads/CritAccessHospfctsht.pdf.

In an acute care record, the outcome of the admission is captured in several places:

- the diagnoses and procedures, telling us what was wrong with the patient and what was done to diagnose or treat the condition;
- the discharge disposition (e.g., home, nursing home, expired), showing whether the patient lived and if he or she went home or for further care elsewhere; and
- the physician's overall explanation of the stay in the discharge summary.

Often, the patient is not fully recovered when discharged and additional follow-up is required. The outcome of the acute care visit may have been favorable because the patient's diseased appendix was removed and he or she was discharged to home for further recovery. However, the patient developed an infection after the operation and died. So, following the patient after discharge is important in understanding the outcome of care for the entire illness, not just the hospital visit. The reasons for unsuccessful outcomes are not necessarily the fault of the attending physician or the facility in which the patient was treated. For example, the patient may not have complied with discharge instructions. Nevertheless, the readmission is attributed to both the attending physician and the facility in the reporting of such data. One example of the shifting emphasis on outcomes and follow-up is the Medical Home model of primary care. *Medical Home* refers to the proactive coordination of patient care by the PCP. The Medical Home model requires coordination and collaboration among all caregivers to ensure that the patient's transition from one setting to another is seamless and is supported by the data collected in the prior settings. In this manner, the PCP would be informed concurrently of the patient's inpatient treatment and discharge instructions so that follow-up would occur promptly, ensuring that the patient understood and was following discharge instructions, potentially preventing unnecessary readmission.

## Clinical Documentation

Physicians, nurses, therapists, and numerous ancillary and administrative departments contribute a wide variety of notes, reports, and documentation of events. As discussed above, such documentation consists of collections of data organized logically into forms or data entry screens that build the health record. This section covers the major data elements that each of these professionals contributes and the traditionally named form into which the data are collected. Fig. 3.9 shows the contributors of health data and the collections of data that they contribute.

The primary purpose of the clinical data is communication. Communication takes place among clinicians before, during, and after the specific episode of care. It is also part of the business record of the hospital and therefore supports both the official record of the care rendered and the documentation of the charges for that care. Therefore accurate, complete documentation is essential for multiple reasons.

## Physicians

When the patient is admitted, the attending physician conducts a medical evaluation. This SOAP format evaluation contains the subjective history, the objective physical examination, the assessment of a preliminary diagnosis or diagnoses, and a plan of care, for which orders are recorded. Medical decision-making is a complex activity that depends on the number of possible diagnoses, the volume and complexity of diagnostic data that must be reviewed, and the severity of the patient's condition. This complexity is reflected in the physician's documentation. Fig. 3.10 illustrates the components of medical decision-making.

### History

A history is taken from the data that the patient reports to the physician regarding the patient's health. These data may

## COMPETENCY CHECK-IN 3.2

### Clinical Flow of Data

Match the physician progress note entry on the left with the SOAP note component on the right.

_____ 1. 60 mg pseudoephedrine every 4 hours; 100 mg Tylenol as needed for pain | A. Subjective

_____ 2. Acute sinusitis with pharyngitis | B. Objective

_____ 3. Patient complains of headache | C. Assessment

_____ 4. Patient's frontal sinuses sensitive to percussion, lungs clear, throat slightly inflamed | D. Plan

5. At registration, patient data are collected that help identify the patient and the payer for the services to be rendered. List as many data items (fields) as you can recall that would be included in an admission record report.
6. Describe the patient registration process.
7. How does the facility know the patient's services will be paid for?
8. How does subjective information differ from objective information?
9. What data element records where the patient went after leaving the facility?

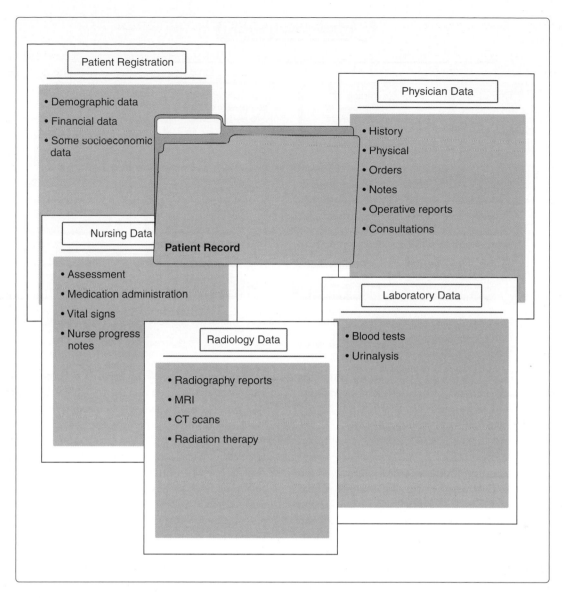

• **Fig. 3.9** Sample data elements in a health record by source. *CT*, Computed tomography; *MRI*, magnetic resonance imaging.

be written by hand, but it is preferable to preserve them in a dictated report that is later transcribed. In a fully electronic **point-of-care documentation system**, either the history could be dictated using a speech-recognition program or data could be collected through menu-driven prompts or templates. In an inpatient setting, the history is usually extensive and comprehensive. The history should consist of the **chief complaint** (the reason that the patient presented for evaluation and treatment), the history of the complaint, a description of relevant previous illnesses and procedures, and a review of body systems. The complexity of the history is directly related to the amount of data that the physician needs to evaluate the patient's problem, measured by the number of body systems that are reported. Table 3.4 lists the data elements that are collected in a history and the levels of complexity.

For example, if a patient visits the ED because of a splinter in a finger, a simple, or problem-focused, history is directed only toward the presenting problem (the splinter), and very little else is discussed or observed. The history would probably contain nothing more than the events surrounding the occurrence of the splinter and possibly an inquiry as to whether the patient had received a tetanus vaccination in the past 10 years.

The finger may appear to be infected, possibly leading to a blood test and thus an expanded review.

Perhaps the patient had fallen beforehand, prompting the physician to suspect possible head trauma or fracture, which would require review of the head and extremities, as well as the abdomen and skin, for possible soft tissue injury or injury to internal organs: a detailed review. The history becomes increasingly complex as the number of body systems involved and the potential threats to the patient's life become more evident.

A patient admitted to an acute care facility requires more substantive evaluation, particularly when the underlying

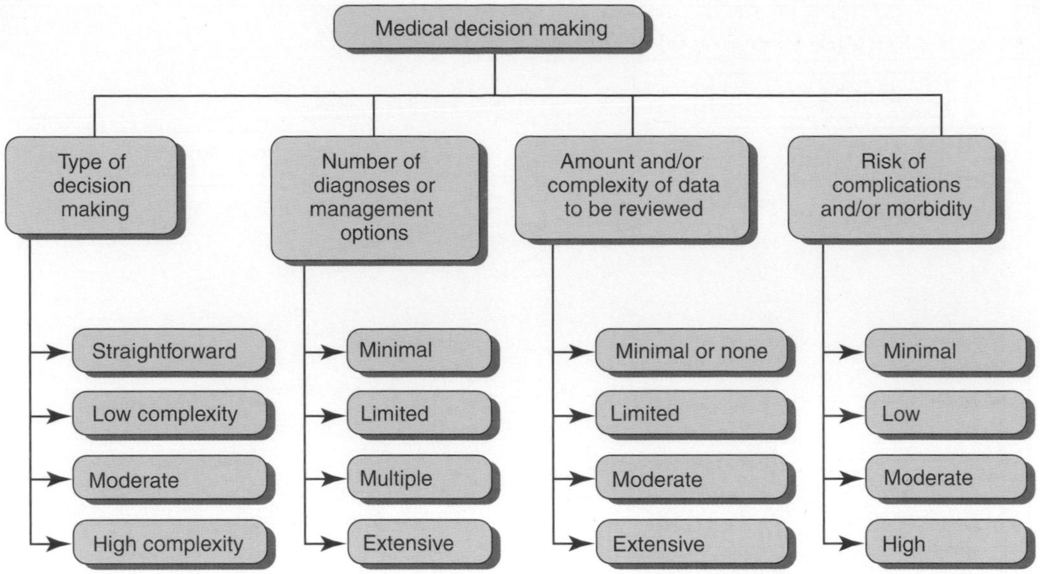

• **Fig. 3.10** Flowchart of medical decision-making. (From Andress AA: *Saunders' manual of medical office management*,1996, Philadelphia, PA, Saunders, pp 96.)

illness is still under investigation. In that case, the physician collects a comprehensive history. The physician makes more detailed inquiries about the patient's entire medical history and asks questions about additional body systems.

### Physical Examination

After collecting the appropriate history data, the physician performs the objective portion of the evaluation: the **physical examination**. Like the history, the physical examination may be dictated and transcribed, dictated through speech recognition, entered through menus/templates, or handwritten. The physical examination (or, more briefly, the physical) includes the physician's examination and observations of every pertinent body system. The term *pertinent* is used because the physician usually follows the same level of complexity as he or she does when collecting the history. For example, the patient with a splinter may require only an examination of the affected finger. In the absence of infection or other trauma, a problem-focused physical examination is appropriate. Moreover, it is not appropriate for the physician to perform a comprehensive physical examination of the patient with a splinter in the absence of a history indicating its necessity. Like the history, the level of detail of the examination is also documented. The physical examination ends with the physician's assessment, also called the *impression*, and the initial plan of treatment. Table 3.5 lists data elements that are collected in a physical.

When the history and physical (H&P) data are collected and reported together in a single, longer report, the report is referred to as the **history and physical (H&P)**. Note that the H&P follows the medical evaluation process previously described. The subjective data (the patient's history) are followed by the objective data (the physical), and then the assessment and the plan of care are recorded.

The data collected in these two reports are critical for patient management; therefore specific rules direct the completion of this data-collection activity. In an acute care facility, CMS (and consequently The Joint Commission [TJC]) requires that the H&P be present in the record no more than 30 days before or 24 hours after admission or registration but prior to surgery or a procedure requiring anesthesia services (Federal Register, 2021b; The Joint Commission, 2012). H&Ps performed more than 30 days prior to admission are not acceptable for the current admission, and a new H&P must be documented. H&Ps performed within 7 days of admission may be accepted as documented; however, H&Ps performed more than 7 days prior to admission must contain an interval note: a brief description by the physician regarding any changes in the patient's condition or the physician's assessment thereof.

The physician creating the H&P must **authenticate** the report, assuming responsibility by signature, mark, code, password, or other means of identification. In teaching hospitals, the H&P may be performed by a resident physician. State law and medical staff bylaws or rules and regulations will specify to what extent an attending physician is required to cosign the documentation of a resident or medical student. Documentation by the first-year residents (also known as *interns*) generally must be cosigned because these residents have not obtained their medical licenses.

### Orders

While the patient is in the facility, the physician makes decisions about the patient's treatment, including those about any further diagnostic testing. For example, a patient who is scheduled for a hemicolectomy (excision of part of the colon) may have entered the hospital with an admitting diagnosis of chronic diverticulitis or colon cancer. The plan

**TABLE 3.4 Data Elements in a History and Level of History**

| Data Element | Explanation | Level of History[a] | | | |
|---|---|---|---|---|---|
| | | Problem Focused | Expanded Problem Focused | Detailed | Comprehensive |
| Chief complaint | The reason for the encounter, usually as expressed by the patient | – | – | – | – |
| History of present illness | The patient's report of the events, circumstances, and other details surrounding the chief complaint | Brief | Brief | Extended | Extended |
| Review of systems | The patient's responses to the physician's questions regarding pertinent body systems, including constitutional symptoms | N/A | Problem pertinent | Extended | Complete |
| | Eyes | | | | |
| | Ears, nose, mouth, and throat | | | | |
| | Cardiovascular | | | | |
| | Respiratory | | | | |
| | Gastrointestinal | | | | |
| | Genitourinary | | | | |
| | Musculoskeletal | | | | |
| | Integumentary | | | | |
| | Neurologic | | | | |
| | Psychiatric | | | | |
| | Endocrine | | | | |
| | Hematologic/lymphatic | | | | |
| | Allergic/immunologic | | | | |
| Past, family, and/or social history | Including the patient's prior illnesses and operations, socioeconomic concerns, and important family illnesses | N/A | N/A | Pertinent | Complete |

[a]All histories contain, at a minimum, the chief complaint and the history of present illness. The history can have four levels of complexity.

Modified from U.S. Department of Health and Human Services, Centers for Medicare and Medicaid Services: *Evaluation and management services guide*, February 2021. https://www.cms.gov/Outreach-and-Education/Medicare-Learning-Network-MLN/MLNProducts/Downloads/eval-mgmt-serv-guide-ICN006764.pdf.

of treatment includes the removal of part of the colon. Other patients enter the hospital with vague or multiple symptoms, and the physician is not entirely sure which of several possible conditions the patient has. In the SOAP note example discussed above, the right lower quadrant abdominal pain could have several different etiologies, or causes, that are investigated while the patient is in the hospital. In an acute care facility, the physician must specifically order the diagnostic procedures that will help reveal the patient's diagnosis.

The physician's instructions for laboratory tests, radiological examinations, consultations, and medication are included in **physician's orders**. No tests or treatment can take place without the physician's order. Orders must be dated, timed, and authenticated by the physician. Only those authorized by the medical staff rules and regulations can write orders, and this authorization can be different for each organization. In some hospitals, physician assistants and midwives may be able to write physician's orders, but in other facilities, only Medical Doctor (MD) and Doctor of Osteopathy (DO) clinicians may do so.

Although each patient is treated individually based on clinical presentation, many conditions call for a predetermined plan of care that guides the health care professional toward best practices in diagnosing or treating the condition. This predetermined plan may include a specific series

| TABLE 3.5 | Data Elements in a Physical Examination |
|---|---|
| **Level of Examination** | **Body Area(s)/Organ System(s)** |
| Problem focused | Affected body area (BA) and organ system (OS) |
| Expanded problem focused | Affected BA and other BAs/OSs |
| Detailed | Extensive affected BAs/OSs |
| Comprehensive | Complete BAs and complete OSs |
| Area | Definition |
| Organ systems | Eyes |
| | Ears, nose, mouth, and throat |
| | Respiratory |
| | Cardiovascular |
| | Genitourinary |
| | Hematologic/lymphatic/immunologic |
| | Musculoskeletal |
| | Skin |
| | Neurologic |
| | Psychiatric |
| | Gastrointestinal |
| Body areas | Head |
| | Neck |
| | Chest |
| | Abdomen |
| | Genitalia, groin, buttocks |
| | Back |
| | Extremities |
| General | Constitutional (vital signs, general appearance) |

Modified from U.S. Department of Health and Human Services, Centers for Medicare and Medicaid Services: *Evaluation and management services guide,* February 2021. https://www.cms.gov/Outreach-and-Education/Medicare-Learning-Network-MLN/MLNProducts/Downloads/eval-mgmt-serv-guide-ICN006764.pdf. https://www.cms.gov/Outreach-and-Education/Medicare-Learning-Network-MLN/MLNEdWebGuide/Downloads/95Docguidelines.pdf, 1995.

of a standard protocol or order set is that for venous thromboembolism prophylaxis (Fig. 3.11). Because virtually every patient admitted to the hospital is at risk for blood clots in the extremities, orders to assess and take preventive measures are an important factor in the quality of care. The order to put a set of protocols into effect comes from the physician, who is still required to authenticate, date, and time the orders.

Orders may be directly entered by the physician or dictated to a registered nurse, who then enters the orders. Orders that are dictated to a registered nurse are called *verbal orders* (VOs). VOs that are communicated over the telephone are called *telephone orders* (TOs). VOs and TOs are sometimes necessary in emergencies and in situations in which the physician is unable to be present at the hospital at the time the orders are required. The recipient of the order must record it, read it back for confirmation, and evidence the read-back. The recipient of the order must sign, date, and time the receipt and method of receiving the order. VOs and TOs must be authenticated by the physician, although they can be executed immediately. The CMS requires authentication of a VO or TO within 48 hours of the communication of the order or in a time frame specified by state law (Federal Register, 2021a). Individual facilities may have stricter requirements. All orders must be dated, timed, and authenticated. Compliance with authentication rules is measured from the time the order is communicated to the nurse to the date and time of the authentication.

The medical staff must clearly define who is eligible to accept a VO or TO, and under what circumstances. Pharmacists, RTs, and radiology technicians, for example, may be permitted to accept a VO or TO specific to their discipline. Tables 3.6 and 3.7 list the data contained in an order.

An important element of a physician's order is the time that it is rendered. The interpretation of the requirement to authenticate VOs as soon as possible is often "within 24 hours." Implicitly, this requires a date and time attached to both the order and the authentication. If the physician personally makes the order, then the date and time of both are the same. If it is a VO, then the nurse taking the order must record the date and time, and the physician logs the appropriate date and time of the subsequent authentication. In a paper-based system, omitting the time of the order is a compliance issue. However, in a computer-based order entry system, the time can be automatically affixed by the computer.

Nursing staff execute the orders, or put them into effect, by notifying the appropriate department or outside agency of the order. For example, medications may be requested from the hospital pharmacy, radiological examinations may be arranged, or a consultant may be contacted. The nurse who executes the order authenticates and dates the activity (Fig. 3.12).

Typically, the first order in the inpatient record is the order to admit. Not surprisingly, the last order is to discharge. Patients should not be released from the hospital without a discharge order. Some orders are constrained

of blood tests, radiographs, and urinalysis (UA). It may also consist of a set of preoperative or pretherapeutic activities. Such predetermined plans are called **protocols** or **order** sets. Protocols arise from evidence-based, best practices as developed and documented by the relevant specialty. They may be applied voluntarily by the facility or they may be mandated for compliance with regulatory or accreditation standards. Protocols may be printed on a paper form or set up as a group of related orders in the CPOE. An example

| Low Risk | Moderate Risk | High Risk |
|---|---|---|
| Ambulatory patient without additional VTE risk factors or expected length of stay <2 days<br>Minor surgery in patient without additional VTE risk factors (same-day surgery or operating room time <30 minutes).<br><br>*Early ambulation | Patients who aren't in either the low- or high-risk group (go to VTE risk factor table)<br><br>Select one pharmacologic* option:<br><br>• Enoxaparin† 40 mg SQ q 24 hours<br>• UFH 5,000 units SQ q 8 hours<br>• UFH 5,000 units SQ q 12 hours (use only if wt <50 kg or >75 years)<br>or<br>• No pharmacologic prophylaxis because of contraindication<br><br>(go to Contraindications table below)<br><br>• No pharmacologic prophylaxis because it is optional in this special population (GYN surgery).<br><br>Sequential compression device aka SCDs (Optional for these patients if they are on pharmacologic prophylaxis, mandatory if not).<br><br>SCDs to<br>• Both lower extremities<br>• Right leg only<br>• Left leg only<br>• Patient intolerant or has skin lesions on both legs, do not use SCDs | Elective hip or knee arthroplasty<br>Acute spinal cord injury with paresis<br>Multiple major trauma<br>Abdominal or pelvic surgery for cancer<br><br>Select one pharmacologic† option:<br><br>• Enoxaparin* 40 mg SQ q 24 hours<br>• Enoxaparin* 30 mg SQ q 12 hours (knee replacement)<br>• Warfarin _____ mg PO daily, target INR 2-3; hold INR >3<br>or<br>• UFH 5,000 units SQ q 8 hours (only if creatinine clearance is <30, SCr >2, and warfarin is not an option)<br>• No pharmacologic prophylaxis because of contraindication<br><br>(go to Contraindications table below)<br><br>and<br><br>SCDs to<br>• Both lower extremities<br>• Right leg only<br>• Left leg only<br>• Patient intolerant or has skin lesions on both legs, do not use SCDs |

\* Go to Contraindications table.
† Enoxaparin should only be used in patients with CrCl>30 and SCr<2; do not use if epidural/spinal catheter is in place.
SCDs should be used in all patients for whom pharmacologic prophylaxis is contraindicated and in all high-risk patients unless patient is intolerant or with contraindications to SCDs.
Note: Enoxaparin is the USCD Medical Center formulary low molecular weight heparin (LMWH); other LMWHs are considered equivalent.
Return to Contents

| Venous Thromboembolism Risk Factors | | |
|---|---|---|
| Age >50 years<br>Myeloproliferative disorder<br>Dehydration<br>Congestive heart failure<br>Active malignancy<br>Hormonal replacement<br>Moderate to major surgery | Prior history of VTE<br>Impaired mobility<br>Inflammatory bowel disease<br>Active rheumatic disease<br>Sickle cell disease<br>Estrogen-based contraceptives<br>Central venous catheter | Acute or chronic lung disease<br>Obesity<br>Known thrombophilic state<br>Varicose veins/chronic stasis<br>Recent post-partum with immobility<br>Nephrotic syndrome<br>Myocardial infarction |

Return to Contents

| Contraindications or Other Conditions to Consider with Pharmacologic VTE Prophylaxis | | |
|---|---|---|
| Absolute | Relative | Other Conditions |
| • Active hemorrhage<br>• Severe trauma to head or spinal cord with hemorrhage in the last 4 weeks<br>• Other _____ | • Intracranial hemorrhage within last year<br>• Craniotomy within 2 weeks<br>• Intraocular surgery within 2 weeks<br>• Gastrointestinal, genitourinary hemorrhage within the last month<br>• Thrombocytopenia (<50K) or coagulopathy (prothrombin time >18 seconds)<br>• End-stage liver disease<br>• Active intracranial lesions/neoplasms<br>• Hypertensive urgency/emergency<br>• Postoperative bleeding concerns†† | • Immune-mediated heparin-induced thrombocytopenia<br>• Epidural analgesia with spinal catheter (current or planned) |

†† Scheduled return to OR within the next 24 hours: major ortho: 24 hours leeway; spinal cord or ortho spine: 7 days leeway; general surgery, status post-transplant, status post-trauma admission: 48 hours leeway

• **Fig. 3.11** University of California, San Diego Medical Center Venous Thromboembolism Risk Assessment and Prophylaxis Orders (paper version of computerized order set). *Note:* Definition of thrombocytopenia (bottom table) is <50,000 platelets per milliliter of blood. *CRCl,* Creatinine clearance, <30mL/min; *GYN,* gynecologic; *INR,* international normalized ratio; *OR,* operating room; *SCr,* serum creatinine concentration, in mg/dL; *SQ,* subcutaneously; *UFH,* unfractionated heparin; *VTE,* venous thromboembolism. (From US Department of Health and Human Services, Agency for Healthcare Research and Quality: Preventing hospital-acquired venous thromboembolism. Appendix B: Sample Venous Thromboembolism Protocol Order/Set. https://www.ahrq.gov/patient-safety/resources/vtguide/guideapb.html.)

**TABLE 3.6   Data Required for an Order Personally Entered by the Physician**

| Data Element | Explanation |
|---|---|
| Patient's name | Full name, including any titles (MD, PhD) |
| Patient's identification number | Number assigned by the facility to this patient |
| Order date | Date the order is rendered |
| Time | Time the order is rendered |
| Order | Medication, test, therapy, consultation, or other action directed by the physician |
| Physician's authentication | Physician's signature or password |
| Executor's authentication | Signature or password of party effecting the order |
| Execution date | Date the order was effected |
| Execution time | Time the order was effected |

**TABLE 3.7   Data Required for a Verbal Order from the Physician**

| Data Element | Explanation |
|---|---|
| Patient's name | Full name, including any titles (MD, PhD) |
| Patient's identification number | Number assigned to the patient by the facility |
| Order date | Date the order is received |
| Time | Time the order is received |
| Nurse's authentication | Signature or password of party receiving the order |
| Order | Medication, test, therapy, consultation, or other action directed by the physician |
| Verification | Note that the order was "read back" to the ordering physician |
| Physician's authentication | Physician's signature or password |
| Physician's authentication date | Date the order is authenticated |
| Physician's authentication time | Time the physician authenticated the order |
| Executor's authentication | Signature or password of party effecting the order |
| Execution date | Date the order was effected |
| Execution time | Time the order was effected |

by rules that are dictated by either the facility or a regulatory or accrediting body. DNR (do not resuscitate) and restraints are examples of special orders that require specific documentation.

### Progress Notes

While treating the patient, the physician continues to make observations and update the assessment and plan. These **progress notes** are important evidence of the care that the patient has received and serve to document the physician's activities and evaluation process. Progress notes are required as often as needed to document treatment provided to the patient, and in acute care they must be written at least daily to validate the need for this level of care. Notes are often documented in the SOAP format; some physicians even write the SOAP acronym on the note. In an inpatient setting, progress notes become critical, because days, weeks, or months may elapse from the time of the H&P obtained at admission to the time of the patient's discharge. Notes must be dated, timed, and authenticated. In a facility in which physician residents are training, the resident may collect and record the data for the note. In many organizations, and always for unlicensed residents, the resident's note must also be authenticated, or **countersigned**, by the attending physician.

### Consultations

Physicians collaborate through the **consultation** process. The attending physician, who is responsible for the patient's overall care, requests a consultation from a specialist, citing the specific reason for the consultation. For example, a patient admitted for treatment of a heart condition may experience severe diarrhea. The attending physician may request a consultation from a gastrointestinal specialist or an infectious disease specialist. A patient undergoing a hemicolectomy may also have chronic obstructive pulmonary disease, emphysema, asthma, or other severe respiratory problem, in which case the attending physician may elect to call in a pulmonologist to evaluate the patient's status before surgery. Some typical consultations that may be performed in an inpatient setting include an endocrinology consultation if the patient has diabetes mellitus; a wound care consultation for a decubitus ulcer or foot wound; a cardiology consultation if the patient has some sort of heart condition; and, as mentioned previously, a pulmonary specialist if the patient has respiratory concerns. Another typical type of consultation is a psychiatric consultation, which would be appropriate if the patient suffers from depression or other behavioral health issues. Table 3.8 lists the data required for a consultation document. The **consultant** evaluates the patient and responds to the request with specific diagnostic or therapeutic opinions and recommendations. The consultant's response is usually dictated and transcribed but may be handwritten if hospital policy permits.

### Discharge Summary

In an inpatient setting, a **discharge summary**, or case summary of the patient's care, is prepared by the attending

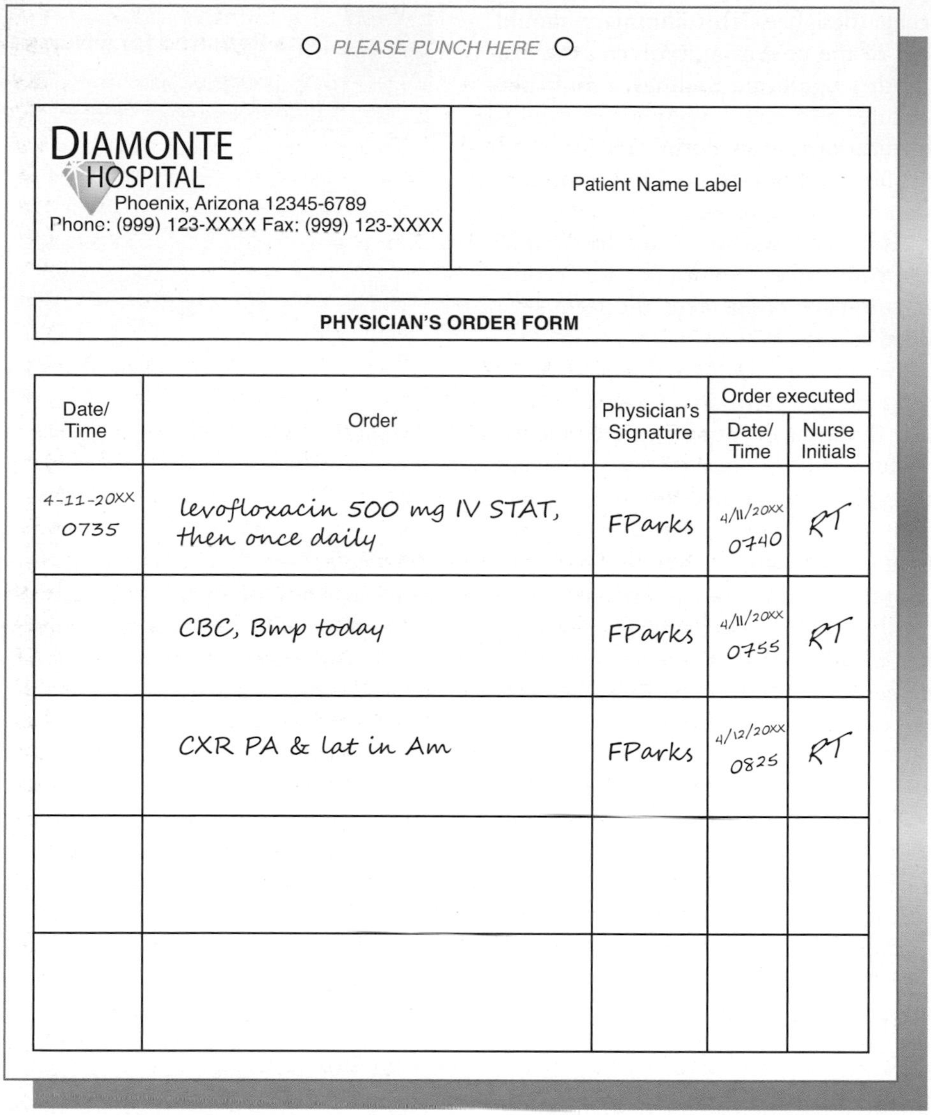

○ *PLEASE PUNCH HERE* ○

**DIAMONTE**
**HOSPITAL**
Phoenix, Arizona 12345-6789
Phone: (999) 123-XXXX Fax: (999) 123-XXXX

Patient Name Label

**PHYSICIAN'S ORDER FORM**

| Date/Time | Order | Physician's Signature | Order executed Date/Time | Nurse Initials |
|---|---|---|---|---|
| 4-11-20XX 0735 | levofloxacin 500 mg IV STAT, then once daily | FParks | 4/11/20XX 0740 | RT |
| | CBC, Bmp today | FParks | 4/11/20XX 0755 | RT |
| | CXR PA & lat in Am | FParks | 4/12/20XX 0825 | RT |
| | | | | |
| | | | | |

• **Fig. 3.12** Nurse execution of a physician's orders.

**TABLE 3.8  Data Required for a Consultation**

| Data Element | Explanation |
|---|---|
| Patient's name | Full name, including any titles (MD, PhD) |
| Patient's identification number | Number assigned by the facility to this patient |
| Physician's order | Required before the consultation is performed (see Tables 3.6 and 3.7) |
| Date of request | Date that the attending physician requests the consultation |
| Specialty being consulted | Cardiology, wound care, gastroenterology, etc. |
| Reason for consultation | Brief explanation of reason that the consultant's opinion is being sought |
| Authentication | Authentication of physician requesting consultation |
| Date of evaluation | When consultant saw patient |
| Consultant's opinion | Diagnosis or recommendations; may be an entire report, similar to an H&P (see Tables 3.4 and 3.5) The opinion will include relevant acknowledgments from the patient's record, such as mention of laboratory values or the attending physician's notes. |
| Report date | Date that consultant prepares report of the opinion |
| Authentication | Authentication of consultant |

physician or his or her designee. This summary should include a brief history of the presenting problem, the discharge diagnosis and other significant findings, a list of the treatments and procedures performed, the patient's condition at discharge, medications given during the stay and those prescribed for at-home administration, follow-up care or appointments, and any instructions given to the patient or patient's caregiver. As with other data, the discharge summary must be dated, timed, and authenticated. The recording of the discharge summary often takes the form of a dictated and transcribed report.

Some inpatient stays do not require a discharge summary, such as that of a normal newborn. Generally, stays of less than 48 hours' duration do not require a detailed discharge summary; a form called a *final progress note/record* may be completed instead. An exception to this occurs when a patient who has been in a hospital for less than 48 hours expires. In such cases, a full discharge summary is required. When a discharge summary is required, TJC mandates that it be on the record within 30 days of discharge. However, in an electronic health record (EHR), a compilation of the components of a discharge summary is typically available once the physician has ordered the discharge.

## Nurses

While the patient is in the hospital, the professionals who perform most of the patient's care, particularly in acute care and LTC facilities, are the nurses and their ancillary staff. Nurses collect and record their own set of data for each patient. As with physician documentation, nursing documentation requires dates, times, and authentication.

### Nursing Assessment

Nurses assess the patient when the patient first enters the facility. The purpose of the nursing assessment is not to diagnose the patient's illness (that is the responsibility of the physician) but to evaluate the patient's care needs. The assessment includes determining the patient's understanding of his or her condition and whether the patient has any concerns or needs that will affect nursing care. The nursing assessment includes an evaluation of the condition of the patient's skin, understanding of his or her condition, diagnosis or reason for admission, learning needs, and ability to perform self-care.

### Nursing Progress Notes

Nurses also must record nursing progress notes. During each shift, the nurse documents particular events or interactions with the patient. Patient complaints and any activities of the nursing staff to address those complaints are noted. The elements of a nursing progress note are given in Table 3.9. In a paper-based record, these notes historically took the form of free text. In an EHR, the documentation may be guided and at least partially menu driven, using templates for required documentation. Some of the

| TABLE 3.9 | Data Required for a Nurse's Progress Note |
|---|---|
| **Data Element** | **Explanation** |
| Patient's name | Full name, including any titles (MD, PhD) |
| Patient's identification number | Number assigned to the patient by the facility |
| Date | Date of the note |
| Time | Time of the note |
| Note | Nurse's comments, observations, and documentation of activities |
| Nurse's authentication | Nurse's signature or password |

documentation remains free text. The organization of the notes may be chronologic or by care plan.

Notes should be written as soon as possible after the activity has occurred. Thus the date and time of the note coincide with the date and time of the occurrence. If a note is written after the fact, the date and time of the occurrence must be separately noted.

In a paper-based system, the note field is generally a large, blank field in which the nurse can comment freely. In a computer-based system, this field may be replaced with a series of fields from which the nurse can compose comments from predetermined menus, in addition to a free field for more specific remarks. The actual content of the note is governed by the patient's condition, nursing professional standards, and facility requirements.

### Vital Signs

Nurses are also responsible for observing and recording the patient's vital signs. Vital signs consist of temperature, blood pressure, pulse rate, oxygen saturation, and respiration. Frequently, vital signs are recorded in a graphic format, which can be referenced easily while the patient is in the facility. Chapter 2 demonstrates how displaying a patient's temperature in a graph or picture facilitates a review of the data (see Fig. 2.3). In an EHR the data are entered into a field that can then be linked to previous data collections to produce a report that is a graphic representation of the cumulative data over time. Electronic recording devices such as cardiac monitors may automatically record the data into the EHR for real-time data review. Other data that nurses collect that are frequently reported in graph format include fluid intake and output and mechanical ventilation readings.

### Medication Administration

One of the most important nursing data collections involves medication administration. The name of the medication, dosage, date and time of administration, method of administration, and name of the nurse who administered it are important data elements. In an electronic medication administration record, the data are captured at each administration, and a report of the administrations can then be printed, if necessary. Fig. 3.13 illustrates a medication-tracking report in a physician's office.

Controls surrounding the administration of medications are focused on the prevention of medication errors. Personnel administering medications are required to identify the patient prior to administration by reviewing the data on the patient's wristband (name, MRN) and comparing it with the data on the medication dispensed by the pharmacy. Ideally, a computer-generated bar code system used both on the wristband and by the pharmacy, linked to the electronic record, can facilitate this process. The nurse can scan the wristband, which brings up the medication order on the computer screen, and then scan the dispensed medication, which matches the order with the drugs (Fig. 3.13). If these elements match, the nurse can complete the administration. If not, the error can be identified and resolved.

## Laboratory Data

In an inpatient setting, the physician frequently orders routine laboratory tests, such as a complete blood count and a UA. When these laboratory tests are performed at the time of the patient's admission, they help identify preexisting infectious conditions. Patient infections identified after 48 hours of hospitalization are attributed to the facility; these are called nosocomial or *hospital-acquired infections*. Laboratory tests are performed only when ordered by the physician. The results of the tests are included in the health record. Laboratory results include both patient-specific data and data comparing the patient's test results with normative ranges of data. For example, the normal hemoglobin range is 12.0–15.0 g/dL for female adults. A female adult patient

whose hemoglobin level is 14.3 g/dL is within normal limits. If a female adult patient's hemoglobin is 6.5 g/dL, the laboratory will flag these results as abnormal.

In an inpatient setting, there may be numerous laboratory tests, depending on the extent to which a patient's condition needs to be monitored or the number of tests required to establish or validate a diagnosis. For some patient conditions, daily blood tests are appropriate. Other conditions may require hourly monitoring. Therefore multiple data fields, in which the results of multiple tests can be recorded, are necessary. As in other situations, the usefulness of an electronic record is evident. Once the test result data are collected, a computer can display them in whole or in part, as well as graphically.

## Radiology Data

Radiology examinations generate two sets of data: the original diagnostic image and the interpretation. The original diagnostic image was historically retained separately from the patient's record. For example, a radiology examination of the chest traditionally produced a large film, which would be retained in a special envelope or file, usually in the radiology department. Facilities are increasingly relying on digital methods of radiographic imaging, recorded in a picture-archiving computer system (PACS). These images are stored in the radiology imaging system, which should be linked to the EHR. Some electronic records can interface with the radiology system and display the radiographic image within the patient's electronic record. These digital images may be downloaded to a disk with the reading software and given to the patient for continuing patient care. The radiologist's interpretation of the image, film or digital, which typically takes the form of a dictated and transcribed report, also becomes part of the patient's record.

| Encounter Type | Medication / Dose | Strength / Form | Route / Frequency | Indication | Status | Entry By | Date |
|---|---|---|---|---|---|---|---|
| Office Visit - Follow-Up/Established Visit 12/05/2018 | Citalopram Tablet - (Celexa)/20mg | 20/Tablet | Oral/Daily | Anxiety | Active | John Tomedi | 12/05/2018 |
| Office Visit - Follow-Up/Established Visit 12/05/2018 | Valsartan/Hydrochlorothiazide 160mg/25mg HCTZ Tablet - (Diovan HCT)/160mg | 160mg/Tablet | Oral/Daily | Hypertension | Active | John Tomedi | 12/05/2018 |
| Office Visit - Follow-Up/Established Visit 12/05/2018 | Esomeprazole Delayed Release Capsule - (Nexium)/20mg | 20/Capsule DR | Oral/Daily | GERD | Active | John Tomedi | 12/05/2018 |

• **Fig. 3.13** The medication report shows that patient Al Neviaser takes Diovan 160 mg daily for high blood pressure. He also takes Nexium 20 mg daily for gastroesophageal reflux disease and Celexa for anxiety. (Courtesy SimChart for the Medical Office, Elsevier, Inc., 2019.)

## Special Records

The previously discussed data elements are very common and occur in one form or another in almost all inpatient health records. The clinical flow of data is similar in every type of health care setting. Depending on the diagnosis and the clinical setting, many other data elements are collected. However, even in an acute care facility, certain clinical situations require additional documentation or variations on the standard documentation described in the previous sections. For example, other types of documentation may include cardiology reports such as electrocardiography (EKG) tracings, neurology reports such as electroencephalography tracings, respiratory therapy diagnostic tests and treatment reports, physical/occupational therapy assessments and treatments, and dietary notes.

### Operative Records

Operative records require detailed data collection of the surgical procedure and the patient's condition before, during, and after the procedure. The record of the patient who undergoes a surgical procedure requires two sets of data: the operative data and the anesthesia data.

#### Operative Data

The operative report is recorded as a detailed, usually dictated and transcribed document. TJC standards call for the dictation to occur immediately following the procedure (The Joint Commission, 2012). Transcribed operative reports are not immediately available to users; therefore a brief operative note in the progress notes is usually written. The operative report lists the preoperative and postoperative diagnosis, the names of the surgeon and surgical assistants, the procedures performed, and a detailed description of the operation, operative findings, estimated blood loss, and specimens removed. As with all physician activities, the operative report is dated, timed, and authenticated. Additional data, such as preoperative checklists, implant information, transfusion record, and instrument counts, are collected and recorded by nursing staff in special forms. In an EHR, this detailed perioperative documentation is collected and recorded with the use of templates. The surgical record system may be separate from the main electronic record system. The perioperative documentation may interface with or be scanned into the EHR.

#### Anesthesia Data

The anesthesia report documents the presurgical evaluation and anesthesia administration of the anesthesiologist. The anesthesiologist performs preoperative and postoperative evaluations of the patient's condition in addition to the continuous recording of the patient's status during the procedure (the intraoperative anesthesia report). The anesthesiology preoperative evaluation is critical to the clearing of a patient for surgery. If the anesthesiologist has concerns about the patient's ability to undergo the administration of anesthesia, the surgery may be canceled. The preoperative and postoperative evaluations may be documented in the progress notes or on a specially designed data-collection device, either paper or electronic. The anesthesiologist is a specially trained physician. Anesthesia may also be administered by a certified registered nurse anesthetist.

### Obstetric Records

Obstetric records differ from the ones already discussed because of the types of data that are collected. When a woman is pregnant and regularly visits a physician's office or clinic for prenatal care, data are collected on the progress of the pregnancy. Specific delivery data, such as the number of previous births, types of deliveries, and conditions of the newborns, are also collected. Shortly before the woman is due to give birth, the data are transferred to the hospital. The data are then incorporated into the inpatient record. On admission for childbirth, pregnant patients are monitored for contractions, fetal activity, and stress during labor. The prenatal record can be considered the H&P for the admission for a normal, uncomplicated vaginal delivery.

### Neonatal Records

Neonatal records for healthy newborns are generally very short. Because these patients are in the hospital solely because of the mother's choice of delivery site, care is focused on promoting the infant's comfort and helping the mother learn how to care for the infant. The contents of a newborn record consist of an admission record, a brief physical examination that includes mention of any congenital anomalies, the birth record, nursing and pediatric progress notes, notes regarding medication administration, a note regarding the circumcision (if applicable), and a record of any testing done, such as a phenylketonuria or hearing test. Newborns who exhibit signs of jaundice also have notes in their records about therapeutic interventions for jaundice, such as phototherapy.

Babies who are born with medical complications require more intensive care. Neonatal intensive care units (NICUs) feature more technological options, specialized caregivers, and specific documentation and data collection for their diagnosis and treatment plans.

### Intensive Care Unit Records

Sometimes patients who are gravely ill when they enter the hospital are sent to special nursing care units called *intensive care units* (ICUs). A patient with a serious heart problem might be cared for in a coronary (or cardiac) care unit (CCU). Because of the intensity of nursing care in ICUs, a large volume of data is collected. In an EHR, vital signs and other data can be recorded either automatically from the equipment that is capturing the data or on data entry screens. Data captured electronically can be displayed in a variety of ways by the user: graphically or in table format, depending on the capabilities of the software. In a paper record, or during computer downtime, such data would be collected on heavy-stock foldout graphs, which can be as large as 8 × 14 in. or 8 × 17 in. and represent 24 hours of care. Vital signs are plotted on graphs that illustrate the patient's progress and the way the patient is being treated.

Unlike standard progress notes, which are completed in the SOAP format, intensive care by physicians requires additional documentation, including details of the specific care given and the amount of time spent at the bedside (for physician billing purposes).

The following are some examples of special care units for close monitoring and care:
- ICU: for medical treatment
- Surgical ICU: for postoperative treatment
- CCU: for cardiac treatment and cardiac monitoring (telemetry)
- NICU: for newborns with medical problems

### Autopsy Reports

Occasionally, patients who expire are subject to autopsy. The *autopsy* is an examination of the deceased, usually to determine the cause of death or other details surrounding the patient's illness at the time of death. The autopsy itself consists of an external and internal examination of the body or a particular organ. Additional testing, such as toxicology and histology (microscopic tissue evaluation), may be performed. The nature and extent of the autopsy are determined by the questions that need to be answered. In the case of an unexpected death from unknown causes in an otherwise healthy person, or if homicide is suspected, an extensive examination and many additional tests may be performed. However, if a confirmation of a suspected condition, such as Alzheimer's disease, is the only question to be answered, then the autopsy will focus on brain tissue.

Autopsies of hospitalized patients are performed according to the policies and procedures of the hospital, at the request of the family, or in compliance with the requirements of the medical examiner. The *medical examiner* is an official whose responsibility is to investigate deaths that occur under specific circumstances. Suspected homicide, unexpected death of unknown cause of a person who is not under the care of a physician, and death from trauma are potential cases for a medical examiner.

Autopsies are performed by *pathologists*: physicians who are specially trained in this type of examination. The autopsy report is a detailed description of the extent of the examination and the findings. This report may take many weeks to prepare, particularly if extensive additional evaluations are required, but it is usually available within 60–90 days of the autopsy. The report becomes a part of the permanent health record.

## Clinical Oversight

In Chapter 1, a collaborative process of patient care involving the physicians, nurses, and other allied health professionals was described. This **patient care plan** is more than just a series of instructions or recommendations for an individual patient. Clinicians typically follow established patterns of care that are based on experience, successful outcomes, and research. The formal description of these patterns of care is the clinical pathway.

### Clinical Pathway

A **clinical pathway** is a predetermined plan for treatment. The plan can come from best practices and **evidence-based medicine**, or the organization can, after studying or reviewing a significant number of health records for patients with a particular diagnosis, develop a guide or plan for patients with that diagnosis. By doing so, a facility can streamline the patient's stay in the hospital, coordinate multidisciplinary care, and ideally eliminate any unnecessary time spent in the facility or at a particular level of care. The goal is to provide high-quality patient care efficiently and effectively. It is important to note that this does not mean that all patients will be treated the same. If the patient's condition warrants a change from the clinical pathway, appropriate treatment is rendered, and ideally, the patient's condition improves. Often, when clinical pathways are utilized, practitioners document only exceptions to the pathway, so daily documentation for standards of care may not be necessary.

Each medical discipline has a specific clinical pathway that describes the appropriate steps to take, given a specific diagnosis or a specific set of signs and symptoms, and based on the answers to critical questions. For example, a patient with high blood glucose (hyperglycemia) must be tested to determine whether the patient has diabetes. If the patient has diabetes, further studies will identify whether the condition is insulin dependent or not. The physician will prescribe the appropriate medications and other regimens based on that determination. Nursing staff will assess the patient's level of understanding of his or her condition and take the appropriate steps to educate the patient and possibly the family. Fig. 3.14 illustrates a clinical pathway.

### Case Management

The responsibility for patient care rests with the provider, but often multiple providers, and possibly multiple facilities, are involved in a patient's care. From the payer's perspective, **case management** is necessary to coordinate the approval of and adherence to the care plan. From the provider's perspective, case managers are necessary to facilitate the continuity of care. Thus a patient may have multiple case managers working from different perspectives, all helping to ensure that the patient is cared for appropriately and efficiently.

Case management is performed by health care professionals, typically nurses or **board-certified social workers (BCSWs)**, within the facility, as well as by the payers who send their employees into the facility to oversee or coordinate care. The health care professional coordinating the care is called a *case manager*. Case management in practice

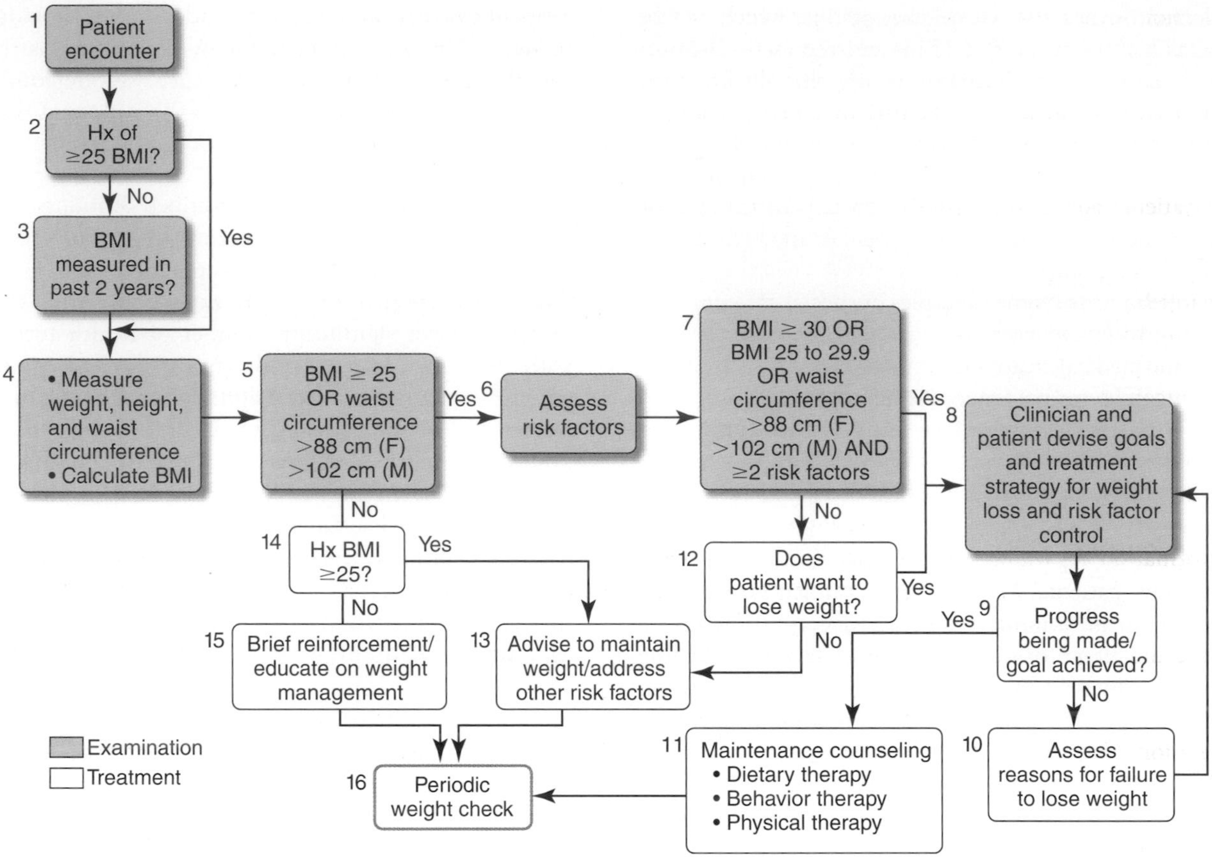

• **Fig. 3.14** Clinical pathway for obesity. (From National Institutes of Health, National Heart, Lung, and Blood Institute, in cooperation with the National Institute of Diabetes and Digestive and Kidney Diseases: *Clinical guidelines on the identification, evaluation, and treatment of overweight and obesity in adults: the evidence report.* NIH Publication No. 98-4083. http://www.nhlbi.nih.gov/guidelines/obesity/ob_gdlns.pdf. September 1998.)

is multidisciplinary. The coordinator interacts with all the health care professionals involved in the patient's care. With such a team, the expectation is that the communication among the disciplines (e.g., physical therapy, occupational therapy, nursing, medical) will facilitate appropriate, effective, and efficient health care for the patient.

The case manager is assigned to the patient when the patient is admitted to the facility. Review of the patient's health information to determine the plan of care happens concurrently. Case management also involves multidisciplinary meetings of health care professionals to coordinate the patient's plan of care and continually update each discipline on the patient's progress.

The team members in this multidisciplinary effort may include, but are not limited to, physicians, nurses, PTs, OTs, RTs, speech therapists, health information management (HIM) coders, and patients (in some settings). Each person on the team attends the case management meeting to discuss the development or progress of the patient's care. The case manager is also concerned with planning for the patient's discharge, making sure that the patient's status is reviewed for appropriate placement in the next health care facility or that care is received via home health or follow-up in the physician's office. Each team meeting is documented

and becomes a part of the patient's health record. When necessary, the plan of care is also updated.

Another type of case management is the coordination of care from the PCP. Ideally, the PCP is aware of and follows up with the patient regarding any care rendered elsewhere, such as during an inpatient admission. The comprehensive implementation of such coordination of care is a key characteristic of the Patient-Centered Medical Home (PCMH) model. The PCMH model requires a PCP, active involvement by the PCP in the coordination of patient care, and high-quality care rendered. Recommendations for implementation of a PCMH were promulgated by the American College of Physicians, American Academy of Family Physicians, American Academy of Pediatrics, and American Osteopathic Association in 2010.

### Utilization Review

Understanding clinical pathways and payer issues enables a facility to evaluate patient care, controls the use of facility resources, and measures the performance of individual clinical staff. In a hospital, the **utilization review (UR)** department works closely with all health care disciplines involved in caring for a patient who has been admitted. UR staff members are responsible, with physician oversight, for performing an admission review that covers the appropriateness of the admission itself, certifying the level of care for an admission (e.g., acute, skilled nursing), monitoring the intensity of services (IS) provided, and ensuring that a patient's LOS is appropriate for that level of care. UR staff members may have daily contact with a patient's insurance company during the patient's admission to verify that the correct level of care payment will be received for the anticipated LOS. UR staff may also make provisions for aftercare once the patient is discharged; this is called discharge planning.

UR is the function or department that ensures appropriate, efficient, and effective health care for patients. It also monitors patient outcomes and compares physician activities.

"Appropriate" may also refer to what is covered by the patient's insurance plan. A health insurance plan may require a specific test before approving a specific treatment or procedure. The expectation is that the test will provide definitive information regarding the necessity of the treatment or procedure. For example, before approving arthroscopy of the knee, an insurance company may require magnetic resonance imaging (MRI). In the past, the physician had sole responsibility for determining the procedures and treatments that a patient would or would not receive. Today, such decisions may be heavily influenced by the third party paying the bill.

CMS and other payers have established efforts to reduce the number of short inpatient LOSs, as these can be costly and may not be medically necessary. For example, when a physician in the ED makes a diagnosis of pneumonia, the Medicare Severity diagnosis-related group (MS-DRG) for pneumonia is sent to the payer either while the patient is still in the ED or shortly after admission. During the evaluation process, use of nationally accepted screening criteria such as InterQual or Milliman provides standards for determining medical necessity, using weights of severity of illness (SI) and intensity of service (IS) for the specific diagnosis to determine the appropriate LOS for the patient and the amount the insurer will reimburse. Given all the factors of a particular weighted DRG, the payer may determine that the patient should have an inpatient stay of 3 days. Because the hospital will not receive payment for an LOS longer than that, UR staff may have to request a recertification of the patient based on changes in his or her condition to justify a longer LOS or risk receiving a payment that does not cover the cost of services.

Payers study historic patient treatment by analyzing patient health records to identify best practices or a specific plan of treatment to identify the best standard of care. The quality improvement organizations that contract with Medicare closely monitor diagnosis data and hospital statistics to limit the potential for overpayment in situations such as short LOSs. For this reason, UR staff work to help physicians move patients through the system efficiently, guiding the screening criteria for admitting diagnoses and the working DRG used during the inpatient stay. This is not to say that physicians do not order tests that payers do

not approve, nor does it imply that payers overrule physician orders. However, there is significant controversy over the influence of payers in medical decision-making.

For example, suppose a patient with Type 1 diabetes mellitus is admitted because the patient performed a self-check at home and could not control the blood glucose level even while taking the prescribed amounts of daily insulin. UR staff members will be notified that the patient has been admitted, and they will perform an admission review. This admission review entails an evaluation of the patient's medical record, including physician orders and any test results. In some cases, the admission will be deemed unnecessary. The admission might be unnecessary if the patient's blood glucose levels were all normal on admission. At that point, UR staff members would not certify the admission for reimbursement; this is called an admission denial.

If UR staff members deem the admission necessary, they will certify the admission. UR staff may contact the patient's insurer, verify the diagnosis of uncontrolled Type 1 diabetes mellitus, and determine that the anticipated LOS for that diagnosis is 2–3 days. The insurer agrees to reimburse the hospital for 3 days of acute care as certified by UR staff. During the hospitalization, UR staff members will discuss the aftercare, or discharge plan, with the attending physician. In this case, perhaps more home health care services are warranted. On the third day, the patient is expected to be discharged. If the patient is not discharged on day 3, members of the UR staff must review the documentation and discuss the case further with the physician to justify additional hospitalization. If the additional days are not justified by the documentation in the health record, the additional days may not be reimbursed by the insurer; this is called a continued stay denial. In these instances, the patient will be notified that he or she no longer needs to be in the hospital, that the insurer will not reimburse the hospital for any additional costs, and that the patient is responsible for all further costs. When a continued stay denial occurs, the physician is also notified. The physician will either concur with the continued stay denial and discharge the patient or provide documentation justifying the additional care.

## Discharge Data Set

Throughout this chapter, specific data elements have been discussed. All of these data fall into one of the four main categories: demographic, financial, socioeconomic, and clinical. Many of these data are used to compile the bill that is sent to the third-party payer or the patient. Certain key data elements are also reported to various regulatory agencies, particularly the state's Department of Health or other agency that governs the licensure of hospitals. Although individual states may require additional data, the specific data elements that are required to be collected and reported by hospitals constitute the **Uniform Hospital Discharge Data Set (UHDDS)**, which is the core data set required by most states. This data set was adopted in 1985 by the US DHHS (US Department of Health and Human Services, 1996). Although many changes have been discussed, the data set has remained stable. Table 3.10 contains a summary of UHDDS data elements and each element's source in the acute care setting.

**TABLE 3.10    Uniform Hospital Discharge Data Set (UHDDS) Data Elements and their Sources**

| UHDDS Element | Description | Typical Recorder/Source of Data |
|---|---|---|
| Personal/unique identifier | The patient's full name and medical record number or another unique identifier | Patient registration |
| Date of birth | The year, month, and day of the patient's birth | Patient registration |
| Gender | Male, female, or unknown/not stated | Patient registration |
| Race and ethnicity | Race<br>American Indian/Eskimo/Aleut; Asian or Pacific islander; Black; White; other; unknown/not stated<br>Ethnicity<br>Hispanic origin; other; unknown/not stated | Patient registration |
| Residence | Full address and zip code of the patient's usual residence | Patient registration |
| Health care facility identification number | Identification number of the facility that treated the patient | Maintained in system files |
| Admission date | The year, month, and day of admission for the current episode of care | Patient registration |
| Type of admission | Was the admission expected or unexpected? | Patient registration |
| Discharge date | The year, month, and day of discharge for the current episode of care | Nursing or patient registration |
| Attending physician's identification number | The unique national identification number assigned to the clinician of record at discharge who is responsible for the discharge summary | Maintained in master physician data file; attending ID entered by patient registration or nursing and verified by HIM |
| Surgeon's identification number | The unique national identification number assigned to the clinician who performed the principal procedure | Maintained in master physician data file; surgeon attributed by HIM in abstract |
| Principal diagnosis | The condition established after study to be chiefly responsible for occasioning the admission of the patient to the hospital (ICD-10-CM code) | HIM |
| Other diagnoses | All conditions that coexist at the time of admission, or develop subsequently, that affect the treatment received, the length of stay, or both (also an ICD-10-CM code) | HIM |
| Qualifier for other diagnoses | For each other diagnosis, was the onset prior to admission? (yes or no) | HIM |
| External cause-of-injury code | The cause of an injury, poisoning, or adverse effect that has been recorded as the principal or other diagnosis (also an ICD-10-CM code) | HIM |
| Birth weight of neonate | If the patient is a newborn, the actual birth weight in grams is reported | Nursing in EHR; HIM abstracts if paper-based |
| Principal procedure and date of procedure | The procedure that was performed for definitive treatment, rather than one performed for diagnostic or exploratory purposes or was necessary to take care of a complication. If more than one procedure qualifies, the one most closely related to the principal diagnosis should be selected (ICD-10-PCS code) | HIM |
| Other procedure(s) and the date(s) of the procedure(s) | All other procedures that qualify | |

*(Continued)*

**TABLE 3.10**   **Uniform Hospital Discharge Data Set (UHDDS) Data Elements and their Sources—cont'd**

| UHDDS Element | Description | Typical Recorder/Source of Data |
|---|---|---|
| Discharge disposition | Disposition of the patient at discharge<br>• Discharged alive<br>• Discharged to home or self-care (routine discharge)<br>• Discharged/transferred to another short-term general hospital for inpatient care<br>• Discharged/transferred to skilled nursing facility (SNF)<br>• Discharged/transferred to an intermediate care facility (ICF)<br>• Discharged/transferred to another type of institution for inpatient care or referred for outpatient services to another institution<br>• Home under care of organized home health service organization<br>• Home under care of a home IV (home intravenous therapy) provider<br>• Left against medical advice or discontinued care<br>• Expired<br>• Status not stated | Nursing in EHR; HIM abstracts if paper-based |
| Expected source of payment | Primary and any secondary source(s) of payment. The primary source is expected to be responsible for the largest percentage of the patient's current bill<br>*Categories of source of payment:*<br>• Self-pay<br>• Workers' compensation<br>• Medicare<br>• Medicaid<br>• Maternal and child health<br>• Other government payments<br>• Blue Cross/Blue Shield<br>• Other health insurance companies<br>• No charge (free, charity, special research, or teaching)<br>• Other<br>• Unknown/not stated | Patient registration |
| Total charges | All charges for procedures and services rendered to the patient during a hospitalization or encounter | Recorded by patient service areas; total cumulated by system |

*EHR*, Electronic health record; *HIM*, health information management; *ID*, identification; *N/A*, not applicable.

## Documentation in Nonacute Care Providers

So far, this chapter has addressed what occurs in an acute care (short-stay) facility, including how data are collected and by whom. Now, let's look at other health care facilities—ambulatory care, LTC, behavioral health, rehabilitation, home health, and hospice in more detail. The most important thing to remember is that the skills and the knowledge presented thus far in this text apply to any health care delivery system. Demographic, financial, socioeconomic, and clinical data are collected in all settings. The volume and types of physician data, nursing data, and data from therapy, social services, and psychology vary significantly, depending on the diagnosis and the setting. In addition to discipline-specific data requirements, health care facilities must also comply with the licensure regulations of the state in which they operate. The regulations may include very specific documentation requirements based on the type of care provided. Further, all facilities seeking full Medicare reimbursement must comply with the Medicare Conditions of Participation (COP). The CMS website should be consulted for detailed information about those requirements. HIM professionals who are employed in special health care settings should become familiar with the unique data requirements of those settings. TJC offers accreditation to all providers discussed in this chapter, either independently or in conjunction with the host facility.

Ambulatory care, or outpatient care, is provided within a brief period, typically in 1 day or in less than 24 hours. This timing distinguishes it from inpatient care, in which the patient is admitted and is expected to stay overnight.

Ambulatory care services are the most frequently utilized patient care service in the health care industry. Changes in reimbursement methodologies and innovations in technology and medicine during the 1980s and 1990s can explain the shift from care provided in acute inpatient to ambulatory settings.

The term "ambulatory care" refers to a wide range of preventive and therapeutic services provided at a variety of facilities. Patients receive those services in a relatively short time. Facilities render services on the same day that the patient arrives for treatment or, in some cases, within 24 hours. So, while we could monitor the number of admissions, the number of discharges, or the number of patients in the bed to determine the volume of patients in an acute care facility, the terms *admission* and *discharge* have little or no relevance in ambulatory care. In the ambulatory care environment, the interaction between patient and provider is referred to as an **encounter** or a **visit**. Ambulatory services are always considered outpatient services for billing purposes.

Visits and encounters may be used synonymously but do not always mean the same thing for counting purposes. For example, think of a patient who goes to a physician's office to see the doctor and undergoes a chest radiograph at the same time in the same facility. The patient interacted with the facility in two ways: an examination by the doctor and a chest radiograph. Think of it another way: The patient *visited* the facility and *encountered* both the doctor and the radiology technician. Thus the visit represents the number of times that the patient interacted with the facility as a whole. The encounter can represent the number of different areas of the facility that were used or services provided. As the different ambulatory care settings are explored in this chapter, think about the ways to count the number of services rendered.

Beyond the time frame stated previously, the services rendered in ambulatory care facilities vary widely. Each type of facility has specific data collection, retention, and analysis needs. However, the general flows of patient care are similar. The patient initiates the interaction; gives demographic and financial data to the facility; meets with the provider, who documents the clinical care; and the patient then implements any follow-up instructions, such as diagnostic testing or a visit to a specialist. Table 3.11 contrasts care events in acute care and ambulatory care settings.

## Physicians' Offices

A **physician's office** is one type of ambulatory care facility. Some physicians do not see patients at all. For example, a pathologist examines tissue samples in a laboratory. Some radiologists examine only radiographs and other types of imaging results. In general, these physicians give the results of those examinations to another physician to discuss with the patient. For this section, only physicians who see patients in their offices are discussed.

### *Settings*

Some physicians have offices attached to their homes. Others have space in office buildings or in a medical mall (a building that contains only health care practitioners in a variety of specialties). Still others are associated with different types of facilities and, as employees, maintain offices in those facilities.

#### Group Practice

Sometimes physicians share office space and personnel with other physicians to reduce the cost of maintaining an office, to share financial risk, to increase flexible time, and to improve continuity of care. This type of physician's office is called a **group practice**. For example, several physicians working together may need only one receptionist. Sharing office space and personnel also provides increased opportunities for professional collaboration among physicians and can improve the continuity of care for the

| TABLE 3.11 | Contrast Between Key Ambulatory and Acute Care Events | |
|---|---|---|
| | **Ambulatory Care (Physician's Office)** | **Acute Care (Hospital)** |
| How to choose | Referral, advertisement, or investigation | Choices limited to facilities in which physician has privileges |
| | Choices sometimes limited by insurance plan | Choices sometimes limited by insurance plan |
| Initiate contact | Call for an appointment; walk-in, if permitted | Emergency department or attending physician orders admission |
| Collection of demographic and financial data | Receptionist, medical secretary | Patient registration, patient access, or admissions department personnel |
| Initial assessment | Vital signs and chief complaint recorded by physician, nurse, or medical assistant | Nursing assessment Physician responsible for history and physical examination |
| Plan of care | Prescriptions, instructions, diagnostic tests, and therapeutic procedures performed on an ambulatory basis | Medication administration, instructions, and diagnostic tests performed on an inpatient basis |

patients served by the practice. Administrative responsibilities of the practice may be shared by all physicians in the practice. Physicians in a group practice share the burden of being on call or available 24 hours a day and are afforded emergency, vacation, and holiday coverage by their colleagues. Physicians in a group practice can distribute the cost of capital investments, innovations, and technology across the practice and reduce the individual financial burdens. Physicians may share a physician's assistant or nurse practitioner. Staffing of this nature may be cost prohibitive in a solo practice.

Group practices may have only one type of physician, such as a group of family practitioners. Frequently, these physicians not only share office space and personnel but also see one another's patients. To help one another with their patient loads, the physicians must also collaborate in developing and maintaining relationships with insurance companies.

Another combination of physicians may consist of several different specialties; this arrangement is called a *multispecialty group*. A family practice physician may be in a group with a pediatrician and a gynecologist, for example. One of the advantages of a multispecialty group practice is the convenience of centralized care that it provides for the patient.

Another administrative advantage of a group practice is the ability to centralize record keeping. Whether the patient records are maintained in paper or electronic form, centralization offers substantial cost savings and efficiency.

Some physicians rely solely on appointments for scheduling office time. Other physicians employ open-access techniques. In open access, some appointments are made, but time is allowed for patients who call for a same-day appointment. Scheduling appointments requires knowledge of time budgeting, and implementation of open-access methods requires a firm understanding of the demand for time in relation to the number of patients per doctor.

### Clinic

A **clinic** is a facility-based ambulatory care service that provides general or specialized care such as those provided in a physician's office. Clinics may be funded or established by charitable organizations, the government, or different types of health care facilities. For example, a community health center is a type of clinic that provides primary or secondary care in a specific geographic area. Many of these centers are located in areas accessible to populations that have challenges with accessing health care. Many acute care facilities have developed clinics that resemble physicians' office services. A hospital may have primary care and specialty clinics that serve particular patient populations, such as an infectious disease clinic or an orthopedic clinic. Clinics may also closely resemble multispecialty group practices. Large teaching facilities may be affiliated with many clinics. The clinic may be part of the physicians' general practice, the physicians may be employees of the parent facility, or they may donate their time, often called *in-kind service*.

### Urgent Care Center

An **urgent care center** provides unscheduled care outside the ED on a walk-in basis. An urgent care center treats injuries and illnesses that need immediate attention but are not life threatening. Urgent care centers are usually standalone facilities equipped with on-site diagnostics and point-of-care medication dispensing. The use of urgent care centers is encouraged by payers and managed care organizations. The centers may be standalone or affiliated with a clinic, group practice, or hospital.

In 2009 the **Urgent Care Association (UCA)**, formally the Urgent Care Association of America, established criteria for urgent care centers. The American Medical Association grants the specialty in urgent care medicine to physicians who choose to specialize in the discipline. Practitioners are licensed in the state in which they operate. Urgent care accreditation is offered by TJC. The Comprehensive Accreditation Manual for Ambulatory Care and National Patient Safety Goals to Reduce Medical Errors guide the accreditation process.

### Services

The following sections describe a hypothetical visit to a physician's office to trace the clinical flow of a patient's data through the office and list the data that are collected. This visit is a general guide to the events that illustrate the flow of health information in the ambulatory care settings as previously mentioned. Fig. 3.15 shows the flow of activities in a typical physician's office.

A patient can usually choose the physician he or she will visit as long as the physician chosen is accepting new patients. The patient may ask friends and family members for recommendations. However, a patient who expects his or her insurance plan to pay all or part of the cost of the visit must take into consideration whether the physician is included in the insurance plan. Many insurers require patients to choose a **primary care provider (PCP)** who participates in the insurance plan. The PCP is a physician or other provider who has been designated by the insurer to deliver routine care to the insured and to evaluate the need for referral to a specialist, if applicable. If the patient needs to see a specialist, such as a cardiologist, some insurance plans require that the PCP refers the patient to a specific physician. Some specialists, such as thoracic surgeons, see only those patients who have been referred by other physicians. Thus the visit is initiated either by the patient or by referral and may be influenced by the patient's insurance plan. Some insurance plans allow patients to self-refer for certain services, such as obstetrics and gynecology.

### Care Providers

After choosing a physician, the patient calls the office for an appointment. Very likely, the patient will speak to someone who works with the physician. The individual who answers the telephone and handles the appointments may be any one of several different allied health professionals, such as a receptionist, a medical secretary, or a medical assistant.

**COMPETENCY CHECK-IN 3.3**

**Clinical Documentation**

**Competency Assessment**

1. Identify the data elements of an inpatient history and physical (H&P).
2. What is the time frame for documenting the following reports?
   a. H&P
   b. discharge summary
   c. operative report
   d. consultation
   e. autopsy report
3. What is The Joint Commission's requirement for the completion of an H&P?
4. What are the clinical components of a patient history report?
5. Why are the H&P data typically collected and reported in a single report?
6. At the end of a hospital stay, a(n) _____ is usually required to be completed as a dictated and transcribed report.
7. List and describe the data elements of the physician's order.
8. What are the components of a discharge summary?
9. In this chapter, we discuss some of the actual data-collection devices that are used in acute care. Table 3.6 lists the key items in a physician's order. List those items as fields and describe them in data dictionary format, as discussed in Chapter 2.
10. Routine documentation of the nurse's interaction with a patient is recorded in the _____.
11. What is a care plan?
12. Explain the difference between case management and utilization review.
13. Explain the difference between an admission denial and a continued stay denial.
14. Sometimes a physician needs to ask another physician for an opinion regarding the care of a patient. The physician asked is referred to as the _____.
15. Identify the appropriate source in the health record of the following data:
    a. patient's name and address
    b. patient's latest blood test results
    c. patient's ability to explain his or her condition
    d. patient/family education activities
    e. plan of treatment on a specific day
    f. whether the patient had a consultation during the inpatient stay

*Match the definition on the left with the vocabulary word(s) on the right.*

| | | |
|---|---|---|
| _____ 16. Acronym that describes the medical decision-making process; also refers to the way physicians organize their progress notes | A. Laboratory tests |
| _____ 17. Analysis of body fluids | B. Medication record |
| _____ 18. Examination of a patient using radiographs | C. Nursing assessment |
| _____ 19. One or more surgical procedures performed at the same time | D. Operation |
| _____ 20. Record of all drugs given to a patient during the hospitalization | E. Operative report |
| _____ 21. The diagnostic, therapeutic, or palliative measures that will be taken to investigate or treat the patient's condition or disease | F. Physical examination |
| _____ 22. The nurse's evaluation of the patient | G. Physician's orders |
| _____ 23. The physician's directions regarding the patient's care; also refers to the data-collection device on which these elements are captured | H. Plan of treatment |
| _____ 24. The physician's documentation of a surgical procedure, usually dictated and transcribed | I. Progress notes |
| _____ 25. The physician's documentation of the examination of the patient, particularly at the initial visit | J. Radiology examinations |
| _____ 26. The physician's record of each visit with the patient | K. Rule out |
| _____ 27. The predetermined, routine orders that have been designated to pertain to specific diagnoses or procedures. Must be ordered and authenticated by the appropriate physician | L. SOAP format |
| _____ 28. The process of systematically eliminating potential diagnoses; also refers to the list of potential diagnoses | M. Order set |

29. Describe the events that will occur when a patient is admitted to an acute care facility for an operation. What caregivers will be involved with the patient throughout this encounter?

## Case Study*
### DISCHARGE SUMMARY
**Eduardo Lopez**
**MRN 4567892**

This 82-year-old man presents in the ED with chills, fever, cough, and congestion and reports shortness of breath for 5 days. He complains that he cannot walk the length of her apartment without being so short of breath that he has to sit down to rest.

HISTORY OF PRESENT ILLNESS: Patient had been a one-pack-per-day smoker for 30 years. Recently, he was diagnosed with mild chronic obstructive pulmonary disease and uses an albuterol metered-dose inhaler for acute episodes; however, this has not been helping. His appetite has decreased, as eating and breathing has become more difficult.

DIAGNOSTICS: Peak flows: 125/175/150 with oxygen saturation of 85%; nebulizer treatment showed minimal improvement with both. Anteroposterior and lateral chest x-ray images show right lower lobe (RLL) infiltrate.

DIAGNOSIS: RLL pneumonia.

HOSPITAL COURSE: Mr. Lopez was hospitalized for 2 days for intravenous antibiotics; nebulizer treatments and supplemental oxygen @ 2 L per nasal cannula.

DISCHARGE INSTRUCTIONS: Discharged to home on amoxicillin for 10 days. Prednisone taper; daily nebulizer treatments and home oxygen therapy 1–2 L by nasal cannula.

Dictated: 04/10/2019

Transcribed: 04/10/2019 mrl

1. Is this a complete, timely, and accurate report? If not, what is missing?

## Case Study
### DISCHARGE SUMMARY
**Karen Carr**
**MRN 5987345**

CHIEF COMPLAINT: Patient is a 23-year-old woman referred to the dermatology outpatient clinic for lesions and neoplasms on her hip, cheek, and nose that have changed in size and shape in the past 6 months.

MEDICAL HISTORY: Patient has no significant history of skin disease except for childhood chickenpox, tinea, impetigo, and a significant history of repeated excessive sun exposure.

CURRENT MEDICATIONS: Medrol dose pack, 1% hydrocortisone cream, Atarax 25 mg tid.

DIAGNOSTIC PROCEDURES: Lesion bx; a combination of cryosurgical and Mohs surgery techniques used.

DIAGNOSIS/TREATMENT: Basal cell carcinoma, benign neoplasm, benign keratotic lesion.

FOLLOW-UP: Surgical incisions healed. Patient is advised to stop deliberate tanning, to use sunblock, and to check skin monthly for new or changed lesions.

1. The above excerpt from a patient's ambulatory surgery discharge summary has been forwarded to you for discussion with the physician. What question(s) do you have about this patient's care?

*Cases studies from Shiland, BJ: *Medical terminology online for mastering healthcare terminology*, 2019, ed 6, St. Louis, Elsevier.

A *receptionist* usually handles the telephones, does some filing, and schedules appointments. A *medical secretary* has a more detailed knowledge of office procedures, scheduling, filing, and billing. A *medical assistant* has all of that similar knowledge and some basic clinical knowledge, such as measuring and recording blood pressure and temperature, changing dressings, and assisting the physician in examining and treating the patient. Medical secretaries and medical assistants have received formal training, particularly if they are certified in their fields.

Other personnel who support the physician include physician's assistants, nurses, and advanced practice registered nurses. Box 3.4 lists some employees common in a physician's office.

### Data-Collection Issues

Suppose that a physician's office has several different staff members and employs a receptionist to handle telephone calls and appointments. When the patient calls for an appointment, the receptionist asks for the patient's name and telephone number and inquires whether he or she is a current patient. The patient's status will be verified, often while he or she is still on the phone. It is very important to know whether the patient is a current patient because a new patient requires more data collection, which takes more of the staff's time, and a longer appointment with the physician. Also, if the physician is not taking new patients, the patient must be directed to another physician. The receptionist also asks why the patient wants to see the physician, information that aids in scheduling. A regular patient coming in for a flu shot takes far less of the physician's time than does a new patient who complains of stomach pains.

Identification of a new versus an established patient is also important for billing physician services. The receptionist will ask the patient whether he or she is insured and who the payer is. If the physician does not accept the patient's insurance, it is preferred that the patient know this before the visit so that the method of payment can be determined or an alternate physician may be chosen. The office staff will verify the patient's insurance before the visit, protecting the patient from incurring unnecessary bills.

When the patient gets to the office, the receptionist asks the patient to fill out some forms. On these forms, the patient provides personal data: name and address, past

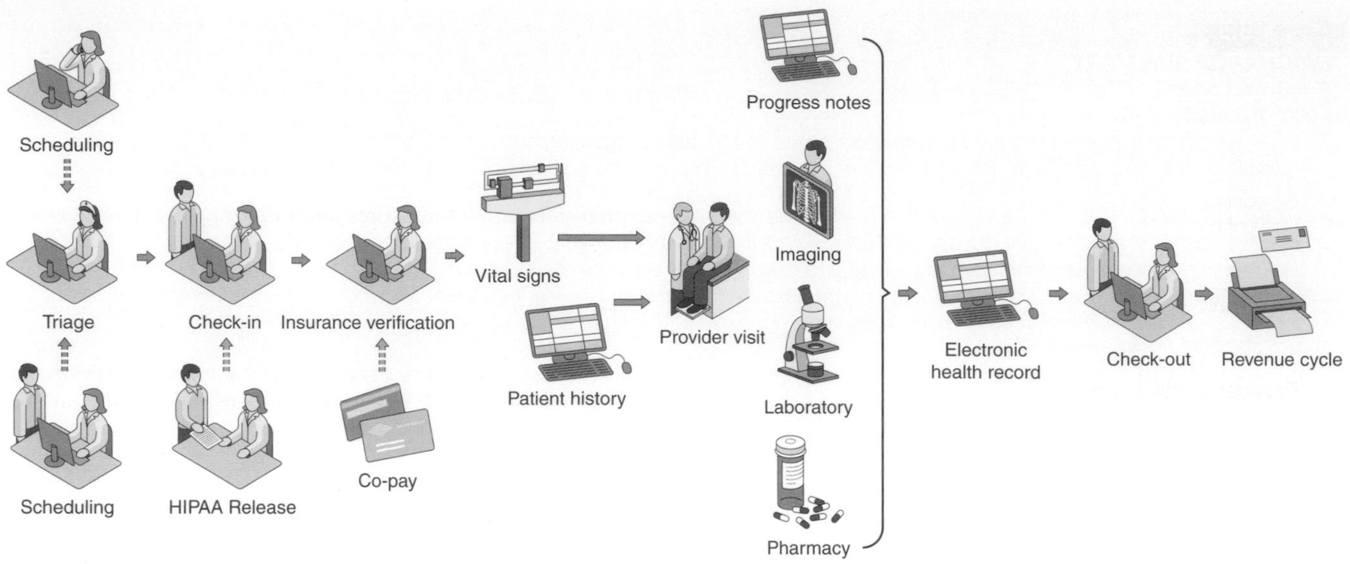

• **Fig. 3.15** Flow of activities in a physician's office. (From Elsevier: *Introduction to health services administration*, 2018, St. Louis, MO, Elsevier.)

---

• **BOX 3.4**　**Employees in a Physician's Office**

**Clinical Care Providers**

- Physician
  - Physician's Assistant (PA)
  - Advanced Practice Registered Nurse (APRN)
  - Registered Nurse (RN)
  - Licensed Practice Nurse (LPN)
  - Licensed Vocational Nurse (LVN)
  - Medical Assistant (MA)
  - Laboratory

**Office Management**

- Office Manager
  - Accountant or Fiscal Manager
  - Medical Secretary
  - Receptionist
  - Maintenance
  - Housekeeping

---

medical history, emergency contact, and how the patient intends to pay for the services. The receptionist or a medical secretary may then enter some or all of these data into the electronic registration system. Some electronic record systems allow the patient to complete the forms online, eliminating the paper and data entry step. Patients will sign forms that authorize the physician to treat them, to release information to their insurance companies, and to acknowledge their receipt of the physician's statement of privacy policies.

In a paper-based environment, a folder is created for each new patient, labeled by name and MRN, and used to hold the personal data form and any other documentation, such as a copy of the insurance card, the clinical notes, and copies of reports and test results. At each subsequent visit, the folder would be retrieved and visit data added. Historically, the folder has been the only record; however, capturing the administrative and clinical data in a point-of-care

information system instead of on paper is becoming increasingly common. Computerization offers options for alerts and reminders for patient health care maintenance and provides easy access for staff and clinicians for patient care and billing purposes.

Once the administrative record-keeping processes are completed, a medical assistant or nurse measures and records the patient's temperature, blood pressure, height, and weight—all data that develop a profile of information about the patient and the visit. If this is the patient's first visit, this profile is called the *baseline*. It is the information against which all future visits will be compared.

Eventually, the physician meets the patient and performs and documents the appropriate level of H&P. A new patient visit requires the provider to perform a more thorough and complex H&P, for which he or she bills at a higher amount. Perhaps the physician recommends tests to determine the extent of disease or to help determine the diagnosis. If the diagnosis is clear, the physician prescribes therapeutic treatment at this visit, which could be medications (prescription), therapy services, diagnostic procedures (radiology, laboratory), or referral to another physician. Before the patient leaves the physician's office, he or she typically remits any required payment for the visit.

### Data Sets

**Minimum data sets** (MDS) are the key data elements regarding the patient and the health care that he or she received. In ambulatory care, the MDS is called the **Uniform Ambulatory Care Data Set (UACDS)**. The UACDS was developed in 1989 by committees working under the auspices of the US DHHS. Reporting of these data is mandatory for facilities that accept Medicare and Medicaid payments. The data set was approved by the National Committee on Vital and Healthcare Statistics in 1989 and is utilized to improve data comparison of ambulatory and

**Section I: Patient Data Items**

1. Personal identification (including name and facility reference number)
2. Residence
3. Date of birth
4. Sex
5. Race and ethnicity
6. Living arrangements and marital status (optional)

**Section II: Provider Data Items**

7. Provider identification
8. Location or address
9. Profession

**Section III: Encounter Data Items**

10. Date, place or site, and address of encounter
11. Patient's reason for encounter (optional)
12. Problem, diagnosis, or assessment
13. Services
14. Disposition
15. Patient's expected source of payment
16. Total charges

outpatient facilities. The data set provides uniform definitions to aid in analyzing patterns of care. Box 3.5 lists the 16 elements of the UACDS; Fig. 3.16 shows the UACDS data elements on the CMS-1500, the standard claim form for physician services.

### Licensure and Accreditation

Practitioners are licensed in the state in which they operate. Ambulatory care accreditation is offered by TJC and the Accreditation Association for Ambulatory Health Care (AAAHC). The AAAHC accredits a variety of ambulatory care organizations, including ambulatory surgery centers (ASCs), community health centers, medical and dental group practices, medical home practices, and managed care organizations, as well as Indian and student health centers (Accreditation Association for Ambulatory Health Care, AAAHC, 2021).

## Emergency Department

### Settings

EDs are unique to hospitals, specifically acute care facilities. They are designed to handle patients in life-threatening situations or crises. Patients arriving in the ED are initially treated as ambulatory care patients because they are expected to be treated (without being admitted) and released. Sometimes, however, the condition of the patient warrants admission to the hospital or placement in observation. In this case, a member of the ED staff contacts the patient registration department to arrange for the change in status and for the patient to be transported from the ED

to a bed on a patient unit. The patient registration department changes the patient's status in the registration system, and an inpatient or observation stay is initiated. Clinical information accompanies the patient to the patient unit. Seriously ill patients may not be able to walk to the patient registration area or to provide required data. Therefore additional data collection often takes place at the patient's bedside or with the assistance of family members.

Although it is often the ED physician who identifies the need to observe or admit the patient, that physician generally does not write the order to do so. The ED physician typically contacts a staff physician, an on-call physician, or the patient's PCP to discuss the patient's condition and issue the order. Acutely ill patients who are admitted to the hospital from the ED will become inpatients.

The Emergency Medical Treatment and Active Labor Act (EMTALA) of 1986 was enacted in response to the practice of hospitals refusing to treat indigent patients and transferring such patients to charity care hospitals. EMTALA requires hospitals with EDs to conduct a medical screening examination on any individual who presents for such a purpose. The hospital is obligated by law to stabilize the patient, which may result in the treatment of the patient's condition. Because EMTALA prohibits the hospital from refusing to treat an emergency patient who cannot pay for the services provided, hospitals comply with EMTALA by deferring the request for insurance information until after the medical screening examination. It should be noted that EMTALA does not prohibit billing the patient after the visit.

### Services

ED services vary dramatically. Broken legs and heart attacks are typical cases. A *trauma patient* is defined as a patient with a serious illness who has a high risk of dying or suffering morbidity from multiple and severe injuries. Trauma patients often are treated first in the ED and are stabilized there before being admitted to the hospital as inpatients. Because the services vary so much, the facility must determine the order in which to treat the patients. The policy of "first come, first served" does not make much sense when the first patient has strained a ligament and the second patient is experiencing a myocardial infarction. Therefore patients are screened as part of the registration process to determine the priority with which they will be treated. This prioritization process is called **triage** and is generally performed by a registered or advanced practice nurse. In some EDs, a separate section of the department is set aside for noncritical services. Noncritical services in this scenario may include minor wound repair, for example.

### Care Providers

The ED is staffed with physicians, nurses, and medical secretaries/unit clerks. The physicians in this department are highly qualified to handle the various types of illnesses and injuries of the patients who seek treatment in the ED. In one room a physician may treat a child with a bead stuck in the ear and in the very next room may diagnose and treat a

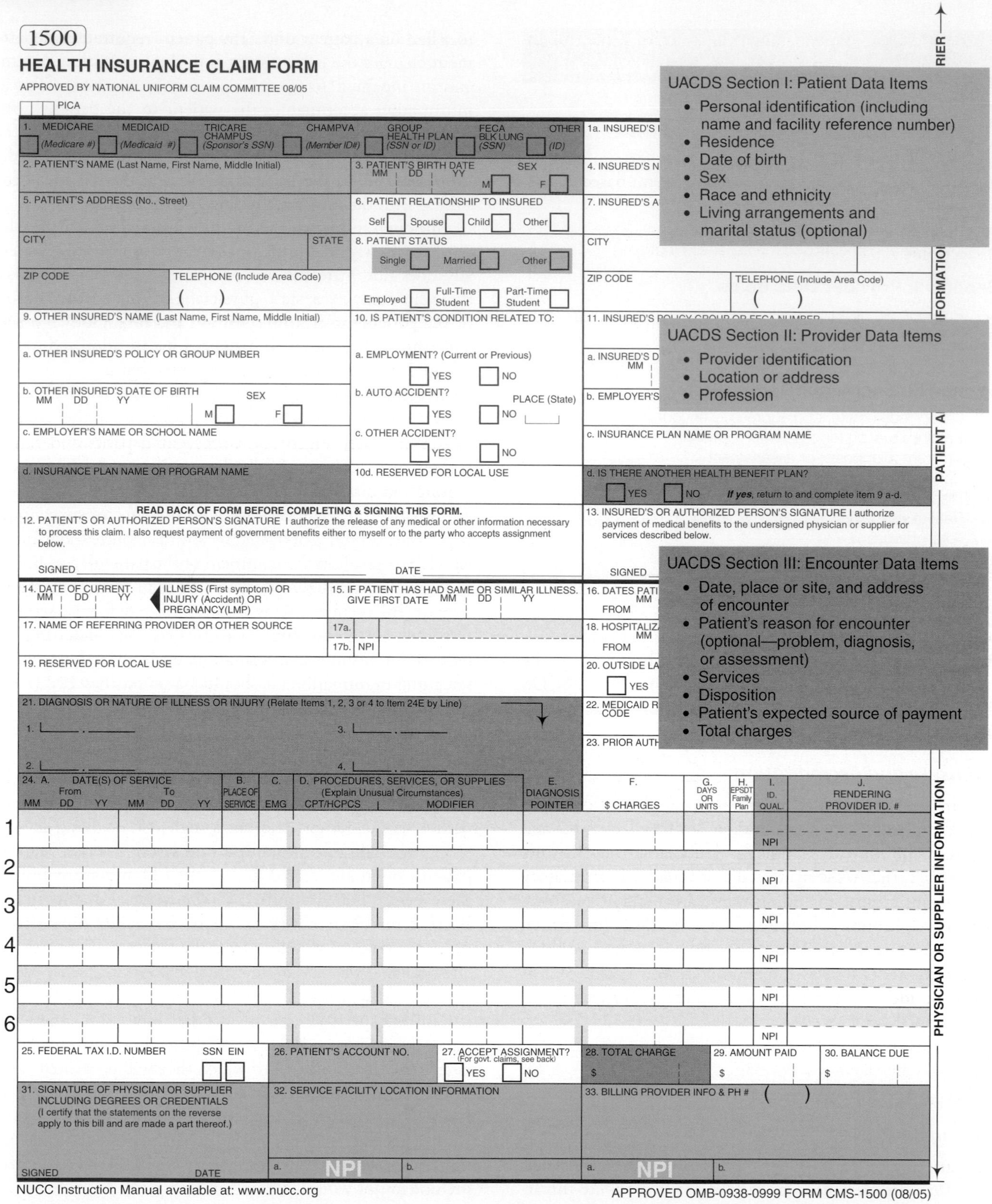

• **Fig. 3.16** UACDS data elements included in the form fields of the CMS-1500 claim form. *UACDS*, Uniform Ambulatory Care Data Set.

patient who was involved in a major traffic accident and is unconscious and bleeding internally. The nurses also have a high level of skills to provide nursing care for these patients. The unit secretary in this department is very helpful in facilitating the flow of patient care, making sure that the

physician's orders are followed in a timely fashion, requesting patient records from the HIM department, and following up with other departments for diagnostic tests that need to be performed or obtaining test results that are needed for diagnosis and subsequent treatment. Because the ED is located within a hospital, other allied health professionals are available for radiology, laboratory, respiratory, and other services required by the patients.

### Data-Collection Issues

Because the pace in the ED is fast, data collection must be fast. In a paper-based environment, menu-based forms have long been the standard for data collection. This menu-driven data collection has facilitated the implementation of electronic data collection in the ED environment. The patient record in the ED may be separate from the hospital system. Integration of the ED record with hospital systems allows orders to flow seamlessly from the ED to the target department and the results to flow back to the ED for easy review. Data collection unique to the ED includes the method and time of arrival.

### Data Sets

The Centers for Disease Control coordinated the development of a uniform data set for EDs. The **Data Elements for Emergency Department Systems (DEEDS)** is not a mandatory data set but rather a set of specifications for the terminology and activities that take place in an emergency setting. DEEDS supports the uniform collection of data in hospital-based EDs and other emergency settings to improve interoperability between ED systems. The Essential Medical Data Set complements DEEDS and provides medical history data on each patient to improve the overall effectiveness of care provided in the ED. In comparison with UACDS, the elements of DEEDS are more concise and specific to the services and treatment provided in the ED.

### Licensure and Accreditation

An ED accounts for most unscheduled admissions to the hospital. The ED is licensed and accredited under the umbrella of its host facility. An ED is licensed according to the types of services available and the capacity to provide trauma services, which is a special level of licensing. Some EDs are actual *trauma centers*, which are specially equipped to treat patients who have suffered traumatic injuries, such as a car accident or a violent assault. Designation of an ED as a trauma center is by state licensure. Additionally, the presence of specific trauma resources may be verified by the American College of Surgeons as either a level I, level II, or level III, with level I trauma centers providing the highest level of care.

## Radiology and Laboratory Services

Some facilities offer a broad range of evaluation services, such as radiology and laboratory services. The radiology department performs and reviews radiographs and other types of imaging, such as CT, MRI, positron emission tomography (PET) scans, and ultrasonography. The laboratory analyzes tissue and body fluids, such as blood. These evaluation services are called *ancillary*, or *adjunct*, services. Many of these services are offered in freestanding (not hospital-based)

facilities. Radiology and laboratory tests require a physician order and diagnosis to support the purpose of the test.

### Settings

Radiology and laboratory services are maintained in acute care and inpatient rehabilitation facilities. These services are often available to the general public and can be obtained through a physician's order. Some of these hospitals do not maintain the services by using their own employees but rather lease the space to organizations that agree to provide the services to the hospitals. Radiology and laboratory services may also be offered in freestanding facilities.

Mobile laboratories are common and began with mobile blood and plasma services. *Mobile diagnostic services* provide convenient access to patient testing and diagnostics, offering convenience and cost efficiency by eliminating unnecessary travel and stress for the patient. These services are widely utilized by older adults and homebound patients because of their convenience. Mobile diagnostics services can provide specialty tests that, due to facility requirements, cannot be performed within a hospital or clinic setting. They can provide radiography, EKG, mammography, ultrasound scanning, Holter heart monitoring, and bone density tests, and some units offer basic blood pressure and cholesterol screenings. Occupational health testing units offer flu shots and private drug screenings. These services are often located near clinics and nursing homes, in rural communities, in heavily populated areas, and near large businesses. Mobile eye and dental units are common in areas where access to care is limited and where demand for convenience is high. These services are covered by federal and private providers. TJC provides accreditation for mobile diagnostic services. Ambulance service is the most common type of mobile diagnostic service.

### Services

Diagnostic radiology services include radiography, CT, MRIs, and PET scanning. Three-dimensional ultrasound scans may be used to visualize a fetus in utero. Therapeutic radiology (also known as radiation therapy) is most closely associated with the treatment of certain types of cancers. Services are provided on the order of a physician.

Laboratory services include examinations of blood, urine, specimens, and other bodily secretions for the diagnosis, treatment, and prevention of disease. Hematology, serology, cytology, bacteriology, biochemistry, and blood and organ banking are functions of the clinical laboratory.

An interesting recent phenomenon, however, is the increased frequency in the marketing of radiology and laboratory services to the general public as a prophylactic diagnostic measure. For example, a PET scan may be advertised as providing the patient with peace of mind. Laboratory tests for vitamin D deficiency may be advocated as a general screening measure. Marketing of health care services of this nature encourages patients to advocate for their personal health and well-being; however, the physician is the arbiter of whether such tests are beneficial in each case, and payers do not necessarily cover such services in the absence of a specific diagnosis or suspected condition.

### Care Providers

Radiologic technologists or radiographers produce images of anatomic structures. Radiographers are typically trained in hospital-based training programs, community colleges, or 4-year baccalaureate degree programs. Their training is accomplished on state-of-the-art equipment that allows them to obtain clear and accurate images. Physicians who work in a radiology department are called *radiologists*. They interpret the images and dictate the reports associated with the interpretation. Front-end voice-recognition software is often used by radiology departments to communicate radiologic findings. The voice-recognition software allows radiologists to review radiology images and speak their findings into the software to create reports, eliminating the need for someone to transcribe the reports.

Laboratories are staffed with a variety of personnel, including pathologists, microbiologists, histotechnologists, cytotechnologists, medical laboratory technicians, and phlebotomists. These lab professionals work with microscopes, computers, and instruments to process body fluids, tissues, and cells that help physicians detect, diagnose, treat, and prevent disease. The phlebotomists draw blood using a procedure called *venipuncture*.

### Data-Collection Issues

Radiology and laboratory services generate various forms of documentation and reports. The original material (radiographic film, digital image, or fluid sample) is retained in the testing department or facility. The report of the analysis or interpretation of the material is maintained in the testing department. A copy of the report is sent to the requesting physician and to the facility that ordered the procedure. The report will become a part of the patient's health record in the facility that ordered the test.

Typically, radiologic images are captured in digital format. These digital images along with the interpretation of the image are captured and shared on the PACS. Images can be given to patients and their physicians on a computer disk along with the program to view the image, integrated into an EHR, or shared over a network. This arrangement facilitates communication with the physician and provides the patient with a valuable tool for developing and maintaining a personal health record, so the patient may retain a copy of the results for future health care encounters.

### Licensure and Accreditation

Facilities are licensed by the departments of health and human services of the states in which they operate and must adhere to the guidelines outlined in the COP. Accreditation is available for these facilities through TJC, AAAHC, and National Integrated Accreditation for Healthcare Organizations (NIAHO). Clinical laboratories are regulated by the CMS under the Clinical Laboratories Improvement

Amendments. For current information about this program, refer to the CMS website: https://www.cms.gov/regulations-and-guidance/legislation/clia.

## Ambulatory Surgery

As health care costs rise, providers are under increasing pressure to offer surgical services more efficiently. As improved surgical technology allows for quicker recovery time, more procedures can be performed on an outpatient basis. A patient can enter a facility, have surgery, and leave on the same day; this process is called **same-day surgery** or **ambulatory surgery**. Because of lower overhead costs, ASCs can perform surgical procedures at lower costs than hospitals.

The CMS maintains a list of surgical procedures that Medicare will reimburse only if they occur in an inpatient setting. All other procedures are designated as appropriate for ambulatory surgery. Although an ASC may operate as a functional unit of a facility, such as a hospital, it is considered a separate entity. The surgery center must maintain individual governance, professional supervision, administrative services, clinical functions, record keeping, and financial and accounting systems. The distinction between an *ASC* and an ambulatory surgery department of a hospital is important. ASCs are individually licensed and accredited.

### Length of Stay

Ambulatory surgery patients technically have a length of stay of 1 day; that is, they are treated and released on the same day. Patients who require additional care beyond the day of surgery may be held overnight under the same-day surgery status, transferred to observation status, or admitted to inpatient status. A hysterectomy, for example, is a common ambulatory surgery procedure; however, if the patient's vital signs are unstable for a significant amount of time post-surgery, the surgeon will write an order to hold the patient overnight for observation or to admit him or her for inpatient care. In a standalone ASC (see the following "Settings" section), the patient would be transferred to an acute care facility and then admitted as an inpatient.

### Settings

Ambulatory surgery may take place in an acute care facility or a freestanding ASC. Sometimes the ASC specializes in a specific type of surgery (e.g., eye operations, orthopedic surgery). Some large health care companies, such as Surgical Care Affiliates, own and operate hundreds of ASCs, both freestanding and located within hospitals. Alternatively, a group of surgeons may form a partnership with one another or may combine with a health care management services company to create an ASC. ASCs look to engage in contractual agreements with hospitals and health systems by providing nonemergency procedures. The ASC can offer the hospital-skilled physicians and state-of-the-art technology, allowing the hospital to stay competitive and to satisfy care requirements imposed by CMS and managed care organizations. In return, the ASC has the support of the hospital, which may include the use of its facilities, staff, and services, if an ASC patient requires admission.

### Services

ASCs provide surgical procedures that do not require inpatient hospitalization. Ambulatory surgery is just that: surgery. The types of procedures performed in this environment are limited only by the postsurgical care required. Cataract removal, colonoscopy, removal of skin lesions, cholecystectomy, appendectomy, and carpal tunnel release are examples of procedures that are typically performed on an ambulatory basis.

### Care Providers

Care providers in this setting are generally limited to:
- physicians
- nurses
- general medical office personnel
- surgical technicians
- anesthesiologists

### Data-Collection Issues

Because of the short recovery time, the volume of data collected for an ambulatory surgery case is relatively low compared with that for inpatient surgical procedures. Preadmission testing may include laboratory work and radiologic services, as well as an anesthesia consultation. The H&P must be completed, but it is shorter than the H&P for inpatient care. The surgical report may be brief and may contain substantial menu-based data. The data are always focused on the reason for the surgical encounter. Anesthesia would include preoperative, intraoperative, and postoperative evaluations and postanesthesia recovery.

For example, an otherwise healthy patient undergoing a screening colonoscopy might require only a brief H&P. The anesthesia and procedural notes might be uncomplicated and therefore quite brief compared with those for a more extensive procedure, such as a colon resection or a hip replacement. The patient recovery time after the colonoscopy might also be very short—perhaps less than an hour—so there is also less postprocedural nursing documentation. On the other hand, many complex surgical procedures, such as hysterectomy and medial meniscus repair, can be performed on an outpatient basis, particularly if they are performed with laparoscopy. These more complex procedures might require extensive documentation. In either event, the data collected and required documentation will be specified by the facility.

### Data Sets

In ambulatory surgery, the UACDS applies (see Box 3.5).

### Licensure and Accreditation

An ASC is considered a separate entity under Medicare and must maintain separate licensure and accreditation, even if it is acting as a functional unit within another facility,

such as a hospital. Outpatient surgical services provided by a hospital are different from an ASC. ASCs are licensed by the departments of health and human services of the states in which they operate. Accreditation is offered by TJC, the AAAHC, the Healthcare Facilities Accreditation Program (HFAP), and the NIAHO.

## Long-Term Care

In addition to length of stay, there are other fundamental differences between **long-term care (LTC)** facilities and acute care facilities. Although both care for inpatients, they differ significantly in focus and delivery of quality health care. Patients receiving LTC are considered residents of the facility; they are not only being treated there—they actually live there. Thus there is a greater emphasis on comfort, **activities of daily living (ADLs)**, and recreational activities, such as games and crafts. Group activities are common ways to facilitate residents' interaction and socialization.

### Length of Stay

Many state licensure documents define an LTC as one in which the average length of stay exceeds 30 days. In practice, the length of stay varies significantly depending on the needs of the patient. It is not unusual for patients to require LTC for months or years.

### Settings

A wide variety of facilities are considered LTC. Some of these facilities, such as assisted living facilities, are not as strictly regulated as others. Table 3.12 contains a brief description of LTC facilities.

These are general categories of care provided to help the reader understand the environment of LTC. Facility, licensure, and regional differences in terminology exist. Many facilities offer multiple levels of care and are not distinguishable as a specific type of facility. For example, some organizations offer lifetime care that transitions from independent to assisted to intermediate to skilled care as the patient's condition deteriorates.

### Services

LTC consists primarily of rehabilitative and supportive services and is typically characterized by the level of nursing care provided, as illustrated in Table 3.12. Nursing care varies from routine care of patients who are in beds to nursing on demand, such as in assisted living. Even within facilities, care varies according to the needs of the patient. In addition to nursing care, LTC facilities typically offer rehabilitation services, such as occupational therapy and physical therapy. While LTC is by definition a residential service, many LTC facilities offer day care or respite care for home-based persons.

### Care Providers

Patients entering an LTC facility are evaluated by a physician to ensure that the facility is appropriate for the patient's optimal care. The physician is responsible for ensuring that the patient meets the goals established by the patient's care plan. Once the patient is admitted, the physician plays a small role in the patient's daily life. Unless there is a change in the patient's medical condition or the patient's care plan, the physician routinely sees the patient only once every month.

The level of nursing care required by the patient is the key to determining what type of facility the patient needs. In an SNF, the patient typically needs 24-hour supervision with skilled nursing personnel at both the registered nurse and licensed vocational nurse (LVN) levels. In an assisted living facility, a resident may need only a nurse on call.

**TABLE 3.12    Examples of Long-Term Care Facilities**

| Facility | Type of Care |
|---|---|
| Independent living | Residents are housed in apartment settings. Health care is provided on site; however, residents are independent in their activities of daily living (ADLs) and do not require medical supervision on a 24-hour basis. Some meals may be provided in a cafeteria or restaurant atmosphere. |
| Assisted living | Assisted living is considered a group living arrangement. It offers help with ADLs and monitors the residents to ensure their health, safety, and well-being. Residents live in apartments that typically have limited kitchen facilities. There are community dining rooms, and residents generally have meal plan options. Most assisted living facilities have worship, entertainment, and personal care services available on site. |
| Subacute care | This is usually a transitional level of care between acute care and either home care or other long-term care (LTC). Subacute care may be offered in acute care facilities or in LTC facilities. Patients require substantial treatment but no longer need the 24-hour supervision of an acute care facility. |
| Transitional | Generally offered in an acute care facility, patients require up to 8 hours of nursing care per day. Average length of stay is within the acute care definition. |
| General | Patients require up to 5 hours of care per day and typically stay from 10 to 40 days in an LTC facility. |
| Chronic | Patients require up to 5 hours of care per day and typically stay from 60 to 90 days in an LTC facility. |
| Long-term transitional | Patients require up to 9 hours of care per day and typically stay more than 25 days in an acute care facility. |
| Intermediate care | Patients do not require 24-hour supervision. Cognitive or motor impairment contraindicates independent living. |
| Skilled nursing | Residents require substantial assistance with ADLs. Frequent therapies from a variety of professionals are needed to maintain status. Skilled nursing facilities (SNFs) are health care facilities that offer both short- and long-term care options for those with temporary or permanent health problems too complex or serious for home care or an assisted living setting. SNFs are designed for very sick patients. Services that an SNF offers may vary, but they normally provide the following: medical treatment prescribed by a doctor; physical therapy; speech therapy; occupational therapy; assistance with personal care activities such as eating, walking, bathing, and using the restroom; case management; and social services. |
| Long-term acute care | Patients require an acute level of care over an extended period. The average length of stay is more than 25 days. Services may be provided in an acute care, LTC, or rehabilitation hospital. Medicare considers this LTC. Long-term acute care (LTAC) facilities focus on treating patients who need special, intense care for a longer time than is customary in an acute care hospital; their stay is usually no less than 25 days. Patients in an LTAC facility could consist of older adults, patients from a nursing home, and those who have serious medical problems, such as patients who need long-term ventilator assistance. |
| Nursing Home | A nursing home is a facility for patients who need constant care and/or help with ADLs but at a lesser level of care than is provided at an SNF. Services are offered to older adults and to individuals who may have physical disabilities. Nursing homes may also offer rehabilitative services after an accident or illness, such as physical therapy and occupational therapy. |
| Board and Care Homes | Board and care homes are basically group living arrangements. The arrangements usually consist of four to six residents whose care is provided by live-in staff. The residents do not need nursing home care but need help with ADLs. Care rendered at many such facilities are custodial in nature as opposed to medical. |
| Continuing Care Retirement Communities | Continuing care retirement communities offer help with the process of aging in place. There are different levels of care, depending on the individual's needs. Considering one's health, residents may be able to live independently when they move in and have more assistance as they age. |

Similar to a rehabilitation facility, LTC facilities maintain physical therapy and occupational therapy professionals to assist residents with maintaining or improving their optimum level of independence in ADLs.

The LTC environment has been slow to transition to electronic records, although some improvement has been made in recent years. Despite this lag, the evidence exists that LTC would benefit from the implementation of EHRs (Kruse et al., 2015).

### Data Sets

LTC facilities seeking reimbursement from Medicare must complete the MDS for each of their patients, currently version 3.0. This lengthy data set is initiated on admission and contains detailed clinical data about the patient. It must be submitted to the facility's state repository within 14 days of admission, updated quarterly for specific sections, and resubmitted at least annually. The MDS is one component of a series of data collected when the health care professional assesses the type of care the patient will need in the LTC setting. Combined with the **Resident Assessment Instrument (RAI)**, the RAI-MDS is a comprehensive assessment that measures physical, psychological, and psychosocial functioning of the resident. Mandated by the Nursing Home Reform Act (1987), this data collection identifies "residents' strengths, weaknesses, preferences, and needs in key areas of functioning. It is designed to help nursing homes thoroughly evaluate residents and provides each resident with a standardized, comprehensive, and reproducible assessment" (U.S. Department of Health and Human Services, 2001). The goal of this volume of documentation is to ensure a high quality of care in LTC settings. Information gathered by this data set can trigger a more detailed assessment using **Resident Assessment Protocols (RAPs)**, which will help establish the patient's plan of care in the LTC setting continuingly, in which the patient's condition is regularly reevaluated. The RAI-MDS is of interest because it illustrates the volume and type of data that are collected in LTC, which is mirrored in other nonacute care settings as well.

### Licensure and Accreditation

LTC facilities are licensed in the states in which they operate. Each state has different licensure and accreditation laws for SNFs, LTACs, and nursing homes, depending on numerous factors. Licensing will define the types of LTC that can be provided, such as skilled, subacute, or rehabilitation services. Each of these specialties and LTC environments requires specially trained personnel and must adhere to specific guidelines. The **Commission on Accreditation of Rehabilitation Facilities (CARF)** accredits LTC facilities offering rehabilitation services; however, not all states require accreditation from that specific organization.

## Behavioral Health Facilities

**Behavioral health facilities** and behavioral health services housed in other types of facilities focus on the diagnosis and treatment of psychological and substance abuse disorders such as drug and alcohol addiction, eating disorders, schizophrenia, bipolar disorders, and chronic cognitive impairment. These services may be residential or nonresidential, ambulatory or inpatient.

### Length of Stay

The length of stay for behavioral health services offered on an inpatient basis depends on the diagnosis and the individual patient's response to the therapeutic plan. Behavioral health services are also offered on an outpatient basis in a day hospital or day treatment program.

### Settings

Behavioral health services are offered in all health care settings. In the acute care setting, services may be provided by consultation; there are also likely to be psychiatrists on staff. In the rehabilitation setting, behavioral health services are vital for cognitive remediation (discussed in more detail later in this chapter). Behavioral health services are also offered in psychiatric hospitals, freestanding outpatient clinics, and physician office settings.

### Behavioral Health Services

Behavioral health services address a wide range of psychological and behavioral disorders. Services include counseling, psychotherapy, occupational therapy, psychological testing, therapy, pharmaceutical interventions, and respite for children and adults.

#### Drug and Alcohol Rehabilitation

Although treatment is referred to as rehabilitation, drug and alcohol abuse or dependence is considered a psychological condition. There are two phases of treatment: detoxification and rehabilitation. *Detoxification* refers to the treatment of a patient who is going through withdrawal of substances from his or her body. This withdrawal may take 3 or 4 days. *Rehabilitation* is the treatment of the patient by psychiatrists, psychologists, drug and alcohol counselors, and social workers that teaches the patient ways to resist drugs and alcohol in the future. Although treatment varies, initial rehabilitation may take weeks or months, with continuing treatment throughout the patient's life. A drug and alcohol rehabilitation facility may be freestanding or connected with another facility, such as a psychiatric hospital or an acute care facility.

### Care Providers

Although some patients in behavioral health facilities may have additional medical conditions that require treatment, the primary thrust of care is delivered by psychiatrists (physicians), psychologists (nonphysician specialists), and social services personnel. Additionally, in an inpatient facility, there may also be a physician known as a *family care physician*, *primary care physician*, or *internist* who is responsible for treating any medical conditions that may occur during the patient's course of treatment.

## Social Workers

Social workers are among the behavioral health specialists who work with individuals with special needs. For example, a patient who leaves the hospital after surgery may need to rest. This is a problem if the patient lives alone and has no caregiver at home. A social worker helps the patient identify and obtain the needed assistance. Social workers also provide education and assistance to individuals with chronic illnesses, including human immunodeficiency virus, and substance abuse problems. The National Association of Social Workers promotes high professional standards and public awareness and administers the credentialing process (National Association of Social Workers, 2021). Some states offer licensure of trained social workers with master's degrees under a variety of different designations. The LMSW (Licensed Master Social Worker) and the LCSW (Licensed Clinical Social Worker), for example, are designations offered by the state of New York (New York State Education Department, 2021).

### Data-Collection Issues

Much of the data collection in behavioral health is free text. Psychology notes tend to be voluminous and detailed and do not lend themselves to menu-driven data collection. Of particular concern are psychology notes and documentation of restraints. Because of changing regulations and the process for billing services, many point-of-care systems are helping to define the content of a clinical note, enabling better management and production of data reports for patient populations.

Psychology notes may include results of testing instruments and extensive interview notes. Many of these notes are retained in the psychology department and do not become part of the patient's legal health record. Confidentiality must be maintained for psychological testing documents as required by the developer/publisher. A summary of the results may be retained in the record. Only specially trained psychology staff may access testing instruments and their scoring and interpretation guidelines. Standards for record retention are established for each state by its DHHS. Accreditation agencies also provide standards for record retention. The facility must have a policy specifically dealing with the storage of, retention of, and access to psychological records. The facility should adopt the standard that is the most stringent if following both state and accreditation guidelines. Separate guidelines may apply to testing instruments and patient records.

Unfortunately, at times, a client may require restraints because he or she would otherwise become harmful to themselves or others and cannot be controlled with less restrictive options. The use of restraints requires a physician's order. Restraints include not only physical restraints but also confinement in protective enclosures or chemical restraint through the administration of strong psychotropic drugs. When the provider orders restraints, documentation of the following is required:

- a complete assessment;
- less restrictive methods attempted;
- interventions attempted;
- consent from the patient for restraints;
- the restraint order specific for type of restraint (e.g., four-point, wrist, ankle, vest, seclusion, type of medication);
- the application of restraints;
- the monitoring of the restrained patient; and
- the timely release from restraints.

Guidelines vary from state to state on the use of restraints. Restraints may be applied for 12–24 hours. Strict guidelines on patient monitoring apply. Some facilities require that patients be checked every 5 minutes. Accreditation and licensure standards offer clear guidelines for the application, use, and monitoring of restraints.

### Data Sets

There is no specific data set unique to behavioral health, so the data collected reflect the setting in which the services are provided. The National Institute of Mental Health offers a limited data set for reporting and surveillance. The CMS inpatient psychiatric facility prospective payment system (IPF PPS) provides a Case Mix Assessment Tool (CMAT). The CMAT includes detailed information about the patient. In the absence of a data set, behavioral health utilizes the **Diagnostic and Statistical Manual of Mental Disorders, 5th edition (DSM-5)**.

The DSM-5 is published by the American Psychiatric Association and provides diagnostic criteria for psychiatric diagnosis to enhance clinical practice. DSM-5 diagnoses are coded using ICD-10-CM, serving as a common language for communicating with third parties such as governmental agencies and insurance companies.

### Licensure and Accreditation

Behavioral health facilities are licensed by the states in which they operate. In addition to TJC, accreditation is available from the CARF and the **National Committee for Quality Assurance (NCQA)**. The **Substance Abuse and Mental Health Services Administration (SAMHSA)** is a governmental agency that provides key resources on behavioral health issues.

An additional layer of regulation in behavioral health is the release of patient information. Release of information is strictly protected by law, over and above the rules that apply to protected health information in general, and release requires special authorization.

## Rehabilitation Facilities

Rehabilitation facilities offer care to patients who need specific therapies as a result of illness or injury. Patients recovering from respiratory failure, cerebrovascular accident, joint-replacement surgery, traumatic head injury, or spinal cord injury are examples of typical rehabilitation patients. Therapies include respiratory therapy, physical therapy, occupational therapy, speech therapy, and *cognitive remediation*. **Cognitive remediation** is used to improve memory, judgment, reasoning, or perception impairments that make it difficult for a person to achieve functional goals. Cognitive remediation includes practice and adaptive strategies to help patients improve memory, attention, and problem-solving skills.

### Length of Stay

The length of stay in a rehabilitation facility will be determined by the patient's diagnosis and care plan. For example, a patient who needs rehabilitation following a total hip replacement may stay only a few days to a week in the facility to improve mobility, function, and range of motion. However, a patient who survived a gunshot wound to the head may need extensive rehabilitation to relearn major motor function and life skills. Rehabilitation is offered on an inpatient or outpatient basis, depending on the needs of the patient. Rehabilitation services are offered in acute care facilities and LTC facilities.

### Settings

To qualify for reimbursement of costs at this level of service, patients must participate in a specific number of hours of therapy. For Medicare patients, 3 hours of therapy daily is required.

Outpatient services may be housed in an inpatient facility, a standalone outpatient facility, or a related facility. For example, a growing number of outpatient rehabilitation services are associated with exercise facilities.

### Services

Respiratory care, occupational therapy, physical therapy, speech therapy, and cognitive remediation are common services utilized by rehabilitation patients. Ventilation and dialysis services are provided at some facilities. Social services are an additional service offered to such patients. They play an important role in helping patients find the additional services that they may need, that is, durable medical equipment (DME) following discharge to the home, home health visits, and assistance with meals. In inpatient facilities, recreation therapy may play a role in helping patients increase their ability to accomplish their ADLs. Social interaction and physical exercise are important aspects of recreational therapy for patient independence and restoration.

A unique aspect of rehabilitation, in comparison to acute care, is the ability of the care providers to focus on preparing the patient to return to the workplace. Industrial rehabilitation, a holistic program of multiple therapies and evaluation techniques, plays an important role in this process. Furthermore, the patient may need to be redirected in his or her employment goals as a result of the sequelae of the illness or injury.

### Care Providers

As with patients receiving behavioral health services, rehabilitation patients may have medical conditions that require treatment while they are in therapy. There is an internist on staff at inpatient facilities to treat these conditions. However, the thrust of treatment is the therapy.

Rehabilitation physical therapy occurs under the direction of a **physiatrist**, a physician who specializes in physical medicine and rehabilitation. RTs, PTs, OTs, speech/language pathologists, social workers, and psychologists participate to varying degrees in the rehabilitation of individual patients.

### Occupational Therapist

OTs are clinical professionals who focus on returning the patient to his or her maximal functions in ADLs. The American Occupational Therapy Association (2021) refers to ADLs as "skills for the job of living," which include but are not limited to self-care, driving, and shopping. OTs are primarily employed in rehabilitation facilities but may work in virtually any health care environment. They serve a wide variety of clients, including those suffering from traumatic injuries, the aftereffects of stroke, and the loss of limbs. OTs may specialize in the treatment of specific conditions or specific age groups. The increasing life span and greater activity of today's older adults are important factors in the demand for OTs.

OTs are required to hold a master's degree in occupational therapy. Certification (registration) can be obtained from the American Occupational Therapy Association. The association defines professional practice domains for education, practice, and licensure. Licensure is required in most states as a prerequisite for practicing occupational therapy.

Occupational therapy professionals also include occupational therapy assistants (OTAs) and aides. OTAs have completed training in accredited programs and have passed a national certification examination. Occupational therapy aides receive on-the-job training and are not eligible for certification or licensing (American Occupational Therapy Association, 2021).

### Physical Therapist

PTs focus on strength, gait, and range-of-motion training to return patients to maximum functioning, reduce pain, and manage illness. They are employed primarily in rehabilitation facilities but may work in virtually any health care environment. A master's or doctoral degree from an accredited program is required to become a PT. To practice, PTs must take a national licensing examination. Practice requirements vary from state to state (American Physical Therapy Association, 2020).

The practices of occupational therapy and physical therapy overlap somewhat, and patients may receive treatment from both in the same period. For example, a patient who has had a hip replacement may undergo physical therapy to learn to walk with the new joint, increase range of motion, and maintain stability. At the same time, the patient might receive occupational therapy to practice getting in and out of a car, making a bed, or bending and stretching to clean house or cook.

### Data-Collection Issues

In a paper-based inpatient environment, the patient's record may travel with the patient from one therapy to the next;

equipment such as walkers, wheelchairs, oxygen, hospital beds, and other supplies.

### Services

Most services available on an outpatient/ambulatory care basis can be provided in the home, including multiple rehabilitation modalities, skilled nursing, and physician care. Table 3.13 lists health care professionals and other caregivers in the home health care setting.

### Care Providers

In addition to nursing and therapies, some home health care providers can also provide para-professional assistance such as companions and housekeepers. In almost all cases, these services are not reimbursed by insurance but are provided on a private pay basis.

### Data-Collection Issues

Before the development of electronic medical records, the accurate collection of data for home health care patients could be challenging. The patient's medical record would be in paper chart form at the Home Health Care Agency office, while representatives of multiple disciplines would visit the patient in his or her home, provide care, and then return to the office to document that care. There was no effective way for one discipline to review the data collected by another without reviewing the in-office chart.

The move to electronic documentation in home health care enables effective data collection and documentation at the time and point of service, which facilitates communication and coordination of services among care providers. It also allows for more effective and timely payment for services rendered.

All orders for home health care must be given by a physician. The physician must review the plan of care every 62 days, or whenever there is a significant change in patient status.

### Data Sets

The **Outcome and Assessment Information Set (OASIS)** applies in home health care. A copy of this data set can be obtained from the Center for Health Services Research, in Denver, Colorado.

### Licensure and Accreditation

Home health care agencies must be licensed in the state in which they operate. The **Community Health Accreditation Program (CHAP)** and TJC both offer accreditation opportunities for home health agencies.

## Telehealth

In some cases, the physician is not present with the patient at all, and care is directed long-distance. **Telemedicine** is the delivery of health care to individuals who are physically remote from the provider through various technologies. The provider may be communicating in real time with the patient via web conferencing or other electronic means. The provider may also be receiving updates on the patient's condition electronically. Telemedicine arose from the need for patients in remote areas to communicate directly with physicians and other clinical personnel. Today, it is available in many settings and for many reasons. For example, an otherwise well-served geographic area may have a sparsity of certain specialists. A patient working with a specialist in another city or state without traveling to that location has become increasingly common.

Telehealth is a broader concept than telemedicine. According to the Health Resources and Services Administration of the US DHHS, telehealth is the "use of electronic information and telecommunications technologies to support and promote long-distance clinical health care, patient and professional health-related education, public health and health administration" (Office of the National Coordinator for Health Information Technology [ONC], 2021). So, beyond the one-on-one patient care are a range of services that are accessible to patients and providers, such as education, online discussion, and public health resources. A useful and interesting source of additional information about telehealth is the Telehealth Start-up and Resource Guide available on the HealthIT.gov website: https://www.healthit.gov/sites/default/files/telehealthguide_final_0.pdf.

### Settings and Services

Telemedicine and telehealth reflect a broad range of services and settings. Telemedicine is not a specific specialty but rather a means of interacting with a patient without physical proximity. A radiologist in Australia may be reading and interpreting radiographs imaged in the United States. A cardiologist in Chicago may be reading EKG output from a patient in a clinic in Alaska. A disaster management group in Louisiana may be consulting remotely with a hospital in Hawaii. Thus telemedicine and telehealth have no specific limitations in terms of setting or type of service. Types of telehealth are listed in Box 3.6.

One type of telehealth is live video, which connects providers and patients through a real-time audiovisual link. Not only is live video quick and cheap, but the geographic distance between a patient and a doctor also does not hinder access to quality care, and it eliminates the time it takes for the patient to travel to the provider, or vice versa (Fig. 3.17). Live video is especially important in cases when time is of the essence or where travel is unrealistic or even impossible. For example, an obstetrician can use videoconferencing to provide prenatal care and counseling to women in rural areas where obstetrical resources are unavailable. Physicians at regional hospitals can use live video to consult with remote neurologists to treat stroke patients in the crucial hours after a stroke.

The use of live video is not limited to matters of life and death, of course. Today, nearly every smartphone, laptop, and tablet sold are equipped with a video camera and a microphone capable of connecting a patient to a health care provider. This makes it possible for providers in primary and

| TABLE 3.13 | Home Health Care Caregivers and Roles |
|---|---|

| Caregiver | Role in Home Health |
|---|---|
| Home care providers | These caregivers deliver a wide variety of health care and supportive services, ranging from professional nursing and home care aide (HCA) care, to physical, occupational, respiratory, and speech therapies. They also may provide social work and nutritional care, as well as laboratory, dental, optical, pharmacy, podiatry, radiograph, and medical equipment and supply services. Services for the treatment of medical conditions are usually prescribed by an individual's physician. Supportive services, however, do not require a physician's orders. An individual may receive a single type of care or a combination of services, depending on the complexity of his or her needs. |
| Physician | Physicians visit patients in their homes to diagnose and treat illnesses just as they do in hospitals and private offices. They also work with home care providers to determine which services are needed by patients, which specialists are most suitable to render these services, and how often these services must be provided. With this information, physicians prescribe and oversee patient plans of care. Under Medicare, physicians and home health agency personnel review these plans of care as often as required by the severity of patient medical conditions or at least once every 62 days. |
| Interdisciplinary teams | Interdisciplinary teams review the care plans for hospice patients and their families at least once a month or as frequently as patient conditions or family circumstances require. |
| Nurses | Registered nurses (RNs) and licensed practical nurses (LPNs) provide skilled services that cannot be performed safely and effectively by nonprofessional personnel. Some of these services include injections and intravenous therapy, wound care, education on disease treatment and prevention, and patient assessments. RNs may also provide case management services. RNs have received 2 or more years of specialized education and are licensed to practice by the state. LPNs have 1 year of specialized training and are licensed to work under the supervision of RNs. The intricacy of a patient's medical condition and required course of treatment determine whether care should be provided by an RN or can be provided by an LPN. |
| Physical therapists (PTs) | PTs work to restore the mobility and strength of patients who are limited or disabled by physical injuries through the use of exercise, massage, and other methods. PTs often alleviate pain and restore injured muscles with specialized equipment. They also teach patients and caregivers special techniques for walking and transfer. |
| Social workers | Social workers evaluate the social and emotional factors affecting individuals with illnesses or disabilities and provide counseling. They also help patients and their family members identify available community resources. Social workers often serve as case managers when patients' conditions are so complex that professionals are needed to assess medical and supportive needs and coordinate a variety of services. |
| Speech/language pathologists (SLPs) | SLPs work to develop and restore the speech of individuals with communication disorders; usually these disorders are the result of traumas such as surgery or stroke. Speech therapists also help retrain patients in breathing, swallowing, and muscle control. |
| Occupational therapists (OTs) | OTs help individuals who have physical, developmental, social, or emotional problems that prevent them from performing the general activities of daily living (ADLs). OTs instruct patients on using specialized rehabilitation techniques and equipment to improve their function in tasks such as eating, bathing, dressing, and basic household routines. |
| Dietitians | Dietitians provide counseling services to individuals who need professional dietary assessment and guidance to properly manage an illness or disability. |
| HCAs/home health aides | These caregivers assist patients with ADLs such as getting in and out of bed, walking, bathing, toileting, and dressing. Some aides have received special training and are qualified to provide more complex services under the supervision of a nursing professional. |
| Homemakers and chore workers | These caregivers perform light household duties, such as laundry, meal preparation, general housekeeping, and shopping. Their services are directed at maintaining patient households rather than providing hands-on assistance with personal care. |
| Companions | These caregivers provide companionship and comfort to individuals who, for medical and/or safety reasons, cannot be left at home alone. Some companions may help clients with household tasks, but most are limited to providing "sitter" services. |
| Volunteers | Volunteers meet a variety of patient needs. The scope of a volunteer's services depends on his or her level of training and experience. Volunteer activities include, but are not limited to, providing companionship, emotional support, and counseling, and helping with personal care, paperwork, and transportation. |

From the National Association for Home and Hospice Care, 2012.

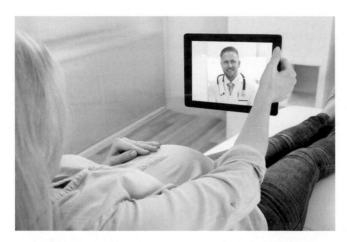

• **Fig. 3.17** A patient communicates with a provider via live video. (Copyright AndreyPopov/iStockphoto.com.)

urgent care to offer *e-visits* for acute, nonemergency situations. Providers can use e-visits to diagnose the most common ailments seen in medical offices, such as conjunctivitis (pinkeye), sinusitis, upper respiratory infections, and UTIs. This functionality makes the delivery of health care available night and day, on weekends, and on holidays.

Other types of services may utilize **store-and-forward** technology, where images or video of a patient is recorded to be viewed by a specialist later. This type of technology is useful in less time-sensitive instances and when the physician does not necessarily need to communicate with the patient. For example, a PCP can take a photograph of a rash or other skin condition and send it to a dermatologist via telehealth technology, who can then diagnose the condition remotely.

**Remote patient monitoring (RPM)** is an increasingly important facet of telemedicine. A patient with congestive heart failure, for example, may need daily monitoring of blood pressure. With a device in the home, the patient can take their blood pressure, press a button, and transmit the results to the physician. It is not a far leap to imagine patients sharing their exercise monitoring device readings to monitor progress. Some systems even run the data through a Clinical Decision Support (CDS) algorithm to alert health care professionals of a change in status or standard of care. RPM technology lowers costs and increases quality by keeping patients out of the hospital, reducing readmission rates, and requiring fewer office visits.

### Care Providers

The purpose of telemedicine is to provide access to physicians and other clinicians that would otherwise be impossible, unrealistic, or excessively burdensome. In general, the care provider is a physician, but it could also be a nurse, physician assistant, or therapist.

### Data-Collection Issues

Several unique issues arise concerning data collection. With home health care, we saw that the provider was with the patient but not where the documentation needed to be filed. With telemedicine, the provider is not with the patient *and* may not be where the documentation needs to be filed. So, the first question has to do with how and where the interaction between the physician and patient will be captured. The answer will vary, depending on the administrative relationships that exist. For a remote patient of a PCP, the PCP would document in the usual way in the PCP's normal record keeping, citing the means of communication. However, if a hospital in Delaware wants to facilitate a relationship between a current patient and a cancer specialist in another state, issues of privileges, licensure, and credentialing may arise. There needs to be a clear understanding of the administrative issues and how they will be solved. How these issues are resolved varies from state to state and facility to facility.

### Data Sets, Licensure, and Accreditation

At the time of this writing, there are no data sets or accreditation issues specific to telemedicine. There may be differences between the states in licensing requirements for telemedicine. Some states require licensure only in the state where the physician practices, while some also require licensure in the state where their patient resides. As of July 1, 2021, 33 states, DC, and Guam participate in the Interstate Medical Licensure Compact that helps qualified physicians become licensed to practice medicine, including telemedicine, in multiple states (Interstate Medical Licensure Compact, 2020).

During the COVID-19 Public Health Emergency, which began in 2020, many states relaxed licensure restrictions to allow interstate telemedicine encounters. Effective from March 6, 2020, the 1135 Waiver and the Telehealth Services During Certain Emergency Periods Act of 2020 temporarily expanded the types of telemedicine encounters for which Medicare paid. Telemedicine could be billed for various services by a variety of providers across the country (CMS, 2020).

## COMPETENCY CHECK-IN 3.4

### Documentation in Nonacute Care Providers

**Competency Assessment**

1. List four different types of ambulatory care.
2. Identify and describe five allied health professions and their principal occupational settings.
3. Describe the difference between the behavioral health care setting and the rehabilitation health care setting, including the type of care provided.
4. What is the difference between occupational therapy and physical therapy? If you have trouble explaining the difference, try finding websites for their national professional associations. What do those sites have to offer the public in terms of information about the profession?
5. Describe home health care and hospice care, including the differences in the type of care provided by each.
6. What services are available on a home health basis?
7. What professionals is the patient likely to encounter in a physician's office? What role do those professionals play in caring for the patient?
8. What role does urgent care play in health care delivery?
9. What services are provided by radiology and laboratory facilities?
10. What services are provided by mobile diagnostics?
11. Define and give examples of ambulatory surgery.
12. What happens in the ambulatory surgery setting when the patient requires "emergency" acute care services?
13. When does a patient require LTC?
14. What services are provided by LTC workers?
15. List three types of LTC.
16. Describe conditions that would require behavioral health treatment.
17. What services are provided by behavioral health workers?
18. When is a patient eligible for rehabilitation?
19. What services are provided by rehabilitation workers?
20. Who receives hospice care?
21. Describe palliative care.
22. When is a patient eligible for hospice care?
23. What role do volunteers play in hospice care?
24. Explain respite care.
25. Describe retail care and medical malls.
26. Explain the care provided by a pain management center and a cancer treatment center.
27. What services are provided by home health care workers?
28. List and describe the data sets unique to nonacute care facilities.
29. List and explain the elements of an admission record.
30. List and describe the elements of the UHDDS and the source of the data elements.
31. List and describe the elements of the UACDS.
32. What is the data set that applies to emergency departments?
33. Describe the unique data-collection issues in radiology and laboratory facilities.
34. Describe the unique data-collection issues in ambulatory surgery.
35. Who accredits ambulatory surgery facilities?
36. Describe the unique data-collection issues in an LTC environment.
37. What minimum data set is associated with LTC?
38. Who accredits LTC facilities?
39. Describe the unique data-collection issues in a behavioral health environment.
40. What minimum data set is associated with behavioral health?
41. Who accredits behavioral health facilities?
42. Describe the unique data-collection issues in a rehabilitation environment.
43. What minimum data set is associated with home health care?
44. Who accredits rehabilitation facilities?
45. Who accredits hospice organizations?
46. Describe the unique data-collection issues in a home health care environment.
47. What minimum data set is associated with home health care?
48. Who accredits home health care agencies?
49. What might be some legitimate reasons to print out an electronically stored report?
50. What health information department policy would support the timely submission of UHDDS data?
51. A physician on staff at the hospital has a habit of printing a patient's lab reports and writing notes on them that are not included in her progress notes. What policy would support the physician continuing this practice?

## Chapter Summary

Health care is delivered in a multitude of inpatient and outpatient settings. Ambulatory care is rendered in physicians' offices, EDs, surgery centers, urgent care centers, radiology and laboratory facilities, rehabilitation facilities, and home care facilities. Specialty therapeutic services are offered both in hospitals and on an outpatient basis, including physical, occupational, and psychological therapies. Health care professionals in every setting contribute to the health record, where data about patient care is collected. From the record, facilities report one of various data sets. Important data sets include UHDDS, UACDS, DEEDS, OASIS, and MDS. In general, health care facilities are licensed in the states in which they operate. Accreditation is offered by TJC, HFAP, ACS, AAAHC, CHAP, and CARF.

All facilities seeking Medicare reimbursement are regulated by the CMS. The CMS website should be consulted for detailed information on those regulations. HIM professionals who are employed in special health care settings must become familiar with the unique data requirements of those settings.

This chapter followed the clinical flow of data through an acute care visit. The clinical flow of a patient's data in an acute care facility starts with the initial assessments: history, physical, and nursing assessment. Various types of clinical data are collected from physicians, nurses, and laboratory and radiology personnel. Most inpatient records contain the assessments, as well as physician's orders, progress notes, and consultations. Nursing progress notes, medication administration, and vital signs are also universal. Some records contain additional information or the same data differently formatted. These records include surgical, obstetric, neonatal, and medical intensive care cases. If the patient expires, an autopsy may be performed, which becomes a part of the patient's health record. Understanding the optimal point of data collection and the most appropriate source of needed data is important. Acute care facilities report the UHDDS, containing key data elements of the inpatient stay.

## Competency Milestone

### CAHIIM Competency

*I.1. Describe health care organizations from the perspective of key stakeholders. (2)*

### Rationale

HIM professionals work in virtually every health care setting. As care is coordinated among settings, it is important that HIM professionals understand not only their own setting but also understand the documentation and data requirements in other settings with which they need to communicate.

### Competency Assessment

1. Compare and contrast the data collected in acute care facilities with data collected in nonacute care facilities.
2. Compare rehabilitation facilities with the various types of LTC facilities, including the specific data-collection issues.
3. What role does patient registration play in ensuring that a facility or other provider is paid for its services?
4. Describe the experiences of a patient in a physician's office. What is the flow of the process of treating patients, and what data are collected at what points in the visit?
5. What role do case management and utilization review play in patient care?

## Ethics Challenge

*VI.7. Comply with ethical standards of practice. (5)*

1. You are a transcriptionist working for a large group of surgeons. Dr. Knowles has limited office hours and spends much of his time at the two hospitals in which he has surgical privileges. He frequently complains that his billing is delayed because his dictations require correction and there is often a lag of 2 weeks between dictation and authentication of the final report. Dr. Knowles has asked you to sign his dictated reports for him after he makes the corrections. He says that since he has already read and approved the final report, this is OK. Is this ethical or not?

## Critical Thinking Questions

1. Fred has been working in acute care facilities for the past 5 years in progressively responsible positions. After he graduated from his associate degree HIM program and passed the Registered Health Information Technician exam, he was offered a position as the HIM manager in his organization's new LTC center, which was recently purchased and is slated to purchase and implement an LTC-oriented EHR within the next 2 years. Fred has heard through the grapevine that the center's records have not been strictly maintained and that the new manager will be expected to organize the records and ensure that the facility's documentation policies are in compliance with all regulatory and accrediting bodies. If Fred decides to accept this position, what can he do to ensure that he is prepared for the challenges of his new position?

2. With increasing electronic health care documentation, *paperless environment* is commonly heard. The term is interesting and potentially misleading. Paperless implies that no paper is used at all. However, consider what happens when a patient's record transitions into the EHR. If admissions data are captured with a computer interface and all forms are generated from the computer, how does the patient sign the admission consent? If your answer included printing the form, how does the form get back into the computer for storage?

3. The physician's H&P report is typically dictated into a software application; the transcriptionist listens to the dictation and transcribes it into the computer using a word-processing program. The physician has to review, correct, and authenticate the report—then it has to be stored electronically in the EHR. What is the most efficient way to facilitate these activities?

4. Think about the order entry system. The CPOE facilitates the entry of the order by the physician. However, when it is received in the pharmacy, the order is often printed out by the pharmacist while he or she is filling it. More paper may be generated when a prescription is transferred to the nursing station for the patient. Still more paper is generated if the order is printed so that it can be filed in the health record. This excessive generation of paper often occurs when a facility is in transition from a paper-based record system to a computer-based system. How can an HIM department manager stop the excessive printing of data that can be viewed on the computer?

5. We focus primarily on regulations and standards that apply throughout the United States. However, it is important to know the state and local standards, if any, that apply where you work. For each of the nonacute care settings discussed in this chapter, locate the licensure standards. What accreditations, if any, are available or required?

## The Role of Health Information Management Professionals in the Workplace

### Professional Profile—Records Manager

#### Medical Records Manager

My name is Francis, and I work in a 120-bed subacute/LTC center. Subacute care centers are rehab and nursing inpatient care facilities that treat patients who no longer need or qualify for acute care but who still are unable to return to their homes or previous care settings because of the severity of their illness or injury. We also accept LTC patients who are on ventilators permanently, as well as those who are considered weanable from ventilators.

My job duties include, but are not limited to, discharge processing, correspondence, utilization review, auditing and thinning of medical records, and general management of the medical records department.

The major differences between working in a subacute care center and working in an acute care center include the absence of large volumes of coding and transcription. We use the MDS for billing purposes. Generally speaking, there is an interdisciplinary team that meets once a week to assess the patient and complete an MDS on the basis of that assessment, which is then electronically submitted to Medicare, Medicaid, or other third-party payers. Also, although our turnover rate is one to two charts per day, our charts are significantly larger than those in a typical acute care hospital. I also have to manage a whole file area for thinned records only (mainly for our LTC patients). We start removing pages from the paper record when the patient has been with us for 3 months. Our rule is to remove nursing documentation that is more than two months old, always leaving the period assessments in place for comparison. Just in case they older pages are needed, we file them by MRN and date.

I enjoy my position because I really feel that I am a part of the team here and I am helping the patients as well as the staff.

#### Career Tip

LTC facilities tend not to be as far along in implementation of the EHR as acute care hospitals. Therefore knowledge of paper-based processing is essential for an HIM professional working in an LTC setting. An associate's degree in HIM is excellent training for this position, although some areas may require a bachelor's degree. Candidates should expect to be working managers and to "do it all."

### Professional Profile—Patient Registration Specialist

My name is Michael, and I am a patient registration specialist at a large medical group practice. My primary responsibility is to register patients when they come into the facility to see a physician or a nurse practitioner. Because we keep all our patient registration information in the computer, I do not have to pull any files to update patient information. We get a lot of walk-ins in addition to patients with appointments, so our office is very busy.

When a patient registers, I make sure that I enter the patient's demographic data (usually from an identification card, such as a driver's license) correctly. I also must record the financial data (the patient's insurance information) so that the office can get paid! In addition to recording the data, I call the patient's insurance company to verify coverage. Every day, I call the patients who have appointments the next day to confirm their appointments. Sometimes they have forgotten, and they really appreciate the reminder.

I started out as a receptionist here when I graduated from high school. I liked the environment and the people, so I enrolled in college to study health information technology. I am about halfway through the program now, and I was promoted to this position last month. I have not decided what I want to do when I graduate, but there are a lot of opportunities here working in the HIM department or patient accounting.

### Career Tip

Medical office administrative jobs such as receptionist and patient registration are good places to look for entry-level positions. Students can take relevant courses in some high schools. Progressive responsibilities can include coding and billing. An associate degree in HIM can help. Also, the American Academy of Professional Coders (AAPC) offers physician office coding credentials that may help leverage employment opportunities.

### Patient Care Perspective

### Maria

I like using Dr. Lewis's medical group because all the types of physicians we use on a regular basis are there. Our insurance changed last year, which I completely forgot about by the time I took Emma for her annual visit. Michael always asks to see our insurance card, even though he has known us for many years. So he caught the change right away and we had no problems with the insurance coverage for the visit.

My mother, Isabel, needed to be in a nursing home for a little while after her stroke last year. I wanted to get a copy of her medical records so that I could work with a private patient advocate to find rehabilitation and home care afterward that met our needs. Because my mother signed herself into the nursing home and did not list me as a contact, I had some difficulty getting the records. I contacted Francis, the medical records manager, who helped obtain consent from my mother to release the records. I really appreciated his compassion in understanding our issues and respecting my mother's dignity and right to privacy.

## Works Cited

Accreditation Association for Ambulatory Health Care (AAAHC): *Accreditation,* 2021. https://www.aaahc.org/accreditation/. Accessed November 7, 2021.

American Occupational Therapy Association: *About occupational therapy,* 2021. https://www.aota.org/About-Occupational-Therapy.aspx. Accessed November 9, 2021.

American Physical Therapy Association: *About PT/PTA careers,* 2020. https://www.apta.org/your-career/careers-in-physical-therapy. Accessed September 24, 2020.

Centers for Medicare and Medicaid Services (CMS). Medicare Telemedicine Health Care Provider Fact Sheet: March 17, 2020. https://www.samhsa.gov/sites/default/files/medicare-telemedicine-health-care-fact-sheet.pdf. Accessed November 14, 2021.

Department of Health and Human Services. Centers for Medicare and Medicaid Services: *hospital inpatient admission order and certification,* 2014. Baltimore, Department of Health and Human Services. https://www.cms.gov/Medicare/Medicare-Fee-for-Service-Payment/AcuteInpatientPPS/Downloads/IP-Certification-and-Order-01-30-14.pdf. Accessed October 18, 2021.

Federal Register: *Code of Federal Regulations,* 42 CFR $482.24 (c)(3)(iv), 2021a.

Federal Register: *Code of Federal Regulations,* 42 CFR $482.24 (c)(4)(i)(A), 2021b.

Garrett P, Seidman J: EMR vs EHR—what is the difference? *Health IT Buzz,* January 4, 2011. https://www.healthit.gov/buzz-blog/electronic-health-and-medical-records/emr-vs-ehr-difference. Accessed October 18, 2021.

Interstate Medical Licensure Compact: *About the Compact,* May 10, 2020. https://www.imlcc.org/a-faster-pathway-to-physician-licensure/. Accessed November 14, 2021.

Kruse CS, Mileski M, Alaytsev V, Carol E, Williams A: Adoption factors associated with electronic health record among long-term care facilities: a systematic review, *BMJ Open* 5(1):e006615, 2015.

National Hospice and Palliative Care Organization: NHPCO's Facts and Figures: Hospice Care in America. 2021 Edition. https://www.nhpco.org/nhpco-facts-figures-2021-edition/ Accessed November 9, 2021.

NHPCS National Hospice and Palliative Care Organization: *NHPCO's facts and figures: hospice care in America,* 2021. https://www.nhpco.org/wp-content/uploads/NHPCO-Facts-Figures-2021-edition.pdf. Accessed November 9, 2021.

New York State Education Department: *Office of the Professions: LMSW license requirements.* http://www.op.nysed.gov/prof/sw/lmsw.htm. Accessed November 9, 2021.

The Joint Commission: *Hospital accreditation standards: record of care, treatment, and services,* 2012. Chicago, The Joint Commission. RC.01.02.01 and RC.02.01.03.

US Department of Health and Human Services: *National Committee on Vital and Health Statistics: Core health data elements report: background,* 1996. https://ncvhs.hhs.gov/rrp/august-1996-ncvhs-report-on-core-health-data-elements/. Accessed October 7, 2021.

US Department of Health and Human Services: *Office of Inspector General: Nursing home resident assessment quality of care*, 2001. http://oig.hhs.gov/oei/reports/oei-02-99-00040.pdf. Accessed November 7, 2021.

## Further Reading

National Hospice and Palliative Care Organization: *Hospice care*, April 3, 2017 https://www.nhpco.org/about/hospice-care. Accessed December 6, 2018.

American Health Information Management Association: Data quality management model (updated), *J Ahima* 83(7):62–67, 2012.

HealthIT.gov: *Official Website of the Office of the National Coordinator for Health Information Technology (ONC): Telemedicine and Telehealth*. https://www.healthit.gov/topic/health-it-health-care-settings/telemedicine-and-telehealth. Last reviewed September 24, 2020. Accessed September 24, 2020.

US Department of Health and Human Services (U.S. DHHS): Centers for Disease Control and Prevention, National Center for Health Statistics (NCHS), *Agency for Healthcare Research and Quality*, n.d. Accessed April 19, 2023. https://www.ahrq.gov/.

# 4

# Data Quality and Management

**LISA REILLY**

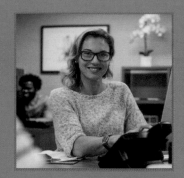

## CHAPTER OUTLINE

**Data Quality**
    Data Quality Characteristics
    Controls
**Postdischarge Processing**
    Identification of Records to Process
    Scanning
    Quantitative Analysis
    Coding
    Master Patient Index Maintenance
    Abstracting
    Tracking Records While Processing
    Transcription
    Workflow
**Record Integrity and Access**
    Storage and Retention
    Retrieval
    Security and Privacy
    Release of Information
    Network Policies
**Uses of Health Information**
    Improving Patient Care
    Education

Support and Collection of Reimbursement
Administration
Prevalence and Incidence of Mortality and Morbidity
National Policy and Legislation
Community Awareness of Health Care Issues
Litigation
Research
Managed Care
Marketing
**Chapter Summary**
**Competency Milestones**
**Ethics Challenge**
**Critical Thinking Questions**
**The Role of Health Information Management Professionals in the Workplace**
    Professional Profile
    Patient Care Perspective
**Works Cited**
**Further Reading**

## CHAPTER OBJECTIVES

*By the end of this chapter, the student should be able to:*

1. Apply policies and procedures to ensure the accuracy and integrity of health data;
2. Explain the flow of postdischarge processing of health information and how those activities support a complete health record according to organizational policies, external regulations, and standards;
3. Discuss organizational policies to safeguard patient records; and
4. List the uses of health information.

## VOCABULARY

| | |
|---|---|
| abstract | exception report |
| abstracting | granularity |
| accuracy | health literacy |
| accessibility | incidence |
| audit trail | indexing |
| batch control form | integrity |
| batch scanning | litigation |
| breach | managed care |
| coding | nonrepudiation |
| completeness | postdischarge processing |
| concurrent analysis | prevalence |
| concurrent coding | preventive controls |
| consistency | probabilistic method |
| corrective controls | protected health information (PHI) |
| countersignature | quantitative analysis |
| data entry | queue |
| deficiencies | release of information (ROI) |
| deficiency system (incomplete system) | registries |
| delinquent | retention |
| detective controls | revenue cycle |
| deterministic method | root cause analysis (RCA) |
| discharge register (list) | timeliness |
| encryption | validity |
| error report | workflow |

### CAHIIM COMPETENCY DOMAINS

I.2.  Apply policies, regulations, and standards to the management of information. (3)

I.4.  Determine compliance of health record content within the health organization. (5)

II.2.  Apply security strategies to health information. (3)

III.2.  Utilize technologies for health information management. (3)

VI.8.  Describe consumer engagement activities. (2)

Previous chapters have focused on the collection of data by clinical practitioners and the organization and storage of those data electronically. This chapter turns attention to the postdischarge processing of patient data, some data quality-control measures, and the role of the health information management (HIM) professional in ensuring data quality, information access, and record retention. We also discuss the many ways health information is used after it has been processed.

This chapter discusses paper-based processing and electronic record processing. Ideally, electronic records replace paper-based records in their entirety. However, it is important to note that facilities must be prepared to conduct business as usual in the event of a computer system "down time": an interruption in service that prevents use of the electronic health record (EHR). System down times can be planned, such as for system upgrades and other system maintenance. Unplanned downtimes, due to hardware failure, software

crashes, malware, and natural disasters, may also occur. Staff must be trained to continue to collect and record data for continuing patient care and patient safety, regardless of the availability of the electronic record. After down time, procedures must also be in place to either backload (enter later) the manually collected data or scan the paper collection into the computer. Thus even in an EHR environment, there is still a need to process paper data collections.

## Data Quality

The process of recording data into a collection device is called **data entry**. Data may be entered onto a paper collection device, such as a form, or into a computer system through a formatted screen. In health care, a patient's life can depend on the quality of the data entered. For example, if an incorrect blood type was recorded and a patient then received the wrong blood type during a blood transfusion, that patient might experience a life-threatening transfusion reaction (agglutination, in which blood cells stick together). This is an extreme example, but errors or delays in recording patient data can affect patient care and lead to poor health care delivery and improper decision-making. Therefore the collection and recording of quality data supports efficient and effective patient care and organizational administration.

The value of data quality cannot be overemphasized. As the health care industry has moved to an EHR, the individual fields are subject to tighter quality review and scrutiny than they were in a paper record. As such, it is critical that those who create, document, and review the data share an understanding of the scope and nature of the data to be collected.

Health records are among the primary documents used by health care facilities to evaluate compliance with the standards set by the accreditation or certification agencies. In brief, health information documentation is analyzed to review the quality of patient care, and this analysis of documentation helps the facility recognize opportunities to improve its performance. This analysis of quality should occur both concurrently (while the patient is in the facility) and retrospectively (after the patient has been discharged).

The HIM department is responsible for monitoring the quality of health information. Each function in the HIM department exists to ensure quality in the documentation; the department, led by a credentialed HIM professional, coordinates review of HIM functions to ensure that the health information is timely, complete, accurate, and valid. The director or manager of HIM must manage the department functions in a manner that promotes useful and accurate information. The director and other personnel ensure quality by reviewing the functions of the HIM department and by developing standards and review processes to monitor competency and compliance with these standards.

## Data Quality Characteristics

You are already familiar with some aspects of data quality. Spelling a patient's name correctly is an example of accuracy. Recording a patient's vital signs as they are being measured is an example of timeliness. But timeliness and accuracy are only 2 of the 10 characteristics of data quality identified by the American Health Information Management Association (AHIMA). AHIMA's Data Quality Management Model reflects the issues in current data quality management (Davoudi et al., 2015). Within that model, the authors list 10 characteristics of data quality. Table 4.1 summarizes these data quality concepts. Although the model as written in 2015 has been retired, these concepts are still useful to help understand the many standards that have evolved over the years, particularly with the development of the EHR and interoperability issues.

### Data Accuracy and Validity

To be useful, the data must be accurate. To understand the importance of data accuracy, think about how irritating it is to receive a telephone call from someone who has dialed the wrong number. Sometimes the person has been given the wrong number; other times, the caller may have recorded the number incorrectly. Either way, the communicated data are

| TABLE 4.1 | Elements of Data Quality | |
|---|---|---|
| Element | Description | Examples of Errors |
| Accuracy | Data are correct | The patient's pulse is 76 beats/min. The nurse recorded 67. That data entry was inaccurate. |
| Accessibility | Data can be obtained when needed by authorized individuals | A health information clerical person was able to change the birth date on a patient's record. |
| Currency | Data are up to date | A dose of medicine depends on a child's weight; the nurse uses the patient's weight from her visit 3 months earlier, rather than her weight today, when calculating the dosage. |
| Consistency | Data are the same wherever they appear | A patient's birth date is 10/7/1954 in the hospital's registration system; however, it is 7/10/1954 in the radiology registration system. |
| Timeliness | Data are recorded within a predetermined period | Operative reports not recorded immediately following surgery. |
| Granularity | Data reflect the needed level of detail | A review of the number of encounters in the emergency department by day includes an unusual circumstance when the department only saw 10 patients all day. Viewing this data by day to determine staffing levels is too granular; a weekly count of encounters would be better for this purpose. |
| Precision | The reason(s) for collecting the data is considered during collection | A foodborne illness is traced to a Sal's Pizza restaurant in Crystal Falls, Minnesota. Asking patients if they were in Minnesota last week is not precise enough to determine their risk. |
| Completeness | Data exist in their entirety | Date, time, or authentication missing from a record renders it incomplete. |
| Definition | Data within the context of the record | The registration field that captures a patient's race allows free text without any parameters of what is acceptable in that field. |
| Relevancy | Data are useful to or needed by the facility | Asking blood donors whether they have a firearm in the home is not relevant. However, this would be a relevant data point when screening patients for suicide risk. |

inaccurate. Receiving misdirected telephone calls is merely an annoyance, whereas receiving someone else's medication could be fatal. If data are not accurate, wrong information is conveyed to the user of the data. Accuracy of health information requires that the documentation reflects the event as it really happened, including all pertinent details and relevant facts. Review of health records for pertinent documentation involves examination of the content of each document.

Accuracy includes the concept of validity. Data **validity** pertains to the data's conformity with an expected range of values. For example, "ABCDE" is not a valid US Postal Service Zip Code, because zip codes in the United States contain only numbers. For health information to be valid, the data or information documented must be of an acceptable or allowable predetermined value or within a specified parameter. This requirement particularly pertains to the documentation of clinical services provided to the patient. For example, there are predetermined accepted values for blood pressure and temperature. 278 °F is not a valid temperature for living human beings. In the electronic record the validity of specific fields can be checked at the time of data entry. Software can be programmed to check specific fields for validity and to alert the user to a potential data-collection error (Fig. 4.1). Electronic forms may contain drop-down menus containing only those values that are valid for the field. Validity checks and menus are common measures to support data quality for dates, gender, race, and ethnicity.

## Data Accessibility

Data **accessibility** means that the data must be able to be obtained by individuals authorized to have it, whenever it is needed, from wherever it is being retained. Think about a library book in a library. In order to access a specific book, one needs to first locate it, then physically go to the book and take it off the shelf. Only one individual can access the book. If the book is checked out of the library, no one else can see it until it is returned. Similarly, paper health records are available to one individual at a time. EHRs allow multiple users to view and work in the same record simultaneously.

In a paper environment, accessibility has traditionally meant that the record is available promptly, as needed, and is securely protected during processing, transportation, and long-term storage from inappropriate viewing and use. Data accessibility is one of the primary benefits of the EHR. Electronic data, if properly captured, are more easily retrieved than paper-based data. The electronic record can improve the speed with which users can obtain patient data and download and manipulate them. However, data access includes the concept of data security. Data must be provided, as needed, but only to those with a legal right to obtain it. Electronic data are not necessarily more secure than physical files and present different problems. Theoretically, one could steal a book from a library; however, human librarians are a deterrent to theft, as are magnetic tags. In an electronic environment, the ability to obtain the data must be restricted, ensuring that only authorized individuals can view and work in the record.

In the EHR, access to electronic data is controlled by requiring a unique login and password for each user. An individual's login grants access to the parts of the computer system necessary to do an employee's job, based on an assigned role. For example, a patient registration clerk's login may allow her to access and edit the demographic data

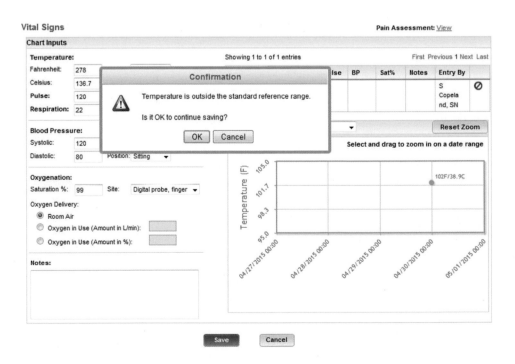

• **Fig. 4.1** Computer prompt indicating that the data entered are not within a valid range. (Courtesy SimChart for the Medical Office, Elsevier, Inc., 2019.)

and financial data of the health record, but she may not be able to view the clinical records or administrative functions of the EHR. The decisions regarding what roles should be granted access to which systems and for what purpose is a data and information governance issue that we will discuss at greater length in Chapter 9.

Access to the health record is monitored using an **audit trail**, which tracks the activity of users in the system. The audit trail logs what information the user accessed and when it was accessed (Fig. 4.2). In addition to the date and time, medical record number (MRN), and patient account number, the audit trail contains a list of the activities, the workstation at which the activity took place, and the user who performed the activity. It usually includes a description of the activity (changed, deleted, and printed information). The audit trail can be a useful piece of evidence showing what a user did while logged into the system, provided a person does not log into the computer under another person's name. It is therefore critical that users do not share their user logins and passwords. Audit trails are discussed in more detail below.

## Data Consistency

Data **consistency** means that the data are the same, no matter where they appear, according to the specifications of the field. For example, if the facility collects birth weight in grams, then all birth weights must be collected and recorded in grams. If the patient registration clerk records a patient's name in the hospital registration system as Martha Jackson, that same patient's name should appear as Martha Jackson in the radiology system and the laboratory system. In order to accomplish this efficiently and effectively, the data should flow from the hospital registration system to the laboratory and radiology systems electronically—without human intervention.

## Data Timeliness

During an episode of care, patient demographic, financial, socioeconomic, and clinical data are collected. Data **timeliness** refers to the recording of data within an appropriate time frame, preferably close to the time the event occurred. Health information should be documented as events occur, treatment is performed, or results are noticed. Delaying documentation could cause information to be

omitted. Reports must be dictated and typed in a timely manner.

Although it makes sense that demographic data are collected at the point of registration, and if the patient is unconscious, that might not be possible. Some financial data are collected at registration; however, in the emergency department, financial data are not collected until after the patient receives a medical screening. In both of these examples, the timeliness of data collection is relative to the situation in which the data are collected.

Other data collection requires specific guidelines. For example, the recording of a patient's vital signs must be done as soon as possible after collection of the readings because monitoring of vital signs is an important aspect of patient care. Similarly, physician documentation of observations and assessments is most useful when it is recorded concurrently with the activity of observing and assessing.

Numerous regulations and guidelines address the issue of when specific data must be recorded. The Joint Commission (TJC), the Centers for Medicare and Medicaid Services (CMS), and state regulations are specific as to the timeliness required for many types of documentation. For example, according to TJC accreditation standards, an operative report must be documented immediately after the operation (The Joint Commission, 2012). A history and physical (H&P) must be completed no more than 30 days prior or 24 hours after admission or before a surgical procedure. The H&P must be placed in the record within 24 hours after admission or prior to a surgical procedure (42 CFR 482.24 2012; The Joint Commission, 2012). Timeliness applies to many other activities, as subsequent discussions demonstrate. Failure to comply with timely documentation requirements is an indicator of lack of quality in the care of patients.

Timeliness is important, particularly in the health care facility's perspective, because the patient's health record is part of the normal business records of the facility. Business records are those that are regularly kept in the normal course of business, recorded at or near the time of the activity by individuals who are knowledgeable of the record's content (see Chapter 8). Therefore data that are being entered into the health record must be recorded as soon as possible after the events that the data describe in order to be considered business records

| | A | B | C | D | E | F |
|---|---|---|---|---|---|---|
| 1 | Username | Last | First | Date/Time | MRN | Action |
| 2 | TFINN | Finn | Timothy | 04/24/20XX 12:10 | 12485635401 | Submitted dictation file |
| 3 | TFINN | Finn | Timothy | 04/24/20XX 12:12 | 12485635401 | Played dictation file |
| 4 | PSTENNET | Stennet | Phillip | 04/24/20XX 14:25 | 12485635401 | Played dictation file |
| 5 | PSTENNET | Stennet | Phillip | 04/24/20XX 14:28 | 12485635401 | Countersigned dictation |
| 6 | SCODY | Cody | Scott | 04/27/20XX 14:03 | 12485635401 | Edited patient demographics information |
| 7 | TFINN | Finn | Timothy | 04/28/20XX 7:10 | 12485635401 | Submitted transcription file |
| 8 | SCODY | Cody | Scott | 04/28/20XX 11:11 | 12485635401 | Viewed record |
| 9 | SCODY | Cody | Scott | 04/28/20XX 18:50 | 12485635401 | Edited patient financial information |

• **Fig. 4.2** This audit trail shows all the users who accessed a patient health record and what actions they took in the record.

(Federal Rules of Evidence: 28a U.S.C. § 803(6) 2015). For example, if a nurse is monitoring a patient at 3:00 p.m., then the note that he or she records in the patient's record must be written very shortly thereafter. Ideally, the note is written concurrently with the observation: point-of-care documentation. Writing that same note at 9:00 p.m., 6 hours after the actual observation, could impair the quality of the recorded note. Can the nurse really remember, 6 hours later, exactly what happened with the patient? Can a physician really remember, weeks later, exactly what happened during an operation well enough to dictate an accurate report?

After the patient has been discharged from an acute care facility, the record must be completed within a specified period of time, usually 30 days. State licensing regulations and medical staff bylaws, rules, and regulations will define the facility's standard for chart completion; however, the maximum is 30 days, by both TJC and Conditions of Participation (COP) standards. In the presence of conflicting standards, the most stringent takes precedence. So, if state licensing regulations require a record to be completed within 15 days of discharge, that shorter time frame takes precedence over 30-day standards. Because timeliness is so important, a significant amount of time and energy is spent facilitating the timely completion of health records. Of course, in an EHR environment, facilities may have a significantly shorter expectation of the amount of time it takes to complete a patient record. With all authorized individuals able to access and work in the record simultaneously, it is not unreasonable to expect clinicians to complete their routine data entry and dictations within 24–48 hours of discharge.

## Data Completeness

If data is not complete, then quality is impaired. **Completeness** refers to the collection or recording of data in their entirety. For example, a recording of vital signs that is missing the time and date is incomplete.

AHIMA refers to completeness as "comprehensive" (Davoudi et al., 2015). Comprehensive health records contain all pertinent documents with all of the appropriate documentation, that is, the H&P, consent forms, progress notes, anesthesia record, operative report, recovery room record, discharge notes, nursing documentation, and so on. Incomplete records can jeopardize patient care, impair correct reimbursement, and skew data used for administrative purposes. For example, a comprehensive physical examination that omits any mention of the condition of the patient's skin condition is incomplete. If a physician's progress note contains the subjective and objective descriptions but is missing the assessment and plan, then it is incomplete. The note may contain all of the SOAP elements, but if it is not signed, dated, and timed, it is incomplete. A progress note that is not authenticated is incomplete.

Comprehensiveness also refers to the compilation of the record from all sources in which it is collected. If multiple systems are involved, then all systems must be accessed to obtain the complete record.

One of the many benefits of an EHR is that the data-collection fields can be programmed to prompt the user to complete all of the fields in a form. For example, a nurse who records the beginning of an intravenous therapy could be prompted to note the site of the venous puncture and the time that the therapy began. Failure to complete the note with the time the therapy ended would leave the record incomplete. The system might then remind the nurse with each login or attempt to sign out that this element is outstanding.

Complete data support the record of care of the patient. If a time is missing from a medication administration record, the hospital cannot provide evidence that the medication was administered on a timely basis. If the physician leaves out the condition of the patient's skin from a physical examination, the hospital may have difficulty claiming that a decubitus ulcer (a progressive wearing away of skin due to pressure—also known as a bed sore) was present on admission.

In order to ensure that data collection and recording are performed with quality elements in mind, health care organizations, such as hospitals and other providers of health care, must develop and implement data quality controls. Review of health records to ensure that each record is complete is called *quantitative analysis*. Concurrent review of records by clinical areas to ensure completeness is an important quality-control activity.

## Data Currency

Data are useful only if they reflect the values that pertain to the period under review. For example, one of the key postdischarge processing functions is coding: assigning the appropriate codes to a patient's diagnoses and procedures. Many code sets are updated at least annually. Therefore using codes in 2023 that were published in 2020 can result in errors because the 2020 codes are not current in 2023. ICD-10-CM, ICD-10-PCS, and Current Procedural Terminology (CPT) are example of commonly used code sets that update at least annually (see Chapter 5).

## Data Precision

For both data collection and reporting purposes, the use of the data drives the precision with which they are represented. For example, it is not useful for billing purposes to know merely that the patient is a resident of a particular state. The exact street address, city, and zip code are also required. However, for analysis of a facility's catchment area, the zip code or county may be the level of precision required.

## Data Definition

In Chapter 2 we discussed the need for a data dictionary in order to clearly define all of the fields to be collected in compiling a patient record. The creation of a data dictionary illustrates the concept of data definition. A data dictionary codifies this effort and provides a reference point for data-collection device creators and users to understand exactly what a field represents and how to collect and record that data. Every field must be clearly defined so that it can be collected consistently and accurately. Definition is important within a system but is further emphasized when sharing data across systems. For example, the Uniform Hospital Discharge Data Set (UHDDS) ethnicity field contains *Spanish origin/Hispanic, Non-Spanish origin/Non-Hispanic,* and *Unknown.* However, data collections may require expanded specificity of ethnicity with many more options in this field, such as subgroups identifying Hispanic countries of origin. Therefore not only does the hospital system have to define the field in which the data is collected, but it also has to map the state's requirements to the UHDDS requirements in order to accurately report its discharge data.

### Data Granularity

**Granularity** refers to the level of detail with which data are collected, recorded, or calculated. For example, a patient's temperature is generally recorded to the nearest 10th of a degree: 98.6°, 101.3°, etc. Many laboratory results are expressed this way. Granularity also applies to reporting as well as recording. For example, the individual length of stay (LOS) for a patient is measured in whole days. However, the average LOS for multiple patients is generally represented with one or more decimal places, such as 4.1 days or 4.13 days. To an administrator using average LOS for control purposes, a movement from 4.1 to 4.14 days could be significant.

### Data Relevancy

Relevancy has two components: should the data be collected at all and, if so, are they being collected in a way that is meaningful in light of the purpose for collecting them? Collection of data should take place only if there is a reason for collecting them that is meaningful in context. For example, hair color has no relevance as a data item to collect regarding a patient entering the hospital for an appendectomy. However, it is a critical data element in reporting to security an individual behaving suspiciously in or around the facility.

## Controls

The primary purpose of documentation is communication. For example, clinical documentation communicates:
- among caregivers for continuing patient care,
- to payers, to justify and substantiate the care provided, and
- to regulatory or accrediting agencies to demonstrate the quality of patient care.

In any communication, there are many opportunities for errors to occur. In clinical documentation, errors may occur, whether handwritten or electronically entered. If an individual's handwriting cannot be read by another health professional, how can those data elements be communicated? How can they be considered valid or accurate? If only the author of the data can decipher the writing, the data is

useless to others. Similarly, if a nurse records a temperature of 98.6°F without the decimal point (986°F), the temperature recorded is not valid and is therefore not useful to other caregivers. Finally, a physician's order that requests 100 mg of a medication instead of 10 mg could have fatal consequences if the larger dose is actually administered. These examples emphasize the need for accuracy.

To ensure that all data—administrative, demographic, financial, and clinical—are accurate, timely, and complete, organizations must have policies and procedures in place to prevent errors, to find errors when they occur, and to correct errors when they are discovered. These policies and procedures include the development and implementation of controls over the collection, recording, and reporting of the data. For example, a provider will have a policy that says that all health records of acute care patients must be completed within 30 days of discharge. In order to ensure that the policy is enforced, the provider will have a set of procedures to review and track the records of discharged patients. This chapter focuses on the collection and recording of data; reporting is discussed in later chapters. There are three basic types of controls over the collection and recording of data: preventive, detective, and corrective (Table 4.2).

### Preventive Controls

**Preventive controls** are designed to ensure that data errors do not occur in the first place. The best example of a preventive control is a software validity check. For example, suppose a user entered a date as July 45, 2019 (i.e., 07/45/2019). If the software is programmed to prevent users from entering invalid dates, it might send a message (an alert) saying, "You have entered an invalid date-please re-enter." It might even make a loud sound or block the character "4" from being typed in the first position of the day field.

Preventive controls are common, both in protocols surrounding clinical care and in paper-based data entry. For

| **TABLE 4.2** | **Processing Controls** | |
|---|---|---|
| **Control** | **Description** | **Example(s)** |
| Preventive | Helps ensure that an error does not occur | Computer-based validity check during data entry; examination of patient identification before medication administration |
| Detective | Helps in the discovery of errors that have been made | Quantitative analysis (e.g., error report) |
| Corrective | Correction of errors that have been discovered, including investigation of the source of the error for future prevention | Incomplete record processing |

example, a nurse checks the patient's identification band and verbally identifies the patient before administering a medication to ensure that the medication is being given to the correct patient. In an electronic medication administration system, bar coding of both the patient wristband (to match the patient record) and the medication itself (bar code medication administration to match the ordered/dispensed drug) is a preventive control. The development of well-designed, preprinted forms to collect data helps ensure that data collection is complete. Some facilities use a combination of paper and bar codes to collect data.

Preventive controls can be expensive and cumbersome to develop and implement. Health care providers might resist the implementation of preventive controls if they are burdensome and time consuming. Therefore the cost of a preventive control must always be balanced against its expected benefits. It is relatively easy to justify checking medications, orders, and patient identification because patient safety is of paramount concern. It is not quite as easy to justify developing a control to prevent errors in recording the patient's preferred language or their ethnicity.

One simple way to prevent invalid data entries is with the use of radio buttons or menus on a printed form or drop-down menus in an electronic record (Fig. 4.3). All of the valid choices are listed so that the recorder merely chooses the correct one for the particular patient. Each of these design elements allows the user to select only one choice from a set of options. This method also prompts the user to complete the form. However, this method does not prevent inaccurate entries because it is still possible to select the wrong item. For example, the staff member may enter the wrong sex for a patient. Because the computer program has no way of "knowing" whether the patient is male or female, it does not prompt a correction. Thus comprehensive, foolproof preventive controls are not guaranteed.

In addition to errors in accuracy are errors in the way documentation is recorded. For example, there are many abbreviations that are discouraged because they can be confusing and lead to medication and other errors in patient care. Drop-down menus do not necessarily prevent all uses of such abbreviations and in paper documentation, only a review afterward will reveal the problem.

Another documentation problem is referred to as "copy/paste." It is extremely tempting for a clinician to copy verbiage from one note and paste it to another note to avoid excessive typing. While the motivation may be benign, this practice is generally prohibited for two reasons. First, it can lead to errors if the pasted verbiage is not customized to the specific event it is describing. Second, it violates the underlying principle that the clinical documentation is specific to the individual patient. Copying documentation from another provider and then billing for the time is another problematic issue. In an EHR, it may be possible to disable the copy/paste function.

### Detective Controls

Detective controls are developed and implemented to ensure that errors in data are discovered. Whereas a preventive control is designed to help prevent the person recording the data from making the mistake in the first place, a detective control is in place to find the data error after it is entered. In the previous date example (7/45/2019), a detective control might generate a list of entries that the software recognizes as problematic. Such a printout is called

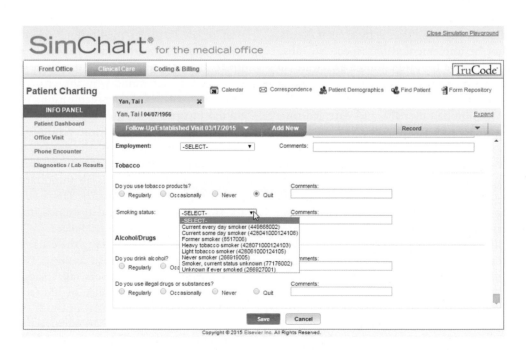

• Fig. 4.3 This drop-down list to enter a patient's tobacco habits limits the recorder to certain valid choices. (Courtesy SimChart for the Medical Office, Elsevier, Inc., 2019.)

an **error report** or **exception report**. Error reports are also generated when the computer or other system encounters a problem with its normal processing. For example, a pharmacy system can be programmed to print an error report to alert the pharmacist that a medication order exceeds the normal dose. Omissions may also be highlighted in an error or exception report. For example, if the medication was ordered but not recorded as administered, this mistake could be detected on an exception report generated by matching orders against medication administrations. Exception reports can also be generated to list potential errors based on customized instructions. In this way, the system can be programmed to list all users who accessed a patient record but who were not either a physician of record on the case or a caregiver assigned to the nursing unit in which the patient is being treated. This type of an exception report is not specifically matching data but rather takes advantage of the ability of an EHR to create an audit trail.

In order to generate an audit trail exception report, the user must initiate the audit process prior to any activity taking place. So, in order to track all of the activities in a specific application for the month of March, the audit function must be set up and running prior to March. Once the audit function is enabled, the system can monitor the target application and create a file (called a log or trail) of every interaction, noting the date, time, user, and action. The log can then be reviewed for errors or inappropriate activity. This audit trail report can assist in determining whether there has been inappropriate access to a patient record, thereby providing a detective control over the "authorized" component of accessibility to data.

An audit trail may be tailored to review specific data elements, such as changing a patient's status from outpatient to inpatient. Because audit trails log user activity as it occurs, an audit trail cannot be implemented retrospectively (after the fact). The system must be programmed to create an activity log that can then be searched only for the data that have been included on the log. Say the system's activity log records the encounter number, user ID, and date and time whenever someone accesses a patient record. We can generate a report of every user who looked at a specific patient's visit; however, we cannot determine what parts of the patient record were viewed. Thus it is extremely important during the design of the system to identify what logs will be useful and what data will be required. Such logs require a significant amount of storage space, which is why systems do not automatically generate logs of every possible viewing event. Audit trails are generally created only for highly sensitive data for which access data could not otherwise be reproduced.

Detective controls are critical in a paper-based environment. Because there is no practical way to prevent erroneous data entry in a paper-based environment, the process of searching for errors is necessary. For example, nursing medication records may be reviewed regularly by nurse supervisors to ensure that medication administration notes are properly entered. Also, if a physician fails to dictate an operative report in a timely manner, a control must be in place to detect the missing report.

Detective controls are frequently the easiest and most cost-effective method to develop and implement, but as with preventive controls, they may be complex. The development of preventive and detective controls requires a thorough knowledge of the process being controlled and of the potential negative impact of data errors. For this reason, a detective control may be performed either facility-wide, under the review of an overall quality improvement plan, or by a specific department. An example of a facility-wide detective control is a newborn amber alert: an alarm sounds when a newborn is removed from the maternity unit, and staff throughout the hospital are mobilized to monitor hallways, stairwells, and exits to detect the abductor. Under a quality improvement plan, management personnel may be charged with periodically reviewing patient care areas for possible violations of regulatory guidelines, patient safety protocols, or hospital policy. In a department, supervisors may review employee time logs to identify violations of attendance policy.

### Corrective Controls

**Corrective controls** may be developed and implemented to fix an error once it has been detected. Corrective controls follow detective controls. In general, identifying an error wastes time and is ineffective if the facility does not correct the mistake. However, corrective controls, by their design, happen after the error has occurred. Thus if an error report identified an invalid date, such as July 45, the date would be corrected after the fact.

Nevertheless, some errors cannot be effectively corrected once they occur. For example, if a patient received an injection of an incorrect medication, the medication cannot subsequently be withdrawn. However, the events leading up to the administration of the drug can be thoroughly examined to determine why the error occurred. Did the physician order the wrong medication? Was the order transmitted incorrectly to the pharmacy? Did the nurse check the patient's wristband before administering the medication? Thus investigation of the error is necessary to determine whether sufficient controls are in place to prevent the error in the future. This is an important component of a *process improvement* or *quality improvement program*. Once the source of the error is determined, the appropriate correction to the process can take place.

The process of determining the cause of an error is often referred to as a **root cause analysis (RCA)**. Facilities in which serious medical errors take place, such as an error that alters a patient's quality of life (such as amputation of the wrong limb) or results in death (which may be due to the administration of an incorrect medication), may be required to report these errors with an RCA and a corrective action plan to the appropriate regulatory agencies. Employee education and disciplinary action are two examples of typical corrective actions that may take place if policies and procedures were in place but not followed. Health care professionals, such as nurses and physicians, can lose their professional licenses if serious patient errors occur once or continue to occur even after the corrective action plan is in effect.

The HIM department plays a role in the detection and correction of certain documentation errors. Earlier in the chapter, an unsigned progress note was used as an example of incomplete data. In a paper-based environment, the HIM professional would have to obtain the record and read all of the progress notes in it to identify the incomplete note. In an electronic record environment, preventive control alerts, such as noises and verbal prompts, can be built into the program to encourage the authentication of the note at the time the note is originally recorded and on subsequent access to the record. As a detective control in an electronic environment, an exception report can identify incomplete notes. In both paper-based and electronic record environments, the corrective control consists of alerting the physician to the omission and giving him or her the opportunity to complete the note.

## Correction of Errors

The correction of errors is an important consideration in patient record keeping because nothing that is recorded should be deleted. Corrections must be made so that the error can be seen as clearly as the modified information. In a paper-based record, errors are corrected by drawing a line through the erroneous data and writing the correct data near it. It is important not to obscure the original entry because doing so may lead to the perception that someone attempted to cover up a mistake. The correction must be dated, timed, and authenticated. In addition, correction of errors cannot consist of destroying entire documents or pages of a record. All of the erroneous documents or pages must be clearly labeled as incorrect; authenticated, timed, and dated; and kept with the correct portions of the record. One important reason that data should not be deleted is that caregivers may have relied on the erroneous data to make decisions about patient care. Leaving that erroneous data for reference helps subsequent caregivers to understand exactly what happened with the patient.

In electronic records, errors can be corrected in several ways depending on the type of error and the data that are being changed. For example, a physician making a correction to a progress note must create an addendum to the record, identifying the error and entering the new note. In both cases, an audit trail should be created to indicate that the correction was made.

As mentioned above, an audit trail is a list of access to an application or patient record, including changes to the patient's record and viewings of the record. In the case of changes to the record, the audit trail also may be programmed to retain the precorrection and postcorrection data. Because the audit trail indicates the user, it can be used to determine whether errors are being made by certain staff members so that retraining can target the correct individuals.

---

### COMPETENCY CHECK-IN 4.1

#### Data Quality

**Competency Assessment**

**Match the characteristic of data quality with its definition.**

_____ 1. Accuracy

_____ 2. Accessibility

_____ 3. Currency

_____ 4. Consistency

_____ 5. Timeliness

_____ 6. Granularity

_____ 7. Precision

_____ 8. Completeness

_____ 9. Definition

_____ 10. Relevancy

A. Data are recorded within a predetermined period

B. Data can be obtained when needed by authorized individuals

C. Data are useful to or needed by the facility

D. Data are the same wherever they appear

E. Data within the context of the record

F. Data exist in their entirety

G. Data are correct

H. Data reflect the needed level of detail

I. Data are up to date

J. The reason(s) for collecting the data is considered during collection

11. The development and implementation of internal controls aid in the protection of data quality and integrity. List and define three fundamental types of internal controls.

## Postdischarge Processing

The understanding of data concepts and control issues is critical for the development and implementation of postdischarge processing procedures (Fig. 4.4). **Postdischarge processing** is what happens to a patient's record after the patient is discharged. In an EHR environment, postdischarge processing consists of ensuring that the record is accurate and complete before being archived. The postdischarge processing of individual records is a part of the larger organizational strategic objectives of data governance and information governance, which we will address in Chapter 9. The goal of *data governance* is to ensure the quality of the data as they are being collected and the integrity of that data over time and among applications. *Information governance* deals with the issues arising from the distribution of the data for analytical, reporting, and legal purposes, for example.

Postdischarge processing is traditionally performed by the facility's HIM department. In a small physician's office

or long-term care (LTC) facility, the entire process may be performed by one person. In a group practice or small inpatient facility, the process may be divided into functions and distributed among several individuals. In a large facility, many individuals may perform each of the separate functions of the process. The data concepts and control issues are relevant to many other health information environments. The following descriptions pertain to inpatient facilities. Although the principles are the same when applied to outpatient facilities, the application of the principles may vary.

### Identification of Records to Process

Postdischarge processing begins with the identification of discharged patients: what records need to be processed. This can be accomplished by reviewing a list of the patients who have been discharged within a specific timeframe: the **discharge register** or discharge list. A discharge register is generated by querying the system to search all encounters

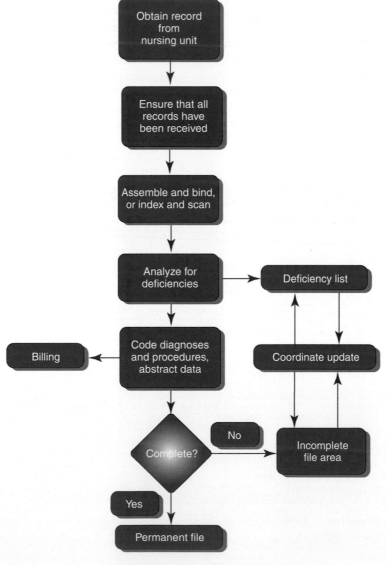

• **Fig. 4.4** Postdischarge processing in an HIM department. *HIM,* Health information management.

with a discharge date within the specified time frame. The report that is typically generated from this query lists the patient account (encounter) number, the MRN, the patient name, the admission date, the discharge date, and often the bed number or nursing unit reference.

As patients are discharged from the facility, their status is updated in the computer system. The discharge date and time are entered in the patient account, which links to the master patient index (MPI). This data entry may be performed by nursing or registration staff because they are the individuals most likely to know exactly when the patient has left. Depending on the needs of the facility, other staff may be assigned to record the discharge. Upon discharge of the patient, bed control is notified, either manually or electronically, that the patient's bed is unoccupied. Housekeeping is notified that the room needs to be cleaned. All three tasks (discharge, notification, and cleaning) must take place in order to admit another patient to that bed. If the patient leaves but the discharge date is not recorded and bed control is not notified, the number of patients in the facility (census) is incorrect and the discharge list is missing a patient. This detailed understanding of the discharge process and how it is performed in one's facility enables users of the discharge register to detect and correct errors. For example, if a record is received but the patient is not on the discharge register, the HIM department must determine what error has been made and notify the correct area to fix the problem.

A corrective control to ensure that the discharge register is correct may involve someone physically visiting all nursing units around midnight, essentially doing a bed check to verify whether all discharges have been recorded and that the census report correctly identifies all of the patients and their locations. Nursing may perform this control function, comparing the patients in the beds with a computer printout of all inpatients as part of the midnight census check. In paper-based facilities, the discharge would be a manual entry into a register, which could be photocopied or manually copied to a list for distribution to departments that use the discharge register, such as HIM. Manual census and discharge registers in a hospital are rare because the MPI and related administrative data collection such as admission and discharge dates have been computerized for decades. In an EHR, flagging the patient status and entering the discharge date and time are performed through computer data entry. However, the discharge register is compiled and it contains a list of the patients who have been discharged on a specific calendar day or during a specific time period. A day is from 12:01 a.m. to 12 midnight, so discharges may include a patient who died at 11:00 p.m. and one who left against medical advice at 5:00 p.m. Fig. 4.5 illustrates a discharge register.

Once the patient has been discharged, the record is no longer needed for direct patient care and documentation should be nearly complete. Theoretically, any paper components to the record could be moved to the HIM department immediately on discharge. Often, however, paper components of records remain on the patient unit until the morning of the day after discharge. This practice gives the clinicians time to complete their documentation and gives the nursing unit personnel time to organize the papers for transportation to the HIM department.

The process by which paper records move from the patient care unit to the HIM department varies by facility. Some of the considerations that determine what process is used include the distance from the patient units to the HIM department, the staffing levels on the patient unit, the staffing levels in the HIM department, and the availability of alternative personnel, such as volunteers. An example of a common practice is as follows: Patient unit personnel remove the records from their binders and leave them in a pile for pickup; the records are then picked up by an authorized person and delivered to the HIM department. Alternatively, the patient unit personnel may deliver the records. Some facilities use physical transportation systems such as pneumatic tube systems, elevators, and even transport robots.

| Admission Date | Patient Identification Number | Patient Name | | Attending Physician | Discharge Disposition | Room Number |
|---|---|---|---|---|---|---|
| | | Last | First | | | |
| 06/02/20XX | 234675 | Johnson | Thomas | Bottoms | Transfer LTC | 313A |
| 06/04/20XX | 234731 | Kudovski | Maria | Patel | Home | 303A |
| 06/04/20XX | 234565 | Kudovski | Vladimir | Thomas | Home | Nursery |
| 05/31/20XX | 156785 | Macey | Anna | Flint | Home | 213B |
| 06/03/20XX | 234523 | Mattingly | Richard | Johnson | Home | 202A |
| 06/05/20XX | 274568 | Ng | Charles | Kudro | Home | 224A |
| 05/15/20XX | 234465 | Rodriguez | Francisco | Benet | Deceased | ICU-4 |
| 06/01/20XX | 198543 | Rogers | Danielle | Patel | Home | 226B |
| 06/02/20XX | 224678 | Young | Rebecca | Muniz | Home | 325B |

• **Fig. 4.5** A discharge register.

Pneumatic tube systems are widely used today at banks for drive-through customers. The customer drives up to a stand that holds a container. The checks or other documents are placed in the container, which is then transported at the press of a button, by forced air, to the teller inside the bank. Larger documents, such as health records, require larger containers. These systems are quick and generally efficient; however, the tendency of containers to get stuck in the tubes and the relatively short range of the system limit their appeal for this purpose. Nevertheless, they may be used within a hospital for transporting physician's orders to the pharmacy, for example. Although theoretically not needed in an EHR, the systems may be retained for use when the electronic system is "down."

Once the record arrives in the HIM department, postdischarge processing can begin. The first step is to ensure that all records have been received. This can be accomplished by checking the records received against the discharge register. If a patient was discharged but a record was not received, the patient unit staff should be contacted immediately so HIM can obtain the record. If a record was received but the patient is not listed on the discharge register, the record may have been sent in error (e.g., the patient may not actually have been discharged). Alternatively, the discharge register may be incorrect (e.g., the patient was discharged but does not appear on the discharge register due to an error in posting the discharge date). The patient unit staff should be contacted to verify the patient's status, and whatever error was made should be corrected immediately.

Other departments also rely on the accuracy of the discharge register. Members of the nutrition or dietary department would not want to deliver meals to patients who are no longer at the facility. The nursing department must know the exact bed occupancy statistics for every unit to ensure appropriate staffing levels. The admitting department must know which beds are open for new admissions. Therefore the facility must have a procedure in place, whether it be telephone, facsimile (fax), Internet communication, or computer-based system, to systematically notify the relevant departments. In an entirely electronic system, manual notifications among departments would be unnecessary because the new status would automatically alert the relevant departments as the patient's status changed. While the concept of a discharge register is not relevant in an outpatient setting, a visit register is useful to ensure that all activities pertaining to a patient interaction are properly completed and billed.

## Scanning

It may seem obvious that an EHR is not paper and therefore there is nothing to assemble. However, quite a bit of paper may be generated from an EHR during the patient's stay, for a variety of reasons. Critical documents, such as dictated reports and laboratory results, may be printed on the nursing unit as a precaution in the event of down time. Also, a document may be generated or received during the patient stay that must be evaluated for inclusion in the record, such

as copies of patient documents from other facilities, patient consent forms, and advance directives. The assembler must evaluate which documents received from the patient unit are original and which documents are printouts (i.e., copies or duplicates) that should be destroyed to prevent confusion. Original documents may contain signatures or indicate in other ways that they are originals. Printouts may need to be retained if they contain written documentation. For this reason, printing out documents from the EHR should be regulated by policy and procedure. Once assembled, these paper components are typically scanned into the computer system through the use of an electronic document management system. Depending on how the documents are developed, they may be directly scanned or batch scanned.

Scanned documents are stored by document type so that users can locate the portion of the record that is needed. The process of assigning the location in which to store a scanned document is called **indexing**. Thus physician progress notes would be indexed so that they are accessible by clicking on a tab or menu for physician progress notes. Users of the EHR will rely on the indexes to find the reports that they need to read. The determination of how scanned documents will be identified and indexed must be made prior to implementation of a scanning process.

If paper records are to be scanned, then the use of bar codes for both the type of form and patient demographics is advantageous. Documents that have bar codes identifying the document and patient demographics may be scanned directly into the system. Using **batch scanning**, many paper documents can be loaded into the scanner at once, after which software sorts the documents into the correct record by bar code. The demographic bar codes can be generated on labels and attached to each form while the patient is in house. In some systems, the demographic bar code is automatically printed out on each report. The bar code indicating the form name is usually preprinted on the form (Fig. 4.6). The bar codes allow for automatic indexing by patient record and report type. Pages are scanned into the computer and linked to the patient's MRN and admission (or encounter).

Documents without bar codes must be scanned with cover sheets to identify them to the system. The scanning operator must enter that data manually, a step that delays processing.

Many reports are generated by systems that interface with the main electronic record system. Laboratory systems, radiology systems, and transcription systems are three examples of systems that generate data or reports and interface directly into the EHR. Just as scanned paper records are indexed, so are these data or reports indexed in the EHR for easy access.

Scanning and indexing are necessary functions with both the hybrid record and the EHR. With the hybrid record, the HIM department may be scanning the whole record or parts of a record. With the EHR, the HIM department may have only a few reports to scan because most data already resides in the EHR, either through direct data entry or by interface from another system. Scanning equipment must be

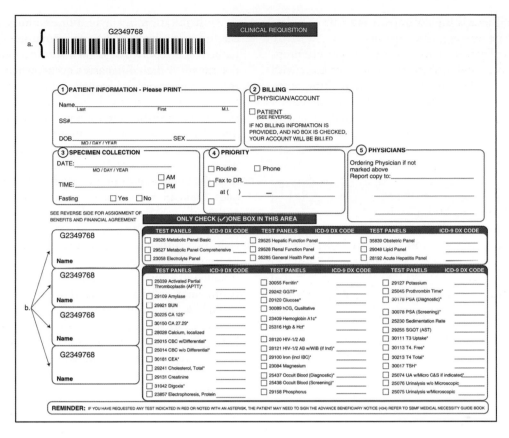

• **Fig. 4.6** An example of a paper document with a bar code, scanned into the patient's record. (From Garrels M: *Laboratory testing for ambulatory settings: a guide for health care professionals*, ed 2, St. Louis, MO, 2011, Elsevier.)

purchased on the basis of the volume of reports (number of pages) to be scanned and the speed of the scanner in mind.

Quality assurance is a critical detective and corrective control function in the scanning process. When a scanning process is initiated, every page must be viewed to ensure that it is legible, properly aligned, and indexed properly. Typically, quality assurance is performed by an individual who did not scan the batch being reviewed. Every page with an error must be rescanned. Over time, as scanning error rates approach zero, the department may make the decision to review only a percentage of the scanned pages rather than all of them. Bearing in mind that the scanned pages are part of the patient's health record, it is critical that all pages be scanned with 100% accuracy.

Pages that have been scanned are held for a period of time, at the discretion of the facility. This holding period is to ensure that the original pages are available should any issues arise with the scanned material. At the end of the holding period, the pages are destroyed.

Participation in the scanning process (assembly, scanning, indexing, and quality assurance) can be a good entry-level position for new HIM professionals. Scanning positions exist both in facilities and outsourcing vendors. HIM departments that do not have the physical area to support a scanning function may contract with outside vendors to perform all or part of the scanning process.

## Quantitative Analysis

Another important detective control that takes place in the HIM department is quantitative analysis. **Quantitative analysis** is the process of reviewing a health record to ensure that the record is complete according to organization policies and procedures for a complete medical record. As previously discussed, *completeness* refers to the entirety of data: Are all of the data elements present? Sample job titles for this HIM professional are *medical record analyst, medical record analysis specialist, health information specialist,* or *health information analyst.*

This professional's responsibility is to review the patient's record and determine whether any reports, notes, or necessary signatures are missing. In general, this analysis occurs after discharge. Review of the chart after the patient has gone home is called a retrospective, or postdischarge, analysis.

The extent of quantitative analysis performed in a facility depends on the type of facility and the rules of its licensure and accreditation. However, there are three guiding principles:

• *Existence*: The record must contain all of the elements required by the licensure and accrediting bodies for the particular type of facility and all of the elements required by the clinical services pertaining to that patient's treatment, as well as the elements common to all patients.

- *Completeness*: The existing documents must be complete and must not be missing data elements.
- *Authentication*: Each element of the record must be properly dated, timed, and authenticated in accordance with the rules and regulations of state or accrediting agencies that apply to the facility, with the authors clearly identified.

The absence of a document, an incomplete document, or a missing authentication are all **deficiencies** in the record.

> **NOTE**
>
> **Qualitative Versus Quantitative**
>
> Where a quantitative analysis reviews the health record to ensure it is complete according to organizational policies, a qualitative analysis is a review of the health record's content to ensure the documentation reflects the care the patient received, and that the services rendered were appropriate. Qualitative analysis is important for facility accreditation and quality initiatives and is explored in more detail in Chapter 10.

### Elements of the Health Record

Different clinical services typically have special forms that pertain to those services, as discussed in Chapters 2 and 3. Physical therapy may have special assessment and progress forms that differ from those used by nursing. The analyst must know which forms are used in each service and must be able to identify any forms that are missing. Again, the complete absence of the data element is easier to identify than the partial absence. For example, an H&P must be documented on every inpatient record. Failure to perform an H&P is a serious error. If either the history portion or the physical portion of the transcribed report is missing, it may not have been performed. More often, however, the H&P was performed, noted in the record, and dictated, but the dictated report has not yet been matched with the chart. The same is true of operative reports and consultation reports. No rule or regulation states that reports must be dictated, so on some records, depending on hospital policy, a handwritten H&P may be acceptable. The analyst must know the rules and must be able to identify noncompliance. The analyst must also be able to identify forms that are incomplete.

The absence of the author's authentication or of identification of authorship is easily recognized as long as the analyst is aware of when and where the authentication must appear. However, the analyst must also know who should have authenticated the document. This knowledge becomes critical if a document has been signed, but not by the correct individual. Perhaps a countersignature is required. A **countersignature** is authentication by an individual in addition to the author. For example, an unlicensed resident may write (author) a progress note, which the attending physician must then countersign to provide evidence that the resident was supervised.

Authentication in a hybrid or electronic record must be carefully considered. A digitized signature is an original signature on a report that is then scanned into an electronic document. A digital signature occurs when the authenticator uses a password or personal identification number (PIN) to electronically sign a document. In some facilities, the authenticator must use both a password and a PIN to sign. The authentication method must provide a means to identify the user, **nonrepudiation** (a process that provides a positive identification of the user), and integrity of the signature (i.e., the document cannot be altered after the signature has been applied). For example, as discussed in Chapter 3, the author of a verbal order may be a registered nurse, who then authenticates the entry by initialing or signing it. The physician then authenticates the order to prove that it has been reviewed. Because both parties can be identified by their unique signatures, a signature can verify identity, as well as represent an activity, such as review or approval.

Finally, the analyst ensures that the record is complete according to licensure and accreditation rules, as well as hospital policy. For example, the H&P, discharge summary, and progress notes are required elements. These elements must be signed, dated, and timed. Table 4.3 summarizes the major record elements for which quantitative analysis acts as a detective control.

There is more to record completeness than compliance with external standards. Because the health record is part of the hospital's business records, the hospital must determine what constitutes its legal record for the purpose of communication or distribution. The analyst must be aware of the hospital's requirements and ensure that the record is compliant (see Chapter 8).

As the analyst identifies deficiencies, the pages are flagged and the missing elements are noted, along with the party responsible for correction. In many facilities, the policy is to analyze only the physician portions of the record, such as orders, progress notes, and all dictated reports. In other facilities, the policy is to analyze many sections or all of the

| **TABLE 4.3** | **Elements of Quantitative Analysis** | |
|---|---|---|
| **Element** | **Analysis to Determine** | **Common Deficiencies** |
| Existence | Does the data exist? | Missing operative report Missing discharge summary |
| Completeness | Are the data entirely present, or are there missing components? | Missing reason for consultation |
| Authentication | Is the author's or other appropriate signature/ password present? | Unsigned H&P Unsigned discharge summary Unsigned order |

clinical documentation, which would include nursing progress notes.

For a hybrid or electronic record, it must be decided how and when the record will be analyzed. When using a hybrid record, an analysis clerk may still need to review the record and provide the physician with the chart deficiencies electronically. In the EHR, an automated deficiency analysis program may be included with the electronic record system; this program allows the record to be completed at the time of ordering or documenting. Policies and procedures must be established to define what constitutes a deficiency and what constitutes a complete record.

In an EHR, most of the quantitative analysis can be performed by the computer. For example, the analyst would receive a computer exception or error report for follow-up purposes. The report might contain a list of incomplete records by the physician with details about what is missing. Analysts can then turn their attention to the analysis of other data quality issues, such as the correct assignment of physicians to specific cases (attribution). Assignment of physicians to cases—attending, consultants, and surgeons—occurs at several points during the inpatient stay. This attribution is important for billing, the evaluation of patient outcomes, and recredentialing. The assignments are verified and corrected by HIM staff during the **quantitative analysis** process. For example, an attending physician may have requested a consultation from a specific physician; however, that physician was not available and a different physician was chosen. If the requested consultant was added as a physician of record, HIM staff will identify the error and remove that physician, adding the actual consultant, if necessary. It is extremely important, both for administrative purposes and legal purposes, to ensure that only physicians who were involved in the care of the patients are associated with the patient's record. Conversely, it is equally important that all of the physicians involved in a patient's care are accurately associated with the patient's record.

## Deficiency System

Once the discharged patient's record has been reviewed and missing elements have been identified, the corrective control procedure is initiated. The responsible party—that is,

the individual who was responsible for preparing the report or signing the note or report—is notified and asked to complete the record. The most common deficiencies that exist in inpatient records are the absences of a discharge summary, an operative report, a formal consultation report, and signatures. This process of recording, reporting, and tracking missing elements in a record is called the **deficiency system** or, in some facilities, the incomplete system. This system applies to retrospective analysis. Concurrent analysis is not generally recorded and tracked because the clinician is expected to see the flag the next time he or she reviews the record.

Keeping track of "who did not do what" is a classic application for computerization and was one of the first HIM department functions to become computerized in many facilities. To track deficiencies, the name of the clinician and the type of the deficiency must be captured and recorded on the record and reported to the clinician. Fig. 4.7 depicts a deficiency sheet.

When deficiencies are tracked in a computer, screens are usually organized by chart, with different lines or pages for each physician. Reports can be generated that show deficiencies by clinician, patient record, and type of deficiency.

On a regular basis, typically weekly or biweekly, clinicians are reminded of their incomplete records. This report of incomplete records must be compiled monthly for accreditation purposes. TJC-accredited facilities, for example, must comply with rules covering the maximum allowable number of incomplete records. Because acute care records must be completed within 30 days of discharge, all records incomplete after 30 days of discharge are considered **delinquent**. The maximum number of delinquent records that acute care facilities are permitted equals 50% of their average monthly discharges for the past 12 months (The Joint Commission, 2012). Therefore a facility with an average of 2000 discharges per month would be allowed to have 1000 delinquent records at any given point in time. Facilities can track deficiency rates to ensure compliance by using reports within the EHR. Specific deficiencies, such as missing H&Ps and operative reports, are very serious. Some facilities track these deficiencies separately to ensure that the records are completed in a timely manner (e.g., within

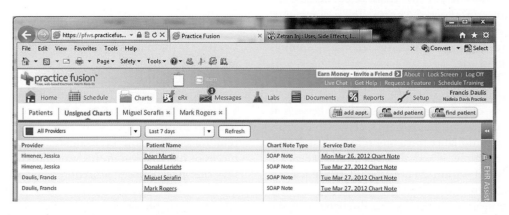

• **Fig. 4.7** A deficiency sheet. (Courtesy Practice Fusion, Inc., San Francisco, CA.)

24 hours of admission or prior to a surgical procedure for H&Ps and immediately after surgery for operative reports).

Each facility has its own policies and procedures for ensuring that records are completed; these depend on the number of incomplete charts, the location of the HIM department, and the historical compliance of clinicians with policies governing record completion.

Electronic records can assist with the tracking of chart completion because the software can identify and report incomplete records. Because certain types of documentation are completed at the point of care, such as physician's orders, nurses' recordings of vital signs, and nursing assessments, authentication is typically affected concurrently with the documentation. Missing components of the documentation can be flagged by alert to the practitioner. Other documentation, such as dictated reports, may be incomplete until it is reviewed and authenticated. In this case, the physician would log into the computer system using a PIN or password, review the document, and give approval for authentication. A report of unsigned documents would help HIMs identify and track incomplete records. Other elements of the medical record, such as progress notes, are more difficult to capture electronically at the point of care. When these elements are still in paper form, some systems allow authentication after scanning; however, the procedure to identify whether the document is complete is manual—whether the analyst is reading a scanned copy of the record or looking at the actual paper. Fig. 4.8 shows a deficiency system on the left prompting the physician to authenticate a scanned progress note on the right.

### Record Completion

Once the deficiencies are identified, the responsible parties are then required to complete the record. The usefulness of requiring clinical staff to authenticate records after discharge is somewhat controversial because the lack of authentication has no clinical significance for patient care. For example, if a physician forgot to sign the progress note of a patient who has already been discharged, what possible impact could the addition of the signature have on the patient 30 days later? Any control function that would have been affected by the physician's signature has been lost. A small benefit may be obtained if the entry is later questioned, because the physician's signature validates the entry. These arguments, of course, are not relevant while licensure and accrediting agencies are still reviewing postdischarge records for compliance with such standards.

On the other hand, an EHR enables some analysis procedures to take place while the patient is still at the facility. This process is called concurrent analysis because it occurs concurrently with the patient's stay. Concurrent analysis facilitates compliance with the intent of authentication rules. For example, if verbal or telephone orders are required to be signed within 24 hours, this deficiency can be identified and corrected within the time frame by concurrent analysis but probably not by postdischarge analysis. In addition, concurrent analysis may speed postdischarge

processing of the record. In an EHR, concurrent flagging of incomplete entries should be automatic. For example, a physician's order entered by the physician will complete itself automatically when the physician finishes the entry. However, a telephone order entered by a nurse on behalf of the physician will be incomplete until the physician's authentication of the order. In a well-designed system, that incomplete order will automatically be flagged and the physician will be alerted on login that there is an order to be signed. Although this automatic flag does not guarantee that the physician will, in fact, review and sign the order on a timely basis, it does alleviate the need to manually review the orders.

It should be noted that concurrent analysis can only look for deficiencies that will have occurred up to that point. For example, 48 hours after admission, the record should certainly contain an H&P, but there will not be a discharge summary because the patient is still in the facility.

The physicians can complete the records electronically and correct their own transcribed documents before signing them. The system can notify the physician that dictation, signatures, and even text are missing. In some facilities, the physician can complete the record remotely: from the private office or even from home. This arrangement eliminates the need for a physician visit to the HIM department. However, it also eliminates the opportunity for HIM personnel to interact with physicians when they visit. When the physician completes the records in the HIM department, procedures are set up to notify the physician of any questions that HIM personnel may have about record completion. Because the physician can complete the EHR from areas other than the HIM department, procedures must be established to notify the physician in some other way about such matters. An alert may pop upon the physician's screen at login or the system may send a secure email alerting the physician that a record needs attention or that someone has a question.

To emphasize the requirement that records be completed properly, Box 4.1 is an excerpt from the CMS State Operations Manual with guidelines for audits of hospitals that describe how an auditor should approach a record review in conformance with regulation.

### Coding

Coding is the representation of diagnoses and procedures as alphanumeric values in order to capture them in the database. Chapter 5 discusses the specific code sets that are typically used for this purpose. For example, diagnosis and procedure codes are used to communicate data about patients among providers, to track and analyze diseases, for reimbursement, and to facilitate research. Standardizing pieces of information in this way allows communication of very specific diagnoses, procedures, and other kinds of clinical data with better control over data quality. For example, an attending physician may request a consultation from a neurologist for evaluation of a patient with Lou Gehrig

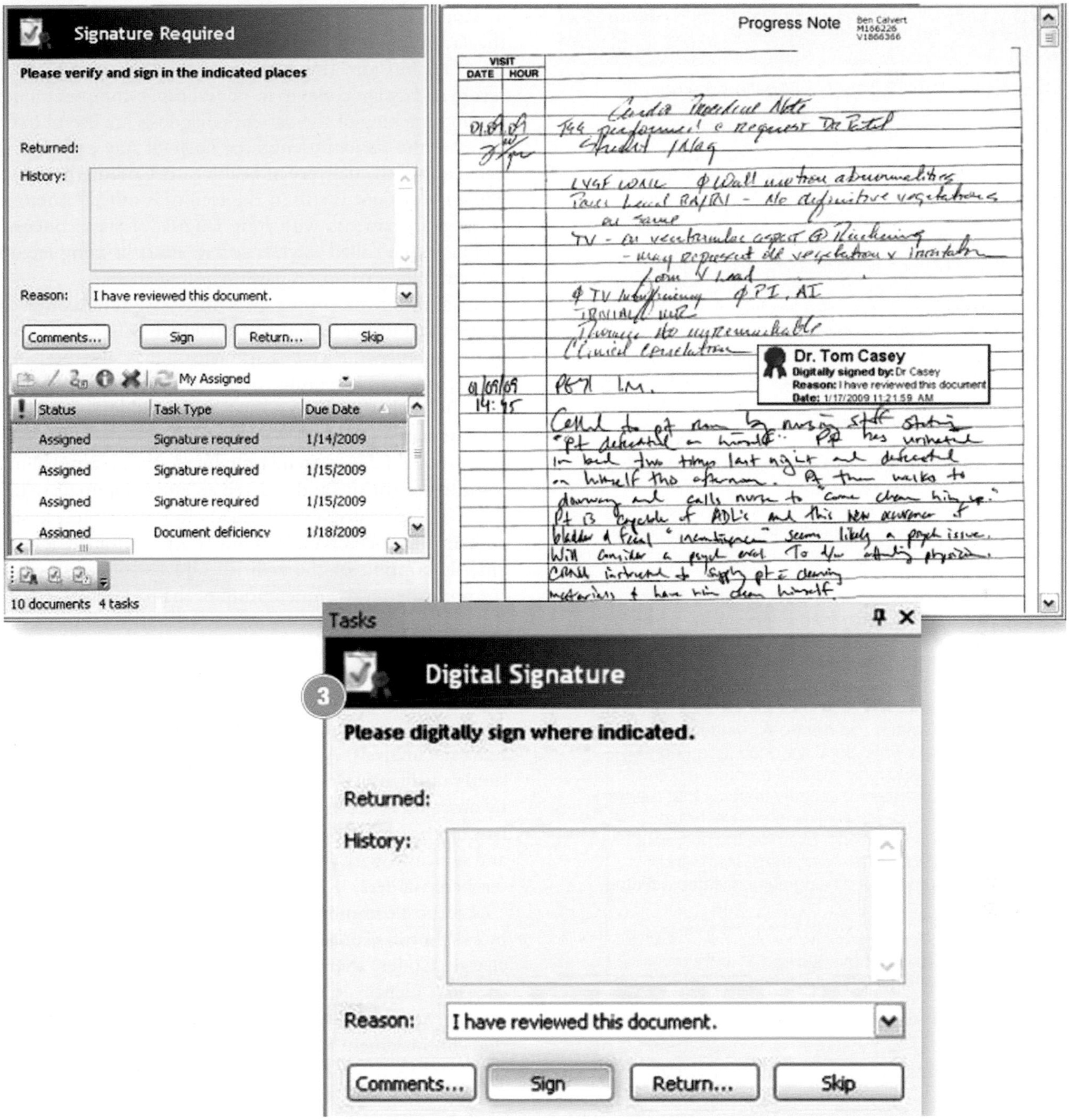

• **Fig. 4.8** The deficiency system alerts the physician to digitally sign a scanned progress note. (Courtesy Perceptive Software, Shawnee, KS.)

disease. At examination, the neurologist diagnoses the patient with amyotrophic lateral sclerosis. Although software can certainly evaluate and match the two names for the same disease, a misspelling of either term could lead to confusion. Assignment of the specific diagnosis code (G12.21) clearly identifies the diagnosis.

There are three times during a patient's encounter with the facility that coding routinely occurs, all of which relate to the physician's development of the diagnosis: on admission, during the stay, and at discharge.

When a patient is being admitted, regardless of the inpatient setting, a physician must state the reason for the admission. The physician's statement of the reason for admission is expressed as a diagnosis—in this case, an admitting or provisional diagnosis. For example, the patient arrives in the emergency department with a complaint, is assessed by the emergency department physician, and is admitted by the attending physician. The emergency department form contains a section for a diagnosis, which is the reason for the emergency department encounter—for example, chest

• BOX 4.1    CMS Guidelines for Complete
Records

*Regulation: 42 CFR §482.24(c)(1) – All patient medical record entries must be legible, complete, dated, timed, and authenticated in written or electronic form by the person responsible for providing or evaluating the service provided, consistent with hospital policies and procedures.* Interpretive Guidelines §482.24(c)(1)

**Survey Procedures**

Review a sample of open and closed medical records.
- Determine whether all medical record entries are legible. Are they clearly written in such a way that they are not likely to be misread or misinterpreted?
- Determine whether orders, progress notes, nursing notes, or other entries in the medical record are complete. Does the medical record contain sufficient information to identify the patient; support the diagnosis/condition; justify the care, treatment, and services; document the course and results of care, treatment, and services; and promote continuity of care among providers?
- Determine whether medical record entries are dated, timed, and appropriately authenticated by the person who is responsible for ordering, providing, or evaluating the service provided.
- Determine whether all orders, including verbal orders, are written in the medical record and signed by the practitioner who is caring for the patient and who is authorized by hospital policy and in accordance with state law to write orders.
- Determine whether the hospital has a means for verifying signatures, both written and electronic, written initials, codes, and stamps when such are used for authorship identification. For electronic medical records, ask the hospital to demonstrate the security features that maintain the integrity of entries and verification of electronic signatures and authorizations. Examine the hospital's policies and procedures for using the system, and determine if documents are being authenticated after they are created.

From CMS Pub 100-7: *State Operations Manual Appendix A Hospitals.* https://www.cms.gov/Regulations-and-Guidance/Guidance/Manuals/downloads/som107ap_a_hospitals.pdf. Accessed December 11, 2018.

pain. The inpatient admitting diagnosis might also be chest pain, or it might be angina or myocardial infarction. The attending physician should state the reason for admission.

In another scenario, a physician sees a patient in his or her office and determines that the patient requires admission, contacts the hospital to make the arrangements for admission, and communicates an admitting diagnosis at that time. At the time of admission, a code should be assigned to the diagnosis so that computer-assisted tracking of the patient's stay can take place. If the admitting diagnosis is expressed only as free text, variations in the expression of the diagnosis impair the ability of the software to match and track the patient's diagnosis with known lengths of stay and clinical treatment plans. Further, if the patient registration staff member merely writes out the words, it is frequently left to the HIM department, after the patient is discharged, to assign a code to the admitting diagnosis.

Codes also may be assigned during the patient's stay in the facility. While the patient is in the facility, there are many reasons for HIM professionals to review the patient's record and assign codes to it. For example, computer matching and tracking of the patient's diagnosis are useful to help estimate the patient's length of hospital stay and thus can help control the delivery of health care. Coding that is done while the patient is still in the facility is called **concurrent coding**. In patients with long lengths of stay, concurrent coding, often called *interim coding*, must be completed for interim billing based on payer requirements.

In addition to coding personnel assigning codes concurrently, another group of individuals, *clinical documentation improvement (CDI)* specialists, may also be reading the records and assigning codes. The fundamental purpose of CDI is to assist physicians in achieving the best possible documentation of their medical decision-making process. Thus a CDI specialist might see that a physician has recorded "arthritis" and ordered an antiinflammatory drug. The CDI specialist would collaborate with the physician to help him or her understand the need for a more specific description of the arthritis and the affected areas of the body. Better documentation of the patient's actual condition, such as "osteoarthritis of the left hip," helps other caregivers understand the patient's needs and helps the coder assign the accurate code for the stay, which facilitates payment from a third-party payer. Furthermore, accuracy of documentation helps to support research and clinical outcome analysis. A CDI specialist's understanding of the needs of all users of clinical data is extremely important in order to function effectively in this role. CDI specialists may be highly experienced coders, nurses, or physicians and typically work in teams and in collaboration with postdischarge coders.

The most common point at which patient charts are coded by HIM professionals is *retrospectively*, after the patient's discharge. Coders then read the entire record and assign the codes to identify the diagnoses and procedures appropriately. In acute care facilities, these postdischarge codes drive the reimbursement to the facility for many payers. Therefore the assignment of postdischarge codes has become a critical revenue cycle function. **Revenue cycle** is the group of processes that identify, record, and report the financial transactions that result from the facility's clinical relationship with a patient (Davis and Doyle, 2016). Fig. 4.9 illustrates the revenue cycle as it relates to an inpatient stay.

In most facilities, the coding function is being assisted by a computer application called an encoder to help assign diagnosis and procedure codes more efficiently and accurately. In order to avoid duplication of effort, such as entering the codes on both the encoder and the abstracting screens, the encoder should interface directly with the abstracting system. The timing of coding is also an issue. In the case of a hybrid record, the coder must use both paper components and electronic record components to identify all of the diagnoses and procedures. If the paper component will be scanned, it might be more efficient for the coding

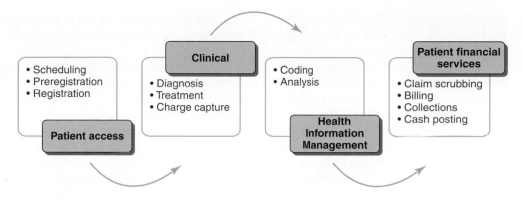

• **Fig. 4.9** A revenue cycle.

personnel to wait until the record is scanned before attempting to code. However, if scanning delays coding beyond the facility's needs, the coders cannot wait for scanning. A fully electronic record eliminates the inefficiency of accommodating paper components and also permits the coding process to migrate to a remote location, as is common with transcription.

When the electronic record is used for coding, the facility may opt to provide large monitors or dual monitors to the coders that give them better visualization of the record and allow them to use two windows at once.

With the availability of electronically captured data, some coding can be automated. As clinicians select diagnoses from drop-down menus, these diagnoses can be captured for billing purposes. Although there is technically no reason for a coder to have to intervene in such a scenario, the reality is that clinicians do not always understand sequencing of codes and billing rules. Therefore review of charts by coders, periodic audits of coded data, and careful attention to billing errors are essential.

For more complex records, *computer-assisted coding* (*CAC*) applications can "read" transcribed documents and assign codes to meaningful phrases. Radiology transcriptions lend themselves to this process, as do operative reports. In a complex inpatient record, a CAC report of coded phrases can facilitate coding by reducing the amount of time a coder has to spend reading detailed reports.

The importance of accurate coding cannot be overemphasized. The capture and reporting of accurate diagnosis and procedure codes enable facilities, payers, government agencies, researchers, and other users to analyze health data over populations and geographic areas. The coded data reported by health care facilities and other providers to payers, government, and regulatory agencies are used to determine reimbursement, monitor patient outcomes, maintain registries, and report quality of care—including adverse events. Knowledgeable individuals, including HIM professionals, who can manage data and can help health care providers identify risks and take preventive action to improve quality, are valuable assets in all of those settings. The process of coding is discussed in greater detail in Chapter 5.

## Master Patient Index Maintenance

As mentioned in Chapter 2, the MPI is the key to locating patient records. The MPI is a database of all patients who have received health care services at the facility.

Data entered into a computerized MPI creates a history for each patient. At registration, the admitting clerk searches the MPI history files to determine whether the patient has been treated at the facility on a previous occasion. If the patient is new, a new history is created. If the patient has been treated at the facility on a previous occasion, the admitting clerk identifies the patient's demographic/financial data history and reviews it to ensure the accuracy of all of the information. Any changes to the patient's address, phone number, or health insurance will be recorded through the registration into the database.

The registration procedure of searching for prior visits is a preventive control. Failure to identify a prior visit will result in the assignment of an additional MRN for the patient. The presence of multiple MRNs for the same patient breaks the continuity of both patient care and billing history. Previous records are not automatically available for review by clinical personnel, and prior outstanding balances on patient accounts will not be noted at registration. Thus despite a patient's assertion that he or she has not visited the facility previously, a registration clerk is required to search for the patient, just to be sure.

In the future, widespread use of person identification systems, such as biometrics (e.g., identification through retinal scanning or fingerprints), may provide improved preventive control against duplicate MRNs. Such systems, although available, are not in widespread use in health care at this time (Harris and Houser, 2018).

Despite the best efforts of registration personnel, duplicate medical records are sometimes mistakenly assigned. The reasons for this are many but are commonly due to clerical errors, spelling issues, and erroneous data entry during the previous registration. Consequently, a detective control must be in place to find duplicates and correct them. The search for, analysis of, and correction of duplicate MRNs for the same patient are typically the responsibility of the HIM department.

Periodically, a search is done to identify duplicate MRNs. The search generally consists of reviewing a report that lists potential duplicates. This report can be a preprogrammed function in the hospital system itself. Alternatively, key administrative and demographic data can be downloaded and analyzed by an external system. There are many external consulting firms that assist with this function. The analysis of the data consists of identifying potential matches in data fields that are unlikely to be identical between two different patients. If the social security number (SSN) is collected and two accounts are associated with the same SSN, then those accounts should be reviewed as being potential duplicates. Key data fields that are compared include name, address, and date of birth. Because addresses and phone numbers change, date of birth is more important than address in predicting a potential duplicate.

Once a list of potential duplicate MRNs is identified, the HIM professional must review the patient records to determine whether they are the same patient. If there is a duplicate, the records are then merged. The merging of two patient records is a serious matter. Although the merge is affected by the press of a button, it is permanent. Therefore extreme care must be taken to ensure that the merge is correct. The decision of which MRN will survive the merge (retain the records) is guided by hospital policy and procedure.

Duplicate MRNs are problematic for individual providers. They become more problematic in the event of a merger of systems. If both systems have a high percentage of duplicate records, merging of the systems is not recommended (Harris and Houser, 2018). Another use for programs that analyze duplicate MRNs is in patient matching. For example, the health information exchange (HIE) storing records from different providers will likely receive patient data from multiple systems. In each of those systems, the patient will have an MRN unique to that patient. Because the MRN is unique to the facility, it cannot be used as a match between different organizations. Therefore the HIE must use a patient-matching algorithm to identify all of a patient's data.

Patient-matching algorithms, such as identifying matching patient demographic data, are an important component of interoperability. Exact matching of patient demographic data is an example of the deterministic method of patient matching. The deterministic method requires that there be unique fields to match, such as SSN, MRN, or account number. This method works fairly well when linking data generated within the facility or by contributors to the patient record, such as external transcription services. It does not work as well between different organizations where the patient's record is not necessarily available for comparison. For example, a blood test result can be transmitted electronically to a physician office or other provider. The recipient does not necessarily have sufficient detail in the transmission to make an automatic match with the patient, necessitating manual intervention to research. Further,

deterministic matching may miss potential matches due to errors (such as spelling and last name) on either side of the transaction.

A matching method that broadens the search for a match is the probabilistic method. This type of algorithm looks for matches not just on exact matches in certain fields but also on the probability of the patients being the same due to other characteristics being the same or similar. For example, two patients with the same name but different birthdates might be matched if the birthdates are similar: 2/12/67 versus 12/2/67. A higher probability of a match would be assigned if the patient addresses also matched. A low probability of a match would be assigned if the patient addresses and other demographic data did not match.

## Abstracting

HIM professionals are uniquely trained to perform functions that require identification of the best source of data. Coding is one such function. Abstracting is another. The term abstracting refers to a number of activities in which specific data are located in the record and summarized in another document or database. The necessity for abstracting arises for various reasons, including data transfer, volume reduction, discharge data sets, and analysis. Two activities are called abstracting. One occurs during postdischarge processing, after coding. The other occurs as a data-retrieval activity.

### Abstracting as a Component of Postdischarge Processing

Patient health data are gathered at admission and throughout the course of the patient's care. In the paper environment, once the patient is discharged, the HIM employee must review key elements in the patient record to ensure that they are present and accurately recorded in the computer system. For example, the MRN, account number, discharge disposition, and admitting diagnosis are typically reviewed and corrected as needed. In an EHR, most of the data is already captured, and the HIM employee verifies the abstract. The abstract can be defined as a summary of the patient's encounter. Verification of the abstract is a detective control. Fixing any noted errors is a corrective control. It provides a brief synopsis of the patient's care that would otherwise require a thorough review of the entire patient record. The abstract typically contains the key demographic field, the physician data, diagnosis and procedure codes, dates of service, and discharge disposition.

To complete an abstract, the HIM clerk must review the health record. The review is necessary to determine the appropriate data element for each field. As previously discussed, the HIM coder must review the record to determine the accurate code (ICD-10-CM/PCS or CPT) to represent the patient's diagnosis and procedures. To make this determination, the coder relies on the documentation in the record and his or her knowledge of coding. In addition to adding codes and related data, the coder will validate some data such as the identification of the attending physician and the discharge disposition.

If the data in a paper-based record are to be transmitted electronically, the data must be transferred from the paper record to the electronic medium. The data are located in the record and copied into the system through data entry. An abstractor reviews the record and enters the desired data into fields in an abstracting form. Sometimes an interim step is performed in which the data are transcribed to a form as they are located and then entered all at once into the computer. Diagnosis and procedure codes are often captured this way, as are surgical procedure dates and physician identification numbers.

Fig. 4.10 is an example of a patient abstract screen. Note the information required in the abstract: patient's name, address, admission and discharge dates, discharge disposition, diagnosis, procedure, procedure date, and physicians' names. The demographic data and financial data are populated into the abstract at registration. Nursing personnel typically complete the discharge date, time, and status. HIM personnel enter the diagnostic and procedural data and validate the existing data before billing.

### Abstracting the Record for Data Retrieval

Another reason for abstracting is to reduce the volume of data. There is often far more data in a health record than is needed for a particular user. For example, a patient keeping a file of his or her health records at home (a personal health record) would not usually need an entire copy of the record. The patient may need only a copy of the discharge summary or the operative records. These data could be abstracted for the patient. In this process, rather than the addition of data to the record, selected parts of the data are copied—to either a paper or an electronic file.

Finally, health data are frequently analyzed for other purposes, such as research and quality measures. In this type of abstracting, patient records are reviewed for specific data elements, which are then recorded on a data-collection sheet for subsequent analysis. One common reason for this analysis is to check whether physicians are following national standardized practices for care, called *Core Measures*, which have been proven to lead to better patient outcomes. For example, all patients with a diagnosis of acute cerebrovascular infarction should receive diagnostic and therapeutic care related to stroke care. The abstracter reviews records of all patients with stroke to identify whether the specific tests were performed and specific medications given. Compliance with the Core Measures is reported to the CMS and TJC for quality review purposes. In this way, patients can compare facilities to see how well each hospital complies with Core Measures. The facilities themselves can look at their compliance over time to see whether they are improving. Agencies such as TJC and CMS periodically review the effectiveness

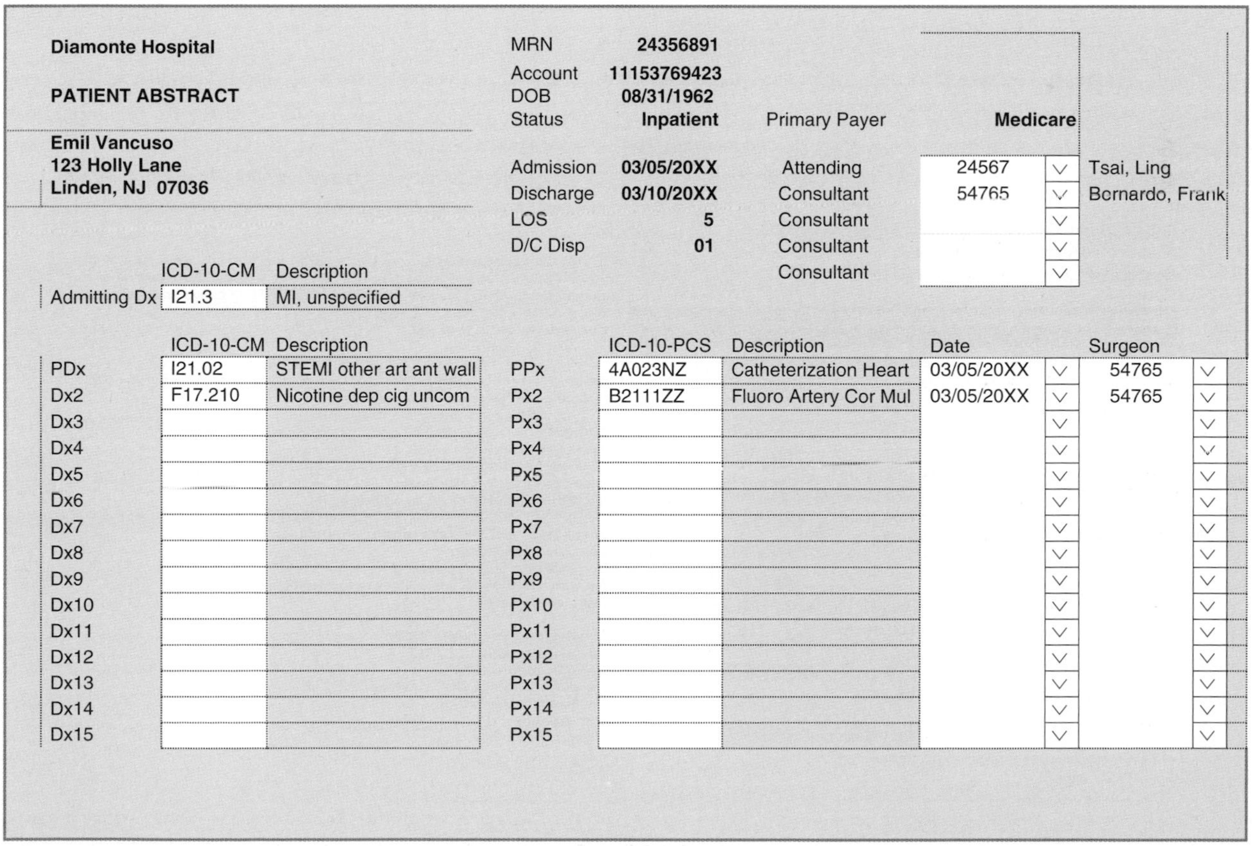

**Diamonte Hospital**

**PATIENT ABSTRACT**

**Emil Vancuso**
**123 Holly Lane**
**Linden, NJ 07036**

| | | | | |
|---|---|---|---|---|
| MRN | **24356891** | | | |
| Account | **11153769423** | | | |
| DOB | **08/31/1962** | | | |
| Status | **Inpatient** | Primary Payer | **Medicare** | |
| Admission | **03/05/20XX** | Attending | 24567 | Tsai, Ling |
| Discharge | **03/10/20XX** | Consultant | 54765 | Bernardo, Frank |
| LOS | **5** | Consultant | | |
| D/C Disp | **01** | Consultant | | |
| | | Consultant | | |

| | ICD-10-CM | Description |
|---|---|---|
| Admitting Dx | I21.3 | MI, unspecified |

| | ICD-10-CM | Description | | ICD-10-PCS | Description | Date | Surgeon |
|---|---|---|---|---|---|---|---|
| PDx | I21.02 | STEMI other art ant wall | PPx | 4A023NZ | Catheterization Heart | 03/05/20XX | 54765 |
| Dx2 | F17.210 | Nicotine dep cig uncom | Px2 | B2111ZZ | Fluoro Artery Cor Mul | 03/05/20XX | 54765 |
| Dx3 | | | Px3 | | | | |
| Dx4 | | | Px4 | | | | |
| Dx5 | | | Px5 | | | | |
| Dx6 | | | Px6 | | | | |
| Dx7 | | | Px7 | | | | |
| Dx8 | | | Px8 | | | | |
| Dx9 | | | Px9 | | | | |
| Dx10 | | | Px10 | | | | |
| Dx11 | | | Px11 | | | | |
| Dx12 | | | Px12 | | | | |
| Dx13 | | | Px13 | | | | |
| Dx14 | | | Px14 | | | | |
| Dx15 | | | Px15 | | | | |

• **Fig. 4.10** An abstract screen.

of such interventions based on data elements related to patient outcomes.

Besides databases for Core Measures, patient records are abstracted for **registries**—collections of data specific to a disease, diagnosis, or procedure. Common registries are the tumor or cancer registry, trauma registry, AIDS registry, birth defect registry, and implant registry. The data are collected specific to the diagnosis, disease, or implant so that users can compare, analyze, or study the groups of patients. A registry is maintained by an agency external to the facility or provider and characteristically requires active follow-up of the reported cases. Participation in the registry may be mandatory or voluntary.

Abstracters comb clinical documentation for data elements related to any of several diseases and disorders, often using laboratory results and progress notes to detect onset of symptoms and changes in patient status. In many cases, this is a completely manual process by the abstractor, but some organizations are beginning to use software to help

summarize longitudinal patient records. In Fig. 4.11, software called HARVEST scans all types of documentation in a patient's record. It creates a "word cloud" of the most commonly documented problems based on their frequency and returns all the documentation that mentions the selected term. In this case, the researcher is looking at any documentation that mentions lupus, or systemic lupus erythematosus (Pivovarov et al., 2016).

HIM professionals are well suited by their training to be involved in these abstracting functions. Although data abstracting is a traditional HIM function, regulatory and research analysis activities are well within the scope of HIM professional capabilities. Knowledge of the components of the record and an understanding of the clinical documentation content are core competencies for HIM professionals. Development of analytical skill sets, including clinical data analysis and regulatory reporting requirements, is useful for professionals who wish to move their careers in this direction.

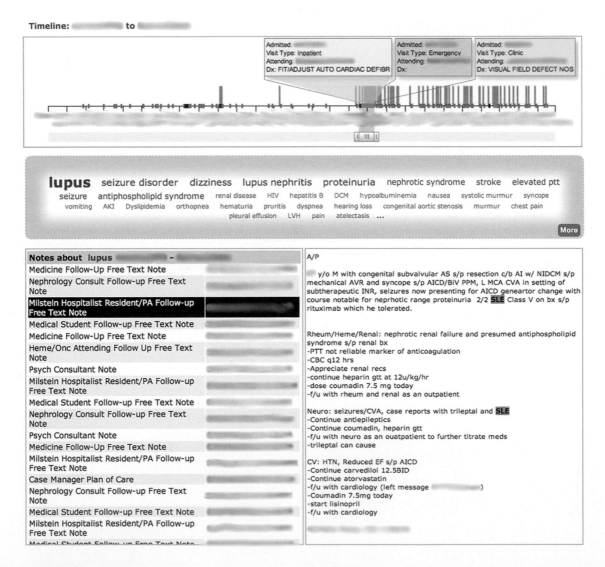

• **Fig. 4.11** The HARVEST software extracts data about lupus from many different pieces of documentation in the health record. (Courtesy Noémie Elhadad, Columbia University.)

## Tracking Records While Processing

While the patient is in the facility, the responsibility for maintaining his or her record rests with clinical staff members, particularly nursing and patient unit clerical staff members. Traditionally, in a paper-based environment, the HIM department assumes control once the patient is discharged. In an EHR environment, a number of departments may control aspects of the record. Because the record never actually moves from the computer, the physical location of the record is not in question. However, a paper-based record moves virtually every time an individual touches it. Therefore keeping track of it requires control procedures.

### Batch by Days

One way to keep track of paper records during postdischarge processing is to batch the records together by day. In this method, all records of discharges from April 15, for example, are gathered and kept together as they are moved as a group through assembly, analysis, and coding. At the end of the process, they are separated according to completion status. Completed charts are moved to the permanent file or scanning area for storage; incomplete charts are moved to the incomplete chart area. This same batch process is used to keep track of paper documents that must be scanned. A **batch control form** lists the processing status of each record. This is particularly helpful if the record must be removed from the processing cycle for any reason.

Records may be removed from the processing cycle for various reasons. The patient may have been readmitted, requiring review of the previous record. The record may need to be reviewed for quality assurance by another department, such as nursing. When the record is removed from the processing cycle, a batch control sheet clearly highlights the status of the record and facilitates its return to the appropriate processing step.

### Efficiency

To facilitate the many uses of the health record, related documents must be processed in a timely manner. It may make sense in some facilities that one must obtain the record in order to assemble it, assemble the record in order to analyze it, and analyze the record in order to code it. In some facilities, all personnel perform all of the steps. In other facilities, the chart is coded before analysis. All facilities process the health record in the way that best suits their particular workflows and revenue cycle needs. For efficient processing, the paper record should be moved as little as possible, and each step should be performed in its entirety before the next step is attempted. In an EHR environment, some processes, such as analysis and coding, can take place concurrently. Many facilities maintain a central staging area, where paper records in process are kept between steps. This approach facilitates the location of records and their movement to the next processing step. Fig. 4.4 illustrates the most efficient postdischarge processing flow, which emphasizes scanning and analysis of the record prior to coding. Ideally, the chart should be complete prior to

coding. By at least scanning and analyzing the record prior to coding, the coder can be more confident of the administrative details, such as physician attribution and discharge disposition, and can focus on the clinical documentation.

## Transcription

The way in which the transcribed report moves to the EHR is an important issue to consider. The hybrid or electronic record will have the transcribed reports available for viewing on the health record as soon as the report is released by the transcriptionist. In some cases, signature deficiencies can be assigned automatically when the document moves from the transcription system to the EHR system. Additionally, with a speech-recognition interface at the point of dictation (front-end), the dictator can view the transcribed document while dictating and make changes concurrently (Fig. 4.12).

Another issue to consider is whether the physicians can correct the transcribed reports electronically. If electronic corrections are allowed, do the different versions of the report need to be saved? Can corrections be made after a digital signature is applied or only before? If such corrections are not allowed, how will corrections be made? For documents with different versions, what type of an audit trail will the system maintain in order to keep track of which version was available at a particular point in time? What about transcribed reports generated from different systems, such as radiology and cardiology? How will these reports be interfaced with the main system? If front-end speech recognition is used, what quality controls will be implemented to ensure complete, properly formatted reports?

Clearly, there are many questions to be answered when dealing with transcribed documents. One key issue when paper-based records are still in use is: Will physicians be required to dictate certain reports or will they still have the option to write out their reports by hand, if desired? For most dictated reports, the cost of transcription is not the issue. The clarity achieved by having a typed document is worth the cost. The author must review the typed document for accuracy, thereby providing an audit of the reports—an important detective and corrective control. However, in a teaching facility where residents are also preparing reports, the cost may become prohibitive. Templates and menu-driven reports may be alternatives to free-form dictation in some cases.

## Workflow

In the paper context, **workflow** refers to the way in which the paper record is processed from one HIM function to another or moved from one desk to another. In the electronic context, workflow describes how the electronic record moves from one electronic component to another. Once a function is completed, the electronic record may automatically be sent to the appropriate work areas. These electronic work areas are called **queues**. An example of an HIM queue would be the coding queue or the analysis queue. Queues can be further defined (e.g., a coding queue may be called an

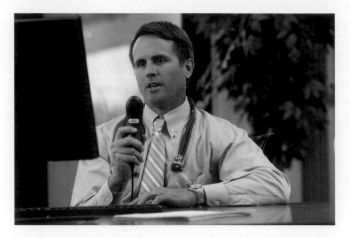

• **Fig. 4.12** A physician dictates directly into the health record at the point of care. (Courtesy Nuance Communications, Inc., Burlington, MA.)

*outpatient coding queue*). Individual coders may be assigned records automatically on the basis of predetermined criteria, such as type of record, may select records from the queue, or may be assigned records manually by the supervisor. These queues are an important workflow distribution tool. Supervisors can manage the workflow among coders, for example, and track the time items spend in queue. Queues are common in coding, transcription, and billing activities.

When an action is completed in a queue, the workflow software sends the electronic record to the next work area or queue. For example, when the coder has completed the abstract, the record may be routed to the coding supervisor for review. If the supervisor identifies an error, the record may then be routed back to the coder for correction. Other possible routing includes postdischarge review by documentation improvement specialists, pending query to physician, or finalize for billing.

Note that the record does not actually move in a completely electronic system. Workflow distribution in this context is a communication tool that alerts a specific user that there is a task to be performed. Once it is performed, the next user is notified. Some users may be able to work concurrently. For example, incomplete chart analysts may be able to work with the record at the same time the record is being coded. Physicians can certainly be reviewing and signing documents while the record is in process. In other cases, tasks may be sequential, such as scanning being followed by coding (particularly if the coder is working remotely).

Workflow issues are complex and must be carefully planned. It must be decided what queues will be included and, more important, which staff members will be responsible for working the numerous queues. *Error* or *pending queues*, for example, are an important control function. A transcribed report goes to the queue when the HIM interface cannot identify the physician's name. HIM personnel review the report and route the report to the correct patient record.

A simple example of workflow in an EHR is shown in Fig. 4.13.

 **COMPETENCY CHECK-IN 4.2**

**Postdischarge Processing**

**Competency Assessment**

1. Summarize the steps in postdischarge processing.
2. Using _____, many paper documents can be loaded into the scanner at once, after which software sorts the documents into the correct record by bar code.
3. In the process called _____, the technician assigns the free text of a nursing progress note into the relevant area of the EHR so that it can be found in the nursing progress notes section of the record.
4. The orthopedic surgeon's physician assistant (PA) records a progress note, which the surgeon must then _____ to provide evidence that the PA was supervised.
5. Because acute care records must be completed within 30 days of discharge, all records incomplete after 30 days of discharge are considered _____.
6. The word _____ means that something is taking place during the patient's stay.
7. In most facilities, the coding function is being assisted with a computer application called a(n) _____ to help assign diagnosis and procedure codes more efficiently and accurately.
8. Cases of birth defects are abstracted and recorded in a(n) _____.
9. The software alerts Ginny that there are three records ready for her to code in the coding _____.
10. Patient matching is important to resolve _____
11. Two algorithms for patient matching are _____.

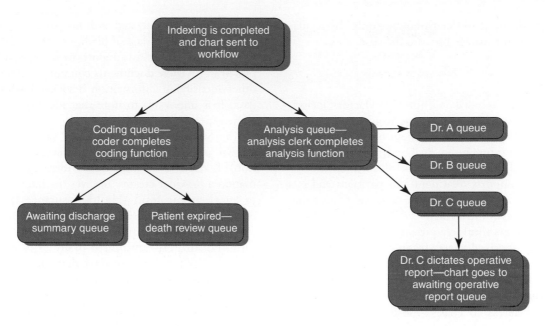

• **Fig. 4.13** A simple example of workflow in an electronic health record.

## Record Integrity and Access

The **retention** of health records, and the ability to retrieve those records efficiently, is traditionally the responsibility of HIM professionals. Retention refers to all of the policies and procedures governing the storage of records, including how long the records will be kept, where and how they will be stored, and how they will be protected. In an EHR environment, storage is electronic, as discussed in Chapter 2. HIM professionals must understand the EHR for the purpose of both using the records for administrative purposes and ensuring the appropriate access to the data therein.

### Storage and Retention

In order to use or access a record, it has to be available. Some parts of a record, such as the MPI, are retained in perpetuity (i.e., forever). However, depending on state regulations and the needs of the organization, some parts of a patient record may be destroyed when they are no longer considered useful.

Key concepts to understand in the retention of records include the following:

*Storage*: maintaining the record appropriately and for the necessary amount of time,

*Security*: preventing accidental destruction or inappropriate viewing or use of records, and

*Access*: ensuring that the record is readily available should it be needed.

Table 4.4 summarizes the components of record retention. Members of the HIM department and facility staff must adhere to requirements for record retention. These requirements vary from state to state (AHIMA).

| TABLE 4.4 | Components of Record Retention | |
|---|---|
| **Component** | **Description** |
| Storage | Compiling, indexing or cataloging, and maintaining a physical or electronic location for data |
| Security | Safety and confidentiality of data (see Chapter 8) |
| Access | Ability to retrieve data; release of data only to appropriate individuals or other entities (see Chapters 8 and 9) |

During conversion to a hybrid or an electronic record, policies and procedures must be established to define what constitutes the legal health record. In a hybrid system, this definition should be specified by hospital policy. In the hybrid record in which a paper chart is generated and then scanned into the electronic record, policies must specify what will happen to the paper record. The policy must address whether the paper record will be destroyed or maintained in offsite storage. Retention issues must be addressed in the policy, such as the length of time that the paper record will be maintained in storage before it is destroyed, as well as how long patient records will be available. As we will see, the patient's health record must be retained for the continuity of care and for reimbursement, accreditation, potential litigation, research, and education purposes.

With the development and implementation of "cloud" storage through offsite servers, there are fewer limitations on the volume of data that can be stored over time. Nevertheless, storage is not free, so an organization that uses offsite storage will need to determine not only the regulatory requirements for storage but also the cost.

## Retrieval

The need for retrieval is based on a number of factors, including continuing patient care. If no one would ever need to look at the record again after the patient has gone home, it would not need to be organized, analyzed, or stored. As previously mentioned, however, the health record is the business record that supports treatment and payment and is a critical communication tool; it will be reviewed many times after the patient leaves the facility.

HIM departments routinely provide health information on request to authorized users. In an electronic environment, access controls are accomplished by login protocols (user ID and password) and the restriction of access based on the user's work (role-based access). Thus business office personnel need access to charges posted in the patient's account but do not necessarily need access to the clinical record. Similarly, a physical therapist would not routinely be given access to the patient's account but would need access to both view the patient's clinical record and create entries in the physical therapy section of the clinical record.

## Security and Privacy

In addition to internal access, the HIM department provides access, including viewing and reporting of data, to external users, including the patient. The Health Insurance Portability and Accountability Act (HIPAA) is federal legislation that ensures equal access to certain health and human services and protects the privacy and security of health information. Any organization that obtains and manages health information must comply with HIPAA privacy and security regulations. These groups are known as *covered entities* and include providers, health insurers, and health care clearinghouses. Business associates must also comply. *Business associates* are those contracted vendors that use confidential health information to perform a service on behalf of the covered entity.

Two major components of HIPAA are known as the Privacy Rule and the Security Rule. These portions of the regulation address how organizations protect health information from unauthorized access while maintaining the integrity of the record. Record **integrity** refers to the idea that regardless of the format, the record is complete, reliable, and consistent. A record that can be accessed and changed by unauthorized persons lacks integrity.

The Privacy Rule recognizes the importance of protecting the confidentiality of patient health information while allowing some information to be shared in the delivery of patient care and in the interest of public health. It limits the communication of all **protected health information (PHI)**, defined as health data that can be connected to an individual. Providers and personnel must keep strictly confidential any information concerning the patient's health status when it is associated with the patient's name, address, telephone number, date of birth, or other identification. A health record, laboratory report, or hospital bill are examples of PHI. These documents contain a patient's name and other identifying information associated with the health data. It is important to note that identifying information alone is not designated as PHI.

The Security Rule focuses on a subset of information known as *e-PHI* (electronic protected health information). It refers to all individually identifiable health information a provider creates, receives, maintains, or transmits in an electronic form (Health Insurance Portability and Accountability Act, 2004). The Security Rule applies only to the transmission of health information in electronic form, not to PHI transmitted orally or in writing. e-PHI encompasses any piece of data that identifies the patient and is considered electronic. If an email is sent, for example, and it includes the patient's name or other identifying information, it is considered e-PHI. The Security Rule requires that facilities identify all systems that contain e-PHI and perform a risk assessment to identify areas that may pose a security risk. This risk analysis enables the organization to evaluate what security measures are necessary and appropriate, and to operationalize those measures effectively through the development, implementation, and maintenance of security protections. It requires health care facilities to have administrative, technical, and physical safeguards in place to ensure privacy and safeguard information whether it is on paper or in an electronic format.

Administrative safeguards include policies and procedures regarding confidentiality and security agreements signed by each staff member and by any nonstaff member users of the medical record. Organizations must also establish personnel responsible for administering security initiatives. This individual is named the security officer.

Administrative safeguards address training personnel on security regulations, including sanctions for violations and continuous evaluation of the security program. The following topics are important and should be included in training:

- How to guard against threats of computer viruses or hackers and where to report suspicious activity.
- Routine performance of audits to ensure that employees are using PHI on a need-to-know basis and that actions have been taken if inappropriate viewing or use of PHI is found.
- Education on how to dispose of PHI on paper or electronic media such as optical disks.
- Management of passwords: how often they will change and sanctions for sharing passwords.

Technical safeguards are addressed in detail in HIPAA's Security Rule. Technical safeguards include controlling access through the use of user identification (user ID) and password creation and maintenance. The organization must train employees in proper protection of their user IDs and passwords. This includes not sharing them with other employees or individuals, refraining from writing the information down, and using proper techniques for changing and resetting passwords. A technical safeguard that can be applied to the entire EHR is automatic log-offs. If a computer idles for more than a specific number of minutes, it will automatically log the user off. Another example of a technical safeguard is a procedure to deny system access immediately upon employee termination. Some facilities may also use encryption of data as a technical safeguard. **Encryption** is computerized scrambling of information to make it unrecognizable except to the intended recipient. To read an encrypted file, you must have access to a secret key or password that enables you to read it. Firewalls (electronic blocks) are preventive techniques that can help prevent unauthorized access as well.

Physical safeguards must be established to protect unauthorized access to areas or systems containing PHI. If a paper-generated record is used, locked doors are used as barriers to protect the information. The following are examples of physical safeguards in an electronic context:

- securing the physical locations of workstations, storage devices, and servers;
- placing sensors on portable devices such as laptops and tablets that sound an alarm if the devices are taken off the premises;
- placing computer monitors in areas that minimize the chance that a stranger could view confidential information;
- controlling the use of portable storage devices such as flash drives, compact disks, and cell phones; and
- using a dark screen monitor cover to prevent passersby from seeing data on the screen (Fig. 4.14).

If an unauthorized user gains access to e-PHI, the event is known as a **breach**. If a breach affects less than 500 patients, the organization must notify the individuals whose information was breached and the secretary of the Department of Health and Human Services (DHHS). In the instance that a breach affects more than 500 patients, the organization is required to notify the individuals, the secretary, and the news media. All reported security breaches affecting more than 500 patients can be viewed on the DHHS website (Health Insurance Portability and Accountability Act, 2004).

## Release of Information

The function of retrieving the health record and providing it, or parts of it, to individuals who need it is commonly called **release of information (ROI)** and requires access to the stored records. We have already discussed authorized access to the data itself. ROI more commonly refers to the provision of patient records to external users, such as the patient, lawyers, and third-party payers.

There are generally five steps to the ROI process:
1. Receive the request for information—usually a form with patient's consent.
2. Validate the request—making sure that requests have the proper consent from the patient or other authorized individual and that the request has all of the proper components.
3. Acquire the information—identifying and printing or downloading the requested information.
4. Distribute information—delivering the information via the requested means (e.g., mailing, electronic transmission).
5. Recording of the details of steps 1–4.

The requirements for ROI are discussed in detail in Chapter 8. For the purpose of this discussion, note that to satisfy the request for information, the HIM professional must understand the contents of the record, where to find it, and whether the record is complete. The completeness of a record is dependent on a number of factors, including organizational policies, regulations, and accreditation standards. As we have been discussing, there are numerous components to a health record. While the quantitative analyst is responsible for identifying missing components, the ROI professional is responsible for ensuring that incomplete records are released within policy, which may dictate special steps if a requested record is incomplete.

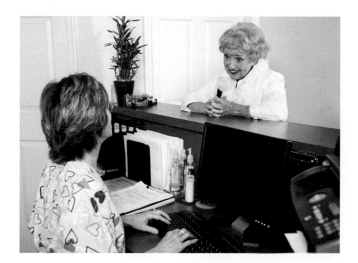

• **Fig. 4.14** Monitors in the medical setting are positioned to minimize the possibility of unauthorized persons seeing what is on the screen. The monitor appears black to anyone but the person sitting in front of the terminal. (Copyright lisafx/iStockphoto.com.)

❖ **COMPETENCY CHECK-IN 4.3**

**Record Integrity and Access**

**Competency Assessment**

1. A(n) _____ is an individual designated to enforce HIPAA compliance in the facility.
2. The _____ Rule requires that facilities identify all systems that contain e-PHI and perform a risk assessment to identify areas that may pose a security risk.
3. Some organizations store all their digital patient records in the _____, which is storage on offsite servers.
4. Before anyone can work at the imaging center, they must attend an orientation that includes several hours of HIPAA training. This is an example of a(n) _____ safeguard.
5. If an unauthorized user gains access to the e-PHI, the event is known as a _____.

## Network Policies

One of the significant effects of the EHR on HIM practice has been the elimination of some traditional roles, such as filing of paper records, and the evolution of new roles, such as scanning. In addition to these effects, the EHR has also freed HIM departments to allow employees to work from home and to contract with vendors who are not present in the facility. Employees who establish appropriate safeguards and work habits at home may find that they enjoy the lack of commute. Vendors may employ staff throughout the country and even the world to provide services remotely to client organizations and other providers.

Any function that is performed electronically can theoretically also be accomplished remotely. The decision to allow a function to be performed remotely is a difficult one. The organization gives up a certain amount of control over the employee or contractor but may gain financially, operationally, or both, as workers may be available at all times, day and night, all year round. For example, ROI contractors no longer have to be present in the facility in order to process requests for information. In addition, coders can do their work effectively and efficiently offsite, with access to the facility's systems from home. We will continue to explore remote workers as we move into more detailed discussions of HIM functions.

One of the key issues that must be resolved in an electronic environment is how to communicate and share data securely. Within the organization, communication among employees and access to important documentation, such as policies and procedures, is often accomplished via an intranet. An intranet is a system that generally requires identification and a password and is used by employees and others who may be acting as employees, such as administrative contractors, who require access to internal documentation. Other individuals who may need access to specific types of information can be granted access through an extranet. An extranet usually requires identification and a password as well, but the types of information that can be accessed are restricted to only that which is needed by the individual. See Chapter 2 for a discussion of assignment of access by role. Intranet and extranet applications and electronic data management can be housed either on a

local server or in the cloud. Intranet access can be restricted to hardwired terminals within the facility or via Wi-Fi on mobile devices. The issue is what level of security is necessary. Using a coder as an example, consider what a coder has to do: review the patient record, assign codes, maybe communicate with a physician, and possibly research a clinical or policy issue. In order to accomplish those tasks, the coder will have to access the EHR, the encoder, the email or intranet, and possibly an Internet browser. The facility has to trust that the coder will not use the Internet inappropriately and will not download or print confidential patient information. To support the organization's trust in the coder, there must be policies and procedures in place to expressly define the rules related to accessing various systems. Some policies that are typically in place include the following:

- The Internet may not be used to access social media.
- Users may not download documents from the Internet.
- Users must not open email from unknown senders.
- PHI may only be communicated via the Secure Mail System.

We will discuss policies and procedures in greater detail in Chapter 9.

## Uses of Health Information

The uses of health information can be classified as internal or external to the health care facility. Here is a list of some internal health care facility uses:

- to improve patient care;
- to support and collect reimbursement;
- to support and prove compliance for licensing, accreditation, and certification;
- to support the administration of the facility;
- to provide evidence in litigation; and
- to educate future health care professionals.

Agencies outside the health care facility (external) use health information for the following reasons:

- to study the mortality rates and the prevalence and incidence of morbidity;
- to support litigation;
- to develop community awareness of health care issues;

- to support the personal health record, patient portal, and health literacy initiatives;
- to influence national policy on health care issues through legislation;
- to educate patients and health care professionals; and
- to develop health care products.

Many of these uses are discussed in more detail later.

## Improving Patient Care

Health information is used to improve the quality of care provided to patients. Many people have been in a health care facility and thought that a few things could have been improved. For instance, did the patient have to wait too long to see the physician? Was communication among the health care professionals inadequate? There may have even been an impression that no one knew exactly what was going on. Historically, HIM professionals have reviewed the documentation of patient health care after the patient is discharged to determine whether patients received appropriate care.

## Education

Health information is used in the education of health care professionals and patients. For example, physicians, nurses, physical therapists, and pharmacists need health information for instruction and examples as they learn how to perform their duties. The documentation of past occurrences provides an excellent opportunity to show others how to handle patient care in the future. Medical institutions use case studies of patients to teach new students about a disease process. Health care professionals are required to earn continuing education credits in their fields to keep their credentials current and to comply with professional standards. These professionals perform case studies on new and intriguing cases or present new technology for the education of their peers.

Likewise, health information is presented to patients and the community to inform them of the prevention, causes, incidence, and treatment for many diseases. This use of health information involves research, statistics, and information on new technology for treatment or prevention of disease.

### Patient Education

Another aspect of education is assisting patients to obtain control of their health care in a variety of ways made feasible by the EHR. As we have mentioned, patients are increasingly able to access their health records through patient portals into the provider's system. These portals allow patients to view their own data, and to send messages and make appointments. Providers typically do not grant access to the entire record, but rather to a subset of the record, which may include laboratory and radiology reports, as well as problem lists.

Payers also offer online access for subscribers to communicate with the payer and also to obtain assistance and information about healthy habits and lifestyle support for those with chronic conditions. Facilitating patient awareness and education in this manner supports health literacy. Health literacy is the ability of a patient to obtain, process, and understand basic information about their condition or that of an individual for whom they are caring. Health literacy is fundamental to compliance with medication and disease-management instructions, for example. Patients with poor health literacy may find it difficult to make lifestyle changes, since they may not understand how their behavior is having a negative impact on their health. A patient with poor health literacy may struggle to understand discharge instructions, which may lead to a relapse or even readmission to the hospital. Furthermore, health literacy is necessary for patient understanding of the risks and benefits of potential treatments.

The federal government has developed an initiative to help increase patients' access to their own health data. The Blue Button Pledge is a voluntary mechanism by which organizations commit to advance efforts to increase patient access to and use of their own health data to improve their health and health care experience. Participating organizations take steps to make a patient's record (or subset of it) available in a secure fashion and encourage consumer engagement with health information (Office of the National Coordinator for Health Information Technology [ONC], 2019).

Access by patients to their data in an HIE is another development. The HIE collects patient data into its system, storing the patient data and making it available to authorized users. Patient access to that data facilitates health care outside the range of the HIE and gives the patient a role in validating the data.

We have discussed the role of mobile technology in collecting and accessing data as it pertains to telehealth. However, there is a growing set of unregulated databases collecting data about individuals' health: exercise and fitness apps. From step counters to heart rate monitors and exercise bikes to diet apps, organizations with no health care regulatory compliance obligation are collecting these data. One burning question is whether these data are useful in the context of the patient's overall care. Can and should these data be a part of the patient's longitudinal record?

## Support and Collection of Reimbursement

Reimbursement refers to the amount of money that the health care facility receives from the party responsible for paying the bill. Health care, although personal in service, has evolved into a large and sometimes impersonal industry. All health care providers have a vested interest in their financial operations. As with any other business, a health care provider offers a service or product and then charges a fee for that service or product. The provider may obtain reimbursement from the patient, an insurance company, a managed care organization, or the state or federal government.

The patient's health record, which contains documentation of all of the patient's care, supports the charges for services and supplies. The health record contains documentation of the type of product or service, the date and time at which the service was provided, and the individual who provided the service to the patient.

HIM coding personnel review the patient's health record to identify the correct diagnoses and procedures and then assign the appropriate ICD-10-CM/PCS and HCPCS/CPT codes. These codes are documented on the Uniform Bill (UB-04) or the CMS-1500 form; they tell the payer why the patient received health care (the diagnosis) and whether any procedures were performed that affect reimbursement. Accurate coding requires a thorough analysis of the complete health record. Inaccurate coding causes the facility to submit false claims for reimbursement. From a compliance perspective, submission of false claims is a crime punishable by law; therefore HIM coders are educated in the review of records and the appropriate assignment of codes for reimbursement. Revenue cycle management, discussed in Chapter 6, ensures timely, accurate submission of patient bills for payment.

## Administration

Administration is the common term used to describe the management of the health care facility. In management of health care, the services that are provided must be evaluated. Managers want to be certain that they are providing health care services in an efficient and effective manner. The administrators responsible for a facility are concerned with personnel, along with the financial and clinical operations of the health care facility. Health information is used in administrative aspects to support reimbursement, make decisions regarding services, and analyze the quality of patient care.

The administrators of the facility rely on the analysis of health information to make decisions regarding the management of the facility. For example, analysis may indicate that improper coding, which affects reimbursement, caused a significant decrease in revenue; that patients who received physical therapy soon after heart surgery recovered in a shorter time; or which cases caused an increase in average LOS, thereby increasing costs. Health information is also used to make decisions about the health care services offered, to formulate policies, and to design an organizational structure.

Administrators also use health information to negotiate and evaluate contracts with managed care companies or other vendors, such as surgical supply companies and laundry services. For surgical supply companies and laundry services, the facility uses statistics from its database to negotiate terms of a contract. The statistics help the facility determine the proper quantities of supplies to purchase.

## Prevalence and Incidence of Mortality and Morbidity

Health care facilities are required to report statistics on communicable and infectious diseases to agencies of the federal government, which will be discussed in Chapter 7. The agencies use this information to aid in the prevention and treatment of these diseases. As you read about this use of health information, it is important to understand some statistical terms. **Prevalence** is the extent to which something occurs, that is, the number of existing cases. **Incidence** is the rate of occurrence, that is, the number of new cases. Prevalence and incidence are very similar terms, but they differ in that incidence captures only new cases of a disease, and prevalence captures all existing cases of the disease. By studying the number of cases and the speed at which a disease is spreading in a given population, the government can target areas for prevention and treatment.

The other statistics that are reported as a result of the review of health information are mortality rates (the frequency of death) and morbidity rates (the prevalence and incidence of disease or sickness). Federal agencies monitor, study, and determine the impact of diseases on American public health. Morbidity rates may also refer to statistics used within the hospital to study the frequency of certain complications, such as infection rates.

Within the US government, the DHHS is responsible for overseeing many agencies that have an impact on health care. The mission of the Centers for Disease Control and Prevention (CDC) is "to protect America from health, safety and security threats, both foreign and in the U.S." (Centers for Disease Control and Prevention, http://www.cdc.gov/about/organization/mission.htm, January 4, 2015). The agencies of the CDC use health information to study diseases and support their mission. The centers, institutes, and offices in the CDC are responsible for a wide variety of health issues, including minority health, human immunodeficiency virus, sexually transmitted diseases, tuberculosis prevention, occupational safety and health, chronic disease prevention and health promotion, infectious diseases, and genetics.

## National Policy and Legislation

Federal and state governments use health information when making decisions related to health care. The federal government makes health care policy influence health care delivery. It uses health information to detect threats to the nation's health, identify disparities in care, and take action to promote individual well-being. As discussed in Chapter 1, Healthy People is a national program that gathers and compiles data on indicators of health. The program collects data on individual behaviors like substance abuse and nutrition; social factors like sexual health and violence; mental health; oral health; and maternal infant and child health, and on the ability of people to access health care and preventative services. Policymakers then create objectives to address the causes of poor health.

The US Surgeon General is an advisor, spokesperson, educator, and leader for many health issues that affect the public. Using the best available data, the Office of the Surgeon General communicates scientific information and sets priorities for the advancement of public health.

Health data is used to create legislation that affects health care delivery. For example, the 2009 American Recovery and Reinvestment Act provided stimulus money for various projects, including health information technology and the implementation of EHR technologies. The 2010 Patient Protection and Affordable Care Act was crafted with the belief that evidence-based health care delivery, rooted in health data, would result in better patient outcomes, which would in turn save costs (HHS.gov).

In other aspects of federal regulation, health information is used to determine the type of coverage that Medicare or Medicaid patients receive. Specifically, the CMS (and other agencies) reviews the history of care provided to its beneficiaries and determines the cost and quality of that care to make decisions and enact legislation. These decisions and the legislation affect future coverage, reimbursement, and availability of services for Medicare and Medicaid beneficiaries.

## Community Awareness of Health Care Issues

For many diseases in our society, people have organized into groups to promote awareness, raise money for research, and increase prevention. Special lapel ribbons are worn to promote awareness of a particular disease. Breast cancer and AIDS awareness groups are quite common. These groups use widely known symbols (i.e., the pink and red ribbons, respectively) to promote public education. Since such groups have become involved in health care, more people are educated about the prevention, detection, and treatment of various diseases. These groups use health information, research, and statistics to inform the public. Health information in this case may relate to different populations' exposure to a disease. Health information about the prevention, cause, and treatment of a particular disease can improve the recognition of the disease in a population. For many diseases, a diagnosis at an early stage is easier to treat, and the patient's prognosis is better.

## Litigation

Litigation is the process by which a disputed matter is settled in court. During litigation, health information is used to support a plaintiff's or a defendant's case. Health records can support or validate a claim of physician malpractice. However, the opposite can be proved if there is complete and accurate documentation showing that the physician was not at fault. The health record, when admissible in court, provides evidence of the events that are alleged in a lawsuit.

Standards of care, expert testimony, and research are other sources of health information that may be used as evidence in a trial. Standards of care provide information about the typical method of providing services to a patient with a particular diagnosis. Expert testimony in health care gives the jury information or an explanation that helps them understand the highly technical language used in the health care profession. Research information furnishes

information that the judge or jury can use to make decisions as well. Health information, whether specific to a patient or a disease, is helpful in litigation that involves a person's health or injury.

## Research

Research is the systematic investigation into a matter to obtain or increase knowledge. Health-related research requires a tremendous amount of investigation of health information. In the health care profession, documentation from previous patient care, combined with the scientific process, allows physicians and other researchers to improve, develop, or change patient care and technology. The intention, of course, is to affect health care by giving patients the treatment they need to live longer, healthier, happier lives.

Researchers review the health information from past or present patient health care. They retrieve data specific to their topic and analyze them to look for trends or suggested ways to enhance a treatment, disease, or diagnosis. They can analyze a patient's response to medication or treatment, a prognosis, and the stages of a disease process, that is, the way in which the disease develops. Health information is documented during the course of the research. Although the health information may not be reported in the traditional form of a health record, it must be organized and stored in a manner that facilitates its retrieval and reference at a later date.

Pharmaceutical companies perform a great deal of research on medications before receiving approval to market them to the consumer. This research involves clinical trials in which patients with a known diagnosis or predisposition are given the medication or a placebo or routine treatment. While receiving the medication, the patients are monitored to determine the impact of the medication on their condition. In later clinical trials, the new medication is administered to a wider group for more extensive study. Results of this monitoring are reported in the patients' health records.

## Managed Care

Managed care is the coordination of health care benefits by an insurance company to control access and emphasize preventive care. Managed care organizations use health information internally and in their relationship with health care providers. A managed care organization chooses to use a health care provider's services on the basis of an analysis of the provider's performance. The managed care organization requires the health care facility to provide information about its services, performance, patient LOS, outcomes, and so on. The managed care organization uses this information to determine whether to include the facility as a provider for the organization's beneficiaries.

This data gathering is part of contract negotiation and evaluation. Before entering into a managed care contract, the managed care organization and the health care provider exchange a great deal of health information. While the facility is providing this information to the managed care organization, it also begins evaluating its own data to determine its ability to provide health care to this group of beneficiaries. With this information, the facility can determine whether the contract is viable.

Managed care organizations can also be accredited by the National Committee for Quality Assurance (NCQA). The NCQA requires that managed care organizations comply with clinical and administrative performance standards, including a requirement for health records. Therefore the use of health information within a managed care organization has an impact not only on the benefits of the group members but also on the accreditation of the organization.

## Marketing

Marketing is the promotion of products and services in the hope that the consumer chooses them over the products and services of a competitor. Health information can be used for

marketing. Many health care facilities are in business to make a profit. Regardless of their status—for-profit or not-for-profit—they must raise enough funds to sustain their business. Facilities routinely involve themselves in situations that allow them to compare their business with that of the competition. They analyze market share and statistical information obtained from health care information databases to determine whether there is a need for new treatment or technology in the community. Perhaps a study reveals that the facility has a significant share of the maternity market. There are methods that the facility can use to promote other services to patients who have used its maternity services. Facilities also analyze trends that show a need for a specific type of health care, such as dialysis care, midwifery, sports medicine, or laser surgery.

The marketing department also uses a successful survey by an accreditation agency as a way to promote the facility in the community. Because the accreditation recognizes compliance with set standards, an accredited facility is perceived as better than one that is not accredited.

### ❖ COMPETENCY CHECK-IN 4.4

#### Uses of Health Information

**Competency Assessment**
1. Each month the tumor registry personnel are required to report the _____ of breast cancer for the facility. They report this statistic by determining the number of new cases of breast cancer for the month.
2. Through the _____, providers grant patients access to a subset of their health record.
3. The number of existing cancer cases reported by the tumor registry is known as _____.
4. Health information may be used in _____ to support the plaintiff's claim.
5. _____ refers to disease within a population.
6. _____ is a national program that gathers and compiles data on indicators of health, using the data to set goals to promote the health of the United States.
7. A reimbursement model that controls access to health care services is called _____.
8. In what ways are health data used to educate health care professionals?
9. Can you think of another use for health information besides those listed in this chapter?

## Chapter Summary

Accuracy, validity, timeliness, and completeness are important data qualities. Prevention, detection, and correction of errors promote data of the best quality. HIM professionals are traditionally responsible for the postdischarge processing of health data. The focus of postdischarge processing of a health record is the preparation of health data for billing and retention (storage, security, and access).

After the patient's discharge, records must be obtained, assembled or scanned, analyzed, coded, and completed.

Once control over the health record has been obtained, the record must be tracked and controlled throughout the postdischarge processing cycle. Ultimately, the record passes to the permanent file area or is finalized electronically. The HIM department is generally responsible for the release of patient information to authorized users. HIM professionals are employed in these traditional functions and also in many other functions throughout the health care industry.

## Competency Milestones

### CAHIIM Competency
*I.2. Apply policies, regulations, and standards to the management of information. (3)*

### Rationale
HIM professionals review certain elements of every record for timeliness, accuracy, and completeness. This process ensures that the facility meets both internal standards and those of outside agencies, such as the CMS and TJC.

## Competency Assessment

1. HIM professionals perform a variety of internal control tasks within the context of postdischarge processing. List and describe one example of each type of control that is performed during this process.
2. On the overnight shift, while the patients are sleeping, the nurses on the behavioral health floor use their manual head counts to make sure the status of all discharged patients is correctly listed in the MPI. What kind of control is this?
3. When babies are born at the hospital and their parents have not yet chosen a name, the nursing staff traditionally recorded the newborn as first name Baby, with the mother's last name, such as Baby Cruz or Baby Pratt. One night a nurse accidentally gave a mother's expressed breastmilk to the wrong baby, since they were both named Baby Jones, even though the bottles of milk are uniquely barcoded. What process will the facility use to figure out how this error happened?
4. It was discovered that the bar codes on expressed breastmilk were affixed to bottles in the nursery, rather than in the mothers' rooms. The hospital writes a new policy requiring the mother's wristband to be scanned, labels to be printed using a portable printer, and labels affixed to the bottles before leaving the mother's hospital room. What type of control is this?
5. A new policy requires that all unnamed neonates must use a more distinct naming convention that includes the mother's full name and the baby's sex in the format [mother's last], [mother's first] [sex], such as "Doe, Jane Girl." Which element of data quality does this reflect?
6. Medical staff bylaws, the COP, and TJC standards all require an H&P to be performed and recorded within 24 hours of an inpatient admission. What data quality element does this reflect?
7. A patient's health record states that she has been taking Prozac, an antidepressant, daily for 2 years. When the nurse asks her about the medication during an annual well visit, the patient is puzzled. "No," the patient says. "I've never taken Prozac in my life! I've never taken anything like that and I have no idea how it got there! Please take it out of my records." Instead of deleting the medication altogether, the nurse amends the record to indicate that the previous entry was incorrect. Why is this important for a complete health record?

## CAHIIM Competency

*I.4. Determine compliance of health record content within the health organization. (5)*

## Rationale

The HIM task of postdischarge processing ensures that the record is accurate and complete, which is important not only for compliance but also to facilitate the delivery of health care across the continuum.

## Competency Assessment

1. Maintaining high standards of data quality is essential for patient care and effective use of health data. Data quality has a number of characteristics, many of which are discussed in this chapter and the preceding chapters. List and define as many characteristics as you can remember.
2. When creating a paper form for new patients to complete at registration in a hospital, you should implement what preventive control to ensure that the patient lists all significant childhood illnesses?
3. The physician accidentally entered an order into the computer to request a cardiology consultation for the wrong patient. A staff nurse noticed the error. How should the correction be handled?
4. What type of control is provided by the first processing step of receiving the records, as previously described?
5. What are the steps in the postdischarge processing of health records?
6. How does the HIM professional know what patient records are ready for postdischarge processing?
7. Explain the principles and process flow of an incomplete record system.
8. You are responsible for reviewing and merging duplicate medical records. Your Duplicate MPI report shows the following:

| MRN 123456 | | MRN 876543 |
|---|---|---|
| Marian | First Name | Marian |
| Sharp | Last Name | Sharp |
| 10/3/1995 | Date of Birth | 10/3/1959 |
| F | Gender | F |
| 101 Mooney Rd | Street Address | 101 Mooney Rd |
| New Paltz | City | New Paltz |
| NY | State | NY |
| 12561 | Zip code | 12561 |

Would you merge these records automatically? Explain why or why not. If not, what would you do in order to determine whether to merge them?

*II.2. Apply security strategies to health information. (3)*

## Rationale

HIM professionals work to ensure the organization's policies and procedures comply with standards for the safeguarding of PHI.

## Competency Assessment

1. A medical receptionist can log into the computers at work to update patient's demographic and financial information, but because of her assigned _____, she cannot access the clinical side of the system.
2. Record _____ refers to the idea that regardless of the format, the record is complete, reliable, and consistent.
3. At the free clinic, patients sign in with their first name on the ledger and then wait to be called to the check-in. The licensed practical nurse typically calls each person's name loudly so everyone in the crowded waiting room can hear. Is this a HIPAA violation? Why or why not?
4. None of the patient access staff have access to the health history section of the patient's health record. This is an example of a(n) _____ safeguard.
5. The housekeeping staff do not clean the file room, and they do not even have a key to get in. This is an example of a(n) _____ safeguard.
6. Doctor Ellison did not receive a copy of Maria Gomez's Operative Report in his office. He has asked you to email him a copy right away for billing purposes. Discuss under what circumstances you would comply with his request.

*III.2. Utilize technologies for health information management. (3)*

## Rationale

Most HIM processes are supported by software; therefore HIM professionals must be proficient in their use.

## Competency Assessment

1. How does the use of bar codes facilitate record assembly?
2. Describe how an analyst uses software to perform quantitative analysis. Identify what systems would be accessed during this activity.
3. What type of software generates a report of phrases and their associated codes from transcribed documents?
4. What kind of software allows the provider's dictation to become digitized text in the EHR?
5. What is an abstract? How is the creation of an abstract from a paper-based record different from abstracting in the EHR?
6. Describe how workflow software facilitates postdischarge processing.

*VI.8. Describe consumer engagement activities. (2)*

## Rationale

Now more than ever, patients want to be active participants and decision makers in their health care. Through patient portal management, the PHR, ROI functions, and health literacy initiatives, HIM professionals ensure patients can access the information they need to make informed health care choices.

## Competency Assessment

1. What is meant by the term "health literacy"? Why is it important?
2. What system allows a patient to schedule appointments and review laboratory results?
   a. Patient portal
   b. HIE
   c. Healthy People
   d. Personal health record
3. Why do providers offer patient health information through a patient portal, as opposed to simply allowing the patient to see the entire record as is?

## Ethics Challenge

*VI.7. Assess ethical standards of practice. (5)*

1. You are a supervisor in the HIM department of a large teaching hospital. You have been conducting a concurrent medical record review of 50 records in compliance with TJC standard regarding completion of H&Ps. You have reviewed 20 so far, of which 8 are not compliant. You have seen the two physicians today in person at the hospital and suggested that they should complete the charts now so that you can mark them as compliant. Both physicians do as you suggested and thank you for calling this to their attention. You marked all eight charts compliant. Is this ethical or not?

## Critical Thinking Questions

1. You are the director of HIM at Community Hospital, a small hospital that has just merged with another hospital in your area. The facilities are roughly the same size. Approximately half of the physicians at your facility also have privileges at the other facility. With some exceptions, the two facilities have similar departments and services. Both facilities have some EHR capabilities and are able to interface because they use the same software vendor. Full computerization will not take place for at least 5 years. The administration of the two facilities would like to standardize the data collection with the goal of reducing the cost of forms and facilitating communication between the two facilities. As the senior director, you have been asked to coordinate this effort. What issues do you think should be addressed first? Who will you ask to assist in the project? What impact does this standardization project have on the HIM department?
2. What could be done to streamline patient matching and facilitate interoperability? Research why your idea has not been implemented. What could be done to move your idea forward?

## The Role of Health Information Management Professionals in the Workplace

**Transcriptionist**

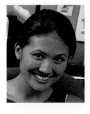

My name is Nicole, and I am a transcriptionist. I work for a large firm that performs transcription services for a lot of different facilities. I could work at home if I wanted to, but I like going into the office. My responsibility is to listen to the physician's dictation and to type exactly what the physician says. I learned transcription and took classes such as medical terminology and anatomy and physiology in the health-related professions program at my high school. I worked in a physician's office for a while and took some additional courses at my local community college.

My job is not just typing. In order to transcribe accurately, I have to understand what the physician is saying and what it means. That means I need to understand and use medical terminology correctly. I need to know the requirements of the various medical reports, such as the H&P and the discharge summary, so that I transcribe them in the right format. I also need to know the regulatory requirements pertaining to the reports. For example, I know that the H&P is more urgent than the discharge summary, so I always transcribe the H&P report first.

Some people think that my job will go away when computers can understand and transcribe human language quickly and accurately. I certainly will not need to type as much, but my skills will become more important in reviewing the clinical reports for completeness, accuracy, and other data quality issues. I am looking forward to that. To better prepare myself for that function, I am studying to become a registered health information technician.

**Career Tip**

Transcription requires a level of speed and accuracy beyond that of the average typist. Transcriptionists need knowledge of medical terminology: not just diseases but also medical equipment, devices, and tools. They must be able to adapt to different styles of dictation and many different accents. Most transcriptionists take career school courses and progress from physician office or clinic dictation to specialized dictation such as radiology. Highly skilled transcriptionists may progress to inpatient dictation. Increasing computerization requires knowledge of computerized workflow distribution. Quality assurance and supervisory positions are logical career progressions.

**Dr. Lewis**

Transcription is important to me, because the reports I dictate are often used by others for legal, billing, and patient care purposes. So they have to be accurate. I can dictate an H&P in about 2 minutes. Within 4 hours, it is waiting in my queue in the hospital system for review and signature. The system allows me to make changes in the document before I sign it. Once I sign it, I cannot make any more changes, but I can dictate an addendum if I realize something is missing or needs to be corrected. Some of my patients like to keep personal health records and I find that a thorough discharge summary is one of their favorite tools to help keep track of inpatient admissions.

## Works Cited

Davis NA, Doyle BM. *Revenue cycle management best practices.* ed 2 Chicago, IL: AHIMA Press; 2016.

Davoudi S, Dooling JA, Glondys B, et al. Data quality management model (2015 Update). *J AHIMA.* 2015;86(10). http://library.ahima.org/doc?oid=107773. Retrieved May 18, 2022.

Code of Federal Regulations (CFR), Title 42, Vol 5, Part 482.24 (c) 2.i.A, 2012.

Federal Rules of Evidence: 28a U.S.C. § 803(6), 2015.

Harris S, Houser HS. Double trouble—using health informatics to tackle duplicate medical record issues. *J AHIMA 2018* 89(8): 20–23, 2018.

Office of the National Coordinator for Health Information Technology (ONC) (2019). *Join the blue button movement, HealthIT.gov: Official Website of the Office of the National Coordinator for Health Information Technology (ONC),* January 29, 2019. https://www.healthit.gov/topic/health-it-initiatives/blue-button/join-the-blue-button-movement. Accessed May 18, 2022.

Pivovarov R, Coppelson YJ, Gorman SL, Vawdrey DK, Elhadad N. Can patient record summarization support quality metric abstraction? *AMIA Ann Symp Proc Arch.* eCollection 1020–1029, 2016. https://pubmed.ncbi.nlm.nih.gov/28269899//. Retrieved May 18, 2022.

The Joint Commission: *Hospital accreditation standards: record of care, treatment, and services,* Chicago, IL, 2012, The Joint Commission; RC.01.02.01, RC.02.01.03, and RC.01.04.01.

The Health Insurance Portability and Accountability Act (HIPAA): Washington, DC, 2004, U.S. Dept. of Labor, Employee Benefits Security Administration.

## Further Reading

AHIMA: *Practice brief "retention and destruction of health information,"* updated October 2013. http://library.ahima.org/xpedio/groups/public/documents/ahima/bok1_049252.hcsp?dDocName=bok1_049252. Accessed May 18, 2022.

Hirsch JS, Tanenbaum JS, Gorman SL, et al. HARVEST, a longitudinal patient record summarizer. *J Am Med Inform Assoc.* 22(2): 263–274, 2015. https://doi.org/10.1136/amiajnl-2014-002945.

The Health Insurance Portability and Accountability Act (HIPAA): Washington, DC, 2004, U.S. Dept. of Labor, Employee Benefits Security Administration.

U.S. Department of Health & Human Services: *HHS.gov: About the Affordable Care Act,* updated March 17, 2022 https://www.hhs.gov/healthcare/about-the-aca/index.html. Accessed May 18, 2022.

# 5

# Coded Data

## TINA CARTWRIGHT

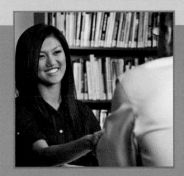

## CHAPTER OUTLINE

**Principles and Applications**
Nomenclature
Classification
Clinical Vocabulary
Taxonomy

**General Purpose Code Sets**
International Classification of Diseases, 10th Revision, Clinical Modification
International Classification of Diseases, 10th Revision, Procedural Coding System
Healthcare Common Procedure Coding System/Current Procedural Terminology

**Special Purpose Classifications and Code Sets**
Systemized Nomenclature of Medicine-Clinical Terms
ICD-O-3
Diagnostic and Statistical Manual of Mental Disorders, Fifth Edition
National Drug Codes
Current Dental Terminology Codes

**Diagnosis-Related Groups**
Diagnosis-Related Group Assignment
Medicare Severity Diagnosis-Related Group Grouper Logic
MDC 05 Diseases and Disorders of the Circulatory System

The Coder's Role in Diagnosis-Related Group (Medicare Severity Diagnosis-Related Group) Assignment

**Coding Quality**
Uses for Coded Clinical Data
Achieving Coding Quality
Computer-Assisted Coding
Coding Compliance
Clinical Documentation Improvement

**Chapter Summary**

**Competency Milestones**

**Ethics Challenge**

**Critical Thinking**

**The Role of Health Information Management Professionals in the Workplace**
Professional Profile—Coder
Patient Care Perspective

**Professional Profile—Corporate Trainer-Coding Specialist Division**

**Works cited**

**Further Reading**

## CHAPTER OBJECTIVES

*By the end of this chapter, the student should be able to:*

1. Explain the purpose and importance of coding in the delivery of health care.
2. List different coding and classification systems and their uses.
3. Apply diagnosis/procedure codes according to current guidelines.
4. Explain diagnosis-related groups and apply grouping codes.
5. Understand the uses for coded information and efforts to improve the quality of coded data.
6. Identify discrepancies between supporting documentation and coded data.

## VOCABULARY

American Medical Association (AMA)
American Psychiatric Association (APA)
case mix
classification
code set
coding compliance plan
coding
Cooperating Parties
Current Procedural Terminology (CPT)
diagnosis-related groups (DRGs)
Diagnostic and Statistical Manual of Mental Disorders, fifth edition (DSM-5)
electronic data interchange (EDI)
evaluation and management (E/M) code
Federal Register
grouper
Health Care Common Procedure Coding System (HCPCS)
hospital-acquired condition (HAC)
Interactive Map-Assisted Generation of ICD-10-CM Codes (I-MAGIC) algorithm
International Classification of Diseases, 10th Revision, Clinical Modification (ICD-10-CM)
International Classification of Diseases, 10th Revision, Procedural Coding System (ICD-10-PCS)
International Classification of Diseases—Oncology (ICD-O)

International Health Terminology Standards Development Organisation (IHTSDO)
major diagnostic category (MDC)
maximization
Medicare Code Editor (MCE)
multiaxial
National Drug Codes (NDCs)
National Library of Medicine (NLM)
nomenclature
Official Guidelines for Coding and Reporting (OCG)
optimization
principal diagnosis
principal procedure
Quality Improvement Organizations
Recovery Audit Contractors (RACs)
reliability
resource intensity (RI)
standards for transactions and code sets
Standards of Ethical Coding
Surveillance, Epidemiology, and End Results (SEER) Program
Systemized Nomenclature of Medicine-Clinical Terms (SNOMED CT)
validity
working MS-DRG

 **CAHIIM COMPETENCY DOMAINS**

I.5. Explain the use of classification systems, clinical vocabularies, and nomenclatures. (2)

IV.1. Validate assignment of diagnostic and procedural codes and groupings in accordance with official guidelines. (3)

IV.1. **RM** Determine diagnosis and procedure codes according to official guidelines. (5)

## Principles and Applications

Coding was discussed in Chapter 4 as an element of postdischarge processing. The activity of coding is a traditional and still very important role that health information management (HIM) professionals perform. This chapter focuses on several of the most commonly used coding systems and their uses and on the activities associated with the coding function.

**Coding** is essentially the translation of documented descriptions of diagnoses (e.g., diseases, injuries, circumstances, and reasons for encounters) and descriptions of procedures (surgical procedures, services, and treatments) into numeric or alphanumeric codes to describe the patient's health and services with the highest accuracy. Coding standardizes the communication of clinical data among users and facilitates electronic transmission of clinical data. For example, if we want to record that a patient has high blood pressure, the diagnosis *hypertension* is translated to International Classification of Diseases,

10th Revision-Clinical Modification (ICD-10-CM) code I10, Essential (primary) hypertension. This precisely and succinctly communicates the patient's diagnosis to other health care providers and payers. From just these three characters, we know not only that the patient has high blood pressure but also that the problem is not caused by some other disease or condition, like a thyroid problem, or pregnancy. As another example, the procedure *laparoscopic total cholecystectomy* is translated to **International Classification of Diseases, 10th Revision, Procedural Coding System (ICD-10-PCS)** code 0FT44ZZ, Percutaneous endoscopic resection of gallbladder. Again, the use of the seven-character code 0FT44ZZ simply communicates the exact procedure: What was removed and how the surgeon removed it.

**Code sets** or coding systems are standardized lists of alphanumeric representations of diagnoses, procedures, data elements, and medical concepts used to communicate health care data. The first standardized code set was proposed by William Farr nearly 200 years ago (Box 5.1). Under the Health Insurance Portability and Accountability Act (HIPAA) of 1996, specific code sets were adopted for use in the electronic transmission of diagnoses and procedures. The HIPAA code sets are:

- International Classification of Diseases, 10th Edition (ICD-10) for transmitting diagnoses and inpatient procedures.
- **Health Care Common Procedure Coding System (HCPCS)** for transmitting outpatient procedures and defining inpatient charges.

• BOX 5.1 **William Farr—Medical Statistician**

William Farr (1807–83) was the first medical statistician in the General Registrar Office of England and Wales. In 1839, at the first Annual Report of the Registrar General, he discussed the principles, still relevant, that should govern a statistical classification of disease and urged the adoption of a uniform classification system, as follows:

*The advantages of a uniform statistical nomenclature, however imperfect, are so obvious, that it is surprising no attention has been paid to its enforcement in Bills of Mortality. Each disease has, in many instances, been denoted by three or four terms, and each term has been applied to as many different diseases: vague, inconvenient names have been employed, or complications have been registered instead of primary diseases. The nomenclature is of as much importance in this department of inquiry as weights and measures in the physical sciences and should be settled without delay.*

Farr proposed a classification system that included the principle of classifying diseases by anatomic site, a concept that was incorporated into early classification systems and that has survived to this day.

- **Current Procedure Terminology (CPT)** for physician medical, surgical, and diagnostic procedures.
- Code on Dental Procedures and Nomenclature (CDT) for dental terms.
- **National Drug Codes (NDCs)** used for defining drugs by name, manufacturer, and dosage.

HIPAA names **standards for transactions and code sets**, which are national standards for exchanging health information electronically. The standards support **electronic data interchange (EDI)** to send and receive patient information between computers in much the same way businesses exchange invoices and purchase orders for goods and services. By using these standards, providers and payers can exchange patient data without human intervention. When health plans, health care clearinghouses, and certain health care providers send health information electronically, the use of these standards is mandatory. Required use of code sets based on EDI improves the efficiency and effectiveness of the nation's health care system. The current version of the standard is called Accredited Standards Committee (ASC) X12 Version 5010. ASC X12 5010 is used for several different kinds of transactions related to health care claims and payments. The electronic version of a Uniform Bill (UB-04), for example, is the 837I, which is sent in 5010 format. We will discuss billing processes in Chapter 6.

Although the coding function is most often associated with payment and reimbursement, coded data are used for other, equally important, purposes. For example, coding professionals are key players in ensuring providers' compliance with official coding guidelines and government regulations. The statistical data collected from complete and accurate coding are necessary to provide a facility or health care provider with the following:

- resource utilization information: volume and disease data;
- databases for maintaining indexes and registries: lists of diagnosis, procedure, and physician data (see Chapter 7);
- physician practice profiling information: physician volume data;
- information to assist in financial and strategic planning: volumes, services, and severity of illness;
- research and clinical trials;
- evaluation of the safety and quality of care;
- quality and outcomes measurements;
- prevention of health care fraud and abuse; and
- other administrative initiatives and activities, such as audits and productivity analysis.

On the patient level, the codes assigned to diagnoses and procedures for an individual patient's encounter or hospital stay may follow that patient throughout the health care delivery system and have an impact on future treatments and insurability. In the quest for fast billing turnaround time and payment, it is sometimes easy to forget that the patient record is a highly personal document, one that often describes a person's last days, and therefore must be treated respectfully concerning the coded data assigned. The American Health Information Management Association (AHIMA) has issued **Standards of Ethical Coding**, guidelines that all coders, regardless of setting, should be aware of and follow (Fig. 5.1).

Many coding systems are in use today throughout the United States and the world. The United Kingdom, for example, uses the *Office of Population Censuses and Surveys (OPCS-4) Classification of Interventions and Procedures*, a coding system comparable to ICD-10; Canada developed an adaptation to ICD-10, ICD-10-CA. Canada has used ICD-10-CA since 2002 for diagnosis coding. ICD-10-CA is very similar to ICD-10-CM but was adapted for use in Canada. For procedure coding, Canada uses the Canadian Classification of Interventions (CCI). CCI resembles ICD-10-PCS in some ways but differs significantly in other ways.

Some coding systems are sponsored and maintained by governmental agencies and others by various medical or health associations in the United States and internationally. In the United States, the coding system used depends on the applicable HIPAA transaction code set used in the provider setting. For example, inpatient hospital-based coders use transaction code sets ICD-10-CM and ICD-10-PCS effective for discharges on or after October 1, 2015.

## Nomenclature

There are two basic types of coding systems: *nomenclature* and *classification*. A **nomenclature** is a system of naming things. Scientific and technical professions typically have their own nomenclatures. A few different nomenclatures are used in medicine. A common nomenclature is found in the **Healthcare Common Procedure Coding System (HCPCS)** and **Current Procedural Terminology (CPT)**.

AMERICAN HEALTH INFORMATION MANAGEMENT ASSOCIATION STANDARDS OF ETHICAL CODING [2016 VERSION]

Standards of Ethical Coding

1. Apply accurate, complete, and consistent coding practices that yield quality data.
2. Gather and report all data required for internal and external reporting, in accordance with applicable requirements and data set definitions.
3. Assign and report, in any format, only the codes and data that are clearly and consistently supported by health record documentation in accordance with applicable code set and abstraction conventions, and requirements.
4. Query and/or consult as needed with the provider for clarification and additional documentation prior to final code assignment in accordance with acceptable healthcare industry practices.
5. Refuse to participate in, support, or change reported data and/or narrative titles, billing data, clinical documentation practices, or any coding-related activities intended to skew or misrepresent data and their meaning that do not comply with requirements.
6. Facilitate, advocate, and collaborate with healthcare professionals in the pursuit of accurate, complete and reliable coded data and in situations that support ethical coding practices.
7. Advance coding knowledge and practice through continuing education, including but not limited to meeting continuing education requirements.
8. Maintain the confidentiality of protected health information in accordance with the Code of Ethics.[3]
9. Refuse to participate in the development of coding and coding-related technology that is not designed in accordance with requirements.
10. Demonstrate behavior that reflects integrity, shows a commitment to ethical and legal coding practices, and fosters trust in professional activities.
11. Refuse to participate in and/or conceal unethical coding, data abstraction, query practices, or any inappropriate activities related to coding and address any perceived unethical coding-related practices.

From AHIMA House of Delegates. "American Health Information Management Association Standards of Ethical Coding [2016 version]" (AHIMA, December 2016) http://library.ahima.org/CodingStandards#.XCTrzVxKhPY. Accessed December 27, 2018.

• **Fig. 5.1** The AHIMA standards of ethical coding. *AHIMA*, American Health Information Management Association.

Nomenclatures facilitate communication because the users have the specific definition of the codes available. For example, HCPCS code G0010 represents administration of hepatitis B vaccine, and HCPCS code G0027 (the next G code) represents semen analysis; presence and/or motility of sperm excluding Huhner. Although many HCPCS codes are related to the next sequential code, there is no global relationship from one code to the next.

## Classification

In addition to nomenclatures, *classification* systems are very important in health care. Classification is the systematic organization of elements into categories. The primary disease classification system used in health care delivery systems, the ICD, is used worldwide and is in its 10th revision (ICD-10). In the United States, it has been modified to increase its level of detail and to add procedural coding.

Classification systems group codes so that coding sequences have logical relationships. For example, ICD-10-CM groups diagnoses by body system and sequences related conditions together. ICD-10-CM codes are organized by categories, subcategories, and valid codes. I25, Chronic ischemic heart disease, is the category of codes for coronary artery disease. A subcategory of I25 is I25.11, Atherosclerotic heart disease of native coronary artery with angina pectoris. A valid code in this subcategory is I25.111, Atherosclerotic heart disease of native coronary artery with angina pectoris with documented spasm.

## Clinical Vocabulary

To communicate, we need to have a common understanding of the meaning of the words we use. This is evident when a person who speaks only French is trying to communicate with a person who speaks only English. The problem of communication is further underscored with a quick reference to a French/English or English/French dictionary. Some words have multiple meanings in translation, and it is only through understanding the context in which the original word is used that one can effectively communicate.

In medicine, the meaning of words is complicated by the user's colloquial expression of the idea, the traditional medical term for the idea, and potential alternative terms.

For example, if renal means "pertaining to the kidney," then why does not renopathy mean "kidney disease"? In a written document, we may have the luxury of consulting a dictionary to identify the meaning (or correct the usage to nephropathy). However, when we are in an electronic health record (EHR) environment sending terabytes of data between systems, we need to be able to communicate in a common language. Clinical vocabulary, very simply, is a listing of preferred terms, their precise definitions, and any alternative terms that may be synonymous. Precision is critical in communication. A fracture of the left arm is not the same as a fracture of the right arm. So, adding a directional qualifier such as left, right, upper, and lower creates a completely different term.

For authoritative information about medical language, review the Metathesaurus. The Metathesaurus is one of the three knowledge sources developed and distributed by the National Library of Medicine (NLM) as part of the Unified Medical Language System project. The Metathesaurus contains information about more than 4 million biomedical concept names from more than 200 controlled vocabularies and classifications used in patient records and administrative health data. It includes vocabularies and coding systems designated as US standards for the exchange of administrative and clinical data, including the Systemized Nomenclature of Medicine-Clinical Terms (SNOMED CT) (https://www.nlm.nih.gov/research/umls/knowledge_sources/metathesaurus/index.html).

## Taxonomy

Taxonomy is the science of classification—a system for naming and organizing things. In coding, it refers to the way a code set is organized. Some code sets are organized by body system, others by type of service. As we will explore later, some code sets, such as ICD-10-PCS, imbue the position of a particular character with meaning. There are seven characters in an ICD-10-PCS code and each character represents a specific value, such as a body system or body part. When using a code set, its taxonomy or organizational structure is important, not just for the purpose of using or assigning a code but also to understand when a code is incorrect. For example, all HCPCS codes have five digits, therefore a four-digit code cannot be a correct HCPCS code.

❖ **COMPETENCY CHECK-IN 5.1**

### Principles and Applications

#### Competency Assessment

1. Distinguish between nomenclatures and classification.
2. Why are taxonomies important?
3. What is a clinical vocabulary?
4. SNOMED CT is an example of:
   a. nomenclature
   b. classification
   c. clinical vocabulary
   d. taxonomy

## General Purpose Code Sets

HIM professionals must be knowledgeable about the coding systems used in the setting in which they are employed. Many HIM professionals are coders; however, a great deal of data analysis and reporting also occurs in health care, much of it in coded format. Therefore students of HIM should pay particular attention to developing sufficient coding skills to enhance their career opportunities. This section discusses the HIPAA code sets and their main uses in health care.

The first classification system, the Bertillon Classification of Causes of Death, was adopted by the International Statistics Institute (ISI) in 1893. Named after Jacques Bertillon, the chair of the ISI committee that developed the system, the Bertillon Classification of Causes of Death was adopted in the United States in 1899. Although some morbidity classifications were being developed at this time as well, it was not until 1948 that the adoption of classifications for disease took root and the sixth revision of the Bertillon Classification was incorporated into the *Manual of the International Statistical Classification of Diseases, Injuries, and Causes of Death* under the auspices of the World Health Congress. This also marked the beginning of the formal international effort to coordinate mortality reporting from national committees of vital statistics and health statistics to the World Health Organization (WHO). The WHO has continued to revise the morbidity and mortality classification system called the ICD-10. With some variations, ICD-10 is used in over 100 countries. The WHO released a working draft of ICD-11 in June 2018 (World Health Organization, 2018). The 72nd World Health Assembly adopted ICD-11 in 2019 and, as expected, it became effective on January 1, 2022. ICD-11 is available electronically at https://icd.who.int/en/.

ICD-10 is a classification of diseases. The United States modifies ICD-10 to provide additional specificity. The United States' modification is called the **International Classification of Diseases, 10th Revision, Clinical Modification (ICD-10-CM)**. This modification process lasted from 1993 to 2015, during which time the United States continued to use its modification of the previous edition, ICD-9-CM. Because so many decades' worth of data is stored as ICD-9-CM, it is not unusual to need a working knowledge of how to map from one code set to the other.

## International Classification of Diseases, 10th Revision, Clinical Modification

ICD-10-CM is mandated by HIPAA for reporting diagnoses and reasons for health care encounters in all settings. Box 5.2 lists some examples of ICM-10-CM codes.

ICD-10-CM codes are alphanumeric; a letter is always the first character in each code. All of the letters of the alphabet are used except the letter *U*, which is reserved for use by the WHO. The WHO provisionally authorized the use of some U codes beginning in March of 2020 for coding COVID-19 cases and vaping-related disorders.

---

**• BOX 5.2    International Classification of Diseases, 10th Revision, Clinical Modification Examples**

- **E10.641** Type 1 diabetes mellitus with hypoglycemia with coma
- **O11.3** Preexisting hypertension with preeclampsia, third trimester
- **O32.1XX2** Maternal care for breech presentation, fetus 2
- **S42.201A** Unspecified fracture of upper end of right humerus, initial encounter for closed fracture
- **T43.8X6D** Underdosing of other psychotropic drugs, subsequent encounter

---

U07.0 Vaping-related disorder

U07.1 Covid-19

U09.9 Post Covid-19 condition, unspecified (referred to as Long Covid)

The organization or taxonomy of ICD-10-CM (Fig. 5.2) is as follows:

- Valid codes range from three to six characters in length.
- The first three characters represent the code category.
- Characters four, five, and six represent etiology, anatomic site, and severity, respectively.
- Certain code categories have applicable seventh characters, the meaning of which depends on the code and chapter where it is required. For example, Code category S00 Superficial injury of head requires that a seventh character be added to each code in that category. The applicable seventh characters for this category are A—initial encounter, D—subsequent encounter, or S—sequela. When a code requiring a seventh character is fewer than six characters in length, a placeholder character, x, is used to ensure that the seventh character is in the seventh character data field (see Fig. 5.2).

ICD-10-CM contains characteristics that were not available in previous versions of the clinical modification of ICD. Other unique features of ICD-10-CM include expanded injury codes, more codes relevant to ambulatory and outpatient encounters, combination codes in which two or more diagnoses are reported using one code, and classifications specific to laterality (right, left, or bilateral body parts). The structure of ICD-10-CM is such that considerable expansion is possible, enabling the addition of new, specific codes as needed without compromising the general code structure.

In the workplace, coders generally have available to them a bound version of ICD-10-CM as well as an interactive electronic version. If you have neither, the current version of ICD-10-CM can be downloaded from the Centers for Medicare and Medicaid Services (CMS) website: https://www.cms.gov/medicare/icd-10/2023-icd-10-cm. With an Internet connection, you can download the code tables and index at no cost and practice applying diagnosis codes right away. The download is in a ZIP file, which contains both PDF (printer-downloadable format) and XML (Extensible Markup Language) formats.

ICD-10-CM consists of the:

- Index to Diseases and Injuries (the main index)
- Neoplasm Table
- Table of Drugs and Chemicals
- Index to External Causes
- Tabular List of Diseases and Injuries

The Index to Diseases and Injuries and the Index to External Causes consist of an alphabetical listing of terms, followed by their corresponding valid (complete) or partial (incomplete) codes and instructional notes that direct the coder to the Tabular List, where the valid or partial codes are located. In the Tabular List, the valid codes are confirmed or the incomplete codes are completed using additional information and instruction notes.

Example 1. The diagnosis is *acute appendicitis*. Appendicitis is the disease/condition; acute is a modifier that tells us the type or quality of appendicitis.

- In the index, look for the main term *appendicitis*, which is capitalized and in **Bold**. Hint: Do not scroll down, and use the search function (the magnifying glass) to find the word. It will appear more than once in your search, so keep going until you find this:

  APPENDICITIS (pneumococcal) (retrocecal) K37
      with
      gangrene K35.891
      with localized peritonitis K35.31
      perforation NOS K35.32
      peritoneal abscess K35.33
      peritonitis NEC K35.33
          generalized (with perforation or rupture) K35.20
              with abscess K35.21
          localized K35.30
              with
                  gangrene K35.31
                  perforation K35.32

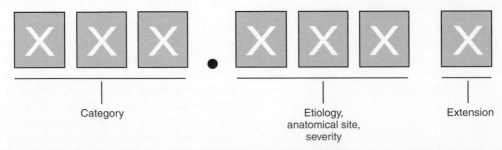

Category

Etiology, anatomical site, severity

Extension

**• Fig. 5.2** ICD-10-CM code format. *ICD-10-CM*, International Classification of Diseases, Tenth Revision-Clinical Modification.

and abscess K35.33
    rupture (with localized peritonitis) K35.32
    acute (catarrhal) (fulminating) (gangrenous) (obstructive) (retrocecal) (suppurative) K35.80

- Notice that all of the terms under the main term are indented.
- Follow the terms that are only indented one space, then look for any relevant terms in the next level.
- In our example, acute appendicitis, notice that acute is a subterm indented one space. We have no other subterms, so we select the code at the end of the entry for acute: K35.80.
- The terms in parentheses are called nonessential modifiers. That means that any of those terms, if they are found in your diagnostic statement, will be included in the code that they modify. So, suppurative appendicitis is included in the coder for acute appendicitis.

Example 2. The diagnosis is *acute, closed nondisplaced traumatic fracture of the posterior column, left acetabulum.* The disease/condition is fracture. Acute, closed, traumatic, and nondisplaced are subterms or modifiers that further describe the fracture. Posterior column, left acetabulum, is the location of the fracture.

- In the Index, find the main term Fracture, traumatic. Under that, find the terms *Acetabulum, column, posterior,* and *nondisplaced.* The code following this term is S32.44-. The dash in the Index indicates that this code is partial or incomplete.

Fracture, traumatic (abduction) (adduction)
    (separation)—see also Fracture, pathological T14.8.
    acetabulum S32.40-
        column
            anterior (displaced) (iliopubic) S32.43-
                nondisplaced S32.436
            posterior (displaced) (ilioischial) S32.443
                nondisplaced S32.44-

- Refer to the Tabular List of Diseases and Injuries, code S32.44. S32.44 is a subcategory (partial, incomplete).
- Recognize from the Tabular List that S32.445, Nondisplaced fracture of posterior column [ilioischial] of left acetabulum, matches the diagnosis.
- In the S32 category, the code is not valid (complete) until a seventh character is added to describe the encounter. In this example, character A for initial encounter for closed fracture.
- Thus the valid code for the diagnosis *acute, closed nondisplaced fracture of the posterior column, left acetabulum* is S32.445A, Nondisplaced fracture of posterior column [ilioischial] of left acetabulum, initial encounter for closed fracture.
- This example illustrates why it is essential to use both the Index and Tabular List for code assignment. In this example, the seventh character needed to complete the code is found only in the Tabular List.

## Official Guidelines

Overall, instruction notes and other elements such as punctuation in both the Index and Tabular List must be followed.

These instruction notes, called *Conventions and Guidelines,* are found in the **ICD-10-CM Official Guidelines for Coding and Reporting (OCG)**. Effective in each October, an updated version is issued by the CMS and the National Center for Health Statistics (NCHS).

Updates are approved by the **Cooperating Parties for the ICD-10-CM**. The Cooperating Parties consist of representatives of the American Hospital Association (AHA), the AHIMA, the CMS, and the NCHS. The Cooperating Parties meet twice yearly, usually in April and October, to hear and discuss proposed code changes or revisions. Anyone can attend these meetings. Notices and agendas can be found on the CMS website https://www.cms.gov/Medicare/Coding/ICD10/ICD-10-Coordination-and-Maintenance-Committee-Meetings. When a proposed code change meets final approval, it can be accessed in the *Federal Register* section as a Final Rule. Coding changes may be approved and issued for use twice yearly, in April and October, although most major changes are effective in October and approved by the Cooperating Parties for ICD-10-CM.

The OCG can be found in its entirety at https://www.cms.gov/files/document/fy-2022-icd-10-cm-coding-guidelines.pdf. Adherence to these guidelines is required under the HIPAA. The following statement is made in the guidelines regarding coding, provider documentation, and incomplete medical records: "The importance of consistent, complete documentation in the medical record cannot be overemphasized. Without such documentation the application of coding guidelines is a difficult, if not impossible, task."

The *OCG* is updated annually along with the code set. They can be located on the same CMS website listed previously. The *OCG* is typically printed toward the beginning of a bound paper code book for easy reference. It contains important directions regarding the conventions used in ICD-10-CM, as well as chapter-by-chapter instructions regarding certain clinical situations. For example, in our fracture example, in the main term for Fracture, traumatic, it says, "see also Fracture, pathological T14.8." *OCG* I.A.16. explains that "a 'see also' instruction following a main term in the Alphabetic Index instructs that there is another main term that may also be referenced that may provide additional Alphabetic Index entries that may be useful. It is not necessary to follow the 'see also' note when the original main term provides the necessary code." (Centers for Medicare and Medicaid Services and the National Center for Healthcare Statistics, 2022).

Since we already knew that the fracture was traumatic, it was not necessary to review pathological fractures.

Section I.B. of the *OCG* contains General Coding Guidelines covering everything from locating a code to acute and chronic conditions and coding for health care encounters in hurricane aftermath. I.B.8. states "If the same condition is described as both acute (subacute) and chronic, and separate subentries exist in the Alphabetic Index at the same indentation level, code both and sequence the acute (subacute) code first" (Centers for

Medicare and Medicaid Services and the National Center for Healthcare Statistics, 2022).

This guideline reminds coders to ensure that all relevant terms are included in the codes that are chosen to describe the encounter.

Section I.C. of the *OCG* discusses Chapter-Specific Coding Guidelines. In some bound paper versions of ICD-10-CM, the chapter-specific guidelines are reprinted in the front of the chapter to which they refer. This alleviates having to flip back and forth between the guidelines and the tabular when coding. Failure to follow the *OCG* is a coding error.

## International Classification of Diseases, 10th Revision, Procedural Coding System

ICD-10-PCS was developed by 3M under contract from the CMS to replace ICD-9-CM, Volume III. At this time, it is commonly used for inpatient procedures only. ICD-10-PCS does not replace the HCPCS or CPT, which are used for procedure coding in outpatient settings. ICD-10-PCS became effective for use at the same time as ICD-10-CM, on October 1, 2015. The CMS is responsible for maintaining ICD-10-PCS, which currently comprises over 78,000 codes. Information, including guidelines for ICD-10-PCS, can be found at the CMS website: https://www.cms.gov/medicare/icd-10/2023-icd-10-pcs. Box 5.3 lists some examples of ICM-10-PCS codes.

ICD-10-PCS consists of 17 sections. The sections contain procedures that pertain to those sections. The Medical and Surgical section contains the most procedure codes and is arranged further by Body System. The Obstetrics section contains the codes for obstetric procedures, such as cesarean sections and vaginal deliveries. The Imaging section contains the codes for radiology procedures.

All ICD-10-PCS codes are composed of seven alphanumeric characters, either letters or digits. Each character has a

---

**• BOX 5.3   International Classification of Diseases, 10th Revision, Procedural Coding System Examples**

*Note*: The first description after the code is the abbreviated or short description that is used in abstracting systems: the second description in brackets is the expanded form.

- **021V09P** Bypass Sup Vena Cava to Pulm Trunk w Autol Vn, Open [Bypass Superior Vena Cava to Pulmonary Trunk with Autologous Venous Tissue, Open Approach]
- **0D5N4ZZ** Destruction of Sigmoid Colon, Perc Endo Approach [Destruction of Sigmoid Colon, Percutaneous Endoscopic Approach]
- **0QS646Z** Reposition R Up Femur with Intramed Fix, Perc Endo Approach [Reposition Right Upper Femur with Intramedullary Internal Fixation Device, Percutaneous Endoscopic Approach]
- **10D00Z1** Extraction of POC, Low Cervical, Open Approach [Extraction of Products of Conception, Low Cervical, Open Approach]

---

character value, and each character value represents a specific option for the general character definition. ICD-10-PCS codes may be found beginning with either the Index or the Code Tables found in each section by selecting the specific character values for each of the seven characters based on the details of the procedure that was performed (Fig. 5.3). Because each character in the code has specific meaning, depending on its position in the sequence, ICD-10-PCS has a **multi-axial** code structure. Each position is an axis, so character 4 in the second character position means something different from 4 in the fifth character position. In the ICD-10-PCS code in Fig. 5.3, character Z in the sixth character position means "No device," while character Z in the seventh character position means "No qualifier."

Each seven-character ICD-10-PCS code comprises a character from each of seven different categories that make up a code. For procedures coded from the Medical and Surgical section, the characters are in the following order: **S**ection, **B**ody System, **R**oot Operation, **B**ody Part, **A**pproach, **D**evice, Qualifier. Sometimes it is easy to use a mnemonic to help remember this order, such as "**S**ally **B**uys **R**oot **B**eer **A**t **D**airy Queen."

For example, Section 1 of the ICD-10-PCS contains the tables for Medical and Surgical procedure codes, which are as follows:

- The first character represents the Section. In the Medical and Surgical section, the first character has a character value of 0 (zero). All codes in the Medical and Surgical section will begin with the character 0.
- The second character indicates the Body System. Each body system has its own character value, such as 2 for Heart and Great Vessels and D for Gastrointestinal System.
- The third character indicates the Root Operation. Assigning the correct root operation to the procedure that was performed is critical to building the correct code. There are 31 different root operations in the Medical and Surgical section. The coder must understand and apply the definitions of each root operation and assign the correct character value. Some Root Operations are as follows:
  - *Excision*: Cutting out of or off, without replacement, a portion of a body part, character value B.
  - *Resection*: Cutting out of or off, without replacement, all of a body part, character value T.
  - *Inspection*: Visually and/or manually exploring a body part, character value J.
- The fourth character indicates the Body Part, the site on which the procedure was performed. These are numerous and may be found in each table.
- The fifth character indicates the Approach, the technique used to reach the site of the procedure. There are seven types of approaches; for example, an Open approach has a character value of 0 (zero).
- The sixth character indicates the Device, of which there are four different categories. The specific types of devices are found in the applicable tables. For example, a

**ODJ**

| Section | 0 Medical and surgical |
|---|---|
| Body system | D Gastrointestinal system |
| Operation | J Inspection: Visually and/or manually exploring a body part |

| Body part | Approach | Device | Qualifier |
|---|---|---|---|
| **0** Upper intestinal tract<br>**6** Stomach<br>**D** Lower intestinal tract | **0** Open<br>**3** Percutaneous<br>**4** Percutaneous endoscopic<br>**7** Via natural or artificial opening<br>**8** Via natural or artificial opening endoscopic<br>**X** External | **Z** No device | **Z** No qualifier |
| **U** Omentum<br>**V** Mesentery<br>**W** Peritoneum | **0** Open<br>**3** Percutaneous<br>**4** Percutaneous endoscopic<br>**X** External | **Z** No device | **Z** No qualifier |

• **Fig. 5.3** Example of table used to build International Classification of Diseases, 10th Revision, Clinical Modification (ICD-10-PCS) codes.

Monitoring Device has a character value of 2. If there is no device, character Z is assigned.

• The seventh character is called the Qualifier and contains unique values for certain individual procedures. For example, assigning character value X to certain procedures in the Qualifier position indicates a biopsy. If there is no qualifier, character Z is assigned.

For example, a colonoscopy is coded in ICD-10-PCS as ODJD8ZZ. Using the table in Fig. 5.3, one builds the PCS code for colonoscopy by assigning the character values from the table, as follows:

0—Section: Medical and surgical, character value 0
D—Body system: Gastrointestinal, character value D
J—Root operation: Inspection, character value J
D—Body part: Lower intestinal tract, character value D
8—Approach: Via natural or artificial opening, endoscopic, character value 8
Z—No device (no device left inside the body after completion of the procedure), character value Z
Z—No qualifier (no unique information specific to the procedure), character value Z

## Healthcare Common Procedure Coding System/Current Procedural Terminology

The HCPCS was developed as a standard coding system for claims processing and is therefore extremely important to physicians and other providers for billing. The HCPCS consists of two levels.

### Healthcare Common Procedure Coding System Level I

Level I is CPT, which stands for Current Procedural Terminology, currently in its fourth version (CPT-4). CPT

is copyrighted, developed, and maintained by the **American Medical Association (AMA)**. CPT codes are composed of five numeric characters (Box 5.4). They are used to report procedures and services performed by physicians and other health care professionals, and in facilities or institutions for services performed in the outpatient setting (e.g., ambulatory surgery centers, emergency departments, clinics, and rehabilitation facilities). There are CPT-4 codes that describe office visits, surgical procedures, radiology procedures, and laboratory tests, for example. There are three categories of codes in CPT: Category 1 for common medical services, Category 2 for performance measures, and Category 3 for new and emerging technology. CPT-4 codes are updated and published yearly by the AMA and become effective for use on each January 1. The code changes and new codes must be purchased from the AMA.

Additions, deletions, and revisions to CPT-4 are determined by the AMA's editorial panel. The editorial panel consists of physicians representing the AMA, the Blue

---

• **BOX 5.4** **Current Procedural Terminology (CPT) (Healthcare Common Procedure Coding System Level I) Examples**

• **43251** EGD c̄ polypectomy snared
• **49320** Laparoscopy, diagnostic (separate procedure)
• **21320** Closed treatment, nasal bone fracture; with stabilization
CPT 2021 American Medical Association. All rights reserved.
CPT is a registered trademark of the American Medical Association.

Cross and Blue Shield Association (BCBSA), the Health Insurance Association of America, the AHA, and the CMS. Providing input to the panel are two advisory committees: The CPT Advisory Committee consists solely of physicians. The Health Care Professionals Advisory Committee is composed of allied health professionals, including HIM professionals. AMA staff review and evaluate requests from the industry for suggestions for new codes. When appropriate, these suggestions are forwarded to the advisory committee for consideration. If the advisory committee agrees that a new code should be added, or if the advisory committee cannot reach an agreement, the issue is referred to the CPT Editorial Panel for resolution. Details of the process may be found on the AMA's website: https://www.ama-assn.org/about/cpt-editorial-panel/cpt-code-process.

### The Current Procedural Terminology's Evaluation and Management Codes

In addition to codes that designate a specific procedure, the CPT utilizes **evaluation and management (E/M) codes** to summarize the various levels of service provided. E/M codes are a method of representing the amount of time and skill needed to treat the patient at that particular visit. As might be expected, the higher the level of time and skill needed, the higher the reimbursement.

For example, CPT's E/M codes assign separate codes for new patients as opposed to established patients. New patients will require more time and documentation, since the collection of demographic data, financial information, and medical history will be more extensive and time consuming. The CPT's E/M code includes the reimbursement formula to capture the additional work required for new patients as opposed to an established patient who only needs to be queried for changes in any of the previous information and the current reason for the visit. In general, established patients are defined as patients receiving medical services from the health care provider or another provider of the same specialty who belongs to the same group practice for the last 3 years.

When determining the level of service or the E/M code, seven components should be considered:

- history
- examination
- medical decision-making
- counseling
- coordination of care
- nature of presenting problem
- time

The first three of these components—history, examination, and medical decision-making—are the key components in selecting the level of E/M services.

As we discussed in Chapter 3, when documenting the patient's history, the E/M services are divided into four levels, from least to most amount of time expended: *problem focused, expanded problem focused, detailed*, and *comprehensive* (Table 3.4). The documentation in the record must support the definition for the particular level. For example, a *problem-focused* history only documents the history of the patient's present illness. A *comprehensive* history needs to have documentation for an extensive history of the present illness along with a review of all body systems and complete family, social, and past medical histories. Regardless, each type of history should include a chief complaint (CC); history of present illness; a review of systems; and past, family, and/or social history.

As shown in Table 3.5, for the examination, the levels of E/M services are based on four types of examinations:

- *problem focused*—a limited examination of the affected body area or organ system,
- *expanded problem focused*—a limited examination of the affected body area or organ system and other symptomatic or related organ system(s),
- *detailed*—an extended examination of the affected body area(s) and other symptomatic or related organ system(s), and
- *comprehensive*—a general multisystem examination or complete examination of a single organ system.

The CPT's definition for a body area is the head, neck, chest, abdomen, genitalia, back, and extremities. Examples of organ systems include the cardiovascular, musculoskeletal, and genitourinary systems. The extensiveness of the examination should be dependent on the presenting symptoms and the provider's clinical judgment. For example, if a patient presents with a suspected fracture of his arm, the examination is limited to one particular body area, and the extent of evaluation is *problem focused*. A *comprehensive* examination is generally a multisystem or complete examination that should include 8 of the 12 organ systems documented.

The third key factor to consider when determining E/M levels is the medical decision-making that is required by the health care provider. The medical decision-making reflects the complexity of making a diagnosis and developing a treatment plan for the patient. The levels of medical decision-making are summarized as: *straightforward, low complexity, moderate complexity*, and *high complexity*. For a visit to be classified as a particular type of medical decision-making, there must be sufficient documentation to support it, such as the number of potential diagnoses or treatment options, the amount and complexity of testing and results to be reviewed, and the risk of CCs or mortality.

To help meet the goals of the 2019 Medicare Physician Fee Schedule final rule, the determination for Office and Other Outpatient Services E/M codes was simplified and effective on January 1, 2021. The new determination is more accurate and less administratively burdensome. Code 99201 was deleted. New Patient codes 99202–99205 and Established Patient codes 99211–99215 all require a "medically appropriate history and/or examination" and one of the four levels of decision-making mentioned previously. Each code includes a range for total encounter time. The appropriate outpatient E/M code is now chosen based on the medical decision-making level or total length of encounter time.

### Healthcare Common Procedure Coding System Level II

Level II codes are generally called *HCPCS codes*. HCPCS Level II codes are reported by regulations that the CMS published on August 17, 2000 (45 CFR 162.10002). They consist of codes used by providers and institutions to report products, supplies, and services not included in CPT. For example, HCPCS Level II codes would be used to submit claims for durable medical equipment and ambulance services. Every HCPCS code is alphanumeric, consisting of a letter followed by four numeric characters. HCPCS Level II codes are maintained jointly by America's Health Insurance Plans, the BCBSA, and the CMS. These same groups also serve on an HCPCS national panel, the functions of which include maintaining national permanent HCPCS Level II codes, as well as additions, revisions, and deletions. According to the CMS, the purpose of the permanent national codes is to provide a "standardized coding system that is managed jointly by private and public insurers. It supplies a predictable set of uniform codes that provides a stable environment for claims submission and processing" (Centers for Medicare and Medicaid Services, 2021). HCPCS Level II codes are updated as needed, usually every quarter, and become effective once announced. Updates can be found on the CMS website. Box 5.5 lists some examples of HCPCS codes.

---

### • BOX 5.5   Healthcare Common Procedure Coding System Examples

- **C1715** Brachytherapy needle
- **J0897** Injection, denosumab, 1 mg
- **T1015** Clinic visit/encounter, all-inclusive

---

## Special Purpose Classifications and Code Sets

### Systemized Nomenclature of Medicine-Clinical Terms

The **Systemized Nomenclature of Medicine-Clinical Terms (SNOMED CT)** was created by the College of American Pathologists and the National Health Service in England. Since 2007 SNOMED CT has been owned, maintained, and distributed by the **International Health Terminology Standards Development Organisation (IHTSDO)**, a not-for-profit association in Denmark comprises representatives from many countries. According to the IHTSDO, SNOMED CT is considered the most comprehensive multilingual clinical health care terminology in the world. It provides the standardized core general terminology for an EHR, enabling better communication and interoperability of the EHR exchange. It is a nomenclature system consisting of more than 1 million medical concepts and attributes arranged in complex hierarchies. SNOMED CT contains codes for diseases and procedures, as well as relational terms that enable the translation of natural language into a classification system, such as ICD-10. SNOMED CT "reads" the natural language and assigns codes to the concepts and relationships that it finds. Although there is not an exact one-to-one translation between SNOMED CT and ICD-10-CM, there is a map that provides the logical choices. An interactive translation demonstration called I-MAGIC was used to create the example in Box 5.6.

The purpose of IHTSDO is to develop, maintain, promote, and enable the uptake and correct use of its terminology products in health systems, services, and products around the world, and to undertake any or all activities incidental and conducive to achieving the purpose of the association for the benefits of the members.

---

## COMPETENCY CHECK-IN 5.2

### General Purpose Code Sets

#### Competency Assessment

1. Provide three examples for which coded data might be used in a facility.
2. What transaction format is used to transfer electronic data?
3. Name three coding systems used for reimbursement.
4. What is the purpose of the Cooperating Parties?
5. What entity is responsible for developing and maintaining ICD-10-CM?
6. What entity is responsible for developing and maintaining ICD-10-PCS?
7. Through what committee do HIM professionals contribute to additions, deletions, and revisions to the CPT?
8. Describe reasons why it is important to have knowledge of ICD-9-CM.
9. What main advantage does ICD-10-CM have over ICD-9-CM?
10. Describe how the structure of ICD-10-PCS enables the addition of new codes.
11. Describe the process of building ICD-10-PCS codes.

| • BOX 5.6 | Systemized Nomenclature of Medicine—Clinical Terms (SNOMED CT) to International Classification of Diseases, 10th Revision, Clinical Modification (ICD-10-CM) Examples |
|---|---|

| Diagnosis | SNOMED CT | ICD-10-CM |
|---|---|---|
| Preinfarction syndrome | 4557003 | I20.0 |
| Cholera | 63650001 | A00.9 |
| Neonatal jaundice | 387712008 | P59.9 |
| Postcholera vaccination encephalitis | 192708007 | G04.02 T50.A95- In this example, a seventh digit to specify the encounter is required |

The IHTSDO seeks to improve the health of humankind by fostering the development and use of suitable standardized clinical terminologies, notably SNOMED CT, to support safe, accurate, and effective exchange of clinical and related health information. The focus is on enabling the implementation of semantically accurate health records that are interoperable. Support of association members and licensees is provided on a global basis, allowing the pooling of resources to achieve shared benefits (SNOMED International, 2022a, b).

The US representative to the IHTSDO is the **National Library of Medicine (NLM)**. Canada's representative is Canada Health Infoway. Both countries use SNOMED CT to facilitate the exchange of clinical data through EHR systems. Two strategic goals Infoway will focus on from 2017 to 2022 are e-prescribing and providing access to digital health information and services (Canada Health Infoway, 2022).

SNOMED CT differs from classification systems such as ICD-10-CM, which are designed to assign codes to patient encounters according to diseases. The output of the coding process is an ICD-10-CM code that is not generally used during, or directly for, patient care. Instead, data generated from ICD-10-CM codes are most useful when aggregated after the encounter and are necessary for reimbursement. Classification systems such as ICD-10-CM are not designed to capture all of the available data and clinical information in a health record that is used by clinicians *during* patient care. SNOMED CT, however, can be applied to free text and, by translating the text or natural language, describe in coded format the diagnosis or activity, such as a procedure. Software "reads" the free text and creates the SNOMED CT code. The SNOMED CT code is then mapped to the ICD-10-CM/PCS or HCPCS code for further processing. Therefore it is a critical link in connecting the data collected in an EHR with the classification or nomenclature system that describes the encounter.

Table 5.1 shows the SNOMED CT codes, ICD-10-CM code, ICD-10-PCS code, and CPT-4 code assigned to the diagnosis *acute lower gastrointestinal hemorrhage* and to the procedure Flexible fiber optic diagnostic colonoscopy. More SNOMED CT diagnoses and procedure codes can be viewed at https://browser.ihtsdotools.org/?.

Because SNOMED CT codes are assigned during patient care, they can be linked with other software programs that can facilitate current patient care. For example, a SNOMED CT code may be assigned with the use of input from a complex set of data extracted from various sections of the EHR. This SNOMED CT code may be programmed to link to a software system to alert the clinician to a life-threatening condition.

Because classification systems and nomenclature systems are designed for different purposes and uses, one type of system cannot entirely replace the other. SNOMED CT is designed to use very specific data, including gender and age, to assign a SNOMED CT code called a *concept*. For example, the SNOMED CT concept, using SNOMED CT terminology, for "a female with a herniated urinary bladder" is 410070006, herniated urinary bladder (disorder)+gender=female. This SNOMED CT concept can be mapped to ICD-10-CM code N81.10, Cystocele, unspecified.

In many instances, there is no direct map from a SNOMED CT concept to an ICD-10-CM code, because the ICD-10-CM code includes information not captured in SNOMED CT. For example, SNOMED CT concept 58149017 (Antepartum hemorrhage) maps by default to the ICD-10-CM code O46.90, Antepartum hemorrhage, unspecified, unspecified trimester. The coder would have to

| TABLE 5.1 | Comparison of Codes for the Diagnosis Acute Lower Gastrointestinal Hemorrhage and the Procedure Flexible Fiberoptic Diagnostic Colonoscopy |
|---|---|

| Code Set | Code | Meaning |
|---|---|---|
| SNOMED CT | 74474003 | Gastrointestinal hemorrhage |
| | 1209098000 | Fiberoptic colonoscopy with biopsy of lesion of colon |
| ICD-10-CM | K92.2 | Gastrointestinal hemorrhage, unspecified |
| ICD-10-PCS | 0DJD8ZZ | Inspection, lower intestinal tract via natural or artificial opening, endoscopic |
| CPT-4 | 45378 | Colonoscopy, flexible; diagnostic, including collection of specimen(s) by brushing or washing, when performed (separate procedure) |

insert the trimester as required in ICD-10-CM to complete the code, but the SNOMED CT concept does not include trimester.

The **Interactive Map-Assisted Generation of ICD-10-CM Codes (I-MAGIC)** algorithm was developed to encode ICD-10-CM codes from computer-generated SNOMED CT codes of clinical problems. I-MAGIC works in real time to decide what user input is needed to assign the correct, detailed ICD-10 code from the SNOMED CT code. Fig. 5.4 illustrates the I-MAGIC algorithm.

The transition to the EHR and SNOMED CT will not eliminate the need for coders in the foreseeable future. The accuracy of the coded data still must be reviewed and verified as the data pertain to each specific patient encounter. Although no electronic system is infallible, the extent to which we can depend on such systems will probably increase with time. Even if the coding function was eliminated in the future, health information professionals with

that knowledge base would assume more complex and advanced roles in, for example, development and maintenance of the code mapping (matching SNOMED CT codes to the correct target code set), quality control of individual patient and aggregate data (making sure coded data are correct and complete), and sophisticated data analysis (including reporting and data presentation).

## ICD-O-3

The **International Classification of Diseases for Oncology (ICD-O)**, currently in its third edition as of January 1, 2001 (ICD-O-3) and second revision as of January 1, 2021 (ICD-O-3.2), is a coding system used to record and track the occurrence of neoplasms (i.e., malignant tumors, cancer). The WHO is responsible for this multiaxial classification system. Its purpose is to be the standard tool for coding neoplasm diagnoses. In a hospital setting, ICD-O-3 is used

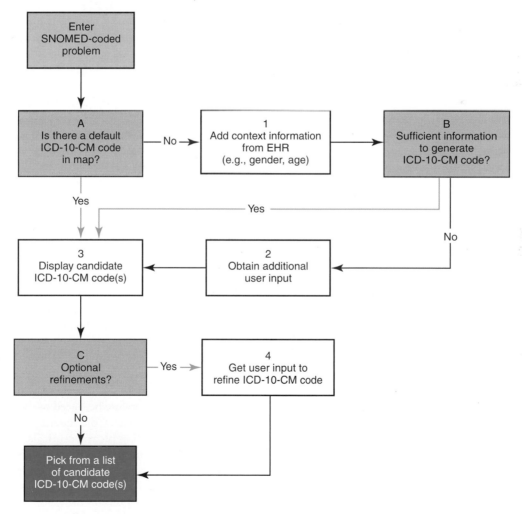

This is an algorithm which utilizes the SNOMED CT to ICD-10-CM Rule Based Map in a real-time, interactive manner to generate ICD-10-CM codes from SNOMED CT encoded clinical problems.

• **Fig. 5.4** The Interactive Map-Assisted Generation of ICD Codes (IMAGIC) algorithm. *EHR*, Electronic health record; *ICD-10-CM*, International Classification of Diseases, 10th Revision-Clinical Modification; *SNOMED CT*, Systematized Nomenclature of Medicine-Clinical Terms. (From National Library of Medicine: Mapping SNOMED CT to ICD-10-CM: Technical Specifications. https://www.nlm.nih.gov/research/umls/mapping_projects/TechnicalSpecifications_SNOMEDCT_ICD10CM_201702.pdf.)

in the pathology department and in tumor (cancer) registries to code the site (topography axis) and the histology (morphology axis) of neoplasms. A *tumor registry* is a central repository of data about cancer, collected from the providers who identified the cancer cases. As an international coding system, it is available in several languages. The codes are the same; only the descriptions and instructional notes are translated where appropriate. ICD-O-3 is not used for reimbursement purposes and is not a transaction code set under HIPAA.

The topography axis uses the ICD-10 classification of malignant neoplasms for all types of tumors as its foundation. For nonmalignant tumors, ICD-O-3 is more detailed than ICD-10. ICD-O also adds topography for sites of certain tumors.

The morphology axis consists of five-digit codes ranging from M-8000/0 to M-9989/3. The first four digits indicate the specific histologic term. The fifth digit after the slash (/) is the behavior code, which indicates whether a tumor is malignant, benign, in situ, or uncertain (whether benign or malignant). A separate one-digit code is also provided for histologic grading and differentiation that indicates how much the cancer cells have changed from normal tissue, or the type of cell lineage for leukemia and lymphoma. So, squamous cell carcinoma (M-8070/3) expressed as "moderately differentiated squamous cell carcinoma with poorly differentiated areas" should be given the grading code "3." The complete code would therefore be M-8070/33 (National Cancer Institute, n.d.).

For example, the diagnosis *neoplasm of the lung and bronchus, small cell carcinoma, fusiform cell* is assigned a code from C34.0 to C34.3 to indicate site (identical to the ICD-10-CM code equivalent) and also 8043/3 to indicate histology. Fig. 5.5 shows the 33–34.3 site codes on a drawing of lung anatomy.

In the United States, the National Cancer Institute's **Surveillance, Epidemiology, and End Results (SEER)** Program collects and compiles cancer statistics, including mortality data, for the United States using ICD-O-3. SEER provides information on incidence, prevalence, and survival from geographic areas in the United States. Tumor registrars use the *SEER Program Coding and Staging Manual* for coding and reporting cancer cases.

## Diagnostic and Statistical Manual of Mental Disorders, Fifth Edition

**DSM-5** stands for *Diagnostic and Statistical Manual of Mental Disorders*, Fifth Edition. Its sponsoring organization is the **American Psychiatric Association (APA)**. DSM-5 is a medical classification of disorders, not a distinct coding classification system. Instead, DSM-5 provides the clinician with a pathway to assigning the ICD-10-CM codes included in the text of the manual for each disorder. The APA planned DSM-5 to be in harmonization with ICD-10-CM and, eventually, with ICD-11-CM. DSM-5 criteria define disorders identified by ICD-10-CM codes and code descriptions.

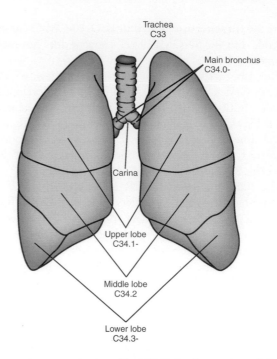

• **Fig. 5.5** Lung anatomy with ICD-O-3 site codes. *ICD-O-3,* International Classification of Diseases-Oncology, Third Edition.

Section II of DSM-5 contains diagnostic criteria, descriptive text, and ICD-10-CM codes for mental disorders and conditions organized into groups and then by specific disorders and conditions. For example, the group "Personality Disorders" contains 14 specific personality disorders including "paranoid personality disorder," "antisocial personality disorder," and "narcissistic personality disorder."

## National Drug Codes

**National Drug Codes (NDCs)** are found in the National Drug Code Directory and serve as universal product identifiers for human drugs. The US Food and Drug Administration (FDA) maintains a list of these identifiers, or codes, on its website https://www.accessdata.fda.gov/scripts/cder/ndc/index.cfm, which is updated daily. NDCs are a transaction code set under HIPAA. They are important for commercial purposes, in selling and purchasing pharmaceuticals. They are also tied to a facility's pharmaceutical system and can therefore be traced to dispensing of medication at the patient level. Consequently, NDCs are critical in the event of a recall of pharmaceuticals.

Medicaid requires NDCs for reimbursement, as do some managed care providers. The NDC is appended to Uniform Bill (UB-04) and gives the payer-specific information regarding the cost of certain drugs.

NDCs contain three segments: labeler, product, and packaging codes. The individual segments are assigned partly by the FDA, which assigns the labeler code, and partly by the labeler, which assigns the product and packaging codes. The labeler may be the manufacturer of the drug or the distributor. For example, a drug manufactured by a pharmaceutical company and sold under that company's name as well as a retail drug store's name would have two different NDCs. The product code describes the strength, dosage, and formulation of the drug. The packaging code defines the packaging size and type.

Examples from the National Drug Code Directory in Table 5.2 show two labelers of acetaminophen: McNeil, which distributes it under the proprietary name Tylenol, and CVS Pharmacy, which distributes a nonproprietary version. Because acetaminophen is not restricted by patent at this time, a search of the NDC Directory yields more than 4000 entries for acetaminophen (U.S. Food and Drug Administration, 2022). In Table 5.2, 50580 is the FDA's labeler code for Johnson & Johnson Consumer Inc., McNeil Consumer Healthcare Division, 783 is McNeil's product code for Tylenol 8 HR Arthritis Pain, and 24, 25, 30, and 32 are various package codes for the configurations listed. The CVS Pharmacy version of acetaminophen is available in different strengths and packaging compared with the McNeil example.

## Current Dental Terminology Codes

The *Code on Dental Procedures and Nomenclature (Code)* (CDT) uses descriptive terms for procedures and treatments unique to dentistry. The American Dental Association owns and holds the copyright to CDT. The CDT code is a transaction code set under the HIPAA and is used for reporting dental services and procedures to payers. The CDT Code is reviewed and revised as needed based on changes in dentistry practice. Prior to 2011, CDT codes were incorporated into the HCPCS code list. Revisions to the CDT code were published and effective biennially, at the start of odd-numbered years (e.g., 2011, 2013). Starting in 2014, the CDT code is updated annually. Box 5.7 lists some examples of CDT codes.

## Diagnosis-Related Groups

With tens of thousands of diagnosis and procedure codes available, it is easy to understand how reviewing, analyzing, and reporting patient and population health data might be unwieldy. A method of classification is needed, then, to

 **COMPETENCY CHECK-IN 5.3**

### Special Purpose Classifications and Code Sets

1. Describe why and how SNOMED CT is used in the EHR.
2. What coding system is used to develop cancer mortality statistics?
3. Explain the terms *topography* and *morphology* as they are applied in ICD-O.
4. What organization sponsors DSM-5?
5. In what patient setting are CDT codes used?

make analysis and reporting of clinical data more useful. **Diagnosis-related groups (DRGs)** are the solution. DRGs are a way of classifying statistically similar patients and their diagnoses to gain insight into the costs incurred by the facility. DRG classifications were originally developed by Yale University in the 1960s as a tool to ensure quality of care and appropriate utilization. In the early 1980s, they became the basis for hospital reimbursement by Medicare and certain other payers, which we will discuss in Chapter 6. DRGs were developed by analyzing the resources used to treat patients, by diagnosis. It was determined that the differences in resources used were related to the number and type of additional diagnoses (if any) present during the admission and to the procedures (if any) performed. The analysis of these relationships continues and has given rise to a few different DRG systems that are in use today. In this chapter and Chapter 6, we will concern ourselves primarily with the Medicare Severity Diagnosis-Related Groups (MS-DRGs).

## Diagnosis-Related Group Assignment

DRGs, including MS-DRGs, were initially developed with some basic characteristics in mind (Fig. 5.6). In general, DRGs classify patients according to diagnosis, treatment, and **resource intensity (RI)**, the demands and costs associated with treating a particular disease or condition. RI depends on what types of resources that type of patient consumes and in some instances factors in the age and gender of the patient.

Put in simple terms, modern DRG grouping software gathers certain demographic data and clinical data and uses those data to assign a DRG, which is represented by a three-digit code. Although there is a documentation manual, the actual process of grouping is performed by the grouper software program.

When a patient is registered for admission, a registrar enters the patient's demographic data, such as his or her age and gender, into the facility's computer system. The patient's gender is entered with a valid range of numeric codes, such as 1–3, in which 1 is male, 2 is female, and 3 is unknown. Entering the clinical data in the form of diagnoses and procedure codes is usually done by the coder and is called *abstracting*. The coder may also be responsible for entering the patient's discharge status. Discharge status is also designated using a numeric assignment, for example, 01 for discharged home, with use of Uniform Hospital Discharge Data Set (UHDDS) standards, as defined for the Uniform Bill (UB-04) by the National Uniform Billing Committee.

The grouper then uses the patient's gender, diagnosis code(s), procedure codes(s), and discharge status to determine the appropriate DRG group. Effective for discharges on or after October 1, 2015, the MS-DRGs are based on ICD-10-CM and ICD-10-PCS codes. Fig. 5.7 illustrates the data elements of MS-DRG grouping.

DRG assignment can proceed once all of the necessary information is abstracted into the hospital's information system. **Grouper** software is used to assign each DRG. 3M Health Information Systems is the grouper contractor for

**TABLE 5.2    National Drug Codes (NDC) Directory for Acetaminophen**

| Product NDC | Product Type Name | Proprietary Name | Nonproprietary Name | Dosage | Route | Labeler | Strength | Package Code | Package Description |
|---|---|---|---|---|---|---|---|---|---|
| 50580-783 | Human OTC drug | Tylenol 8 HR Arthritis Pain | Acetaminophen | Tablet, extended-release | Oral | Johnson & Johnson Consumer Inc., McNeil Consumer Healthcare Div. | 650 mg/L | 50580-783-24 | 1 bottle, plastic in 1 carton/24 tablets, extended release in 1 bottle, plastic |
| 50580-783 | Human OTC drug | Tylenol 8 HR Arthritis Pain | Acetaminophen | Tablet, extended-release | Oral | Johnson & Johnson Consumer Inc., McNeil Consumer Healthcare Div. | 650 mg/L | 50580-783-32 | 1 bottle in 1 carton/100 tablets, extended release in 1 bottle |
| 50580-783 | Human OTC drug | Tylenol 8 HR Arthritis Pain | Acetaminophen | Tablet, extended-release | Oral | Johnson & Johnson Consumer Inc., McNeil Consumer Healthcare Div. | 650 mg/L | 50580-783-25 | 1 bottle, plastic in 1 carton/225 tablets, extended release in 1 bottle, plastic |
| 50580-783 | Human OTC drug | Tylenol 8 HR Arthritis Pain | Acetaminophen | Tablet, extended-release | Oral | Johnson & Johnson Consumer Inc., McNeil Consumer Healthcare Div. | 650 mg/L | 50580-783-30 | 290 tablets, extended release in 1 bottle |
| 59779-484 | Human OTC drug | Pain relief | Acetaminophen | Tablet | Oral | CVS Pharmacy | 500 mg/L | 59779-484-62 | 1 bottle in 1 carton/24 tablets in 1 bottle |
| 59779-484 | Human OTC drug | Pain relief | Acetaminophen | Tablet | Oral | CVS Pharmacy | 500 mg/L | 59779-484-71 | 1 bottle in 1 carton/50 tablets in 1 bottle |
| 59779-484 | Human OTC drug | Pain relief | Acetaminophen | Tablet | Oral | CVS Pharmacy | 500 mg/L | 59779-484-76 | 1 bottle in 1 carton/120 tablets in 1 bottle |

OTC, Over-the-counter.

CMS. Inpatients covered by Medicare are grouped into MS-DRGs. Patients that self-pay or have other insurance may be grouped into a different DRG grouping system, such as the AP-DRG. For statistical analysis of risk of mortality and severity of illness, APR-DRGs may be used. APR-DRGs are particularly useful in comparing patient data when multiple DRG classifications are used for reimbursement. Medicare uses MS-DRGs; the use of other DRG groupers, including Medicaid, varies from state to state. Table 5.3 compares various DRG grouping systems. Notice how the DRG changes (or does not) in each example as the diagnosis codes change.

---

**• BOX 5.7 CDT Examples**

- **D0120** Periodic oral evaluation-established patient
- **D2710** Crown-resin-based composite (indirect)
- **D5410** Adjust complete denture-maxillary

---

**NOTE**

The abbreviation CC means Chief Complaint and it also means Comorbidity or Complication. The context in which the abbreviation appears is your guide to which term the abbreviation is referring.

---

| Characteristics | Explanation |
|---|---|
| "The patient characteristics used in the definition of the DRGs should be limited to information routinely collected on hospital abstract systems." | This information consists of the patient's principal diagnosis code, secondary diagnosis code or diagnoses codes, procedure code or codes, the patient's age, sex, and discharge status. In some DRG groupers, a newborn's birth weight must also be included. |
| "There should be a manageable number of DRGs which encompass all patients seen on an inpatient basis." | The point of this is so that meaningful comparative analyses of DRGs can be performed and patterns detected in case mix and costs. |
| "Each DRG should contain patients with a similar pattern of resource intensity." | Clinical coherence means that patients in a particular DRG share a common organ system or condition and/or procedures, and that typically a specific medical or surgical specialty would provide services to that patient. For example, one would expect a psychiatrist to treat all patients in DRGs created for mental diseases and disorders. |
| "Each DRG should contain patients who are similar from a clinical perspective (i.e., each class should be clinically coherent)." | This is so that a hospital can establish a relationship between their case mix and resource consumption. |

• **Fig. 5.6** Characteristics of diagnosis-related groups. (From All patient refined diagnosis related groups [APR-DRGs], methodology overview, version 20.0. 3M Health Information Systems: Wallingford, CT; 2003.)

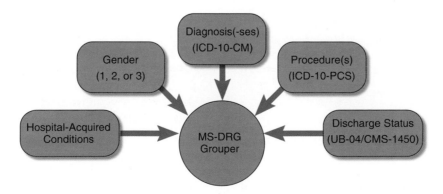

• **Fig. 5.7** Data inputs for an **MS-DRG** grouping program. *MS-DRG*, Medicare Severity Diagnosis-Related Group.

| TABLE 5.3 | Comparison of Diagnosis-Related Group Groupers for a Specific Diagnosis, Heart Failure, and Shock, in a 60-Year-Old Woman | | |
|---|---|---|---|

**First Example**

| Principal diagnosis | Combined Systolic And Diastolic Heart Failure, Acute on Chronic | |
|---|---|---|
| Secondary diagnoses | Pneumonia, Not Otherwise Specified | |
| | Obstructive Chronic Bronchitis With Acute Exacerbation | |
| MS-DRG | 291 | Heart Failure & Shock W MCC |
| AP-DRG | 544 | CHF & Cardiac Arrhythmia W Major CC |
| APR-DRG | 194 | Heart Failure |
| | | 2 Moderate Severity of Illness |
| | | 1 Minor Risk of Mortality |

**Second Example**

| Principal diagnosis | Combined Systolic And Diastolic Heart Failure, Acute on Chronic | |
|---|---|---|
| Secondary diagnosis | Obstructive Chronic Bronchitis With Acute Exacerbation | |
| MS-DRG | 292 | Heart Failure & Shock W CC |
| AP-DRG | 127 | Heart Failure & Shock |
| APR-DRG | 194 | Heart Failure |
| | | 2 Moderate Severity of Illness |
| | | 1 Minor Risk of Mortality |

**Third Example**

| Principal diagnosis | Combined Systolic & Diastolic Heart Failure, Acute on Chronic | |
|---|---|---|
| Secondary diagnosis | No Secondary Diagnosis | |
| MS-DRG | 293 | Heart Failure & Shock W/O CC/MCC |
| AP-DRG | 127 | Heart Failure & Shock |
| APR-DRG | 194 | Heart Failure |
| | | 1 Minor Severity of Illness |
| | | 1 Minor Risk of Mortality |

*AP*, All patient; *APR*, all patient refined; *CC*, comorbidity or complication; *CHF*, congestive heart failure; *DRG*, diagnosis-related group; *MCC*, major comorbidity or complication; *MS*, Medicare severity; *w/o*, without.

## Medicare Severity Diagnosis-Related Group Grouper Logic

The MS-DRG grouper software follows a process referred to as *grouper logic* and can be thought of as a decision tree. DRG grouper programs vary depending on the DRG system in use, but some generalizations may be made about the basic formats.

The process most often begins with an examination of the **principal diagnosis** code. The principal diagnosis is defined in the UHDDS as "that condition established after study to be chiefly responsible for occasioning the admission of the patient to the hospital for care." In the *OCG*, it is quoted at the beginning of Section II, Selecting the Principal Diagnosis, in which inpatient coding is discussed.

ICD-10-CM codes must be currently valid and accepted as a principal diagnosis code by the **Medicare Code Editor (MCE)**, software that checks for illogical or inconsistent diagnoses on billing claims. The MCE is primarily a preventive control against billing errors. Box 5.8 shows a list of the main edits:

Once the principal diagnosis code is accepted as a valid code, the grouping process begins. The first step is to screen the case for extremely resource-intensive procedures, such as organ transplants of the heart, lung, or liver. These patients are assigned into MS-DRGs based on the **principal procedure** code, not the principal diagnosis code, and are directly assigned to each respective MS-DRG. Examples of these MS-DRGs include:

- MS-DRG 002, Heart transplant or implant of heart-assist system
- MS-DRG 013, Tracheostomy for face, mouth, and neck diagnosis

| • BOX 5.8 | Medicare Code Editor Examples |
|---|---|
| **Edit** | **Example** |
| Invalid diagnosis or procedure code | Code is missing one or more required digits or code does not exist in the current code set. |
| External causes of morbidity codes as principal diagnosis | Codes that describe the reason for a trauma, such as "passenger in an automobile collision" are not acceptable principal diagnoses. |
| Age conflict | Use of a code associated with a newborn, such as newborn jaundice, with a teenager. |
| Sex conflict | Use of a gender-specific diagnosis or procedure with a patient of a different gender, such as an ovarian cyst when the patient is male. |
| Manifestation code as principal diagnosis | Manifestation codes are always listed AFTER the underlying condition, so they can never be principal. |
| Unacceptable principal diagnosis | Certain diagnoses are unacceptable in an inpatient setting, because Medicare considers their treatment to be outpatient. Encounter for physical examination for employment is not an inpatient visit. For example, many "Z codes" are on this list, such as ICD-10-CM code Z85.3, history of breast cancer-not a reason for an inpatient admission. |

These first MS-DRGs are considered pre-MDC (major diagnostic category). The next step in the grouping process, then, is to assign the case into its **major diagnostic category (MDC)**. There are 25 MDCs in the Medicare MS-DRG grouper that resemble the chapters in ICD-10-CM, although not necessarily in the same order. To follow a consistent example, consider that we are assigning an MS-DRG to the case of a patient with *acute diastolic heart failure* (I50.31) and no additional diagnoses.

The MDCs are listed in Table 5.4. The complete list and the appendices can be seen on the CMS website: https://www.cms.gov/icd10m/version39.0-fullcode-cms/fullcode_cms/P0001.html. Our patient will group to MDC 05, Diseases and Disorders of the Circulatory System.

Once the patient is assigned to an MDC, the grouper examines any procedure codes. Most MDCs have two main sections, one for medical patients and another for surgical patients. The two sections are referred to as medical partitioning and surgical partitioning. Once a case is assigned to an MDC, the case is sorted or assigned to one of these main sections. Not all procedure codes are used for MS-DRG assignment. For example, codes for ultrasound examinations are diagnostic radiology and are essentially ignored during the grouping process. Procedure codes that are recognized and used for grouping are categorized as either OR (operating room) or non-OR. An OR procedure code indicates that the patient has undergone a procedure usually requiring the use of an OR, for example, a gastric bypass or open fracture reduction. Non-OR procedures include procedures or treatments such as paracentesis or nonexcisional debridement. The designation of an OR procedure versus a non-OR procedure for the purpose of grouping is made by the CMS during its annual MS-DRG update process. The grouper effectively asks the question: Did the patient have an OR procedure? If the answer is yes, then the correct MS-DRG is found in the surgical partition. If the answer is no, then the correct MS-DRG is found in the medical partition. Our patient did not have an OR procedure, so we will be grouping to the medical partition of MDC 05.

For cases sorted into the medical partition, the grouper may look for, depending on the MDC, the patient's age. The MCE detects instances in which a patient's age does not correspond with the principal or secondary coded diagnoses. For example, an 80-year-old woman with pregnancy codes would not pass the edit and would not be grouped until a correction was made in abstracting.

The next step in the grouping process is to identify the cluster of MS-DRGs into which a specific principal diagnosis is grouped. At this point, it might be useful for you to look at the MS-DRG definitions manual at https://www.cms.gov/icd10m/version39.0-fullcode-cms/fullcode_cms/P0001.html. Here, you can confirm that the principal diagnosis is listed under the DRG. Remember that it changes every year, so you might find a more recent version as you are reading this.

**TABLE 5.4 Major Diagnostic Categories for Medicare Severity Diagnosis-Related Group**

| MDC Number | Description |
|---|---|
| 01 | Diseases & Disorders of the Nervous System |
| 02 | Diseases & Disorders of the Eye |
| 03 | Diseases & Disorders of the Ear, Nose, Mouth, & Throat |
| 04 | Diseases & Disorders of the Respiratory System |
| 05 | Diseases & Disorders of the Circulatory System |
| 06 | Diseases & Disorders of the Digestive System |
| 07 | Diseases & Disorders of the Hepatobiliary System & Pancreas |
| 08 | Diseases & Disorders of the Musculoskeletal System & Connective Tissue |
| 09 | Diseases & Disorders of the Skin, Subcutaneous Tissue, & Breast |
| 10 | Endocrine Nutritional & Metabolic Diseases & Disorders |
| 11 | Diseases & Disorders of the Kidney & Urinary Tract |
| 12 | Diseases & Disorders of the Male Reproductive System |
| 13 | Diseases & Disorders of the Female Reproductive System |
| 14 | Pregnancy, Childbirth, & the Puerperium |
| 15 | Newborns & Other Neonates with Conditions Originating in the Perinatal Period |
| 16 | Diseases & Disorders of Blood, Blood Forming Organs, Immunological Disorders |
| 17 | Myeloproliferative Diseases & Disorders, Poorly Differentiated Neoplasm |
| 18 | Infectious & Parasitic Diseases, Systemic or Unspecified Sites |
| 19 | Mental Diseases & Disorders |
| 20 | Alcohol or Drug Use or Induced Organic Mental Disorders |
| 21 | Injuries, Poisonings, & Toxic Effects of Drugs |
| 22 | Burns |
| 23 | Factors Influencing Health Status & Other Contacts with Health Services |
| 24 | Multiple Significant Trauma |
| 25 | Human Immunodeficiency Virus Infections |

*MDC*, Major diagnostic category.
From Centers for Medicare and Medicaid Services: *ICD-10-CM/PCS MS-DRG v39.0 Definitions Manual.* Available at: https://www.cms.gov/icd10m/version39.0-fullcode-cms/fullcode_cms/P0001.html Accessed January 29, 2022.

## MDC 05 DISEASES AND DISORDERS OF THE CIRCULATORY SYSTEM

### Heart Failure and Shock

| MCC | CC | DRG |
|-----|-----|-----|
| Yes | n/a | 291 |
| No | Yes | 292 |
| No | No | 293 |

Heart failure and shock group to the cluster MS-DRG 291-293.
DRG 291: Heart failure and shock with MCC
DRG 292: Heart failure and shock with CC
DRG 293 Heart failure and shock without CC/MCC

### Principal diagnosis[a]

| | |
|---|---|
| I09.81 | Rheumatic heart failure |
| I11.0 | Hypertensive heart disease with heart failure |
| I13.0 | Hypertensive heart and chronic kidney disease with heart failure and stage 1 through stage 4 chronic kidney disease, or unspecified chronic kidney disease |
| I13.2 | Hypertensive heart and chronic kidney disease with heart failure and with stage 5 chronic kidney disease, or end stage renal disease |
| I50.1 | Left ventricular failure, unspecified |
| I50.20 | Unspecified systolic (congestive) heart failure |
| I50.21 | Acute systolic (congestive) heart failure |
| I50.22 | Chronic systolic (congestive) heart failure |
| I50.23 | Acute on chronic systolic (congestive) heart failure |
| I50.30 | Unspecified diastolic (congestive) heart failure |
| I50.31 | Acute diastolic (congestive) heart failure |
| I50.32 | Chronic diastolic (congestive) heart failure |
| I50.33 | Acute on chronic diastolic (congestive) heart failure |
| I50.40 | Unspecified combined systolic (congestive) and diastolic (congestive) heart failure |
| I50.41 | Acute combined systolic (congestive) and diastolic (congestive) heart failure |
| I50.42 | Chronic combined systolic (congestive) and diastolic (congestive) heart failure |
| I50.43 | Acute on chronic combined systolic (congestive) and diastolic (congestive) heart failure |
| I50.810 | Right heart failure, unspecified |
| I50.811 | Acute right heart failure |
| I50.812 | Chronic right heart failure |
| I50.813 | Acute on chronic right heart failure |
| I50.814 | Right heart failure due to left heart failure |
| I50.82 | Biventricular heart failure |
| I50.83 | High output heart failure |
| I50.84 | End-stage heart failure |
| I50.89 | Other heart failure |
| I50.9 | Heart failure, unspecified |
| R57.0 | Cardiogenic shock |
| R57.9 | Shock, unspecified |

From Centers for Medicare and Medicaid Services: *ICD-10-CM/PCS MS-DRG v39.0 Definitions Manual*. Available at: https://www.cms.gov/icd10m/version39.0-fullcode-cms/fullcode_cms/P0001.html. Accessed January 30, 2022.
[a]Amended for clarity by adding periods, which do not typically appear in official documentation.

Next, depending on the MDC, the grouper will search the secondary diagnosis codes for a comorbidity or complication (CC) and major comorbidity or complication (MCC). The list of CCs and MCCs can be seen on the CMS website listed previously, in Appendix G, Diagnoses Defined as Complications or Comorbidities, and Appendix H, Diagnoses Defined as Major Complications or Comorbidities. MCC codes are complications or comorbidities of greater severity than CC codes. MCC codes, when applied in the MS-DRG calculation, "adjust" the DRG assignment and reimbursement to account for this greater severity. Our example patient has no CC or MCC. According to the table, we answer "No" to the question of where there was an ECMO and "No" to both the CC and MCC. Therefore this case groups to MS-DRG 293.

In this context, a comorbidity is a condition that was present on admission (POA), whereas a complication is a condition that arose during the hospitalization. This distinction is significant for reimbursement purposes, as we discuss later in this chapter and in Chapter 6. If a secondary diagnosis code, when matched with a certain principal diagnosis code, is statistically proven to extend a patient's length of stay by at least 1 day in 75% of cases, that secondary diagnosis is considered a CC in combination with that principal diagnosis. For example, suppose our patient has a principal diagnosis of *acute diastolic heart failure* (I50.31) and also has *hyponatremia* (E87.1). It has been statistically demonstrated that 75% of patients with a secondary diagnosis of hyponatremia typically remain in the hospital at least 1 day longer than patients without hyponatremia. Therefore E87.1 is considered an applicable CC code when I50.31 is the principal diagnosis code, and this case groups to MS-DRG 292.

The lists of CC and MCC codes are reviewed and revised each year by the CMS and published in the *Federal Register* and on the CMS website previously listed, usually at the same time as any MS-DRG revisions.

Not all CC codes appearing in the CC or MCC list apply in all instances. Certain CC codes are not considered CCs with certain principal diagnoses codes because the secondary diagnosis code is a condition that has been determined to not significantly affect length of stay or treatment. A list of all CC codes and MCC codes can be seen in Appendix C (of the *definitions manual*), Complications or Comorbidities Exclusion List. Each CC or MCC code listed is followed by a code or codes that, when assigned as principal diagnoses, exclude that CC or MCC from affecting MS-DRG assignment. For example, I09.81, Rheumatic heart failure, is a CC. If I09.81 is assigned as a secondary diagnosis code with a principal diagnosis of I50.1, Left ventricular failure, it will not "count" as a CC because I09.81 is on the CC exclusion list for code I50.1. Therefore this case groups to MS-DRG 293. If you are following along in the Definitions Manual, select Appendix C and find I09.81 toward the bottom of the G codes. Next to I09.81, there is a link to the 30 codes that, in combination, convert a CC/MCC to a non-CC.

Cases assigned to the surgical partitioning section of an MDC essentially follow the same format for MS-DRG assignment as those in the medical partitioning section but must account for instances in which more than one procedure is performed (from the OR or non-OR list) on the same patient during the same admission. Only one MS-DRG is assigned for each admission, even if multiple procedures are performed. In these cases, the grouper reviews all of the procedure codes assigned and identifies the single procedure that required the most RI. Each surgical partition is sequenced according to a surgical hierarchy. When multiple procedures have been performed, the procedure code that is highest in the surgical hierarchy is selected by the grouper for MS-DRG assignment. On the MDC tree diagram, the surgical hierarchy lists procedures in descending order, with the procedure requiring the greatest RI at the top of the list. For example, assume that a patient in MDC 8 (diseases and disorders of the musculoskeletal system and connective tissue) undergoes a total hip replacement. This case would group to MS-DRG 470, Major joint replacement or reattachment of lower extremity without MCC. In another case, a patient undergoes a shoulder arthroscopy. That case would group to MS-DRG 512, Shoulder, forearm or shoulder procedure excluding major joint procedure without CC/MCC. Now, suppose that a patient who was admitted for and underwent total hip replacement later complained of severe shoulder pain and was returned to the OR during the same admission for a shoulder arthroscopy. The MS-DRG for this admission would be MS-DRG 470 because a total hip replacement is higher on the surgical hierarchy than a shoulder arthroscopy. The arthroscopy has no influence on MS-DRG assignment in this case because it is superseded by the total hip replacement in RI. When abstracting a case, even if the arthroscopy were listed first as principal procedure, the grouper would still select the total hip replacement for MS-DRG assignment. This is a major difference from cases in the medical partition, in which the principal diagnosis selected by the coder drives the MS-DRG assignment.

In addition to the cases grouped directly into a pre-MDC MS-DRG, there are other exceptions in which a case is grouped directly to an MS-DRG, without first being assigned to an MDC. Unusual, unpredictable, or unique circumstances occasionally occur during hospitalization, making such cases exceptions to the usual rules of MS-DRG assignment. These exceptions are categorized into the following MS-DRGs:

DRG 981, extensive OR procedure unrelated to principal diagnosis with MCC, DRG 982, extensive OR procedure unrelated to principal diagnosis with CC, and DRG 983, extensive OR procedure unrelated to principal diagnosis without CC/MCC: An example would be a patient admitted for a myocardial infarction. During her hospitalization, a breast lump is noticed, the patient is found to have breast cancer, and a mastectomy is performed. The myocardial infarction as principal diagnosis is not associated with or related to the mastectomy, so the case is grouped to DRG 983.

DRG 998, *Principal diagnosis invalid as discharge diagnosis*: A code, such as Z93.8, Colostomy status, was submitted as principal diagnosis for an inpatient admission.

DRG 987, nonextensive OR procedure unrelated to principal diagnosis with MCC, DRG 988, nonextensive OR procedure unrelated to principal diagnosis with CC, and DRG 989, nonextensive OR procedure unrelated to principal diagnosis without CC/MCC: These DRGs are similar to DRGs 981 to 983, except that the procedure is, as it states, nonextensive. An example would be if the previously mentioned patient with a myocardial infarction had a breast biopsy instead of a mastectomy. The myocardial infarction as principal diagnosis is not associated with or related to the breast biopsy, and the breast biopsy is a nonextensive procedure, unlike the mastectomy, so the case is grouped to DRG 989.

A complete list of DRGs and related information is published yearly, in late summer, as a Final Rule in the *Federal Register* on the CMS website in conjunction with ICD-10-CM/PCS updates, effective on each October 1. To see the entire list, look for Table 5.5 in the CMS web page for the current version: https://www.cms.gov/medicare/acute-inpatient-pps/fy-2022-ipps-final-rule-home-page#Tables.

Understanding how DRGs are assigned helps coders to properly sequence their code assignments and focus on the correct principal diagnosis. Even though the coder is using encoder software to find the codes and grouper software to assign the MS-DRG, it is important to pay attention to ensure that the MS-DRG assignment makes sense. If the MS-DRG assignment does not seem correct, there may be an error in the coding. Box 5.9 summarizes the steps in DRG assignment.

### The Coder's Role in Diagnosis-Related Group (Medicare Severity Diagnosis-Related Group) Assignment

The coder must be able to properly apply current coding rules and coding conventions to each case. Although this section focuses on Medicare usage, all cases, regardless of payer, should be coded with equal care, even if payment is not affected, if a hospital's statistics are to be accurate and useful. As previously emphasized, complete and accurate coding is necessary to generate data and statistics beyond MS-DRGs and other DRG grouper assignments.

It is unethical and fraudulent to deliberately code a case incorrectly so that it may be placed into an MS-DRG with a higher reimbursement rate. This practice is sometimes referred to as *upcoding*, maximizing, or *DRG creep*. Some coding software includes prompts that alert the coder that a case would group to a higher paying MS-DRG if a CC or MCC were added or if a different principal diagnosis were assigned. The coder may wish to review the medical record to search for a CC or MCC or confirm that there is no CC or MCC. Under no circumstances should the coder simply add a CC or MCC without confirming that the CC or MCC is documented in the medical record. Likewise, the principal diagnosis code should not be changed unless an error was made in the original assignment. The coding

| TABLE 5.5 | Comparison of Current Coding Systems | |
|---|---|---|
| **Acronym** | **Full Name** | **Use** |
| SNOMED CT[a] | Systemized Nomenclature of Medical Clinical Terms | Extensive clinical vocabulary, machine-readable terminology for potential use in an electronic health record (EHR) |
| ICD-O-3 | International Classification of Diseases for Oncology, Third Revision | Coding of neoplasm/cancer diagnoses for tumor reporting |
| DSM-5 | Diagnostic and Statistical Manual of Mental Disorders, Fifth Edition | Classification of mental and behavioral disorders, coded using ICD-10-CM |
| ICD-10-CM[a] | International Classification of Diseases, 10th Revision-Clinical Modification | Coding and reporting diagnoses for patient encounters. Used for reimbursement |
| ICD-10-PCS[a] | International Classification of Diseases, 10th Revision-Procedure Coding System | Coding and reporting procedures for inpatient encounters. Used with ICD-10-CM for reimbursement |
| HCPCS/CPT-4[a] | Healthcare Common Procedure Coding System and Current Procedural Terminology, Fourth Version | Coding and reporting for reimbursement for outpatient and physician office procedures |
| CDT[a] | Current Dental Terminology | Used to report dental services and procedures to dental plans for reimbursement |
| NDC[a] | National Drug Codes | US Food and Drug Administration (FDA) list of drugs used by humans |

[a]HIPAA Transaction Code Set.

software prompts are intended to assist the coder in ensuring proper coding and sequencing; this process is sometimes referred to as optimizing. The prompts should never be interpreted as directives to code or sequence a certain way simply to obtain higher reimbursement when no supporting documentation exists.

In all cases, without exception, coding and sequencing must be supported by documentation in the medical record. To code otherwise is considered fraudulent by the federal

**Assignment of the Diagnosis-Related Group**

Most cases in various grouper programs follow the following format:

1. Search for clinical procedures: transplants, ventilators, and tracheotomies, and group immediately to the appropriate DRG, if detected.
2. The principal diagnosis code assigns a case to MDC.
3. The grouper reviews all diagnoses and procedure codes and then assigns the case to either the medical or surgical portion of the MDC.
4. The grouper, using the Medicare code edits, makes sure that the principal diagnosis code is appropriate for an inpatient admission.
5. The grouper, using the Medicare code edits, makes sure that the patient's age and sex are appropriate for the diagnoses and procedures assigned.
6. The grouper may further process the case according to the patient's age.
7. The grouper reviews all secondary diagnosis codes for the presence of a CC.
8. If the case is surgical, the grouper reviews all procedure codes assigned and bases the DRG selection on the procedure code highest in the surgical hierarchy.

*DRG*, Diagnosis-related group; *MDC*, major diagnostic category.

**• BOX 5.10  Present on Admission Indicators**

| Code | | Reason for Code |
|------|------|------|
| Y | Yes | Diagnosis was present at the time the order for admission was written. |
| N | No | Diagnosis was not present at the time the order for admission was written. |
| U | Unknown | Documentation insufficient to determine if the condition was present at the time of inpatient admission. |
| W | Undetermined | Provider unable to clinically determine whether the condition was present at the time of inpatient admission. |
| | Unreported/Not used | Exempt from POA reporting. This code is equivalent to a blank on the UB-04; however, it was determined that blanks are undesirable when submitting this data via the 4010A. |

From Centers for Medicare and Medicaid Services, https://www.cms.gov/Medicare/Medicare-Fee-for-Service-Payment/HospitalAcqCond/Coding, Accessed January 29, 2022.

government under the Civil False Claims Act and may subject the hospital to considerable monetary penalties if a pattern of fraud and abuse is demonstrated.

Usually, medical records are coded and MS-DRGs are assigned after the patient is discharged. The hospital cannot submit a claim for reimbursement until after the patient is discharged. To minimize the time between discharge and claim submission, some facilities perform coding concurrently, that is, while the patient is still in the hospital. The coder may review the medical record when the patient is admitted and every day or every other day thereafter until discharge. Temporary codes are assigned along with a temporary MS-DRG. This concurrently assigned MS-DRG is often referred to as a **working MS-DRG**. The coder has the opportunity to question the physician about documentation and potentially facilitate coding and MS-DRG assignment accuracy; these efforts may shorten the time between discharge and claim submission. Coding concurrently does present some disadvantages, however. More coding staff may be needed, and some necessary information, such as pathology reports, may not yet be available. In effect, concurrent coding may be a duplication of effort since the postdischarge coding must still take place.

### Present on Admission

In addition to assigning the principal diagnosis, the coder must also assign to each diagnosis code on an inpatient admission an indicator that identifies whether the diagnosis was POA. That is, did the patient already have the disease or condition at the time of admission or did it occur during the patient's stay? This indicator is captured in a separate field but is directly associated with each diagnosis. The codes for the POA indicator can be found in Appendix I of the Official Coding Guidelines and are listed in Box 5.10.

The assignment of a POA indicator is critical in determining the MS-DRG for a case, because the MS-DRG is not only a resource utilization tool, it is also used for payment.

Examples:

- Patient admitted with dizziness, confusion, and left-sided hemiparesis is diagnosed with a cerebrovascular accident. On day 2 of the admission, the patient fell out of bed and broke her arm. The coder will assign POA indicator "Y" to the CVA and POA indicator "N" to the fracture, which happened in the hospital after admission.
- Patient admitted with shortness of breath and a history of *Type I diabetes mellitus*. The patient is diagnosed with *acute exacerbation of chronic asthma*. The coder will assign POA indicator "Y" to both asthma and diabetes because they were both POA.
- Single, live newborn delivered by cesarean section in the hospital. The coder will assign POA indicator "Exempt" because newborns are exempt from POA assignment.

The Unknown and Clinically Undetermined POAs may require a discussion with the physician prior to coding. Discussions with physicians that may lead to an amendment to the patient record or additional documentation should take place in a formal, written query (see Physician Query Process section later). Detailed examples of how to assign POAs under various scenarios are included in the OCG.

### Hospital-Acquired Conditions

The assignment of a POA indicator is a component of the CMS **Hospital-Acquired Condition (HAC)** regulation, which has been in effect since fiscal year 2009. This regulation enforces a component of the Deficit Reduction Act of 2005 in which CMS is directed to identify conditions that:

(a) are high cost or high volume, or both;

(b) result in the assignment of a case to a DRG that has a higher payment when present as a secondary diagnosis;

(c) could reasonably have been prevented through the application of evidence-based guidelines (Centers for Medicare and Medicaid Services, 2021).

HACs are conditions that are generally considered to be preventable. Therefore in the calculation of the MS-DRG, conditions that are on the HAC list are ignored for the purpose of MS-DRG assignment when they are not POA (i.e., when they are nosocomial). Effectively, this means that an HAC, developed during the hospital stay, representing the only CC or MCC on a case would be ignored and the MS-DRG assigned to the case would be "without CC or MCC." As we will see in Chapter 6, this results in lower payment to the hospital. The payment impact of each POA indicator is described below.

| Code | Payment |
| --- | --- |
| **Y** | CMS will pay the CC/MCC DRG for those selected HACs that are coded as "Y" for the POA indicator |
| **N** | CMS will not pay the CC/MCC DRG for those selected HACs that are coded as "N" for the POA indicator |
| **U** | CMS will not pay the CC/MCC DRG for those selected HACs that are coded as "U" for the POA indicator |
| W | CMS will pay the CC/MCC DRG for those selected HACs that are coded as "W" for the POA indicator<br><br>HACs should not be coded as exempt from POA assignment. CMS will not pay the CC/MCC DRG for those selected HACs that are coded as exempt from POA assignment |

HACs that the CMS considers in the MS-DRG assignment are identified in an official list that is published annually with any revisions along with the updated MS-DRG list. The categories of conditions that represent HACs when not POA are:

- Foreign Object Retained After Surgery
- Air Embolism
- Blood Incompatibility
- Stage III and IV Pressure Ulcers
- Falls and Trauma
- Catheter-Associated Urinary Tract Infection (UTI)
- Vascular Catheter-Associated Infection
- Surgical Site Infection (SSI)—Mediastinitis After Coronary Bypass Graft
- Manifestations of Poor Glycemic Control
- Deep Vein Thrombosis/Pulmonary Embolism (PE) with Total Knee or Hip Replacement
- SSI—Bariatric Surgery

**COMPETENCY CHECK-IN 5.4**

**Diagnostic-Related Groups**

**Competency Assessment**

1. Define present on admission.
2. Define HAC.
3. The patient was admitted to the hospital with chest pain and shortness of breath. The patient was diagnosed with congestive heart failure (CHF) via X-ray and was treated for asthma. No new signs or symptoms arose during the stay. The final diagnosis is CHF with acute exacerbation of chronic asthma. What is the POA?
   a. POA for the CHF and asthma is Y.
   b. POA for the CHF is Y; the asthma is N.
   c. POA for the CHF is Y; the asthma is W.
   d. POA for the asthma cannot be determined and the physician should be queried.
4. A recent coding audit has revealed that Coder B has been assigning POA Y to all diagnoses. Comment on this finding, explaining any concerns, and describe any action you would take.

- SSI—Certain Orthopedic Procedures of Spine, Shoulder, and Elbow
- SSI Following Cardiac Implantable Electronic Device Procedures
- Iatrogenic Pneumothorax with Venous Catheterization (Centers for Medicare and Medicaid Services, 2022)

To illustrate the impact of HACs, consider the following example:

Patient is admitted with osteoarthritis of the knee for a total knee replacement and suffers a PE on day 2 of the admission. Osteoarthritis is POA indicator "Y." PE is POA indicator "N." PE is an MCC. This case would group to MS-DRG 469 if the PE were not on the HAC list. Because it is on the HAC list, and it was not POA, the case groups to MS-DRG 470. As we will see in Chapter 6, MS-DRG 470 pays 37% less than MS-DRG 469.

## Coding Quality

The accuracy of coded clinical data is essential. As we have seen throughout this chapter, there are many rules, guidelines, and procedures that must be followed for high-quality coding. In this section, we will explore some of how we get to that high quality.

### Uses for Coded Clinical Data

Coded clinical data are used for a variety of purposes by many different users. Therefore the quality of the data is critical to ensure that all users can rely on the data. Some common uses of coded data are case mix analysis, reporting, comparative analysis, and reimbursement. Table 5.5 lists the code sets discussed in this chapter and their applications.

Case mix analysis looks at groups of patient data to determine what types of patients are treated in a particular setting. For example, some hospitals treat a large number of maternity and newborn cases; other hospitals treat a large number of trauma patients. Even within a particular facility, a hospital may see that there is a trend over time: less cataract surgery being performed this year than last year, or more complicated cases treated in the first half of the year than the last.

Case mix analysis can be used to identify coding errors. If there is a sudden change in the number of complicated cases, the coders (or one coder) may be missing complicating diagnoses. Hospitals often pay close attention to case mix and perform routine audits to ensure accurate coding, which produces coded data that accurately reflect the case mix. The CMS also looks at case mix within the Medicare population and may initiate an audit of a hospital, the case mix of which shows an inexplicably high number of complications over time.

As discussed in previous chapters, coded data are used for reporting purposes. Hospitals report the UHDDS, for example, which provides the states and subsequently the federal government with details of inpatient stays. Coded data are also provided to accrediting agencies and the CDC (to report infectious diseases).

Internally, coded data may be used to identify quantities of procedures performed for physician credentialing purposes and service area volume analysis. Many reports that are generated internally from the hospital system pull the data based on the desired coded data element, such as diagnosis or procedure code. These reports can be used internally for administrative, clinician credentialing, and other purposes.

Coded data are used to compare facility-specific, regional, national, and international health care observations. For example, CMS publishes aggregate (general, not patient-identifiable) data that can be used to compare hospital performance. So a facility can review their MS-DRG mix and compare it to overall Medicare results.

One of the most common uses of coded data today is reimbursement. HCPCS/CPT codes, for example, were developed specifically to communicate to payers information about services rendered by the provider. With the evolution of DRG systems, Medicare has expanded the use of clinical data to drive reimbursement to include most settings. Inpatient rehabilitation, inpatient behavioral health, skilled nursing, and home health, for example, are all reimbursed based on some form of coded data collection. Chapter 6 discusses reimbursement in detail.

## Achieving Coding Quality

### Timely Processing

The timeliness and completeness of the postdischarge processing of a record are important. In addition to charge capture, all pertinent medical record data must have been collected for correct assignment of codes, and the processing cycle must facilitate efficient, timely coding. For example, if the paper components of a health record must be assembled, scanned, and analyzed before it is given to a coder, and if the assembly, scanning, and analysis sections are 5 or 6 days behind the current discharge date, then medical records may not be coded until 7 days after the discharge date. Even factoring in the bill-hold period, a week is a long time for a facility to go without dropping a bill for a patient's stay. Facilities sometimes choose to code the record before it is assembled or analyzed so that the bill may be dropped more quickly. Although this sequence expedites payment, it can also lead to coding errors if the medical record is incomplete, because missing elements are not clearly identified or if important reports are misplaced in the wrong sections of the record.

The issues surrounding a paper-based medical record will generally be reduced with the EHR. The EHR will permit access to patient information immediately on its entry. Information cannot be lost once it is entered into the EHR. Coders may access the EHR at any point after patient admission and after discharge. In addition, computer-assisted coding (CAC) programs embedded in the EHR may facilitate the coding process in terms of speed and accuracy.

Coding must be reliable and valid, both individually and collectively within a facility or group. A coder or group of coders is said to demonstrate reliability when codes are consistently assigned for similar or identical cases. Validity of coding refers to the degree of accuracy of the codes assigned.

### Coder Training

Forty years ago, when computerized collection and storage of coded data was in its infancy, it was fairly common to hire individuals with limited knowledge and experience to assign codes to the discharged cases. Tales are told of coders sitting around debating how to code thorny cases and many coders learned on the job, following rules developed within the facility or imposed by payers who did not all agree. Today, with the increasing complexity of the coding process and pressure from administration for accurate reimbursement, it is rare to find an employer willing to hire a completely untrained coder.

Coders are required to know medical terminology, anatomy and physiology, pathophysiology, pharmacology, coding and classification systems, and computer software. Knowledge can be obtained through formal training programs available in schools or through some employers. Table 5.6 lists the resources needed for the coding process.

### Accuracy

Assigning the correct code to the documented diagnoses and procedures is the most important element of coding quality. Accurate coding is necessary for optimization of reimbursement and is best achieved through coding from a complete medical record. Optimization occurs when the coding results in the MS-DRG that most accurately represents the facility's utilization of resources, based on the diagnoses and procedures, and is completely substantiated by documentation. Maximization is simply assigning and sequencing codes to obtain the highest paying MS-DRG.

## TABLE 5.6    Coding Resources

| Code Books | ICD-10-CM<br>ICD-10-PCS<br>HCPCS<br>CPT |
|---|---|
| Specialty Systems | Abstracting Module in facility system<br>Encoder<br>Grouper<br>Computer-Assisted Coding software |
| Clinical References | Anatomy and physiology<br>Pharmacology<br>Surgical procedures |
| Code Set references | Coding Clinic<br>CPT Assistant<br>AHA ICD-10-CM/PCS Coding Handbook |

Optimization is highly desirable; maximization is illegal and unethical. Patterns of maximization could be considered abuse. Patterns of maximization that intentionally result in excessive payments to the provider are considered fraud. Under the US government's National Correct Coding Initiative (NCCI), and their fraud and abuse audits, patterns of maximization, if proved, can result in the criminal prosecution of facility administrators and individual complicit employees.

### Volume

Also important in measuring coding productivity is volume: the speed with which the coder can assign accurate codes. Although accuracy is critical, it is not financially advantageous to the organization for a coder to take an entire 8-hour day to code one chart. Assuming there are 30 discharges a day, the hospital would need more than 30 coders to keep up with the workload. Volume productivity expectations are difficult to quantify as a rule because facilities vary significantly in their processes, coder job descriptions, and work environment. To illustrate, imagine a coder sitting in a quiet room with no distractions, on a very fast computer system, using an EHR in which all of the codable components are easily accessible from a single source and an encoder that interfaces seamlessly with the abstracting module. Now think about a coder sitting in the middle of a department using an EHR with multiple modules that require separate logins and screens and an encoder that is separate from the EHR so that every data point must be entered manually. This coder also must cover the phones. Obviously the first coder is going to be able to complete more records in a day than the second coder. Logically it would take longer to code a complicated inpatient record than it would to code a normal newborn or an ED visit for a simple fracture. Despite these variances, HIM managers will define volume productivity standards for their facility. Collecting actual volume data from coders for a period, and discussing with them the reasons for day-to-day variances, is the best place to start.

## Computer-Assisted Coding

As mentioned earlier, electronic documentation can be interpreted by SNOMED CT to result in the assignment of ICD-10-CM/PCS codes. The assignment is called CAC, and software that affects this assignment can be interfaced with EHRs and groupers to assist the coding process. Because there is not always a one-to-one relationship between the SNOMED CT-coded concepts and a particular diagnosis or procedure code, human intervention is required to ensure that a case is coded correctly.

A CAC program will present the coder with a list of suggested codes that it gleaned from the EHR. CAC programs can link the codes to the location in the record from which it obtained the concept. The coder is responsible for accepting, modifying, or rejecting the codes as relevant to the case. The coder is also responsible for ensuring that all relevant codes are identified, including any that were not displayed by CAC.

CAC should improve coder productivity volume because it reduces the need to look up all of the codes every time. However, the responsibility for coding accuracy rests with the coder. The HIM department should have policies and procedures in place that describe the extent to which coders must validate CAC-assigned codes and search for codes not identified by the CAC program. CAC programs that link the code to the documentation are valuable for audit purposes as well as to ensure that code assignment is transparent.

Another reason that CAC programs do not produce 100% of the codes accurately is that they do not necessarily recognize a diagnosis or a procedure that was mentioned in the record but resolved or performed in the past. So, the history and physical (H&P) or problem list may discuss a hernia with repair that the CAC will identify and code; however, the diagnosis was resolved with the procedure years ago and does not pertain to the current encounter. The coder will need to check the coding for relevance and accuracy. Here is an example:

> The patient was admitted with a myocardial infarction. In the H&P, the physician notes a history of pneumonia and Type I diabetes mellitus. Past surgical procedures were tonsillectomy and appendectomy. The patient underwent angioplasty on Day 1 of the stay and was discharged to home on Day 4. The operative report has not yet been transcribed and the discharge summary is not dictated yet.

The CAC program presented the coder with the following:

> Myocardial infarction not otherwise specified
> Pneumonia
> Type I diabetes mellitus without complications

> CODER ACTION:
> Review the chart for greater specificity in the myocardial infarction code.
> Review the chart for any treatment for pneumonia; otherwise, delete.

*Read the operative report when available for details of the angioplasty to code.*

## Coding Compliance

As mentioned earlier, facilities and payers were historically able to set their own rules regarding how and what to code. Even within a facility, there might be individual variation. For example, some facilities always coded blood transfusions; others did not. Some facilities stopped coding when the number of codes assigned reached the maximum number of spaces available on the Uniform Bill. In early versions, the Uniform Bill had space for nine diagnoses and six procedures. Today, there are multiple programs in place both federally and by payers to monitor coding quality. We have already mentioned the *NCCI*. Since many of these programs affect reimbursement, we will address them in Chapter 6. Of particular interest here are the *Official Guidelines for Coding and Reporting* and the *Office of Inspector General Compliance Plan*.

Under the auspices of the US Department of Health and Human Service's Office of the Inspector General (OIG), the federal government released *Compliance Program Guidance for Hospitals*, which addresses coding issues. Coders should be familiar with this publication, as well as with their own hospital's compliance program. The OIG published a Work Plan every year that included coding projects focused on particular MS-DRGs and patterns of MS-DRG assignment. Starting on June 15, 2017, the OIG Work Plan is available on a website and is updated monthly.

A comprehensive **coding compliance plan** is an important part of a facility's corporate compliance plan. The coding compliance plan should include regular internal audits and audits performed by objective external reviewers who have no vested interest in the facility's profit margin. Coding audits performed by payers are not necessarily useful in determining coding accuracy because their overall goal is to find only those coding errors that adversely affect the payer. In any type of audit, however, results should be shared and discussed with the coding staff.

There are two fundamentally different approaches to coding audits: general reviews of all records of all payer types to identify potential problems and targeted reviews of known or potential problem areas. In general reviews, records are selected by a statistical method or by any method that captures a representative sample of records. All coders, all record types, and all payers should be included in a general review. The audit results can be used to determine coding error rates by coder or more generally. Both upcoding (coding to a higher paying DRG than is supported by the documentation) and downcoding (coding to a lower paying DRG) are problematic from a payer's standpoint. Only consistently accurate code assignment will produce consistently accurate reimbursement.

## COMPETENCY CHECK-IN 5.5

### Coding Quality

#### Competency Assessment

1. Why is the timing of postdischarge processing important to a coder?
2. What is a coding compliance plan?
3. Explain the difference between optimization and maximization.
4. Name two types of coding audits. When would you use each?
5. Describe and discuss an example of an unethical coding practice.
6. Compare and contrast two different approaches to high-quality coding audits.

#### Case Study

PATIENT NAME: ALEXANDER POWELL
MRN: 1215613
Patient, 57 years of age, first reported discomfort and hesitancy with urination and lower abdominal pain. Acute abdominal pains are sporadic. Vital signs: pulse 72 bpm; temperature 98.6 °F; respirations 16 breaths/min.
HISTORY: History of gallbladder excision 14 years ago, kidney stones 7 years ago, and late-onset type 2 diabetes and chronic UTIs before lithotripsy.
FAMILY HISTORY: Grandfather and father, late-onset type 2 diabetes. Grandfather, history of glaucoma. Father, nonfatal prostatic carcinoma.
DIAGNOSIS: Recurrence of UTI ruled out by specimen analysis. Early-stage prostatic carcinoma indicated by CT scan.
TREATMENT/PROGNOSIS: Outpatient treatment with implanted radiotherapy. Patient released with prescription analgesic. Prognosis: full recovery.

1. What is the patient's chief complaint?
2. What is the patient's current diagnosis? (List all that apply to this encounter)
3. Does the patient have any family history relevant to the current diagnosis? (List, if any)
4. What tests support the patient's diagnosis?
5. Do you have any questions for the physician to further clarify the patient's diagnosis, treatment, or discharge plan? (List, if any)

## Case Study

PATIENT NAME: MITCHELL BURKOVICZ
MRN: 2018001

### History and physical

HISTORY OF PRESENT ILLNESS: Patient seeks a physical examination, which is required before running a marathon. Reports no current complaints except shin splints.

REVIEW OF SYSTEMS: Denies any recent change in weight, mood, or energy; physical history suggests normal metabolism and homeostasis. Denies headaches, vertigo, or changes in hearing or vision. Denies chest pain, palpitations, or syncopal episodes. Positive for SOB while running; denies cough and history of asthma or pneumonia and does not use tobacco products. Denies heartburn, melena, or hemorrhoids. Denies muscle cramps but is positive for shin splints. No history of fractures.

SOCIAL HISTORY: No current problems. Patient is married and living with wife and small child. Is a full-time student employed as a medical library aide.

FAMILY HISTORY: Arthritis (type unknown): father, PGM; type II DM: MGF; breast CA: MGM (deceased); HTN/heart disease: father; negative family history for COPD, glaucoma, or CVA.

MEDICAL HISTORY: Age 3 pneumonia; 2002 appendicitis; 2005 optic nerve changes and shin splints.

### Physical examination

GENERAL: Well-groomed man, NAD.
HEIGHT: 5 ft, 11 in.
WEIGHT: 165 pounds.
VITALS: Temp: 97.9°F. BP: 120/78 mm Hg
HEENT: Head normocephalic atraumatic. PERRLA and EOMs intact. Bilateral TMs intact without inflammation. Nares patent; pharynx pink without drainage or inflammation. Good dentition noted. No lymphadenopathy noted or enlargement of thyroid. Scar noted right side of trachea medial aspect 2 cm in length from childhood accident.
LUNGS: Bilateral breath sounds clear and equal both, A & P. No cyanosis noted.
HEART: RRR (reg. rate rhythm) with normal S1 S2, no murmurs or gallops noted. No bruits detected; capillary refill less than 3 seconds and no peripheral edema.
GI: +BS (bowel sounds) throughout, and nontender, no masses or organomegaly noted.
GENITALIA: Negative for lesions, drainage, inflammation, or hernia.
MS: MAEW (moves all extremities well); strength 5+ upper/lower extremities. FROM (full range of motion) upper/lower extremities and spine. Positive for pain in dorsal aspect of lower extremities with straight leg raises. Small abrasion (epithelial tear) noted on posterior aspect of left calf, healing well.
1. What is the patient's chief complaint?
2. What is the patient's current diagnosis? (List all that apply to this encounter)
3. Does the patient have any family history relevant to the current diagnosis? (List, if any)
4. What tests support the patient's diagnosis?
5. Do you have any questions for the physician to further clarify the patient's diagnosis, treatment, or discharge plan? (List, if any)

## Case Study

PATIENT NAME: LARRY SIMON
MRN: 4448724
PHYSICIAN'S REPORT
CHIEF COMPLAINT: Patient complains of polyuria, polydipsia, diaphoresis, shakiness, polyphagia, and fatigue.
HISTORY OF PRESENT ILLNESS: Patient is a 40-year-old man, generally in good health, but reports recent weight gain over a 12-month period. General symptoms are consistent with hypoglycemia.
SIGNIFICANT VITAL SIGNS: BP 127/82 mm Hg
MEDICAL HISTORY: No significant illnesses.
ALLERGIES: None.
CURRENT MEDICATIONS: None.
LABS: The patient had RBC count to rule out anemia. FBS was elevated, indicative of DM.
DIAGNOSIS: Patient diagnosed with Type 2 DM.
AFTERCARE AND DISPOSITION: Patient was started on oral sulfonylurea with the goal to decrease or discontinue if dietary habits indicate adequate control in 6 weeks. Patient is referred to a dietitian for training in dietary modifications and the use of a glucometer.
FOLLOW-UP: At 6-week and 3-month follow-up visits, patient's blood glucose levels remained consistently below 250 mg/dL. Sulfonylurea subsequently discontinued with a reminder to the patient to have regular triglyceride and FBS checks, and to maintain appropriate diet modifications.
1. What is the patient's chief complaint?
2. What is the patient's current diagnosis? (List all that apply to this encounter)
3. Does the patient have any family history relevant to the current diagnosis? (List, if any)
4. What tests support the patient's diagnosis?
5. Do you have any questions for the physician to further clarify the patient's diagnosis, treatment, or discharge plan? (List, if any)

*Case Study health records from Shiland BJ: *Medical terminology online for mastering healthcare terminology*, ed 7, St. Louis, 2023, Elsevier.

Targeted reviews may be aimed at specific coders, codes, DRGs, MS-DRGs, or other factors or elements of coding. For example, the OIG develops a list of so-called targeted MS-DRGs, which are MS-DRGs that have a history of aberrant coding (i.e., inaccurate coding leading to Medicare overpayments). **Quality Improvement Organizations** monitor and assess facility data and may perform reviews of cases assigned to these targeted MS-DRGs. **Recovery Audit Contractors (RACs)** are another group that reviews cases on behalf of CMS. RACs request records based on targeted cases, including the DRG assignment and medical necessity. RACs review all providers, including physicians, durable medical equipment providers, and hospitals. Regardless of audit findings, coding error rates do not apply to targeted reviews because such audits are not based on a random selection.

## Clinical Documentation Improvement

Clinical Documentation Improvement (CDI) is a constellation of activities that center around ensuring that the documentation in the patient's record supports the diagnoses, treatments, and surgical procedures.

### Purpose

The primary purpose of CDI activities is to improve the quality of clinical documentation. As we mentioned in Chapter 4 and illustrated in our coding discussion, code sets yearn for specificity. A patient does not just have CHF. The patient has systolic, diastolic, chronic, acute, or any combination of these. If the clinician documents CHF, the coder may be obligated to ask the physician for further specificity. That query may not be answered for days, preventing the coder from completing the record and sending it off to billing (more on that in Chapter 6). A CDI specialist reviews the patient's record DURING the visit and works with the physician before discharge to identify these opportunities to improve documentation. Therefore CDI activities can facilitate efficient postdischarge coding.

### Staffing

CDI specialists need to have a strong foundation in clinical documentation, pharmacology, pathophysiology, and medical coding. Their understanding of the medical decision-making process supports their ability to communicate with the documenting clinician. CDI specialists generally have a strong background in nursing, medical coding, or a related discipline. A CDI team that includes both nurses and coders is particularly strong, as they can support each other in identifying opportunities to improve the final coding of cases.

Another important member of the CDI team is a physician champion. A physician champion assists with communication, clinician education, and resolving conflict when there are doubts about the documentation of the plan of care. Remember that the plan of care is in response to or in pursuit of a diagnosis. A clinician who documents *sepsis* should be responding to specific signs and symptoms, as well as laboratory results. The CDI specialist will be looking for a plan of care that addresses *sepsis*. In the absence of documentation of signs, symptoms, lab results, and an expected plan of care, the CDI specialist may approach the physician to discuss documentation. The physician champion may be involved if the CDI specialist is unsuccessful in that conversation.

Remembering that outpatient services are communicated via coded data, there is also opportunity for improvement in outpatient records. The Association of Clinical Documentation Improvement Specialists (ACDIS) discusses a variety of ways in which facilities can support their outpatient programs, such as the emergency department and infusion centers, by assigning CDI specialists to focus on the accuracy of facility ED-level charges, improved documentation of infusions and injections, and improved documentation supporting observations services (Association of Clinical Documentation Improvement Specialists (ACDIS), 2016).

Both AHIMA and ACDIS have developed and implemented educational pathways and certification processes for CDI specialists. AHIMA offers the Certified Documentation Improvement Practitioner (CDIP). ACDIS offers the Certified Clinical Documentation Specialist (CCDS). The prerequisites for both credentials include multiple years of CDI experience and relevant existing credentials.

### Physician Query Process

Sometimes, CDI specialists can have an in-person discussion with a physician to discuss a case and the need for improved documentation, such as increased specificity in a diagnostic statement or rationale for a diagnosis or treatment. These discussions can be documented in the specialist's notes for follow-up. At other times, the physician is not available. In either case, a formal, written query may be provided to the physician. A physician query is a structured communication that describes the documentation as it exists, including clinical indicators, tests, and treatment for a diagnosis, and asks the physician to provide clarification or documentation of that diagnosis.

There are two major considerations in the development of a query. First, the CDI specialist should not diagnose the patient and tell the physician what to write. The assumption is that the physician is the clinical expert. The CDI specialist is assisting the physician to clearly document the physician's own work to ensure that the patient's record is accurate and complete. Second, the hospital decides whether the query itself and, particularly, the physician's reply become part of the patient's record as opposed to requiring the physician to document the reply in the appropriate section of the record. Since coding can only be applied to documentation in the record, this is not a small question.

The AHIMA has published extensive guidance in the development and implementation of physician queries. This guidance is available in the following documents:

CDI Toolkit

https://bok.ahima.org/PdfView?oid=301829

Physician Query Examples: Guidelines for Achieving a Compliant Query Practice https://bok.ahima.org/doc?oid=301700#.Yf_6w5bMJaQ

Updated 2016.

AHIMA Practice Brief. Guidelines for Achieving a Compliant Query Practice (2019 Update). Updated May 2021.

According to the AHIMA Practice Brief:

*Queries are utilized to support the ability to accurately assign a code and can be initiated by either coding or CDI professionals. Queries may be necessary in (but are not limited to) the following instances:*

- to resolve conflicting documentation between the attending provider and other treating providers (whether diagnostic or procedural);
- to support documentation of medical diagnoses or conditions that are clinically evident and meet UHDDS requirements but without the corresponding diagnoses or conditions stated;
- to clarify if a diagnosis is ruled in or out;
- to seek clarification when it appears a documented diagnosis is not clinically supported; and
- to support appropriate POA indicator assignment.

For common or problematic queries, the CDI specialist in collaboration with coding management and clinical staff may develop a set of standard compliant queries. Written queries typically use the open-ended, multiple-choice, or yes/no format. During the patient visit, the CDI specialist will present queries to the physicians as needed. After discharge, the coder assigned to the record may also present queries and the CDI specialist may continue to follow up on existing queries. For an efficient and effective query process, the CDI specialist and coders should collaborate as needed to complete the coding process on a timely basis.

## Monitoring

If a patient is in the hospital for a week, it is easy to see that the CDI specialist has plenty of time to review the documentation, meet with the physician, and follow up before the patient is discharged. However, more commonly, patients are in the hospital for 2 or 3 days. CDI specialists need to hit the ground running on new admissions as soon as possible to achieve maximum benefit. Furthermore, CDI specialists need to be able to distribute workload among themselves efficiently and reach out to physicians quickly and efficiently. The manager responsible for CDI activities needs to be able to identify the activities of the individual specialists, including their documentation reviews, interactions with physicians, and follow-up interactions with the coding staff. Technology is of assistance in this regard. CDI

software that allows the specialist to document their activities, communicate with clinicians and coders, and track the results of their activities is optimum.

## Outcomes Reporting

The success of a CDI program can be measured in several ways. While there is a temptation to focus on how documentation improvement affects reimbursement, the activities themselves are all about the documentation. The outcome of CDI activities is most appropriately measured by indicators that reflect changes in documentation and the effort expended to effect those changes. Table 5.7 lists some indicators that are useful in this regard.

| TABLE 5.7 | Clinical Documentation Improvement Outcome Reporting |
|---|---|
| Initial record reviews per day | **Productivity Measure**. The initial record review familiarizes the specialist with the case. In cases with a short LOS, this may be the only review. |
| Subsequent record reviews per day | **Productivity Measure**. This measure helps explain low initial record reviews on days in which they occur. |
| Number of documentation queries Sorted by topic Sorted by physician | **Productivity Measure**. Theoretically, this volume starts out high upon initiation of a program and levels off at a lower rate. **Improvement Measure**. Recurring or high-volume topics are subjects for clinician training. **Improvement Measure**. Recurring or high-volume queries to a physician are subjects for intervention by the physician champion. |
| Percentage of queries that resulted in documentation changes | **Effectiveness Measure**. Low volume of effective queries may indicate a process problem such as failure to communicate effectively with clinicians. Tracking by target clinician can identify subjects for intervention by the physician champion. |
| Number of documentation queries that resulted in a change in DRG | **Effectiveness Measure**. A change in principle diagnosis, present on admission indicator, or surgical procedure has the potential to change the DRG on the inpatient case. |

**COMPETENCY CHECK-IN 5.6**

**Clinical Documentation Improvement**

**Competency Assessment**

1. Download the ACDIS white paper on Outpatient CDI https://acdis.org/system/files/resources/outpatient-cdi-intro.pdf. Compare and contrast inpatient and outpatient CDI.
2. The CDI specialist wrote the following query to the attending physician on an inpatient case:
   a. Doctor A: Please add Acute Diastolic Heart Failure to your list of diagnoses for this patient, consistent with the echocardiogram.
   b. Comment on this query and rewrite it as needed.
3. Using the clinical indicators for a specific diagnosis and published guidelines, develop a standard query form for that diagnosis.

## Chapter Summary

Coding is an increasingly important function in health care. Guided by a strict code of ethics, coders in a variety of settings use different nomenclature and classification systems to facilitate communication among providers, payers, and other users of health care data. These systems include ICD-9, ICD-10-CM, ICD-10-PCS, HCPCS/CPT-4, ICD-O-3, DSM-5, and current dental terminology. Because these systems are required for use in EDI, the coder assumes the important role of ensuring that the data derived from the systems are complete and accurate.

Other systems without direct coder involvement include SNOMED CT and NDCs. These systems are important because of their use in the EHR and as HIPAA transaction code sets. Different coding systems currently in use satisfy the need to capture coded data for different uses by different providers. Some systems are very specialized, whereas some systems, such as SNOMED CT, are far more comprehensive, with a broader range of users. Each system has its own unique uses. In most provider settings today, such as physician offices and acute care hospitals, there are three important coding systems currently in use: ICD-10-CM, ICD-10-PCS, and HCPCS/CPT.

Coders are an integral part of maintaining the quality of a facility's coded clinical data, ensuring compliance with regulatory mandates, and facilitating optimal reimbursement. DRGs classify patients according to diagnosis, treatment, and RI into statistically similar categories to understand the costs of caring for patients. Assignment begins with the principal diagnosis and takes into consideration any complications or comorbidities. Accurate coding results in proper DRG assignment and ethical, honest reimbursement.

Medical coding work aims for timeliness and completeness in the interest of optimizing reimbursement and staying compliant. Coding must be reliable and valid, both individually and collectively within a facility or group. CDI is a process to ensure that documentation about the patient accurately supports the diagnoses, treatments, and surgical procedures of clinical professionals.

Throughout this chapter, the importance of the coding function and reimbursement has been emphasized. The essence of being a professional coder entails training and development; continuous education; knowledge and application of current rules, regulations, and guidelines; and ethical conduct, despite daily challenges and pressures. Performing the coding function well makes the professional coder a valuable member of the health care team.

## Competency Milestones

### CAHIIM Competency

*I.5. Explain the use of classification systems, clinical vocabularies, and nomenclatures. (2)*

### Rationale
HIM professionals frequently encounter classification systems, clinical vocabularies, and nomenclatures, whether actively coding or in some other role.

### Competency Assessment
1. List and describe the classification systems discussed in this chapter.
2. Describe four uses of classification systems.
3. List and describe two nomenclatures discussed in this chapter.
4. How do clinical vocabularies support communication and interoperability?

CAHIIM Competency
*IV.1. Validate assignment of diagnostic and procedural codes and groupings in accordance with official guidelines. (3)*
*IV.1. RM Determine diagnosis and procedure codes according to official guidelines. (5)*

### Rationale

Whether an HIM professional is actually a coder or not, the ability to use coded data is a skill that permeates HIM practice. Note that in this competency assessment, you will practice looking up and applying ICD-10-CM, ICD-10-PCS, and HCPCS Level II codes, but only one CPT code. This is because the basic tools to use ICD-10 code sets are freely available from the CMS, while the CPT code set is owned by the AMA. No-cost resources are limited. The AMA offers a free app that includes a 14-day full access trial. Continued use of the app requires a year's activation or in-app purchases. You can access their code lookup tool at https://www.ama-assn.org/practice-management/cpt/need-coding-resources.

### Competency Assessment

1. If patients are grouped into the same MS-DRG, it is because they have what three criteria in common?
2. What is meant by the term *resource intensity*?
3. Describe how a case is assigned to an MDC.
4. After assignment of the MDC, what occurs next in the grouping process?
5. What patient attributes are important to grouper assignment?
6. What is a CC code, and why is it significant?
7. What is the difference between a comorbidity and a complication?
8. What is an MCC code, and why is it significant?
9. What coding classification or nomenclature system is used to indicate medical necessity?
10. What does the MCE do?
11. Describe two types of coding errors that may affect MS-DRG assignment.

### Coding Application: International Classification of Diseases, 10th Revision, Clinical Modification

If you do not have a code book, download the Code Tables and Index from the CMS website: https://www.cms.gov/medicare/icd-10/2023-icd-10-cm

*Assign the correct code for each diagnostic statement. Next to the code(s), describe the index path, any tabular notes, and any guidelines that you followed to get to the code.*

1. Hydrophthalmos
2. Newborn jaundice
3. Type 2 diabetes mellitus with gastroparesis
4. Gestational diabetes
5. Traumatic nondisplaced spiral fracture of the shaft of the right humerus
6. Pneumonia due to aspiration of food
7. Acute and chronic asthma
8. Baby's chart: Normal newborn, single live birth, born in hospital by cesarean section
9. Mother's chart: Single live birth delivered by cesarean section for cephalopelvic disproportion
10. Patient with malignant neoplasm of left lower lobe of lung is admitted for chemotherapy

### Coding Application: International Classification of Diseases, 10th Revision, Procedural Coding System

If you do not have a code book, download the Code Tables and Index from the CMS website: https://www.cms.gov/medicare/icd-10/2022-icd-10-pcs

*Assign the correct ICD-10-PCS code for each of the following procedural statements.*

1. Laparoscopic appendectomy
2. Open removal of the entire left lobe of the thyroid gland
3. Endoscopic biopsy of the bronchus, right middle lobe
4. Uncomplicated delivery of single live newborn
5. Fitting for a new monaural hearing aid
6. CT scan of the liver and spleen with and without low osmolar contrast
7. Removal of a bean from a child's nose with forceps
8. Closed setting of a fracture of the right tibia
9. Esophagogastroduodenoscopy with biopsy of pyloric antrum
10. Transcatheter aortic valve replacement procedure with a synthetic substitute

## Coding Application: Healthcare Common Procedure Coding System

The index and code files for HCPCS Level II codes can be found at: https://www.cms.gov/Medicare/Coding/HCPCSReleaseCodeSets/HCPCS-Quarterly-Update

*Assign the correct HCPCS code for each of the following medical devices.*

1. Ambulatory surgical boot
2. Manual breast pump
3. Albuterol, compounded, 1 mg unit dose
4. Continuous positive airway pressure device and headgear
5. High-strength lightweight wheelchair, detachable arms desk or full length, swing away detachable elevating leg rests

## Accuracy of Diagnostic and Procedural Coding

1. The final diagnoses for an inpatient stay were chronic CHF, hypertension, and Type 2 diabetes mellitus with no diabetes-related complications. Is this record coded correctly? Explain.

   I50.2 Systolic (congestive) heart failure

   I10 Hypertension

   E11.9 Type 2 diabetes mellitus without complications

## Case Study

1. Refer to the record for **Alexander Powell, MRN 1215613** on page 179 of this chapter.
   a. The coder assigned these diagnoses and procedures to this record. Is this record coded correctly? Explain.
   b. Diagnoses: CA prostate (C61), UTI (N39.0), late-onset Type 2 diabetes (E11.9)
   c. Procedures: CT scan (BV23ZZZ), implanted radiotherapy (Table DV1; additional information required in order to code)
2. Refer to the record for patient **Mitchell Burkovicz, MRN 2018001** on page 179 of this chapter. Apply a CPT code to this outpatient visit.

## Grouping Application

To complete the following exercises, open:

* the free grouper software at http://www.ipgmr.com/indexing.htm
* the current MS-DRG Grouper Manual. The version 39 manual is at: https://www.cms.gov/icd10m/version39-fullcode-cms/fullcode_cms/P0001.html
* Tables 6I and 6J from the CMS website. The 2022 tables are available at: https://www.cms.gov/medicare/acute-inpatient-pps/fy-2023-ipps-final-rule-home-page#Tables

*Case #1*  Principal Diagnosis: I21.4 Non-ST elevation (NSTEMI) myocardial infarction

   Secondary Diagnosis: I10

1. Into which MDC does this case fall?
2. Does this case group to a medical or surgical partition?
3. Is I10 a CC or MCC with I21.4?
4. What MS-DRG should be assigned to this case?
5. What is the cluster of MS-DRGs into which this case falls?
6. What would cause this case to be grouped into a different MS-DRG in the cluster?

*Case #2*  The patient was admitted with a chief complaint of shortness of breath not relieved by rescue inhaler. During the inpatient stay, the patient's diabetes was monitored closely and insulin was administered per a sliding scale. The patient's acute asthma was resolved and the patient was discharged home with a change in asthma medication. The coder assigned the following, which grouped to MS-DRG 074.

   Principal Diagnosis: E10.43 Diabetes, type II, with gastroparesis

   Secondary Diagnosis: J44.1 Asthma, chronic, with exacerbation (acute)

1. Evaluate the accuracy of the coding/grouping of this case.

*Case #3*  The patient presented in the ED in active labor and was admitted for delivery. The patient was prepped for a cesarean section for known cephalopelvic disproportion and was delivered via cesarean section of a normal newborn with Apgars of 10/10. Mother and baby were discharged with instructions for outpatient follow-up.

   The coder has assigned the following codes, but the grouper is coming up with an error instead of grouping to the expected MS-DRG.

   Principal Diagnosis: O33.9 (Delivery, cesarean, cephalopelvic disproportion)

   Secondary Diagnosis: Z38.01 (Newborn, born in hospital, by cesarean)

1. Evaluate the problem and assign the correct MS-DRG.

**Clinical Documentation Improvement Application\***

*Patient Name: Owen Seagraves*
*MRN: 7797132*
*Surgical Patient*

*Patient History: Patient, a 34-year-old man, in whom TUR was performed for BPH 4 years ago and who has remained symptom free until 6 weeks ago. Patient visited the clinic 9 days ago complaining of side pains related to interstitial nephritis, which was treated with a corticosteroid. Patient reported diminished force, dysuria, urinary frequency, and hesitation. Urethral stricture ruled out.*

*Chief Complaint: Patient admitted to ER with worsening, severe bilateral side pain, radiating to the back, profuse sweating, nausea, and vomiting.*

*Lab Values: Increased serum potassium, increased BUN, and decreased creatinine clearance.*

*Vital Signs: Blood pressure 124/80 mm Hg, pulse 75 bpm, temperature 100.6 °F.*

*Procedure and Findings: Nephrolithiasis both kidneys confirmed. Acute renal failure confirmed. IVU was performed, followed by ESWL. Patient was given IV calcium, glucose, insulin, and oral potassium exchange resin. BP brought back under control.*

*Aftercare and Disposition: Patient was discharged in good condition with instructions to rest and restrict fluid intake and comply with temporary dietary modifications. When normal activities are resumed, patient should return for BUN test to determine course of action for secondary ARF. Continue monitoring blood pressure, monitor sodium intake, and develop plan of physical exercise.*

1. The CAC program presents the following coding for Owen Seagraves. For each code, accept or delete the code as written. If the code needs to be modified, show the modified code. Insert the POA Indicators. What is the principal diagnosis? Do you need any clarification from the physician?

| Code | Description | POA Indicator | Documentation | Coder Action (Accept/Delete/Modify) |
|------|-------------|---------------|---------------|-------------------------------------|
| R11.2 | Nausea and vomiting | | Chief complaint | |
| N12 | Interstitial nephritis | | History | |
| R30.0 | Dysuria | | History | |
| N20.0 | Nephrolithiasis | | Procedure and findings | |
| N40.1 | BPH | | History | |
| 0TF3XZZ; 0TF4XZZ | ESWL | | Procedure and findings | |
| BT04YZZ | IVU | | Procedure and findings | |

## Ethics Challenge

*VI.7. Assess Ethical Standards of Practice (5)*

1. You are a coder in a small community hospital. You sent a query to Dr. Smith because you are coding one of her patients who was admitted with bacterial pneumonia for the second time in the last 2 months. He also has a secondary diagnosis of oral thrush. Because you also code outpatient clinic records, you recognize that he is also a patient in the infectious disease clinic and was diagnosed HIV positive there last year. You are aware that, per CDC guidelines, multiple admissions for bacterial pneumonia and a diagnosis of oral thrush in an HIV patient are both indicators for acquired immune deficiency syndrome (AIDS); however, Dr. Smith has not made any reference in the record to HIV or AIDS. Dr. Smith has now come to see you in person and is telling you in no uncertain terms that it is not your business to tell her how to diagnose a patient and to just leave it off. Because Dr. Smith did not document the diagnosis, you comply and do not assign any code for HIV or AIDS to the record. Is this ethical or not?

## Critical Thinking Questions

1. AHIMA's *Standards of Ethical Coding* was first published in 1999 as a statement of principles that reflected the expectations of a professional coder. In 2016, the *Standards of Ethical Coding* was revised to reflect the current health care environment and modern coding practices. These standards are intended to be relevant to all health care settings and applicable to all coders, regardless of whether they are members of AHIMA.

---

\*Health record from Shiland BJ: *Medical terminology online for mastering healthcare terminology*, ed 7, St. Louis, 2023, Elsevier.

By following the *Standards of Ethical Coding*, the coding professional agrees to ethical principles that may have legal and reimbursement implications. If you were the coding supervisor, what emphasis would you put on the *Standards of Ethical Coding* in your area? Would you include the *Standards of Ethical Coding* in your policy and procedure manual? Would you review the *Standards of Ethical Coding* on a regular basis? If yes, how often? What disciplinary action would you take if you found that a coder violated the *Standards of Ethical Coding*? Would the severity of the disciplinary action depend on which standard was violated? Why or why not?

2. You are a coder in a small community hospital. Your employer required your Certified Coding Specialist (CCS) credential as a condition of employment. However, other than circulating the AHA Coding Clinic to read, there is no budget for coder continuing education. To maintain your CCS, you need to obtain and report continuing education. How many credit hours are needed to maintain a CCS credential? What opportunities do you have locally to obtain continuing education? Develop a plan for the current year that represents your most economical and efficient way to obtain 10 hours of continuing education.

# The Role of Health Information Management Professionals in the Workplace

## Professional Profile—Coder

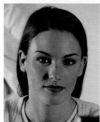

My name is Olga, and I am a coder in the HIM department at Diamonte Hospital. There are six coders in our department: four inpatient coders and two outpatient coders. In addition, there is a coding supervisor who trains us and checks our work.

I started out as a scanner in the department. I indexed and scanned records for a year. I had to learn the postdischarge order of the record and how to scan and index miscellaneous paperwork (aka, loose sheets). When an opening came up in the analysis section, I applied for it and was promoted. I enjoyed analysis but I also began to understand the importance of the data contained in the records. I was really interested in the clinical data and decided to go to school to learn about coding, because coders work with the data.

Our local community college has an HIM department, and I enrolled in their coding certificate program. I studied medical terminology, health record development and retention, anatomy and physiology, and disease pathology. I took several coding courses, learning ICD-10-CM and CPT. While I was a student, the coding supervisor allowed me to study completed records so that I could practice coding. When I finished the program, I was promoted to outpatient coder. I kept practicing inpatient coding with the completed records, and I asked a lot of questions. Now I code inpatient records most of the time and help out with the outpatient records.

After 2 years as an inpatient coder, I sat for and passed the CCS examination that is offered by the AHIMA. I am now a CCS! I really enjoy coding. It is challenging and interesting, and there are a lot of opportunities for me as I learn more about clinical data and how to manage health information.

## Career Tip

There are many opportunities for coders from physician offices to hospitals to consulting firms and even software developers. Knowledge of medical terminology, anatomy and physiology, pathology, and coding is essential. On the physician-based side, the American Academy of Professional Coders offers focused courses that lead directly to specific coding credentials. This training can lead to opportunities in physician offices or hospital outpatient settings. For inpatient coding, courses from a certificate program approved by the AHIMA or from AHIMA itself are optimum. A degree in HIM is helpful for individuals who want to progress to supervisory or management roles.

Many health information professionals choose to specialize in cancer coding and cancer registries and obtain the credential Certified Tumor Registrar. Those professionals working in Tumor Registries use ICD-O-3 to code cancer cases, similar to the way inpatient coders use ICD-10-CM. Depending on the facility, in an inpatient setting, a patient with cancer will have been coded using both ICD-O-3 and ICD-10-CM, usually by different professionals in different departments, with each distinct case and code set reported electronically to entirely separate databases.

## Patient Care Perspective

### Sara Brady

I see my Primary Care Physician every 6 months for a checkup, because I have several chronic conditions that need regular monitoring and routine laboratory tests. When I went into the doctor's patient portal to make my next appointment, I noticed that there was a new diagnosis of *congenital iodine-deficiency syndrome* on my record. I was shocked and really worried at first, because the doctor had never mentioned it to me. When I called the office, I found out that it was a "coding error." I have had uncomplicated diabetes for years and they tell me that someone typed E00.9 instead of E10.9. I hope they fix it soon.

### Professional Profile—Corporate Trainer-Coding Specialist Division

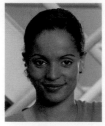

My name is Charlene, and I am employed in the Corporate Training Department of a large, multicampus medical center. In addition to our six inpatient facilities, we see hundreds of patients on a daily basis in our outpatient clinics, including behavioral health, and our same-day surgery centers. We are also affiliated with a dental school.

The Coding Specialist Division of the Corporate Training Department provides the coding training for all of our facilities, clinics, and outpatient programs. As a trainer within this division, I am responsible for training all new employees on the specific code sets they need to learn for their jobs and training existing employees on coding updates and changes in coding regulation.

Because we offer so many services in different settings, I must know ICD-10-CM, ICD-10-PCS, CPT-4, HCPCS, DSM-5, and CDT. I need to have an in-depth knowledge of all of these code sets in order to be an effective trainer. I must keep abreast of all changes and revised coding and reporting guidelines for all the services the medical center provides and provide in-service training to all of our coders accordingly.

I also act as a resource for the Patient Financial Services Department when there are code-based reimbursement issues. When Chargemasters are updated, I am part of a team that reviews all new and revised codes to ensure they are current and correctly applied. This may sound tedious, but our work is extremely important if our medical center is to receive the reimbursement that we are entitled to for services provided.

I was promoted to this position because of my years of experience coding in one of our inpatient facilities and in several outpatient clinics. I am a Registered Health Information Technician (RHIT), Certified Coding Specialist (CCS), and Certified Coding Specialist-Physician Based (CCS-P).

I enjoy my job very much because my needed knowledge base is so varied, even though it is all coding. It is personally rewarding to be able to share my enthusiasm with the new coders and set them on the right track for a successful career with our medical center.

### Career Tip

Inpatient coding experience and experience coding in a variety of settings is essential for a position in coder training. A college degree in a related field and supervisory or management experience are competitive advantages. To expand your skill set, offer to guest lecture in a local coding program or to speak at a local professional association meeting. Take continuing education courses that teach training and professional development leadership skills. Consider a master's degree in education, focusing on adult learning.

## Works Cited

Association of Clinical Documentation Improvement Specialists (ACDIS): *CCDS Program Requirements and Prerequisites*, 2021. Association of Clinical Documentation Improvement Specialists (ACDIS) website. https://acdis.org/certification/ccds/requirements. Accessed February 12, 2022.

Canada Health Infoway: *Summary Corporate Plan 2020–2021: Driving Access to Care*, 2021. Canada Health Infoway website. https://www.infoway-inforoute.ca/en/component/edocman/resources/i-infoway-i-corporate/business-plans/3793-summary-corporate-plan-2020-2021?Itemid=101. Accessed February 12, 2022.

Centers for Medicare and Medicaid Services and the National Center for Healthcare Statistics: *ICD-10-CM Official Guidelines for Coding and Reporting, FY 2022*, 2022. CMS.gov: Centers for Medicare and Medicaid Services website. https://www.cms.gov/files/document/fy-2022-icd-10-cm-coding-guidelines-updated-02012022.pdf. Accessed February 12, 2022.

National Cancer Institute: *Coding Rules for Topography & Morphology*. National Cancer Institute, n.d. SEER Training Modules website. https://training.seer.cancer.gov/coding/guidelines/. Accessed February 12, 2022.

SNOMED International: *Our Organization*, 2022a. SNOMED International website. http://www.snomed.org/our-organization/our-organization. Accessed February 12, 2022.

SNOMED International: *SNOMED International SNOMED CT Browser*, 2022b. SNOMED CT International Browser website. https://browser.ihtsdotools.org/?.

U.S. Food and Drug Administration: *National Drug Code Directory*. https://www.accessdata.fda.gov/scripts/cder/ndc/index.cfm. Accessed February 29, 2022.

World Health Organization: *WHO Releases New International Classification of Diseases (ICD 11)*, June 18, 2018. World Health Organization website. https://www.who.int/news-room/detail/18-06-2018-who-releases-new-international-classification-of-diseases-(icd-11). Accessed February 12, 2022.

## Further Reading

AHIMA House of Delegates: *American Health Information Management Association Standards of Ethical Coding [2016 version]*, December 2016. http://library.ahima.org/CodingStandards. Accessed January 26, 2022.

American Dental Association: *Publications: CDT Coding*. http://www.ada.org/en/publications/cdt. Accessed February 12, 2022. Copyright 2022.

American Health Information Management Association (AHIMA): *Certified Documentation Improvement Practitioner (CDIP)*, 2021. AHIMA website. http://www.ahima.org/certification/cdip. Accessed February 12, 2022.

American Psychiatric Association: *Psychiatrists: Practice: DSM-5*, http://www.psychiatry.org/practice/dsm/dsm5. Accessed February 12, 2022. Copyright 2022.

Association of Clinical Documentation Improvement Specialists (ACDIS): *Forums: Outpatient Clinical Documentation Improvement*

(CDI): An Introduction, 2016. https://forums.acdis.org/uploads/editor/rv/37tx4ko1seo0.pdf. Accessed February 6, 2022.

Canadian Institute for Health Information: CCI Coding Structure. https://www.cihi.ca/en/cci-coding-structure. Accessed February 12, 2022. Copyright 1996–2022.

Center for Medicare and Medicaid Services: Healthcare Common Procedure Coding System (HCPCS). Level II Coding Procedures. https://www.cms.gov/Medicare/Coding/MedHCPCSGenInfo/Downloads/2018-11-30-HCPCS-Level2-Coding-Procedure.pdf.

Centers for Disease Control and Prevention, National Center for Health Statistics: Classification of Diseases, Functioning, and Disability: International Classification of Diseases, Tenth Revision, Clinical Modification (ICD-10-CM). http://www.cdc.gov/nchs/icd/icd10cm.htm. Updated February 11, 2022. Accessed February 12, 2022.

Centers for Medicare and Medicaid Services: Statute Regulations Program Instructions, CMS.gov: Centers for Medicare and Medicaid Services website. https://www.cms.gov/Medicare/Medicare-Fee-for-Service-Payment/HospitalAcqCond/Statute_Regulations_Program_Instructions.html. Modified December 1, 2021. Accessed February 6, 2022.

Centers for Medicare and Medicaid Services: Hospital-acquired Conditions, CMS.gov: Centers for Medicare and Medicaid Services website. https://www.cms.gov/Medicare/Medicare-Fee-for-Service-Payment/HospitalAcqCond/icd10_hacs. Modified December 1, 2021. Accessed February 6, 2022.

Centers for Medicare and Medicaid Services: Code Sets Overview, CMS.gov: Centers for Medicare and Medicaid Services website.

https://www.cms.gov/regulations-and-guidance/administrative-simplification/code-sets. Updated December 17, 2021. Accessed February 12, 2022.

Centers for Medicare and Medicaid Services: ICD-10 PCS. https://www.cms.gov/Medicare/Coding/ICD10/2019-ICD-10-PCS.html. Accessed February 12, 2022.

Centers for Medicare and Medicaid Services: Adopted Standards and Operating Rules. https://www.cms.gov/Regulations-and-Guidance/Administrative-Simplification/HIPAA-ACA/AdoptedStandardsandOperatingRules.html. Modified December 1, 2021. Accessed February 12, 2022.

Centers for Medicare and Medicaid Services: HCPCS. Level II Coding Process & Criteria. https://www.cms.gov/Medicare/Coding/MedHCPCSGenInfo/HCPCSCODINGPROCESS.html. Modified December 1, 2021. Accessed February 12, 2022.

Fung KW, Fung KW: I-MAGIC: Using 202109 Release of the SNOMED CT to ICD-10-CM Map, n.d. I-MAGIC Demo website. https://imagic.nlm.nih.gov/imagic/code/map.

U.S. National Institutes of Health, National Cancer Institute: Surveillance Epidemiology and End Results. http://seer.cancer.gov/. Accessed February 12, 2022.

World Health Organization: History of the Development of the ICD. http://www.who.int/classifications/icd/en/HistoryOfICD.pdf. Accessed February 12, 2022.

World Health Organization: Classifications: International Classification of Diseases for Oncology, 3rd Edition (ICD-O-3). http://www.who.int/classifications/icd/adaptations/oncology/en/index.html. Accessed February 12, 2022.

# 6

# Financial Management

LISA REILLY

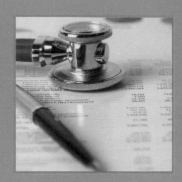

## CHAPTER OUTLINE

Insurance
   Assumption of Risk
   Types of Health Insurance
   Self-Insurance
Entitlements
   Medicare
   Medicaid
   Federal Coverage for Specific Populations
   Tax Equity and Fiscal Responsibility Act of 1982
Fee for Service
   Charges
Discounted Fee for Service
Capitation
Prospective Payment
   Diagnosis Related Groups (DRGs)
   Case Mix Index
   Ambulatory Payment Classification
   Inpatient Psychiatric Facility Prospective Payment System
   Inpatient Rehabilitation Facility Prospective Payment System
   Long-Term Care Hospital Prospective Payment System
   Home Health Prospective Payment System
   Skilled Nursing Facility Prospective Payment System and Resource Utilization Groups
   Resource-Based Relative Value System

Comparison of Reimbursement Methods
Patient Financial Services
   Chargemaster (Charge Description Master)
   Charge Capture
   Impact of Coding on Reimbursement
   The Uniform Bill
   CMS-1500
   Claim Rejections
   Claim Denials
   Error Correction
   Collection
Financial Accounting
Management Accounting: Budgets
   Strategic Budget
   Capital Budget
   Operational Budget
Chapter Summary
Competency Milestones
Ethics Challenge
Critical Thinking Questions
Professional Profile
   Practice Manager
   Patient Care Perspective
   Patient Care Perspective
Works cited
Further Reading

## CHAPTER OBJECTIVES

*By the end of this chapter, the student should be able to:*

1. Discuss types of health insurance and government payers;
2. Compare the major health care reimbursement methodologies;
3. Evaluate the revenue cycle management process and the role of coding in this process; and
4. Explain accounting methodologies, plan budgets, and calculate budget variances.

## VOCABULARY

accrual basis
amortization
balance sheet

billing
blended rate
capital budget

capitation
case mix index (CMI)
case mix
cash basis accounting
cash flow
charge capture
charge
Chargemaster
claim
coinsurance
copay
deductible
depreciate
diagnosis-related groups (DRGs)
discounted fee for service
encounter form
entitlement program
expenses
fee for service
fee schedule
financial accounting
fiscal intermediaries
fixed expense
gatekeeper
group plan
group practice model HMO
grouper
guarantor
health maintenance organizations (HMOs)
income statement
indemnity insurance
independent practice association (IPA) model HMO
insurance
insurer
local coverage determination (LCD)
managed care
Medicaid
Medicare
Medicare Administrative Contractor (MAC)
minimum data set (MDS)

modifier
national coverage determination (NCD)
network
operational budget
outlier payment
Outpatient Prospective Payment System (OPPS)
patient assessment instrument (PAI)
payback period
payer
preferred provider organization (PPO)
premium
primary care provider (PCP)
prospective payment system (PPS)
provider number
reimbursement
relative weight (RW)
reliability
Resident Assessment Instrument (RAI)
resource-based relative value system (RBRVS)
resource intensity (RI)
resource utilization group (RUG)
return on investment (ROI)
revenue code
revenue cycle management (RCM)
revenue
risk
self-pay
staff model HMO
superbill
Tax Equity and Fiscal Responsibility Act of 1982 (TEFRA)
third-party payer
TRICARE
Uniform Bill (UB-04)
usual, customary, and reasonable (UCR) fee
validity
variable expense
variance
wraparound policies

## CAHIIM COMPETENCY DOMAINS

IV.2.  Describe components of revenue cycle management
       and clinical documentation improvement. (2)
IV.2.  **RM** Evaluate revenue cycle processes. (5)
IV.3.  Summarize regulatory requirements and
       reimbursement methodologies. (2)
IV.3.  **RM** Evaluate compliance with regulatory
       requirements and reimbursement methodologies. (5)
VI.5.  Utilize financial management processes. (3)

Patients and providers were, historically, the two main parties involved in a health care relationship. Patients were free to seek whatever services they were able to afford, and providers could charge whatever the market would bear. This one-on-one relationship has been split into a complex multiparty system. In previous chapters, we have been discussing how health care is delivered and how the components of the system communicate with each other. This chapter explores the way health care services are paid for. In order to

fully understand the health care system in the United States, it is good to remember that health care is an industry with many components. Some of those components are not-for-profit, as we discussed in Chapter 1. Other components are for-profit. Regardless of the organization's tax status, it is unlikely that any component of the industry would exist indefinitely without at least bringing in as much in earnings as it expends in providing those services. Thus we need to understand how health care is financed.

## PAYING FOR HEALTH CARE

The party (person or organization) from whom the provider is expecting payment for services rendered (reimbursement) is called the **payer**. The payer is frequently an insurance company. It may also be a government agency, such as Medicare or Medicaid. The term **reimbursement** is generally used today to refer to the payment provided to a physician or other health care provider in exchange for services rendered.

With respect to reimbursement in health care, one of the following two reimbursement scenarios typically occurs:

1. A patient pays a health care provider directly for services rendered and then that patient requests reimbursement from the insurance company (the insurer).
2. The health care provider renders services and requests payment (reimbursement) for those services directly from the insurer (the payer).

In a hospital setting, for example, a hospital provides services and supplies to a patient, thus incurring costs, under the assumption that it will be reimbursed for these costs after the patient has been discharged. The payer is billed at a later date. Insurance plans today do not typically require a patient to pay a hospital and then submit a **claim** to the insurance company for reimbursement. Patients without some form of third-party payment relationship are called **self-pay** patients and are billed directly for services rendered.

Reimbursement takes many different forms. In the past, it was not uncommon for a physician to be "paid in kind." For example, a physician might have made a house call to treat a patient and then received chickens as compensation. These types of bartering arrangements were mutually acceptable to both physician and patient. Reimbursement today is generally monetary, especially for hospitalization services, but in many parts of the world and in the United States, bartering for health care services is common and acceptable.

Historically, a physician did not necessarily receive the payment that he or she charged but rather the payment that the patient thought the physician's services were worth. In the early 20th century, this practice changed to paying what the physician charged. More recently, the amount of compensation given to the physician or health care provider is decided not by the patient or physician but by the **third-party payer**, an entity that pays for some or all health care services on behalf of the patient. Third-party payers have assumed the risk that a particular group of patients will require health care services and therefore incur the cost of paying for the services. In recent years, third-party payers are focusing not just on the services themselves but also on the quality of care, as we shall see. In the following discussion, reimbursement is categorized according to the control that the health care provider exerts over the fees that are charged.

## Insurance

**Insurance** is a contract between two parties in which one party assumes the risk of loss on behalf of the other party in return for some, usually monetary, compensation. The **insurer** receives a payment for coverage under a policy called a **premium**, often on a monthly basis. In return, the insurer pays for some or all of the contracted amount for health services rendered. Table 6.1 contains definitions of several terms that are useful during any discussion of health insurance.

Many patients have more than one payer. The primary payer is billed first for payment. A secondary payer is approached for any amount that the primary payer did not remit, and so on. For example, patients who are covered by Medicare may have supplemental or secondary insurance with a different payer. The physician first sends the bill to Medicare. Any amount that Medicare does not pay is then billed to the secondary payer.

Ultimately, the patient or other responsible party, such as the parent, is financially responsible to pay for services that he or she has received. Depending on the type of insurance, the patient may have cost sharing responsibilities, such as *copays*, *coinsurance*, or *deductibles*. These are sometimes called "out-of-pocket" costs. A **copay** is a fixed amount that a patient remits at the time of service. Copays vary according to the service rendered. For example, a copay may be $20 for a physician visit and $100 for an emergency department (ED) visit. **Coinsurance** is the percentage of the payment for which the patient is responsible. The payer may have 80% responsibility for the payment and the patient 20%. A **deductible** is a fixed amount of patient responsibility that must be incurred before the third-party payer is responsible. For example, if the patient has a $500 deductible, then the patient must spend $500 for health care services first. After $500 is expended, the third-party payer will begin to reimburse for services rendered. Health insurance plans with higher copays, coinsurance, and deductibles typically have lower monthly premiums. Plans with higher premiums have lower out-of-pocket costs.

In all cases, payment by third-party payers depends on the contractual relationship between the third party and the patient. Third-party payers will only reimburse for services that are covered in that policy.

If the patient is a dependent, a person other than the patient may be ultimately responsible for the bill. The person who is ultimately responsible for paying the bill is called the **guarantor**. For example, if a child goes to the physician's office for treatment, the child, as a dependent, cannot usually be held responsible for the invoice. Therefore the parent or legal guardian is responsible for payment and is the guarantor. Fig. 3.3 illustrates financial data required by a health care provider.

Many Americans today obtain health care coverage through an employer. This system of "employer-sponsored" health care began after World War II, when employers began offering their employees certain benefits, including health insurance. Benefits packages became useful in enabling employers to hire and retain employees. Employees benefited because they did not need to spend money on premiums, and employers benefited because health insurance benefits were a relatively low-cost way to attract quality employees. Insurance companies benefited from an increased client base. However, this thrust a fourth party into the provider/patient relationship: the employer.

Originally, the focus of insurance was on the coverage of services at the health care provider's fee. If the provider raised the fee, the insurance company raised its premiums to cover these fees. As health care costs increased, premiums also increased dramatically, becoming too expensive for many employers to pay in full. Currently, many employers

of "in-network" doctors, nor does it require referrals from primary care providers (PCPs) to specialists; it will reimburse a set percentage of any covered service from any provider once the deductible is met and after any copayments. Indemnity insurance was the predominant type of health insurance for many years. Today, very few patients elect for this coverage.

Indemnity plans usually require the subscriber to meet a deductible before paying claims. Depending on the insurance company plan, a deductible could apply for every encounter, every visit, or every hospitalization, or it could be applied on an annual basis. If the insurance plan covers a whole family, the deductible could be per person or per family. Routine health care costs often do not exceed the deductible amount. Thus the insurance company ultimately covers and pays for only unusual or extraordinary expenses. In addition, indemnity contracts often specify limits for certain covered services. If the benefit limit is $3000 for physician office visits and the patient's care (after the deductible) costs $4000, then the patient is responsible for the additional $1000.

### Managed Care

Indemnity insurance plans led to an increase in the amount of money spent on health care. In a simple physician–patient relationship, the patient bears the cost of the care and therefore has some influence on the fees. Individuals may choose not to go to the physician in the first place because they feel the fee is too high and they cannot afford it, or they might be able to afford only some services. Indemnity insurance plans, even with the deductible, reduced the out-of-pocket expense to the patient. Consequently, people sought health care services more frequently and increased the number of services they received. In addition, physicians had no incentive to be conservative in their diagnostic and treatment plans, because ultimately, the insurer reimbursed the patient for any services the physician provided. The costs rose still further with advances in diagnostic and therapeutic technologies, many of which are extremely costly in their initial phases. As these technologies become more widely used, the cost of providing health care increases.

In addition to the medical technology–driven expenses, health care costs have risen because a small portion of the health care community provided an excessive number of services to their patients. Two radiographs may have been taken when one would have sufficed, or computed tomography or magnetic resonance imaging was used when a simple radiograph would have been sufficient to achieve the same diagnostic goal. Often it is not entirely the provider's fault when these excesses occur. Some patients may feel entitled to the newest technologies even if they are not necessary, and so they pressure their physicians into ordering them. The physician may not want to lose the patient's business or to be subjected to a lawsuit for failure to use all available diagnostic means.

To meet the rising costs of health care, insurance companies raised health care premiums. However, insurance becomes less attractive under these circumstances.

Employers began imposing higher deductibles and strictly limiting the numbers and types of covered services to help lower the cost of premiums. Many employers began shifting the cost of insurance to the employees. Other employers solved the escalating premium problem by hiring more part-time employees, who were not eligible for benefits. Still other employers hired outside contractors to perform noncritical functions. Eventually, some employers could no longer afford to offer health insurance as a benefit.

With costs rising and insurers losing customers, health insurance companies had to find ways to control their expenses. The insurance industry responded to these circumstances and factors, opening the door to the concept of managed care plans. The term **managed care**, in general, refers to the control that an insurance company or other payer exerts over the reimbursement process and over the patient's choices in selecting a health care provider.

In the pure physician–patient relationship, the patient uses the physician of his or her choice. The patient arrives at the office with a medical concern, and the physician determines a diagnosis and develops a treatment plan. The patient agrees (or declines) to undergo the treatment plan, the physician bills the patient, and the patient pays the physician.

Under managed care, the insurer (payer) and the health care provider have a contractual arrangement with each other. Providers apply to be included in insurers' **network** of providers. Insurance companies negotiate with the provider to determine the services that apply to that provider, how much the insurer will pay for those services, and under what circumstances the provider may render those services. Once they participate in a particular managed care plan, the provider is under contract with the managed care plan insurer to provide services to the insurer's patients. Under the contract, the provider agrees to be compensated certain amounts for services to patients of the managed care company, theoretically at prices lower than the provider would charge patients who are not in the plan.

Patients must choose their health care providers from the network of those participating in the managed care plan. Even though the physician earns less for his or her services, being in-network is attractive because it offers the physician a steady pool of patients.

Managed care patients are referred to, depending on the insurer, as *members*, *enrollees*, or *covered lives*. The primary insured member is the subscriber, with those covered under the subscriber's policy referred to as dependents or additional insured. The scope of services paid for is determined by the insurer's contract with the subscriber (or the subscriber's employer or group manager).

Because subscribers are encouraged to choose from the list of in-network providers, being on multiple lists is theoretically a good business decision for providers. However, if insurers reduce payments and restrict services, providers may decide to avoid these payer relationships entirely. In fact, some physicians may elect not to accept insurance at all, requiring patients to file cumbersome claims for reimbursement with their insurers.

In a managed care scenario, the patient goes to the **primary care provider (PCP)**, whom the patient has chosen from a list of participating physicians and qualified providers. The PCP diagnoses and treats the patient according to the guidelines from the managed care plan. The patient may pay the PCP a copay. The PCP bills the managed care insurer directly for the visit.

The PCP treats a wide variety of conditions but also identifies whether a patient requires the services of a specialist. The process of sending a patient to another physician, usually a specialist, is called a **referral**. Most managed care insurance plans require a referral from the PCP for the patient to see a specialist, further controlling the circumstances under which a patient uses health care services. After examination and discussion with the patient, the PCP must justify the necessity for the involvement of a specialist and must refer the patient to a specialist participating in the plan. For example, the PCP may identify a suspicious mole and refer the patient to an in-network dermatologist—the patient cannot simply go to the dermatologist first. Similarly, patients cannot access allied health services such as imaging centers or physical therapy without an order from the physician. The primary care system where a PCP limits access to other parts of the health care delivery system is called a **gatekeeper** model.

The managed care insurer may refuse to pay the physician if the physician does not obtain preapproval or authorization for some treatments, such as hospitalization. If the patient sees a physician outside the plan, the patient may not be covered at all and may have to pay the physician himself or herself.

Managed care organizations seek to reduce costs by controlling as much of the health care delivery system as possible. The underlying rationale for managed care is to reduce overall costs by eliminating unnecessary tests, procedures, visits, and hospitalizations through financial incentives if the plan is followed and financial penalties or sanctions if the plan is not followed. A major controversy in this strategy lies in the definition of what constitutes "unnecessary" health care and who makes this determination. Traditionally, physicians have determined the care that they provide to patients, whereas managed care has shifted that determination somewhat to the insurer. Decisions about the medical necessity of specific services are made by the managed care organization. For example, a participating physician writes an order for a blood test to determine whether the patient has a vitamin D deficiency, which could explain the patient's gloomy mood. The managed care organization, however, has determined that it will pay for vitamin D blood tests only if the patient is known or suspected to have a bone loss condition, such as osteopenia or osteoporosis. Without the suspected bone loss condition, the insurer will not pay for the blood test, which may result in the patient not having the blood test. This result causes some to feel that managed care rules are limiting the physician's freedom to practice in the way he or she thinks best for his or her patient's health. To emphasize, the managed care organization does not dictate what care will be rendered; it dictates what care it will pay for. It is the prohibitive cost of care that drives a patient to elect only that care for which third-party payment is available.

It should be noted that managed care plans employ physicians who assist in making determinations. These physicians evaluate care plans based on current research and patient outcomes. For example, at one time, many managed care insurers did not consider preventive care such as screenings to be necessary and would not pay for it. It was only through years of study, investigation, and trial and error that they discovered that preventive care was one of the best ways to reduce health care costs. This fact is particularly salient with regard to obstetric care. The costs of treating a pregnant woman through prenatal testing, education, and regular examinations, with the goal of delivering a healthy newborn, are significantly less than those of treating a newborn or new mother with complications that could have been prevented or treated earlier at less cost. The same holds true for dental care. Theoretically, if teeth are examined and cleaned routinely, expensive fillings and root canal treatments will not be needed because the dentist will help detect and treat those problems early.

Individuals who change jobs are often forced to find new health care providers if their previous physicians are not included in the new insurer's plan. The same may be true if the employer changes insurers. Patients who live on the outskirts of a plan's primary service area may be required to travel unacceptably long distances to receive covered health care services.

Physicians may feel a loss of control in the treatment process. They are sometimes frustrated by the emphasis on medical practice standards, what some call *cookbook medicine*, and resistance to what they may see as individualized, alternative approaches to care. Managed care organizations focus heavily on statistical analysis of treatment outcomes and scrutinize physicians whose practices appear to vary significantly from the norm. Managed care has forced physicians to become more aware of and active in managing their own resources by employing reimbursement methods that shift some financial risk to the physician.

Despite controversy and criticism, managed care has become an important presence in the health care arena. In fact, most of the exchange plans available under the ACA are managed care plans. Managed care takes a number of different forms, and there are many variations in the relationship among managed care organizations and physicians and other health care providers who deliver their services. At the heart of managed care is the idea that the insurer can gain better control over the cost of health care by actively engaging with the provider in determining the services to be rendered.

## Health Maintenance Organizations

The US Congress supported the managed care concept as early as the 1970s. The Health Maintenance Organization Act of 1973 encouraged the development of **health** maintenance organizations (HMOs) and mandated certain employers to offer employees an HMO option for health care delivery.

An HMO is a managed care organization that has ownership or employer control over the health care provider. Essentially, the HMO is the insurer (payer) and the provider. Members must use the HMO for all services, and the HMO will generally not pay for out-of-network services without prior approval. In some plans, approval to obtain health care services outside the plan is granted only in emergency situations.

In the staff model HMO, the organization owns the facilities, employs the physicians, and provides essentially all health care services. In a group practice model HMO, the organization contracts with a group or a network of physicians and facilities to provide health care services. Finally, in an independent practice association (IPA) model HMO, the HMO contracts with individual physicians, portions of whose practices are devoted to the HMO. Regardless of the HMO model, an HMO generally does not reimburse for services provided by providers who are not in the HMO's network.

### Preferred Provider Organizations

A preferred provider organization (PPO) is another managed care approach in which the organization contracts with a network of health care providers who agree to certain reimbursement rates. It is from this network that patients are encouraged to choose their PCP and any specialists. If a patient chooses a provider who is not in the network, the PPO reimburses in the same manner as an indemnity insurer: for specified services, with specific dollar amounts or percentage limits, and after any deductible is paid by the insured.

A PPO is a hybrid plan that gives patients the option of choosing physicians outside the plan without totally forfeiting benefits. In addition, PPOs may offer patients a certain degree of freedom to self-refer to specialists. For example, some plans allow patients to visit gynecologists and vision specialists directly, without referral from the PCP.

### Affordable Care Act

In an effort to increase the number of individuals who can obtain health insurance, the Patient Protection and Affordable Care Act (PPACA), conventionally abbreviated as ACA, was passed into law in 2010. This legislation was designed to improve patient outcomes, increase access to health insurance, and lower costs. It requires all health plans—whether offered by private carriers or government agencies—to cover certain services, called minimum essential coverage (MEC) (Box 6.1). It also prohibits insurers from denying coverage to those with preexisting conditions.

While these provisions increase costs overall, the ACA seeks to offset premium increases by enlarging the risk pool. To accomplish this larger pool, the law created health insurance exchanges, which enable individuals who do not have

---

> **• BOX 6.1   Minimum Essential Coverage's Essential Health Benefits**
>
> All health plans sold or offered in the United States must have coverage for:
> - ambulatory patient services
> - emergency services
> - hospitalization
> - pregnancy, maternity, and newborn care
> - mental health and substance use disorder services, including behavioral health treatment
> - prescription drugs
> - rehabilitative and habilitative services and devices
> - laboratory services
> - preventive and wellness services and chronic disease management
> - pediatric services, including oral and vision care

---

coverage through an employer-sponsored group policy to obtain health insurance at rates that are lower than they could obtain on their own. The underlying premise of the exchanges is that a wide variety of individuals would theoretically create a sufficiently diverse risk pool to reduce the insurance company's risk and enable the insurance company to offer lower rates. The ACA also originally required all individuals to obtain health coverage through their employer and entitlement programs or by purchasing it privately through the newly formed marketplace or state-based exchanges. Lower-income individuals qualify for lower monthly premiums through tax subsidies, making health insurance more affordable to more people, and it expanded Medicaid to cover all adults with incomes below 138% of the Federal Poverty Level.

The mandate that all individuals be insured was eliminated by Congress in 2017; however, the exchanges, MEC requirements, and many other provisions remain. For example, the ACA mandates that employers with 50 or more full-time employees offer insurance and requires that plans allow dependents of the subscriber to stay on the policy until age 26. Providers must demonstrate high-quality outcomes before receiving full payment rendered for services to federally funded patients. Because the ACA includes requirements that affect all health insurance (e.g., coverage of preexisting conditions), you are encouraged to stay abreast of this law at: www.healthcare.gov.

### Self-Insurance

Although not specifically a type of insurance, self-insurance (or self-funded insurance) is an alternative to purchasing an insurance policy. The term *self-insurance* should not be confused with patients who "self-pay" or those who have no insurance or coverage plan at all. Self-insurance is really a savings plan in which an individual or employer puts aside funds to cover health care costs. In this way, the individual or company assumes the financial risk associated with health care. Because the assumption of risk rests with the company or the individual, this is not so much a type of insurance as it is an alternative to shifting the risk to an insurer.

An employer may choose to self-insure for all health care benefits, or it may self-insure to provide specific benefits that its primary insurance plan does not cover. For example, an insurance plan may cover preventive care, hospital and physician services, and diagnostic tests. However, it may not cover vision or dental care. The employer may designate to each employee a certain dollar amount with which the employee may then be reimbursed for these other services. Ordinarily, if the annual dollar amount is not spent, it is lost to the employee. Because the issue of confidentiality is so important, employers may choose to contract with an insurer to process health care claims, even if the employer self-insures.

Individuals may self-insure by contributing money to an account designated for health care expenses. One formal plan that enables individuals to save in this manner is a *health savings account (HSA)*. Paired with a high-deductible health plan, HSAs allow individuals to set aside funds for health expenses. Any monies contributed to the HSA are excluded from the person's taxable income. Money in the account can be spent on health-related "qualified expenses," from prescription drugs, to office copays, to contact lenses. Funds in an HSA can be invested and earn interest. When obtained through the employer, a set amount determined by the employee can be deposited routinely into HSA through payroll deduction.

Many employers offer a similar savings vehicle called a *flexible spending account (FSA)*, into which the employee can designate a certain amount of money from each paycheck. The funds are withdrawn from the individual's salary on a pretax basis, thereby reducing the individual's income tax liability. FSA contributions are exempt from payroll taxes in addition to income tax. These funds can then be drawn on to pay out-of-pocket health care and some child care expenses. Unlike an HSA, FSAs do not need to be paired with a high-deductible health plan. Funds in the FSA are not invested but rather remain with the employer. Unused funds are forfeited at the end of the year.

Some interesting strategies have evolved. First is the independent physician–patient contract, sometimes called *concierge medicine* or *retainer medicine*. In this strategy, a physician who is independent of other health care system relationships contracts with individuals at a flat rate paid monthly, biannually, or annually. In exchange, the physician provides primary care services, which may include some labs, radiology, and medication. The patient has unlimited access, as needed, to the physician. The physician has a pool of patients that may be significantly smaller than that normally experienced when a payer contract is involved. The physician has no third-party payer paperwork to complete, because any insurance held by the patient is the responsibility of the patient. While many patients also have insurance, their plan may have a very high deductible. There are critics who argue that independent physicians in this model impair access for the general population, because they see fewer patients. In areas where physicians are in short supply, this is particularly problematic. Other critics argue that, since many of the patients also carry insurance, the patient is effectively double-paying for their health care. Advocates of this model point to the reduced stress of the independent physicians and increased patient satisfaction. It remains to be seen whether this is a growing trend.

---

❖ **COMPETENCY CHECK-IN 6.1**

**Insurance**

**Competency Assessment**

1. Match the definition on the left with the health insurance terminology on the right.

| | |
|---|---|
| _____ 1. Amount of cost that the beneficiary must incur before the insurance will assume liability for the remaining cost | 1. Beneficiary |
| _____ 2. Contractor that manages the health care claims | 2. Benefit |
| _____ 3. One who is eligible to receive or is receiving benefits from an insurance policy or a managed care program | 3. Claim |
| _____ 4. Party who is financially responsible for reimbursement of health care costs | 4. Deductible |
| _____ 5. Payer's payment for specific health care services or, in managed care, the health care services that will be provided or for which the provider will be paid | 5. Fiscal intermediary |
| _____ 6. Payment by a third party to a provider of health care | 6. Payer |
| _____ 7. Request for payment by the insured or the provider for services covered | 7. Reimbursement |

2. Health insurance involves the assumption of the risk of financial loss by a party other than the patient. Describe how insurance companies can afford to assume such risk.
3. In this section you learned about different types of health insurance. List them, and describe how they are different.
4. The physician charged the patient $75 for the office visit. The patient paid the physician $5, and the patient's insurance company paid the physician $70. The patient's portion of the payment is called the _____.
5. What are the financial risks in health care delivery for providers, third-party payers, and patients?
6. Explain the ways managed care plans seek to lower costs.
7. Name various vehicles for self-insurance.

Another emerging self-pay strategy is a health sharing plan. These plans are not insurance, per se, but rather a cooperative agreement with other individuals to share medical costs. All health sharing plans have a few things in common:

- a religious component,
- a community comprises healthy individuals initially, and
- a community of individuals committed to a healthy lifestyle.

The religious component exempts the plan from the rules of the ACA, specifically the law's requirements that health plans cover preexisting conditions. Bearing in mind our previous discussion of risk, you can see that only accepting healthy individuals into the plan significantly lowers risk. In a health sharing plan, members of the cooperative pay a shared amount (similar to a premium) and are responsible for an "unshared" amount (similar to a deductible) before the cooperative begins to share costs. Shared amounts are distributed according to need of other members of the community (Liberty Healthshare, 2018).

## Entitlements

Although the United States does not have universal health care (i.e., government-subsidized health care for all citizens), the various levels of government do serve as the largest payer for health care services. Because eligibility for certain government-sponsored programs is automatic, which is based on age, condition, or employment, they are called **entitlement programs** rather than insurance. The federal and state governments administer a variety of plans that are available to specific populations. Table 6.3 provides a summary of this involvement.

## Medicare

Title XVIII of the Social Security Act established the Medicare program in 1965. Originally enacted to provide funding for health care for older adults, **Medicare** has grown to include individuals with certain disabilities or with end-stage renal disease requiring dialysis or kidney transplantation. Medicare represents more than 50% of the income of some health care providers. Medicare is an extremely important driving force in the insurance industry because many insurance companies follow Medicare's lead in adopting reimbursement strategies. For example, if Medicare decides that a particular surgical procedure will be reimbursed only if it is performed in the inpatient setting (as opposed to ambulatory surgery), other insurance companies may choose to enforce the same rule.

The Medicare program, although funded by the federal government and administered by the Centers for Medicare and Medicaid Services (CMS), does not process its own claim reimbursements. Reimbursements are processed by **Medicare Administrative Contractors (MACs)** located in different regions throughout the country.

Medicare coverage applies in four categories: Parts A, B, C, and D. Part A covers inpatient hospital services and some other services, such as hospice. Part B covers physician claims and outpatient services. Part C is a voluntary managed care option. Part D, implemented in 2006, is a prescription drug program.

**TABLE 6.3    Summary of Federal Government Involvement in Health Care**

| Acronym | Description | Covered Lives |
|---|---|---|
| Medicare | Title XVIII of the Social Security Act (1965) | Older adult, disabled, renal dialysis, and transplant patients |
| | | Part A: inpatient services |
| | | Part B: outpatient services and physician claims |
| | | Part C: managed care option |
| | | Part D: prescription drug benefit |
| Medicaid | Title XIX of the Social Security Act (1965) | Low-income patients |
| TRICARE | Medical services for members of the armed services, their spouses, and their families | Administered by the Department of Defense and applying to members of the Army, Air Force, Navy, Marine Corps, Coast Guard, Public Health Service, and National Oceanic and Atmospheric Administration |
| VHA | Veterans Health Administration | Health services for veterans |
| CHAMPVA | Civilian Health and Medical Program of the Department of Veterans Affairs (CHAMPVA) | Programs administered by the US Department of Veterans Affairs (Health Administration Center) for veterans and their families |
| IHS | Indian Health Service | Provides or assists in providing and organizing health care services to American Indians and Alaskan Natives |

Because there are limits to Medicare coverage, many beneficiaries choose to purchase additional insurance; such plans, called **wraparound policies** (supplemental or Medigap policies), are aimed at absorbing costs not reimbursed by Medicare. Many end-of-life hospital stays generate costs in the hundreds of thousands of dollars. Therefore wraparound policies can help preserve estates and save surviving spouses from financial ruin. Medicare may also be the secondary payer for enrollees who are still employed and covered primarily by the employer's insurance plan.

Medicare beneficiaries also may enroll in a Medicare HMO program, called Medicare Advantage. Different HMOs have contracted with the federal government under the Medicare Advantage program to provide health services to these beneficiaries.

## Medicaid

In 1965 Congress enacted Title XIX of the Social Security Act, which authorized **Medicaid**, a formal system of providing funding for health care for low-income populations. Also administered by CMS, Medicaid is a shared federal and state program. The federal government allocates funds to states through the Federal Medical Assistance Program according to the average income of the residents of the state. The federal government specifies minimum requirements for Medicaid programs, beyond which states may choose to expand coverage. Unlike Medicare, which reimburses through **fiscal intermediaries**, Medicaid reimbursement is handled directly by each individual state. Medicaid coverage and reimbursement guidelines vary from state to state. Some states have contracted with insurers to offer HMO plans to Medicaid beneficiaries. One of the provisions of the ACA was to expand Medicaid coverage, thereby increasing the number of eligible individuals. This expansion was not mandatory, but it was temporarily funded 90% by the federal government. Some states declined to participate in the expansion partly because the economic burden of the expansion shifted to the states after 3 years.

Unlike eligibility for the Medicare program, which is based on age, disability, or the need for renal dialysis, eligibility for Medicaid is based primarily on economic circumstances, as determined by the individual states. Individuals with limited resources may be eligible for Medicaid, including some children whose parents may not personally be eligible. The eligibility rules and application process vary by state. Funding for Medicaid is shared between the federal government and the state. The federal government mandates that the following services be included in each state's program:

- inpatient hospital services,
- outpatient hospital services,
- EPSDT: Early and Periodic Screening, Diagnostic, and Treatment Services,
- nursing facility services,
- home health services,
- physician services,
- rural health clinic services,
- federally qualified health center services,
- laboratory and X-ray services,
- family planning services,
- nurse midwife services,
- certified pediatric and family nurse practitioner services,
- freestanding birth center services (when licensed or otherwise recognized by the state),
- transportation to medical care, and
- tobacco cessation counseling for pregnant women.

(See the Medicaid website for more information: http://www.medicaid.gov/medicaid-chip-program-information/by-topics/benefits/medicaid-benefits.html)

States vary in their provision of health care benefits to special populations, such as children. The Children's Health Insurance Program provides free or low-cost health care coverage to eligible children and other family members. The program may be known by different names. For example, in Delaware it is the Delaware Healthy Children Program; in Arizona, it is called KidsCare.

In addition to Medicaid, states provide funding for a variety of programs supporting the health care needs of individuals who do not have the resources to pay for care. For example, all hospitals that maintain an ED are required to evaluate patients prior to obtaining information about the patient's ability to pay for care. If the patient has an emergency, such as a stroke, the hospital could admit and treat the patient without knowing whether the patient could pay for the services rendered. If the patient has no resources with which to pay for the services and is not eligible for other government programs, the hospital may obtain some reimbursement from the state's uncompensated care program.

*Uncompensated care*, also called "charity care," refers to the value of services rendered to patients who have no ability to pay for those services. Financial assistance policies help provide free or discounted medical services to patients who meet certain eligibility standards and are unable to pay for medical care or treatments. Patients may be eligible for Medicaid or some other state-funded program, for which they must apply and from which the hospital may obtain some level of payment. The state may also provide payments to hospitals, which are not specifically tied to individual patients but are based on the quantity of uncompensated care rendered as a percentage of total care provided. For example, a state may determine that a hospital rendering 20% of its total dollar value of care to indigent patients will be reimbursed by the state for 10% of that dollar value. If the value of care to indigent patients is $60 million, then the hospital would receive $6 million from the state.

## Federal Coverage for Specific Populations

In addition to Medicare and Medicaid, the federal government administers **TRICARE**, which provides health benefits for military personnel, their families, and military retirees. The federal government provides health services to veterans through the Veterans Health Administration (VHA). The Civilian Health and Medical Program of the Department of Veterans Affairs (CHAMPVA) was created in 1973 to provide health services for spouses and children of certain deceased or disabled veterans. TRICARE, VHA, and CHAMPVA are service benefits, not insurance, and are included here to illustrate the extent of the federal government's financial involvement in health care. (See the TRICARE and CHAMPVA websites for additional information.)

The Indian Health Services (IHS) provides care for American Indians and Alaska Natives. The IHS provides a comprehensive health service delivery system for approximately 2.56 million of the nation's estimated 5.2 million American Indians and Alaska Natives, who belong to 573 federally recognized tribes in 37 states (Department of Health and Human Services, Indian Health Service, 2019).

## Tax Equity and Fiscal Responsibility Act of 1982

With the federal government's entry into the reimbursement arena, more citizens had access to health care services than ever before. The use of health care services rose accordingly, in turn driving health care costs upward at an alarming rate. Improved access for older adults meant better care and therefore longer life expectancy, which further increased costs. Thus cost containment became a critical issue. In the early 1970s Professional Standards Review Organizations (PSROs) were established. PSROs conducted local peer reviews of Medicare and Medicaid cases for the purpose of ensuring that only medically necessary services were being rendered and appropriately reimbursed. Under the Peer Review Improvement Act of 1982, PSROs were replaced by Peer Review Organizations (PROs) through a federal law called the **Tax Equity and Fiscal Responsibility Act of 1982 (TEFRA)**. TEFRA included a broad array of provisions, many of which had nothing to do with health care. For example, TEFRA raised taxes by eliminating previous tax cuts. In 2002 PROs were replaced by (or, more accurately, renamed) Quality Improvement Organizations (QIOs). Many health information management (HIM) professionals are employed in QIOs because certain specialized skills, such as data analysis and coding expertise, are necessary to support various federal initiatives delegated to QIOs. TEFRA's impact on health care included a modification of Medicare reimbursement for inpatient care to include a **case mix** adjustment based on diagnosis-related groups (DRGs). In 1983 Medicare adopted the *prospective payment system (PPS)*, which uses the DRG classification system as the basis of its reimbursement methodology. PPSs are discussed at length later in the chapter, but in the broadest terms, they operate on the assumption that patients with the same diagnoses will require roughly the same level of care, therefore consuming roughly the same resources and incurring roughly the same costs. Of course, the focus of treatment, patient length of stay, and the individuals involved in the care plan differ from setting to setting. Because prospective reimbursement systems are based on just these types of factors, different systems were developed for each health care setting.

Paying for health care is an ever-changing subject. HIM professionals must be aware of new developments that pertain to their practice and keep abreast of general reimbursement issues.

## COMPETENCY CHECK-IN 6.2

### Entitlements

#### Competency Assessment
1. What is the difference between Medicare and Medicaid?
2. What is the difference between the VHA and TRICARE?
3. Who benefits from the Indian Health Services?
4. Explain the impact of TEFRA on health care.
5. An 82-year-old patient came to the physician's office for a routine physical examination. He gave the receptionist two cards proving his primary, government-funded insurance plan, which pays for most of the bill, and an additional private plan that covers the remaining charges. The patient's primary insurance is most likely _____. The patient's secondary insurance is called a(n) _____.

## REIMBURSEMENT METHODOLOGIES

This section provides a general discussion of how reimbursement is accomplished in the health care industry, who is involved in the reimbursement process, what methodologies are used to calculate reimbursement, and how HIM professionals are involved in the process. One of the most visible roles that HIM professionals play in health care today involves the reimbursement process (e.g., as coding professionals or clinical data managers).

## Fee for Service

As previously mentioned, a physician or other health care provider does not necessarily need to receive money as compensation. Perhaps chickens, bread, or other food are acceptable under certain circumstances. In other circumstances, services might be bartered (e.g., "You treat my pneumonia, and I will take care of your plumbing."). This is known as an *exchange of services*, or *reciprocal services*. The parties involved decide the value of each service (e.g., how many hours of plumbing would be equal in value to how many hours of physician treatment). However, monetary compensation is the generally accepted reimbursement method in the United States. **Fee for service** is the exchange of monies, goods, or services for professional services rendered at a specific rate, typically determined by the provider and associated with specific activities (such as a physical examination). There are several different ways to reimburse on the basis of fees for services rendered.

### Charges

A physician or other provider decides the price for services rendered. For example, a patient goes to, or visits, the physician's office because of a runny nose. The physician examines the patient and determines that the patient is allergic to a house pet. This service, which comprises an office visit and examination, is billed at $100. This $100 is the *fee*. Suppose this same patient also needs an allergy shot, and this shot has a fee of $20. In this case, the total fee for the visit is $120. As this example shows, fees correspond to the services rendered, or fee for service. Health care provider fees are also called **charges**. Note that costs and charges are different. Cost is what the health care provider expended in the process of rendering services. Costs include time, supplies, salaries, and expenses such as rent and utilities. Charges are the fees that are billed for the services. In order to stay in business, the provider must charge (and receive payment) for more than the cost of services. The term *cost* is often used to refer to the overall expenditures for health care, but the correct accounting definition is used for this discussion. A self-pay patient checking out after an examination will likely be asked to pay the total charges for the visit. However, these charges are not necessarily what will be reimbursed by a third-party payer.

Comparing the fees charged by physicians in a particular state or geographic area, one finds that the fees for services are similar. Ignoring the very high and very low fees, one would be able to determine the **usual, customary, and reasonable fees (UCRs)** charged by physicians in that area. To determine the UCR amount, it is necessary to compare not only the services but also such issues as the specialties of the physicians providing the services, the cost of living in the geographic area, and the cost of malpractice insurance. The term *usual and customary fees* commonly appears in the language of insurance contracts because this is the fee that third-party payers are willing to reimburse for services. For example, a physician may decide to charge $100 for an office visit, but the insurer will reimburse only $80, if $80 is the UCR for that specialty in that area.

## Discounted Fee for Service

Within this category of reimbursement are other negotiated fees. In a typical **discounted fee for service** arrangement, the third-party payer (in this case, the managed care insurer) negotiates a payment that is less than the provider's normal rate. Providers are willing to discount their charges in order to obtain business from the payers—the result of being included in the payer's "network." For example, the provider may charge $100 for a service. The insurer assumes that the volume of patients added to the provider's business would warrant a 10% discount from the normal rate. Therefore the payment for the service would be $90. To a certain extent, discounted fees are negotiable and are increasingly dependent on the quality of services rendered by the provider.

Some insurers reimburse at flat rates, known as *per diem* (daily) rates, for service. A per diem rate is basically a flat fee, negotiated in advance, that an insurer will pay for each day of hospitalization. For inpatient health care providers or facilities, per diem rates may represent a significant discount from the actual accumulated fees for each service performed, but again, the provider or facility benefits by gaining that payer's business. Per diem rates are most commonly negotiated with providers who serve a limited patient population, such as providers of rehabilitation services.

## Capitation

Reimbursement does not have to be based on services rendered. **Capitation** requires payment to a health care provider regardless of whether the patient is seen or how frequently the patient is seen during a given period. For example, a physician might receive $10 a month for each patient under an insurance plan whose patients choose him or her as their PCP. If 100 patients choose this physician as their PCP, the physician receives $1000 a month for those patients—even if no one comes in for a visit. If all 100 patients are seen in 1 month, the physician still receives $1000. Generally, however, the more patients who choose this physician under

There are 20 patients in the physician's panel
No one received treatment in June

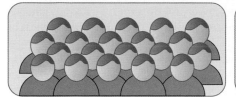

In July, 2 of the 20 patients receive treatment

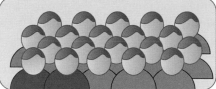

All 20 patients come in for treatment

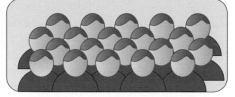

The payer pays $10 for each
patient this month.

Physician receives $200
with no expenses

The payer pays $10 for each patient in July,
regardless of whether they came in for a visit.

If each visit costs $12,
the physician receives
$176 in July

| $10 × 20 patients | = | $200 |
| $12 × 2 patients seen | = | −$ 24 |
| | | $176 net profit |

The rate does not change in August. The
payer pays a total of $200 for the panel.

Because the physician's expenses
outweigh his payment for August,
the physician loses $40 this month

| $10 × 20 patients | = | $200 |
| − $12 × 20 patients seen | = | − $240 |
| | | $40 net loss |

• **Fig. 6.2** Capitation scenarios with a pool of 20 patients.

a capitation plan, the greater the odds that that physician will receive adequate overall payment for his or her services, especially if that group of patients is relatively healthy and does not make many office visits. The insurer will still benefit if it is less expensive to pay a known monthly capitation fee rather than reimburse an unpredictable amount of money to the physician each month (Fig. 6.2).

## Prospective Payment

A **prospective payment system (PPS)** is a method of determining the payment to a health care provider on the basis of predetermined factors, not on individual costs for services. Although technically a "fee for service" payment in the sense that it is tied to a particular health care event, PPS payments are determined by the payer rather than the provider, so we are discussing them separately. Numerous insurers and government agencies use PPSs for reimbursement, most notably the Medicare PPS, which is discussed in detail later in this chapter. PPSs are based on the statistical analysis of large quantities of historical health care data for the purpose of evaluating the resources used to treat specific diagnoses and effect certain treatments. On the basis of this evaluation, it has been determined that certain diagnoses and procedures consume sufficiently similar resources, such that reimbursement to the facility for all patients with such diagnoses and undergoing such procedures should be the same. For this purpose, resources are measured in both costs and days. Essentially, the provider receives a payment that is based on the historical cost of treating patients with that particular combination of diagnoses and procedures.

For example, suppose a review of 10,000 uncomplicated appendectomies reveals that the patients were hospitalized for an average of 2 days. The statistical average cost for these hospitalizations, based on the 10,000 uncomplicated appendectomy cases, is $5000. An insurer who uses a PPS to reimburse a facility may agree to pay that facility $5000,

regardless of how long a given patient who received an uncomplicated appendectomy was actually hospitalized or what the actual charges were. If the charges for that hospitalization were actually $4500, the facility would still receive $5000. If the charges for that hospitalization were actually $5500, the facility would still receive $5000. The use of the term *prospective* in this type of reimbursement system means that both the facility and the insurer know, in advance, how much each type of case will be reimbursed.

From the payer's perspective, prospective payment can be an extremely effective budgeting tool. Utilization trends can be followed, types of cases can be analyzed in groups, and reimbursement costs can be better controlled through rate setting for each type of case. From the perspective of the provider or facility, there is greater motivation to keep costs under tight control. If there are inefficiencies within the facilities or among physicians, facilities may lose income. In contract negotiations with a payer, a hospital may agree to accept the $5000 for the appendectomy but might press for a higher-than-average amount for a knee replacement due to its variability in cost. Critics of PPSs, including some physicians, maintain that prospective payment focuses only on the financial aspects of treating a patient and does not take into consideration individual, case-by-case clinical management.

## Diagnosis Related Groups (DRGs)

PPSs, as they apply to inpatient acute care, are based on **diagnosis-related groups (DRGs)** that we discussed in Chapter 5. Medicare inpatients under PPSs are grouped, and hospitals reimbursed, through the use of the MS-DRG **grouper**. The MS-DRG grouper is a DRG grouper that incorporates a patient's medical severity (MS) into its assignments and reimbursement calculation. The MS-DRG grouper is one of several DRG groupers. For example, the AP-DRG grouper and APR-DRG grouper are groupers used by some payers other than Medicare. "AP" stands for All Payer, and "APR" stands for All Payer Refined. In general,

DRGs classify, or group, patients by common type according to diagnosis, treatment, and resource intensity (RI). The statistical foundation of DRGs is based on the assumption that the same diagnosis requires the same type of care for all patients. The term **resource intensity (RI)** generally refers to demands and costs associated with treating specific types of patients: How much it costs to treat a particular disease or condition, depending on what types of resources that type of patient consumes and in some instances factoring in the age and gender of the patient. For example, if a patient is being treated in the hospital for congestive heart failure and nothing else, then that patient will probably consume the same amount of resources, have the same procedures performed, require the same number of consultations, and have the same intensity of nursing care as any other patient coming into the hospital with the same diagnosis, barring complications. Statistically, on the basis of review of hundreds of thousands of records, this assumption proves to be true, allowing for the classification of the patient's stay into a DRG assignment.

Classifying types of patients into DRGs and predicting their expected resource consumption provide the basis for assigning monetary amounts for each MS-DRG in the Medicare PPS. For example, even though a patient admitted with new onset of atrial fibrillation (an abnormal heart rhythm) and a patient admitted for an elective carotid endarterectomy (surgery to clear a blockage in a carotid artery) may both stay in the hospital for 3 days, the patient treated with medications for atrial fibrillation will not consume as much in the way of resources as a patient who required use of the operating room and postoperative care. Both patients, having different diagnoses and treatments, would be assigned to two different MS-DRGs, with the amount reimbursed for the patient with atrial fibrillation's hospitalization less than the amount reimbursed for the patient who had the carotid endarterectomy.

DRG classifications were separate from reimbursement until the late 1970s, when the New Jersey Department of Health mandated use of the system for reimbursement. In New Jersey, DRG-based methodology reimbursement applied to all patients and all payer classifications; DRG reimbursement classifications were adopted with the goal of containing overall inpatient health care costs, which were rapidly increasing. Because the DRG classification system in New Jersey applied to all inpatients and payers, even self-pay patients, it has been referred to as an "all payer" PPS. (This is a historical reference, as the New Jersey systems have since changed.)

In Chapter 5, you learned how patients are classified into groups according to the DRG classification system, with coding being the main critical element. Without assigned codes for each patient, there cannot be a DRG assignment. Without a DRG assigned, a hospital cannot receive reimbursement. When the coding function became linked to reimbursement, coders and HIM personnel (e.g., medical records staff) made enormous gains in importance and stature. There was a saying at the time that medical records

professionals came "out of the basement and into the boardroom." For the first time ever, a national health care publication featured a medical records director on its cover, when it published a feature article about DRGs. With the advent of the DRG system, HIM professionals basked in the national health care spotlight and embraced their new leadership roles and responsibilities.

Again, the coding function had comparatively fewer pressures before the implementation of PPSs and DRGs. Coders were focused on assigning codes for statistical purposes, such as analysis of resource utilization in the facility. The accuracy of codes, although important, was not so closely scrutinized, and coders were under less pressure to perform their tasks in a timely manner. Most hospital administrators would try to complete the previous month's cases no later than 2 weeks into the following month. Coding was considered just another function in a medical records department, perhaps on par with the analysis function. Coders were trained primarily by their employers, and some were credentialed as either registered record administrators (RRAs) or accredited record technicians, which were the only two credentials offered by the American Health Information Management Association (AHIMA) at the time. People earning either credential did not specialize in coding but rather took one or two courses in coding. Today, coding has become a highly specialized and desirable profession in itself, with several credentials offered solely for coding by different organizations. Coders play a valuable role in the health care industry by accurately selecting codes for proper reimbursement. The coder helps to maintain compliance for providers and health care facilities by adhering to government regulations and coding guidelines. When selecting a coding credential, consider the type of services you want to code and the type of setting where you want to work. The AHIMA offers a Certified Coding Specialist and Certified Coding Assistance Credential; the American Academy of Professional Coders offers credentials as a Certified Professional Coder, Certified Outpatient Coder, Certified Inpatient Coder, and Certified Risk Adjustment Coder (CRC).

With the evolution of coding and the coding profession, tremendous changes occurred in hospital computer systems. In the late 1970s most medical records departments did not have computers or even access to their hospital computers. In some instances, DRG grouping was actually done by using a large paper manual that outlined the DRG grouper program. In most cases, however, coders dialed into a system off-site, entered codes and other data elements for each patient, and received a DRG assignment over the telephone connection. This was not even an Internet connection but rather a telephone modem connection to an off-site computer, originally at Yale University, where DRGs were developed. One advantage (possibly the only one) in grouping cases this way was that the coder truly understood the software program and could therefore provide feedback and suggestions. Because today grouping is computerized, coders may not be as familiar with all of the nuances and elements of grouping. On the other hand, computerized grouping is certainly far more accurate than grouping with a paper manual. In any event, coders not only began to take greater responsibility for timely and accurate coding because of the DRG system but also learned more about information technology and health information. Eventually, computerization and the data collection activities required to support coding, DRG assignment, and reimbursement moved facilities closer to what is or will eventually become an EHR.

Overall, the impact of DRGs and the PPS on health care was enormous. In addition to New Jersey, a number of states soon adopted PPSs, or "all payer" systems, requiring all payers, including Medicare, to use DRGs as a reimbursement methodology for hospital inpatients. Because the PPS was a completely new reimbursement model, its adoption had a dramatic financial impact on facilities during the initial years. Patients were also affected because lengths of stay were gradually decreased. Before the adoption of PPSs, there were no financial incentives to reduce a patient's length of stay. For example, it was once common for a new mother and baby to stay in the hospital for a week; today it would be unusual for a healthy mother and baby to stay more than 2 or 3 days.

### Diagnosis-Related Group (MS-DRG) Reimbursement Calculation

Medicare reimbursements for MS-DRGs are based on two components: the national numeric value, or **relative weight (RW)**, of each MS-DRG and each hospital's **blended rate**. The blended rate consists of the hospital-specific rate, which is based on historical financial data provided annually to CMS by the hospital, and additional factors such as regional labor costs and graduate medical education. The blended rate is expressed in a dollar amount specific to each hospital. All hospitals are reimbursed on the basis of the same national RW for each MS-DRG multiplied by the individual hospital's blended rate. For example, suppose MS-DRG 999 (fictional) has a national RW of 3.0000. Hospital A has a blended rate of $5000, and hospital B has a blended rate of $4500. Hospital A will receive $15,000 for each case in MS-DRG 999 (3.0000×$5000). Hospital B will receive $13,500 for each case in MS-DRG 999 (3.0000×$4500).

There are variations to this basic calculation for cases incurring extraordinarily high costs. These cases may qualify for **outlier payment**. "To qualify for outlier payments, a case must have costs above a fixed-loss cost threshold amount (a dollar amount by which the costs of the case must exceed payments in order to qualify for outliers)" (Centers for Medicare and Medicaid Services, Outlier Payments, 2021). Several calculations to determine outlier payments depend on the hospital's specific operating and capital cost factors.

The fact that each MS-DRG has its own RW used to calculate reimbursement makes the importance of correctly assigning codes for each case to group into the correct DRG apparent. For example, suppose that you are a coder at Hospital A. Your fictional MS-DRG 924 has an RW of 3.0000. MS-DRG 924 happens to be a pair MS-DRG (i.e., there is another similar MS-DRG, MS-DRG 925, that resembles MS-DRG 924 except MS-DRG 925 denotes that

a CC code is present). Suppose MS-DRG 925 has an RW of 4.0000. If you do not correctly code and do not include the CC code for MS-DRG assignment, the case would group to MS-DRG 924. If the CC code were included, the case would group to MS-DRG 925. In this example, the absence or presence of the CC code would have the following effect on reimbursement with Hospital A's blended rate of $5000:

$$\text{MS-DRG 925 "With CC" RW} : 4.0000 \times \$5000$$
$$= \$20,000 \text{ reimbursement}$$

$$\text{MS-DRG 924 "Without CC" RW} : 3.0000 \times \$5000$$
$$= \$15,000 \text{ reimbursement}$$

Consider how the MS-DRG grouper assigns cases to an MS-DRG and the great importance of assigning the correct principal diagnosis. If the incorrect principal diagnosis is assigned, it is highly likely that the MS-DRG will also be incorrect. The resultant incorrect MS-DRG assignment may be reimbursed at either a higher or lower rate than the correct MS-DRG assignment would have been. In either case, the hospital will not receive the appropriate reimbursement. When such errors in MS-DRG assignment are found, the hospital must rebill or reconcile the reimbursement amount with Medicare and other affected providers. In addition, the hospital's statistics will be negatively affected if cases are not correctly assigned. One important statistic is the hospital's case mix index (CMI).

### Case Mix Index

A hospital's **case mix index (CMI)** is the average of the DRG RWs over a period of time, which can be used to measure the complexity of the diagnoses of its patients. A hospital uses the CMI to monitor its performance and calculate the amount of money it will receive for the patients currently being treated. The higher the number, the greater the reimbursement received. Fluctuations in CMI indicate incorrect coding, changes in patient populations, changes in physician practices and personnel, or other conditions.

The CMI number is derived by adding the RWs of all of the actual MS-DRG cases and then dividing by the total number of cases discharged in a given period. For example, Hospital A discharged 54 patients in January. Each of the 54 MS-DRG RWs is added together, with a combined total of 43.9675. To calculate its CMI for January, Hospital A divides 43.9675 by 54; the CMI for January is 0.81421. Hospital A then decides to do a 6-month comparison and calculates its CMI for June. In June 47 patients were discharged with a combined RW of 41.5482. The CMI for June is calculated by dividing 41.5482 by 47; the CMI for June is 0.88400. Hospital A must decide whether the difference in the CMI from January to June is significant enough to warrant further investigation. Remember that the CMI is a measure of RI, so the hospital had fewer but more resource-intensive patients in June compared to January. In this example, the CMI was higher in June than January, so the hospital received more reimbursement on average per patient in June. We can obtain a dollar amount for the average patient by multiplying the CMI by the hospital's blended rate of $8000.

$$\text{January: } \$8000 \times 0.81421 = \$6513.68$$

$$\text{June: } \$8000 \times 0.88400 = \$7072.03$$

The CMI for all hospitals is published yearly by CMS on its website in the Public Use Files. Each hospital has its own unique **provider number** that can be referenced on a chart. The chart notes the total number of Medicare cases discharged in the previous fiscal year (FY) and the CMI for that FY. The federal FY begins October 1 and ends September 30. The chart is useful in that hospitals can use it as a reference to compare their CMIs with those of other hospitals that have a similar number of cases. The provider number must be known in order to identify a specific hospital. For example, an employee at Hospital A checks the chart and goes to the hospital's provider number, 000099. The chart shows that Hospital A had 4082 Medicare cases discharged in the previous FY and that Hospital A had a CMI of 1.023784 for that period. Next, the Hospital A employee checks the chart for hospitals that had a similar number of discharges and sees that provider number 000054 had 4120 cases and a CMI of 2.371271, significantly higher than that of Hospital A. The employee reviews the chart again and in each instance notes that the CMI for similar providers is higher than the CMI for Hospital A. After they determine that the comparison hospitals appear to offer similar services, Hospital A administrators may elect to perform an internal investigation, such as a coding audit.

One way to obtain both the advantages of concurrent coding and the resolution of physician queries prior to discharge is through a Clinical Documentation Improvement (CDI) program, as discussed in Chapter 5. In a CDI program, improving the quality of the physician's documentation is the primary goal. Developing a working MS-DRG is important; however, the entire chart is not coded. A CDI program can be an effective and efficient way to ensure that the documentation accurately reflects the patient's severity of illness and the medical decision-making involved in directing the care of the patient. This effort can support both case management, ensuring the documentation of the medical necessity of the case, and postdischarge coding, obtaining the highest degree of specificity in the documentation. Complete and accurate documentation supports accurate coding, which results in accurate and defensible reimbursement. Thus, although reimbursement is not at the heart of a CDI program, it is clearly affected by an effective CDI program.

## Ambulatory Payment Classification

As is true for inpatient services, the costs for outpatient, or ambulatory, services have risen. In addition, many patient care services have shifted from inpatient to outpatient settings, thus increasing the amount of reimbursement from outpatient/ambulatory services. In ambulatory health care, a number of different reimbursement methodologies apply; fee for service and discounted fee for service are most commonly used. A number of insurers are participating in capitation as well.

In the 1990s the federal government was spending billions of dollars on outpatient services using a cost-based system. In an attempt to cut or at least control the costs of these services and as part of the Balanced Budget Act of 1997, Congress mandated that CMS (at that time the HCFA) develop a PPS for Medicare outpatient services, referred to as the **Outpatient Prospective Payment System (OPPS)**. Just as DRGs are used for reimbursement for Medicare inpatient services under PPS, the OPPS uses ambulatory payment classifications (APCs) to reimburse for Medicare outpatient services. APCs are updated annually to include additions, deletions, and modifications. Updates occur each CY.

The APC system uses the Healthcare Common Procedure Coding System (HCPCS)/Current Procedural Terminology (CPT) procedure, service, or item codes to group patients. ICD-10-CM codes are used not for grouping but to indicate the medical necessity of the procedure, service, or item provided. For example, if a claim were submitted for reimbursement of an electrocardiogram, there should be a logical corresponding cardiac ICD-10-CM code that indicates the reason that the electrocardiogram was performed. ICD-10-PCS (procedure) codes are not used in the OPPS and the APC system, although they are sometimes assigned.

Under the APC classification system, patients are grouped on the basis of clinical similarities and similar costs or resource consumption. There are approximately 2000 APCs, a figure subject to change depending on the yearly modifications. APCs are categorized as follows:
- significant procedures, therapies, or services;
- medical visits;
- ancillary tests and procedures;
- partial hospitalization;
- drugs and biologicals; and
- devices.

Consideration of these categories makes it easier to envision how one outpatient visit can result in the assignment of multiple APCs. That more than one APC can be assigned per visit is a major difference between APCs and MS-DRGs, in which only one MS-DRG is assigned per inpatient hospitalization. For example, suppose a man is found unconscious on the sidewalk and brought to the hospital's ED by the police. The ED physician performs a workup, discovers that the patient is in a diabetic coma, and gives him insulin to bring his glucose level under control. In addition, the emergency physician notes that the patient injured his arm after falling on the sidewalk and orders a radiograph to rule out a fracture. In such a scenario, there will be an APC for the emergency visit, an APC for the administration of the drug insulin, and an APC for the radiograph. Each APC has its own payment. The facility is reimbursed in an amount equal to all three APCs added together or, in some instances, receives a reduced or discounted payment for one of the services. For example, if a patient requires the use of a minor surgery suite for multiple procedures, the patient probably uses fewer resources overall than if the procedures were performed separately at different times. Therefore a reduced payment is warranted. By the same logic, if a procedure is terminated or discontinued, the payment is reduced or discounted, depending on whether anesthesia was started.

Final payment for APCs is based on a complex set of edit and payment rules that include, for example, HCPCS/CPT codes, code modifiers, and revenue codes. The coder is usually responsible only for assigning the HCPCS/CPT codes and modifiers, and the other billing elements are the responsibility of other departments where charges have been incurred.

A code **modifier** is a two-digit number added to an HCPCS/CPT code that provides additional information regarding the procedure or service performed. A modifier may be used, for example, to indicate a right, left, or bilateral body part; a specific appendage; extent of anesthesia; limited or reduced services; and other situations or circumstances. A **revenue code** is a three-digit code that denotes the department in which a procedure, service, or supply item was provided. Revenue codes are in the *Chargemaster*, which is discussed later in this chapter. Some modifiers are classified as "pricer modifiers"; others are considered "informational" or "statistical" modifiers.

On the basis of the HCPCS/CPT code or codes, each APC is assigned a payment status indicator (SI) that determines reimbursement under OPPS. For example, SI T indicates "significant procedure, multiple-procedure reduction applies." SI V indicates "clinic or ED visit," and SI X indicates "ancillary service." The entire list of APCs and each SI can be found on the CMS website along with the RW for each APC, each payment rate, national unadjusted copayment, and minimum unadjusted copayment. CPT/HCPCS codes and APCs are updated each CY; therefore it is important to note any changes because reimbursements may be affected.

Coding professionals in various settings, from ambulatory hospital settings to physician offices, are frequently responsible for ensuring the accuracy of coding for billing purposes. As noted in this brief overview of APCs, the system undergoes changes yearly and is complicated on several levels, from coding to billing. When claims are submitted through the MACs, the claims are subjected to a number of edits that include the outpatient code editor (OCE) and National Correct Coding Initiative (NCCI) edits. The OCE and NCCI edit flag coding errors in the claims. Until the errors are corrected, the claim is rejected and reimbursement is denied for that claim.

Avoidance of payment denials or claim rejections is of paramount concern because income is adversely affected. One way to avoid these rejections is to understand the reasons for the rejections. Each MAC uses a **local coverage determination (LCD)** definition to determine if a service is covered for payment. These LCDs are derived from the CMS (Medicare) **national coverage determination (NCD)**. The NCD is a general discussion of the service and what it is useful in determining. The LCD lists the specific diagnosis codes that justify the medical necessity of the service. The LCD is available to providers, usually on the MAC's website. The LCD is extremely useful in that the policy defines covered services and details concerning exactly what diagnosis codes are needed for a service, procedure, or item to be deemed medically necessary. Coders familiar with the LCD, and with the OCE and NCCI edits, can be proactive in avoiding payment denials and claim rejections.

For example, a general medical examination is not sufficient justification for Medicare to pay for a blood test for vitamin D deficiency. Osteoporosis and osteopenia, on the other hand, will justify the vitamin D test. A provider who is performing the laboratory test on a physician's order must query the physician to determine the reason for the test. If the diagnosis does not meet the LCD requirement for performing the test, then the provider should obtain a signed Advance Beneficiary Notice (ABN) from the patient. Completion of an ABN obligates the patient to pay for the test if Medicare does not. It is important to note that there is no prohibition on performing the test itself. If the physician feels the test is necessary and the patient is willing to pay for it, then the provider can certainly perform it.

OCE and NCCI details can be found on the CMS website in the Medicare section under OPPS. LCDs are issued by the regional MACs and are described in detail on the MACs' websites.

---

**◆ NOTE**

**Ambulatory Surgery Coding Notes**

Diagnosis Code is ICD-10-CM.
Procedure Code is HCPCS/CPT®.
*Example:*
- **K35.80** Unspecified acute appendicitis
- **44970** Laparoscopic appendectomy

Bill format: UB-04
CPT is a registered trademark of the American Medical Association.

ᵃCPT copyright 2023 American Medical Association. All rights reserved.

---

## Inpatient Psychiatric Facility Prospective Payment System

CMS recognized that providing services for psychiatric patients is unique and not readily comparable to providing services for medical or surgical patients. The psychiatric setting is often more difficult to manage in terms of resources and length of stay. The Inpatient Psychiatric Facility Prospective Payment System (IPF PPS) was designed to address these issues beginning January 1, 2005. Under the IPF PPS, payment is made on a per diem rate based on a federal rate.

The federal rate is based on various factors and adjustments. There are two levels of adjustments: patient level and facility level. The patient level includes length of stay and patient age, and the facility level includes the geographic location of the facility and whether the facility is a teaching hospital.

IPF PPS is based on ICD-10-CM coding, and, as was the case under MS-DRGs, all of the coding rules will apply. A difference that coders will notice is that CC codes play a larger role in determining payment than in the psychiatric MS-DRGs in the PPS MS-DRG system. The addition of these CC codes under IPF PPS will cause a case to fall into additional adjustment categories. It is important for psychiatrists to fully document all secondary diagnoses, including all medical diagnoses, in addition to psychiatric diagnoses.

bowel continence, impairments, infections, and pressure ulcers. Two sections of the IRF-PAI require the use of ICD-10-CM codes. Patients are grouped into case mix groups (CMGs). Each CMG has four possible weights; the final weight is determined by the patient's comorbidities.

Unique to the IRF PPS is that two types of coding practices are applied: one type for the IRF-PAI and one type for billing. The IRF PPS requires coding of the etiology diagnoses, essentially the same diagnoses that would have been coded in the acute setting even though the patient is no longer receiving acute care. For reporting purposes on the UB-04, standard coding rules and conventions are applied. For example, suppose a patient admitted to the hospital was diagnosed with Type 1 diabetes mellitus with severe peripheral angiopathy and gangrene and had to have his leg amputated. The ICD-10-CM diagnosis code assigned for the inpatient stay is E10.52, Type 1 diabetes mellitus with diabetic peripheral angiopathy with gangrene. After the amputation, the patient was transferred to an IRF to learn how to use an artificial leg. The same code, E10.52, would be used for the IRF-PAI, but a rehabilitation code, code Z47.81, Encounter for orthopedic aftercare following surgical amputation would be reported as the principal diagnosis on the UB-04.

---

◆ *NOTE*

**Inpatient Behavioral Health Coding Notes**

Diagnosis Code is ICD-10-CM.
Procedure Codes are ICD-10-PCS.
*Example:*

- **F10.20** Alcohol dependence, uncomplicated
- **HZ2ZZZZ** Detoxification services for substance abuse treatment
- **HZ33ZZZ** Individual counseling for substance abuse treatment

Bill format: UB-04

**Outpatient Behavioral Health Coding Notes**

Diagnosis Code is ICD-10-CM.
Procedure Code is HCPCS/CPT®.
*Example:*

- **F33.2** Major depressive disorder, recurrent, severe without psychotic features
- **90870** Electroconvulsive therapy
- Bill format: usually UB-04 for facility-based; CMS-1500 for practitioner

CPT is a registered trademark of the American Medical Association.

---

## Inpatient Rehabilitation Facility Prospective Payment System

The PPS for Inpatient Rehabilitation Facilities (IRF PPS) became effective on January 1, 2002, replacing a cost-based payment system. It reimburses on a per-discharge basis and addresses both the costs of inpatient rehabilitation services and the unique needs of each patient that a facility admits. A comprehensive **patient assessment instrument (PAI)**, called the *Inpatient Rehabilitation Facility Patient Assessment Instrument* (IRF-PAI), is used to assess each patient with the intent that patients with greater needs will be identified and that the facility will receive higher payment for these individuals. The IRF-PAI includes sections on, for example,

---

◆ *NOTE*

**Inpatient Rehabilitation Facility Coding Notes**

Diagnosis Code is ICD-10-CM.
Procedure Codes are ICD-10-PCS.
*Examples:*

- **I69.351** Hemiplegia and hemiparesis following cerebral infarction affecting right dominant side
- **F021DYZ** Neuromotor development assessment of neurologic system upper back/upper extremity
- **F022DYZ** Neuromotor development assessment of neurologic system upper back/upper extremity

Bill format: UB-04

**Outpatient Rehabilitation Coding Notes**

Diagnosis Code is ICD-10-CM.
Procedure Code is HCPCS/CPT®.
*Example:*

- **I69.951** Hemiplegia due to cerebrovascular accident, affecting right dominant side
- **97535** Self-care/home management training

Bill format: UB-04 for facility and CMS-1500 for practitioner

---

## Long-Term Care Hospital Prospective Payment System

Medicare regulations define long-term care hospitals (LTCHs) as hospitals that have an average inpatient length of stay greater than 25 days. Patients in LTCHs have multiple acute and chronic complex conditions and may need, for example, comprehensive rehabilitation services, respiratory therapy, cancer treatment, and pain management. The Long-term Care Prospective Payment System (LTCH-PPS) is based on DRGs, but these DRGs are modified to reflect patient acuity and the greater costs involved in treating the complex conditions of these patients, which require longer lengths of stay. This modification is accomplished through the identification of a resource utilization group (RUG) category. A minimum data set (MDS), which includes the MS-DRG, is completed for the patient at various intervals during the stay. The data are entered into a grouper that determines the RUG.

## Home Health Prospective Payment System

The Home Health Prospective Payment System (HH PPS) applies to reimbursement for services rendered by home health care providers. Payments are in units, each unit being a 60-day episode, and are distributed to the provider in two split payments. The case mix system used is called *Home Health Resources Groups* (HHRGs), and the level of the HHRGs determines the payment. A comprehensive patient assessment tool, OASIS (Outcomes and Assessment Information Set), is used with ICD-10-CM codes to group these patients into HHRGs.

---

### NOTE

**Long-Term Care Facility Coding Notes**

Diagnosis Codes are ICD-10-CM.
Procedure Codes are HCPCS/CPT®.
Limited procedures, usually therapies and charge items.
MDS RUG Code is reported.
Global billing—most services covered by PPS payment.
*Examples:*
- **M62.82** Rhabdomyolysis
- **J18.9** Pneumonia, unspecified organism
- **I10** Hypertension
- **97001** PT Eval
- **97110** PT Therapy
- **97116** PT Gait training
- **G9679** Treatment of Acute care pneumonia (HCPCS)
- **RUB01** RUG code
Bill format: UB-04

---

### NOTE

**Home Health Care Coding Notes**

Diagnosis code is ICD-10-CM.
Diagnosis is a component of the patient assessment, which is the foundation for the Health Insurance Prospective Payment System (HIPPS) codes.
Bill format: UB-04
Z48.01 Encounter for change or removal of surgical wound dressing

---

## Skilled Nursing Facility Prospective Payment System and Resource Utilization Groups

RUGs are the basis of payment for skilled nursing facility (SNF) services for Medicare patients. RUGs are currently in their fourth version and are referred to as *RUG-IV*. Unlike DRGs and APCs, RUGs are not a retrospective reimbursement system for an entire stay or visit. Reimbursement based on RUGs is a daily, or per diem, rate based on the admission assessment of the patient. A review of data sets may help in a discussion of this concept.

As discussed in Chapters 2 and 3, specific data sets are abstracted and reported retrospectively for both ambulatory and hospital care: the UACDS and the UHDDS, respectively. In long-term care, the MDS is collected as part of the Resident Assessment Instrument (RAI). The MDS, currently in version 3.0, contains far more data than the UHDDS or the UACDS. It includes the patient's cognitive and medical condition, as well as his or her ability to perform self-care and other activities of daily living. Assessment is performed periodically during the patient's stay, not just at the end. Reimbursement is then based on the patient's care needs, consisting of 1 of 44 groups within seven broad categories: rehabilitation, extensive services, special care, clinically complex, impaired cognition, behavioral problems, and reduced physical function. Although there are other RUG systems in existence, Medicare reimbursement is determined using the RUG-IV system.

In most SNF settings, much of the information collected has been under the domain of the nursing department. Nursing staff members usually collect and record the MDS data, largely composed of diagnostic statements and including the ICD-10-CM codes associated with the patient's medical condition. This is not to imply that health information professionals are incapable of performing this task.

---

### NOTE

**Hospice in Skilled Nursing Facility Coding Notes**

Diagnosis Codes are ICD-10-CM.
Procedure Codes are HCPCS/CPT®.
*Examples:*
- **C43.8** Malignant melanoma of overlapping sites of skin
- **C79.81** Secondary malignant neoplasm of breast
- **C79.51** Secondary malignant neoplasm of bone
- **G89.3** Neoplasm-related pain (acute) (chronic)
- **96374** Injection, intravenous push
- **J2271** Injection, morphine
- **Q5004** Hospice care in skilled nursing facility (HCPCS Level II)
Bill format: UB-04 for facility and CMS-1500 for practitioner

---

PPSs continue to evolve and expand into various patient settings, primarily as a result of legislation and instruction from Congress. Although these PPSs are initiated and

| TABLE 6.4 | Summary of Prospective Payment Systems | | |
|---|---|---|---|
| **System** | **Setting** | **Code System** | **Basis of Reimbursement** |
| Medicare Severity Diagnosis-Related Groups (MS-DRG) | Short-stay facility, inpatient acute care, Medicare patient | ICD-10-CM diagnosis and ICD-10-PCS procedure codes | Diagnoses and procedures Single MS-DRG assignment Retrospective |
| Ambulatory payment classification (APC) | Ambulatory care, outpatient services, emergency departments | CPT-4 HCPCS ICD-10-CM diagnosis codes | Procedures Diagnoses used for validation May have multiple APCs Retrospective |
| Inpatient psychiatric facility (IPF) PPS | Inpatient psychiatric facility | ICD-10-CM | Per diem and federal rate |
| Inpatient rehabilitation facility (IRF) PPS | Inpatient rehabilitation facilities | ICD-10-CM | Per discharge Inpatient Rehabilitation Facility Patient Assessment Instrument (IRF-PAI) Case mix groups |
| Long-term care hospital (LTCH) PPS | Hospitals with average length of stay >25 days | ICD-10-CM | DRGs Patient acuity |
| Home health care (HH) PPS | Home health care providers | ICD-10-CM | Home Health Resources Groups (HHRGs) Payment units OASIS |
| Resource Utilization Group, version 4 (RUG-IV) | Medicare skilled nursing facility services | ICD-10-CM | Per diem rate Not retrospective Minimum data set data |

developed for reimbursing services for Medicare patients, other payers and insurers often use or modify these systems for their patients as well. To code accurately and in compliance with regulations, all coding professionals should be aware of what PPSs apply, and to whom, in the setting in which they are employed. Table 6.4 contains a summary of the previously discussed PPSs.

## Resource-Based Relative Value System

The **resource-based relative value system (RBRVS)** is the basis of reimbursement to physicians for services rendered to Medicare patients. Because the reimbursement is for physician services, the location where services were provided can be the physician's office, a hospital, or a nursing home—essentially anywhere that a patient can be treated. Physicians submit claims for reimbursement using HCPCS/CPT codes. Each HCPCS/CPT code has three relative value units (RVUs). Each RVU corresponds to the complexity of the service provided, the consumption of resources incurred by the service provided, and the relation of the service provided in comparison with other services provided. Physicians receive reimbursement on the basis of a national Medicare physician **fee schedule** that is adjusted according to the physician's geographic location. Physicians located in different areas of the United States receive varying reimbursement amounts for identical services because Medicare recognizes that operating costs vary by location.

| TABLE 6.5 | Comparison of Reimbursement Methods |
|---|---|
| **Method** | **Description** |
| Fee for service | Payment for services rendered |
| Discounted fee for service | Payment for services rendered but at a rate lower than the usual fee for a service |
| Prospective payment | Payment of a flat rate on the basis of diagnoses, procedures, or a combination of the two |
| Capitation | Payment of a regular, flat rate to the provider regardless of whether services are rendered |

There are numerous variations on these methods, and exceptions to a normal method of payment are made under certain circumstances. For example, under prospective payment, additional compensation can sometimes be obtained if it is medically necessary for the patient to be hospitalized far in excess of the average length of stay for the diagnosis or procedure.

## Comparison of Reimbursement Methods

Table 6.5 summarizes the four methods of reimbursement previously discussed: fee for service, discounted fee for service, prospective payment, and capitation. To distinguish among these methods, remember the previous example of the patient's visit to the doctor's office for an allergy shot. Say the charge for that visit, under charges, is $100. Under discounted fee for service reimbursement, a contract may be negotiated for payment based on a discount of 10% of the charges; therefore the charge for the same visit would still be $100, but the reimbursement would be $90. The $10 difference is a contractual allowance, enabling the provider to keep track of the discount for accounting purposes. Under a PPS, the insurance company may reimburse the physician $85 on the basis of a statistical analysis of costs associated with office visits for allergy shots. Under capitation reimbursement, the insurance company would not pay the physician anything for a particular visit, paying instead $10 each month for that patient. The total reimbursement for that patient under capitation amounts to $120 annually: a financial advantage to the provider if the patient visits once or not at all but a disadvantage if the patient visits more than once.

These methods vary widely, and exceptions to a normal method of payment are made under certain circumstances. For example, under PPS, additional reimbursement can sometimes be obtained if it is medically necessary for the patient to be hospitalized far in excess of the average length of stay for the medical service.

## REVENUE CYCLE MANAGEMENT

To be reimbursed for services rendered to a patient, a facility must alert the payer that payment is due. This is accomplished by filing a claim with the patient's health insurance carrier, which is also called **revenue cycle management (RCM)**. In an acute care facility, the **billing** function is performed in a department that is often called *patient accounting* or *patient financial services*.

Coding and billing are key components of the RCM process. RCM is composed of all the activities that connect the services being rendered to a patient with the provider's reimbursement for those services. The revenue cycle begins with the patient appointment and ends with the collection of the payment for services. Patient access plays a key role in RCM, because registrars are responsible for collecting the demographic and financial data relevant to each encounter. If the insurance data is incorrect, billing will be incorrect, and the provider's payment will be delayed until the correct data is submitted. Therefore data accuracy at the point of registration includes the verification of insurance

data. Clinical staff play a key role in RCM, because they record the services they render, which are linked in the computer system to the charges for those services through the Chargemaster. Even in a PPS, it is important to capture the charges for services rendered so that the provider can compare reimbursement to charges and costs. The HIM department is important because the diagnosis and procedure codes assigned are included on the bill and drive the reimbursement itself. Thus there are many players in the RCM process before billing actually takes place.

## Patient Financial Services

The patient financial services department is responsible for ensuring that accurate claims are sent for each patient's account, that they are sent in the correct format to the correct payers, and that the facility receives the correct reimbursement. A patient's bill includes a compilation of charges for items used and services rendered. Each patient is assigned an account number for items received and services rendered during a particular visit or stay. The account number, unlike the patient's medical record number, changes for each visit or stay. In this way, charges can be accurately assigned, or posted, to each specific visit so that the bill reflects the charges for each individual account. For example, a patient may visit a hospital three times in 1 month: once as an inpatient, then as a clinic patient, and later as an ED patient. The hospital does not combine all three visits into one monthly bill. Instead, a different account number is assigned for each encounter, and a separate bill is sent for each account that reflects the charges incurred for each individual visit. On the other hand, certain services such as outpatient physical therapy may hold the bill for all visits in a month and bill only once at the end of the month. A bill that is produced and sent is called a *dropped*, or *final*, bill. A bill that has been dropped is pending payment. Once the dropped bill has been paid, the account is closed to any further activity.

To use an acute care inpatient as an example, three key steps must happen in order to produce and drop a bill: (1) the patient's charges must be entered into, or posted to, the account; (2) the patient must have been discharged so that the account reflects the charges accumulated for the patient's entire length of stay; and (3) the medical record must be coded. Whether or not payers use MS-DRGs or another DRG grouper as a method of reimbursement, they still want to see the ICD-10-CM and ICD-10-PCS codes related to the clinical stay, and these codes must appear on the UB-04, a billing form discussed later in this chapter. It is through the coding of the diagnoses and procedures that the payer often gets the first impression of what actually should have happened in terms of services rendered.

Beginning at discharge and until a final bill is dropped, hospitals monitor the accounts that have not been billed. This list of undropped bills is called by a variety of names, including the *unbilled list* or the DNFB (discharged, no final bill, or discharged, not final billed). Regardless of the name used, this list of delayed payments can add up to millions of dollars. Because the delays are partially due to the fact that coding has not occurred on some of the accounts, the HIM department proactively and aggressively monitors the DNFB on a regular basis. Management of the coding function and the DNFB is often complex, with many factors contributing to uncoded medical records that then result in unbilled accounts such as missing charges, coding errors, and mismatched diagnoses/procedures. Because the patient accounting and HIM departments both have the same goal of reducing or eliminating unnecessary unbilled accounts, the departments ideally assist each other in reducing the factors contributing to payment delays.

## Chargemaster (Charge Description Master)

Whether a facility is reimbursed using PPS or another system, a variety of procedures must be in place to ensure the accurate accumulation of charges and the accurate coding of the clinical data. Charges are the facility's individual fees, or the dollar amount for items or services provided to a patient and owed to the facility. Each item or service is assigned a charge, which is usually reviewed and adjusted or changed annually. Charges may be set on the basis of fee schedules or contractual arrangements with certain payers or may be determined internally through the use of the facility's cost accounting system. The actual charges are not always equal to the amount that the payer reimburses a facility; the payment received depends on contractual agreements and may be discounted accordingly, as discussed earlier in this chapter. A facility compares its charges with actual reimbursements to determine the impact of contractual arrangements and whether they allow the facility to operate profitably (i.e., earn more money than it spends).

The database that contains a facility's charges or costs for services and items is called a Chargemaster. Other terms that are sometimes used include *Charge Data Master* and *Charge Description Master* (CDM). Table 6.6 illustrates key data fields that usually appear in a Chargemaster. The Chargemaster must be updated regularly so that fees and costs are accurate. Because HCPCS/CPT codes are included in the Chargemaster, these codes must also be updated

| TABLE 6.6 | Sample Fields in a Charge Description Master |
| --- | --- |
| **Field** | **Description** |
| General ledger code | Internal code used by the facility's accounting department to track revenue and expenses |
| HCPCS/ CPT code | Billing code for transmission to the insurer |
| Cost basis | The cost of the item to the facility |
| Charge | The amount that the facility charges for the item or service |
| Description | Definition or description of the item or service |
| Date | Date of the most recent update of the aforementioned fields for the item or service |

*HCPCS/CPT,* Healthcare Common Procedure Coding System/Current Procedural Terminology.

when changes or revisions occur. All the services that a facility provides, from adhesive bandages to intravenous drips and room and board, must appear on the Chargemaster, or they cannot be billed. Coding professionals often initiate or assist in making the updates to the CDM and informing departments about changes.

## Charge Capture

As previously discussed, charges must be posted to a patient's account in order for proper billing to occur. This process is called **charge capture**.

In an inpatient hospital setting, charges are usually posted to the patient's account electronically, using order-entry software, each time a service or item is provided. If the hospital does not use order-entry software or does not use the software for all types of charges, these charges still must be captured on a paper form called a *charge ticket*. All charge tickets must be forwarded to the accounting or billing department at the end of each business day and manually posted to the correct account. As one can imagine, manual charge capture is extremely laborious and vulnerable to human error.

Depending on factors such as length of stay, each account may have hundreds of posted charges. Most facilities allow time between discharge and submission of the bill so that all charges can be posted. This period, called the bill-hold period, usually ranges from 1 to 5 days after discharge, perhaps longer for outpatient or ambulatory services. In smaller facilities, posting delays may occur because of reduced staff on weekends. Charges posted after the final bill drops are considered late charges. Because late charges must be submitted separately and some insurers do not pay late charges at all or only after a certain time, it is essential that charges be posted no later than the end of the bill-hold period.

**PATIENT VISITS**

| X | DESCRIPTION | CODE | AMOUNT |
|---|---|---|---|
| | **NEW PATIENT** | | |
| | Problem focused Hx | 99201 | |
| | Expanded prob/Focused Hx | 99202 | |
| | Detailed Hx | 99203 | |
| | Comp Hx/Moderate complex | 99204 | |
| | Comp Hx/High complex | 99205 | |
| | **ESTABLISHED PATIENT** | | |
| | Minimal | 99211 | |
| | Problem focused Hx | 99212 | |
| | Expanded prob/Focused Hx | 99213 | |
| | Detailed Hx | 99214 | |
| | Comprehensive Hx | 99215 | |
| | **CONSULTATION** | | |
| | Problem focused Hx | 99241 | |
| | Expanded prob/Focused Hx | 99242 | |
| | Detailed Hx | 99243 | |
| | Comp Hx/Moderate complex | 99244 | |
| | Comp Hx/High complex | 99245 | |
| | **NURSE SPECIALIST** | | |
| | Computer analysis | 99090 | |
| | Group health ed | 99078 | |
| | Skills management (15 min.) | 97535 | |
| | **PROCEDURES** | | |
| | Accucheck/One Touch | 7182948 | |
| | EKG w/interpretation | 93000 | |
| | IV infusion, up to 1 hr. | 90780 | |
| | IV infusion, each add'l hr. | 90781 | |
| | Immunization administration | 90471 | |
| | Two or more vaccines/toxoids | 90472 | |
| | Therapeutic/diagnostic injection Specify: med/dose | 90782 | |
| | Injection of antibiotic Specify: med/dose | 90788 | |
| | Occult blood (guaiac) | 82270 | |
| | ANS | 95937 | |
| | 24 hour cardiac monitor | 93230 | |
| | Pap smear | 88150 | |
| | Thyroid fine needle asp. (proc.) | 7190357 | |
| | Group counseling, 30 min. | 99411 | |
| | Group counseling, 60 min. | 99412 | |

**PROCEDURES cont.**

| X | DESCRIPTION | CODE | ALPHA | AMOUNT |
|---|---|---|---|---|
| | Preventive counseling, 15 min. | 99401 | | |
| | Preventive counseling, 30 min. | 99402 | | |
| | Preventive counseling, 45 min. | 99403 | | |
| | Preventive counseling, 60 min. | 99404 | | |
| | **DIABETES/LIPID** | | | |
| | Cholesterol, HDL | 7190053 | HDL | |
| | C-peptide | 7190219 | CPEP | |
| | Glucose serum | 7182947 | GLU | |
| | HGB A1 C | 7190057 | HA1 | |
| | Insulin | 7190343 | INS | |
| | Lipoprotein panel A | 7175004 | | |
| | Micral, random | 7190335 | MLBU | |
| | Protein, urine 24 hr. | 7195011 | PROU | |
| | **GONADAL** | | | |
| | Estradiol | 7190044 | ESD | |
| | FSH | 7190048 | FSH | |
| | LH | 7190069 | LH | |
| | Progesterone | 7190078 | PROG | |
| | PSA | 7190079 | PSA | |
| | SHBG | 7190622 | SHBG | |
| | Testosterone | 7190086 | TEST | |
| | Testosterone, Free | 7190322 | FTES | |
| | PSA, Free | 7184999 | | |
| | **PROFILES** | | | |
| | Basic metabolic panel | 7180049 | CH7 | |
| | Comp. metabolic panel | 7180054 | CMP | |
| | Electrolyte panel | 7180051 | ELEC | |
| | Hepatic function panel | 7180058 | HFPA | |
| | Hepatitis panel | 7180059 | | |
| | Lipid profile 2 | 7190257 | LPP2 | |
| | **THYROID** | | | |
| | Antimicrosomal antibody | 7190213 | TM | |
| | TSI | 7190476 | TSIG | |
| | Thyroglobulin | 7190584 | THY | |
| | T4 - Thyroxine | 7190047 | FT4 | |
| | T3 uptake | 7190292 | TU | |
| | Total T3 | 7190095 | T3 C | |
| | T3-Free | 7190595 | FT3 | |
| | TSH (Thyroid stim hormone) | 7190253 | TSH | |

**CALCIUM/BONE/KIDNEY**

| X | DESCRIPTION | CODE | ALPHA | AMOUNT |
|---|---|---|---|---|
| | Calcium, ionized | 7190821 | ICAL | |
| | Calcium, serum | 7190311 | CAL | |
| | Calcium, urine 24 hr. | 7190222 | CALU | |
| | Creatinine, clearance ht. ___ wt. ___ | 7194754 | CRCP | |
| | Microalbumin, urine 24 hr. | 7190335 | MLBT | |
| | Magnesium, serum | 7190317 | MAG | |
| | Parathyroid hormo | 7190387 | PTH | |

**ADRENAL/PITUITARY**

| X | DESCRIPTION | CODE | ALPHA | AMOUNT |
|---|---|---|---|---|
| | ACTH | 7190005 | ACTH | |
| | Aldosterone, serum | 7190204 | ALD | |
| | Androstenedione | 7190336 | AND | |
| | Cortisol, serum | 7190032 | COR | |
| | DHEA | 7190341 | DHEA | |
| | DHEA S serum | 7190312 | DHES | |
| | Human growth hormone | 7190379 | HGH | |
| | Prolactin | 7190316 | PRL | |
| | 17OH Progesterone | 7190479 | HY17 | |
| | 17OH Pregnegalone | 7190480 | LONE | |
| | Urine catecholimine 24 hr. | 7190021 | CATU | |
| | Urine cortisol 24 hr. | 7190033 | CORU | |
| | Urine metanephrines 24 hr. | 7190475 | METU | |
| | Urine potassium 24 hr. | 7190077 | POTU | |
| | Urine sodium 24 hr. | 7190261 | SODU | |
| | Urine VMA 24 hr. | 7190534 | VMAU | |

**CHEMISTRY/HEMATOLOGY**

| DESCRIPTION | CODE | ALPHA |
|---|---|---|
| CBC w/diff & platelets | 7190327 | CBC1 |
| Erthrocyte sed rate | 7190330 | ESR |
| Potassium, serum | 7184813 | POT |
| Urine culture | 7190041 | BACTI |
| Urinalysis, routine | 7190334 | URTN |
| Urinalysis, dipstick | 7190384 | URCH |
| Venipuncture | 7190323 | VENI |
| GGI | 7184773 | |
| HCE | 7190329 | |

**AUTHORIZATION #**
**DIAGNOSIS**
**SPECIAL INSTRUCTIONS**

**REFERRING MD**

| | |
|---|---|
| Tax ID # | 62-1162462 |
| Previous bal. | |
| Amount paid | |
| Today's chrg | |
| Amount paid | |
| Total rec'd | |
| Balance due | |
| Check one: | |
| □ Cash | |
| □ Check, M.O.# _____ | |
| □ MC □ VISA | |
| □ Care Card # _____ | |

Physician signature:     Date:

I authorize release of any medical information necessary to process this claim. I also authorize the direct payment of any benefits due me for the described services to _____ I understand I am financially responsible for paying any unpaid balance and will be responsible for the entire bill if this claim is not covered. **Medicare Patients:** The Medicare program requires that all diagnosis be ICD 9 coded. We are unable to provide this service to you at the time of your visit, and therefore, require that you permit us to file an insurance claim with your Medicare carrier.

Patient (Beneficiary) signature:     Date:

98381 7/99

• **Fig. 6.3** Ambulatory care encounter form/superbill. (From Abdelhak M, Grostick A, Hanken MA, Jacobs H: Health information: management of a strategic resource, 2nd ed. Philadelphia, 2001, Saunders: 244. CPT copyright 2023 American Medical Association. All rights reserved. CPT is a registered trademark of the American Medical Association.)

In an ambulatory setting, charges are often captured, by service, on an **encounter form**, or **superbill**. An encounter form may be in electronic format or a single sheet of paper, sometimes double-sided, that contains a list of the most common patient complaints, diagnoses, procedures, and services provided by the facility. The paper form must be transferred into an electronic billing format in order to submit the claim electronically. Some insurers provide their own encounter forms. A comprehensive encounter form includes ICD-10-CM diagnosis codes and HCPCS procedure codes. Encounter forms facilitate communication between the physician or other health care provider and the administrative personnel who are responsible for coding and billing. Because it is not the encounter form but the health record that supports the reimbursement claim, care must be taken to ensure that the health record indicates all services provided. Fig. 6.3 is an example of an encounter form (superbill).

In a physician's office, the process of obtaining reimbursement may rest with the administrative personnel (e.g., the medical secretary, medical assistant, or practice manager). The role of these employees is to determine which services were provided for which patient and which insurer or insurers should receive a bill and to ensure that all services provided are billed correctly.

In some situations, such as in a solo practitioner's office, the physician may file the claims directly to the insurer for payment. Because the insurance industry is so complex and there are many different types of payers, all with their own rules, many physicians rely on billing services to perform the administrative tasks of charge capture and billing. Performing all of these tasks is critical to accurate and timely reimbursement.

## Impact of Coding on Reimbursement

In any discussion of the revenue cycle, the importance of accurate ICD-10-CM, ICD-10-PCS, and HCPCS/CPT-4 coding cannot be overstated. Because the codes determine the payment and facilitate the claim, the accuracy and timeliness of the coding function are critical.

In addition to charge capture, all pertinent medical record data must have been collected for correct assignment of codes, and the processing cycle must facilitate efficient, timely coding. For example, if a record must be assembled/indexed and analyzed before it is routed to a coder, and if the assembly and analysis sections are 5 or 6 days behind the current discharge date, then records may not be coded until 7 days after the discharge date. Even factoring in the bill-hold period, a week is a long time for a facility to go without dropping a bill for a patient's stay. Facilities sometimes choose to code the record before it is assembled or analyzed so that the bill may be dropped more quickly. Although this sequence expedites payment, it can also lead to coding errors if the medical record is incomplete because missing elements are not clearly identified or if important reports are misplaced in the wrong sections of the record.

Although the EHR will permit analysts, coders, and others to access records simultaneously, there are occasions in which a coder cannot complete a record without documentation, such as an operative report. Therefore timely completion of records, for revenue cycle purposes, imposes an urgency not implied by the CMS/TJC 30-day chart completion guidelines. Therefore, in the EHR environment, facilities may impose stricter timelines. In addition, computer-assisted coding programs embedded in the EHR may facilitate the coding process in terms of speed and accuracy.

Coding must be reliable and valid, both individually and collectively within a facility or group. A coder or group of coders is said to demonstrate reliability when codes are consistently assigned for similar or identical cases. Validity of coding refers to the degree of accuracy of the codes assigned.

## The Uniform Bill

The National Uniform Billing Committee (NUBC) is responsible for developing and implementing a single billing form and standard data set to be used nationwide by providers/hospitals and payers/insurers for handling inpatient health care claims. The NUBC comprises representatives from all the major provider and payer organizations, including the American Hospital Association and Medicare, the public health sector, and electronic standards development organizations.

The first standard Uniform Bill (UB) appeared in 1982 and was referred to as the UB-82. Representatives from across the country were surveyed to seek improvements on the UB-82, and the UB-92 was the result of their efforts. At this time, claims are submitted electronically using the UB-04, also known as *Form CMS-1450*. Although the UB was originally used for claims reimbursement only, the NUBC has recognized that it contains a wealth of data that can be used for additional purposes. The data captured on the UB are now also used by health researchers to gauge the delivery of health care services to patients and to set future policy.

Fig. 6.4 shows a UB-04 form. Notice that the Uniform Bill itself is composed of the UHDDS demographic and financial data elements, as well as many additional data fields that are useful for communication between the provider and the payer. Coding professionals should be aware that fields on the UB-04 form include the admitting diagnosis code, distinct fields for the patient's reason for visit, and expanded diagnosis and procedure fields to accommodate ICD-10-CM and ICD-10-PCS codes. The UB-04 is the paper representation of the electronic 837I billing file.

UHDDS definitions allow standardized reporting of specific data elements collected by all acute care short-term hospitals. These data elements and their definitions can be found in the July 31, 1985, *Federal Register* (Health Information Policy Council, 1985). Fig. 6.5 illustrates the data elements of the UHDDS and their relationship to the fields of the UB-04.

## CMS-1500

The CMS-1500 form is the paper data collection form used for transmittal of billing information for ambulatory/outpatient claims and physician's office claims. The CMS-1500 form has fewer fields than the UB-04, but it contains much of the same information. Fig. 6.6 shows a CMS-1500 form. The CMS-1500 is the paper representation of the 837P electronic billing file.

## Claim Rejections

Optimally, the facility or provider has recorded all of the required billing data accurately, and the claim drops to the payer without human intervention. However, the potential for human error requires that all claims be reviewed prior to being submitted to the payer. The provider, or provider's billing service, will examine the claims for errors such as missing fields, LCD errors, and invalid data. Claims that are rejected must be corrected prior to resubmission.

An example of a claim rejection is the failure to combine an outpatient account with an inpatient visit that occurs within 3 days prior to the inpatient visit. Consider a patient who is treated for congestive heart failure in the ED and is admitted to that hospital 2 days later—also for congestive heart failure. Because the admission is within 3 days, Medicare will not pay separately for the ED visit. All diagnostic testing and all related therapeutic services must

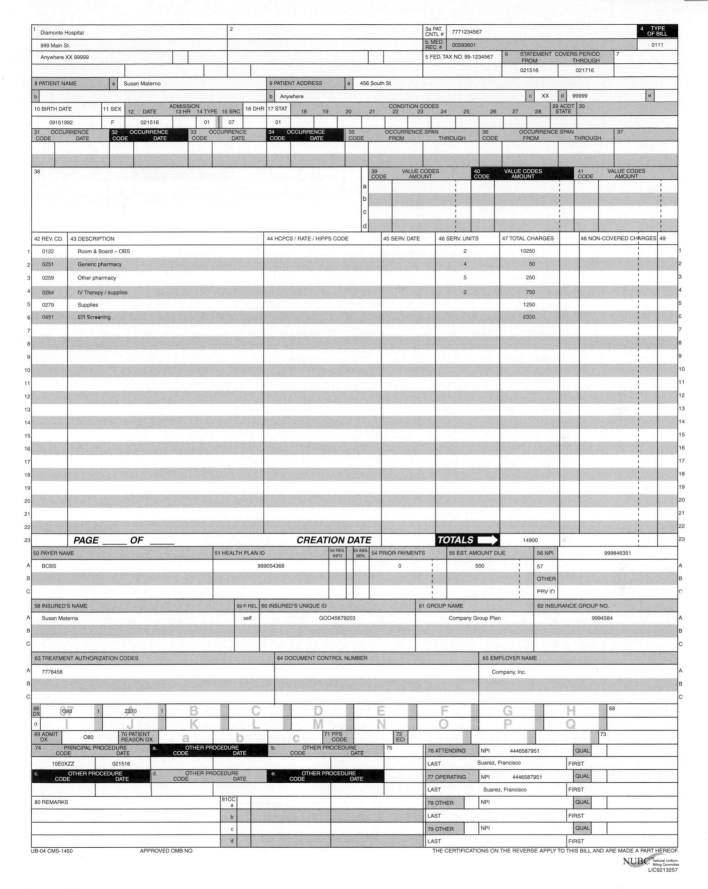

• **Fig. 6.4** UB-04.

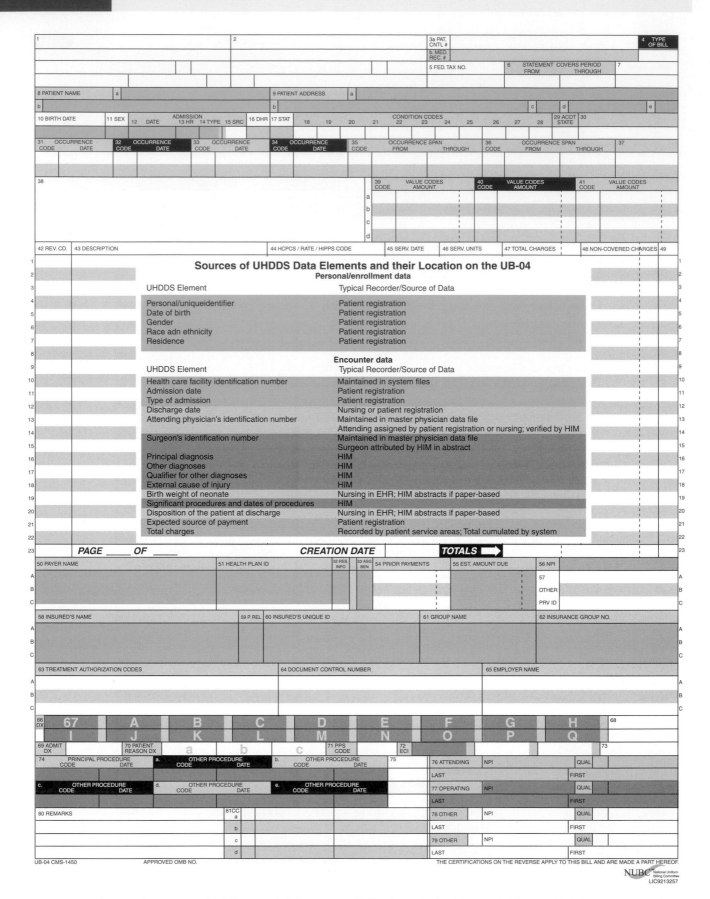

| 1 | | 2 | | | 3a PAT. CNTL # | | 4 TYPE OF BILL |
|---|---|---|---|---|---|---|---|
| | | | | | b. MED. REC. # | | |
| | | | | | 5 FED. TAX NO. | 6 STATEMENT COVERS PERIOD FROM   THROUGH | 7 |
| 8 PATIENT NAME | a | | 9 PATIENT ADDRESS | a | | | |
| b | | | b | | | c | d | e |
| 10 BIRTH DATE | 11 SEX | 12 DATE ADMISSION 13 HR 14 TYPE 15 SRC | 16 DHR | 17 STAT | 18 19 20 21 CONDITION CODES 22 23 24 25 26 27 28 | 29 ACDT STATE | 30 |

**Sources of UHDDS Data Elements and their Location on the UB-04**

**Personal/enrollment data**

| UHDDS Element | Typical Recorder/Source of Data |
|---|---|
| Personal/uniqueidentifier | Patient registration |
| Date of birth | Patient registration |
| Gender | Patient registration |
| Race adn ethnicity | Patient registration |
| Residence | Patient registration |

**Encounter data**

| UHDDS Element | Typical Recorder/Source of Data |
|---|---|
| Health care facility identification number | Maintained in system files |
| Admission date | Patient registration |
| Type of admission | Patient registration |
| Discharge date | Nursing or patient registration |
| Attending physician's identification number | Maintained in master physician data file |
| | Attending assigned by patient registration or nursing; verified by HIM |
| Surgeon's identification number | Maintained in master physician data file |
| | Surgeon attributed by HIM in abstract |
| Principal diagnosis | HIM |
| Other diagnoses | HIM |
| Qualifier for other diagnoses | HIM |
| External cause of injury | HIM |
| Birth weight of neonate | Nursing in EHR; HIM abstracts if paper-based |
| Significant procedures and dates of procedures | HIM |
| Disposition of the patient at discharge | Nursing in EHR; HIM abstracts if paper-based |
| Expected source of payment | Patient registration |
| Total charges | Recorded by patient service areas; Total cumulated by system |

• **Fig. 6.5** UHDDS data elements on the UB-04 and their sources. *EHR*, electronic health record; *HIM*, health information management (department); *UHDDS*, Uniform Hospital Discharge Data Set.

## 1500

# HEALTH INSURANCE CLAIM FORM

APPROVED BY NATIONAL UNIFORM CLAIM COMMITTEE 08/05

| | PICA | | | | | | PICA | |

| 1. MEDICARE | MEDICAID | TRICARE CHAMPUS | CHAMPVA | GROUP HEALTH PLAN | FECA BLK LUNG | OTHER | 1a. INSURED'S I.D. NUMBER (For Program in Item 1) |

(Medicare #) (Medicaid #) (Sponsor's SSN) (Member ID#) (SSN or ID) (SSN) (ID)

2. PATIENT'S NAME (Last Name, First Name, Middle Initial)

3. PATIENT'S BIRTH DATE MM DD YY SEX M F

4. INSURED'S NAME (Last Name, First Name, Middle Initial)

5. PATIENT'S ADDRESS (No., Street)

6. PATIENT RELATIONSHIP TO INSURED Self Spouse Child Other

7. INSURED'S ADDRESS (No., Street)

CITY STATE

8. PATIENT STATUS Single Married Other

CITY STATE

ZIP CODE TELEPHONE (Include Area Code) ( )

Employed Full-Time Student Part-Time Student

ZIP CODE TELEPHONE (Include Area Code) ( )

9. OTHER INSURED'S NAME (Last Name, First Name, Middle Initial)

10. IS PATIENT'S CONDITION RELATED TO:

11. INSURED'S POLICY GROUP OR FECA NUMBER

a. OTHER INSURED'S POLICY OR GROUP NUMBER

a. EMPLOYMENT? (Current or Previous) YES NO

a. INSURED'S DATE OF BIRTH MM DD YY SEX M F

b. OTHER INSURED'S DATE OF BIRTH MM DD YY SEX M F

b. AUTO ACCIDENT? PLACE (State) YES NO

b. EMPLOYER'S NAME OR SCHOOL NAME

c. EMPLOYER'S NAME OR SCHOOL NAME

c. OTHER ACCIDENT? YES NO

c. INSURANCE PLAN NAME OR PROGRAM NAME

d. INSURANCE PLAN NAME OR PROGRAM NAME

10d. RESERVED FOR LOCAL USE

d. IS THERE ANOTHER HEALTH BENEFIT PLAN? YES NO If yes, return to and complete item 9 a-d.

**READ BACK OF FORM BEFORE COMPLETING & SIGNING THIS FORM.**

12. PATIENT'S OR AUTHORIZED PERSON'S SIGNATURE I authorize the release of any medical or other information necessary to process this claim. I also request payment of government benefits either to myself or to the party who accepts assignment below.

SIGNED _____ DATE _____

13. INSURED'S OR AUTHORIZED PERSON'S SIGNATURE I authorize payment of medical benefits to the undersigned physician or supplier for services described below.

SIGNED _____

14. DATE OF CURRENT: ILLNESS (First symptom) OR INJURY (Accident) OR PREGNANCY(LMP) MM DD YY

15. IF PATIENT HAS HAD SAME OR SIMILAR ILLNESS. GIVE FIRST DATE MM DD YY

16. DATES PATIENT UNABLE TO WORK IN CURRENT OCCUPATION FROM MM DD YY TO MM DD YY

17. NAME OF REFERRING PROVIDER OR OTHER SOURCE 17a. 17b. NPI

18. HOSPITALIZATION DATES RELATED TO CURRENT SERVICES FROM MM DD YY TO MM DD YY

19. RESERVED FOR LOCAL USE

20. OUTSIDE LAB? YES NO $ CHARGES

21. DIAGNOSIS OR NATURE OF ILLNESS OR INJURY (Relate Items 1, 2, 3 or 4 to Item 24E by Line)
1. __ . __  3. __ . __
2. __ . __  4. __ . __

22. MEDICAID RESUBMISSION CODE ORIGINAL REF. NO.

23. PRIOR AUTHORIZATION NUMBER

| 24. A. DATE(S) OF SERVICE | | B. PLACE OF SERVICE | C. EMG | D. PROCEDURES, SERVICES, OR SUPPLIES (Explain Unusual Circumstances) | | E. DIAGNOSIS POINTER | F. $ CHARGES | G. DAYS OR UNITS | H. EPSDT Family Plan | I. ID. QUAL. | J. RENDERING PROVIDER ID. # |
|---|---|---|---|---|---|---|---|---|---|---|---|
| From MM DD YY | To MM DD YY | | | CPT/HCPCS | MODIFIER | | | | | | |
| 1 | | | | | | | | | | NPI | |
| 2 | | | | | | | | | | NPI | |
| 3 | | | | | | | | | | NPI | |
| 4 | | | | | | | | | | NPI | |
| 5 | | | | | | | | | | NPI | |
| 6 | | | | | | | | | | NPI | |

25. FEDERAL TAX I.D. NUMBER SSN EIN

26. PATIENT'S ACCOUNT NO.

27. ACCEPT ASSIGNMENT? (For govt. claims, see back) YES NO

28. TOTAL CHARGE $

29. AMOUNT PAID $

30. BALANCE DUE $

31. SIGNATURE OF PHYSICIAN OR SUPPLIER INCLUDING DEGREES OR CREDENTIALS (I certify that the statements on the reverse apply to this bill and are made a part thereof.)

SIGNED _____ DATE _____

32. SERVICE FACILITY LOCATION INFORMATION a. NPI b.

33. BILLING PROVIDER INFO & PH # ( ) a. NPI b.

APPROVED OMB-0938-0999 FORM CMS-1500 (08/05)

CARRIER

PATIENT AND INSURED INFORMATION

PHYSICIAN OR SUPPLIER INFORMATION

• **Fig. 6.6** CMS-1500 health insurance claim form.

be combined into the inpatient visit. It is the responsibility of the hospital to support the rationale for not combining therapeutic visits. An example of therapeutic services that might not be combined is an ED visit for a broken leg, which would likely not be combined with a subsequent unrelated inpatient visit for pneumonia (CMS Three Day Payment Window, 2021).

## Claim Denials

Once the claim is submitted, there is an additional layer of review by the payer. The payer may refuse to pay the claim for a variety of reasons; examples are services not covered by the patient's insurance plan, service overlapping another provider's bill, codes submitted on the bill do not match the preauthorized services, lack of medical necessity for the services provided, and untimely filing.

Some errors, such as untimely filing and lack of medical necessity, cannot be corrected. Such claims will be adjusted to a zero balance and the provider will receive no payment for the services. If the provider has obtained an ABN or waiver from the patient in advance of the services, the patient may be billed for the services directly. In some cases, the provider may file an appeal with the payer to challenge the payer's denial. There may also be the opportunity for the patient to appeal.

## Error Correction

There is a great deal of pressure on both HIM professionals and billing professionals to submit claims that will be paid. Great care must be taken to ensure that only accurate, verifiable, and valid data are submitted on claims. If a claim is denied for codes submitted that do not match the preauthorized services, the case could be sent to a coding supervisor for review. Perhaps the case was coded incorrectly. If the coder made an error, the case can be recoded, reabstracted, and rebilled. However, in some cases the codes provided to the payer at preregistration are not the codes for the services that were ultimately provided. For example, an ambulatory surgery case may have been preauthorized for dilation and curettage without indicating that intrasurgical decision-making could result in a hysterectomy. If the hysterectomy

is performed and that is what the coder entered, then the case cannot be recoded, because there was no coding error.

## Collection

Coding and billing processes may take place without error and yet the provider has one major step left in the revenue cycle process: follow-up and collections. Medicare and most major commercial payers remit payment on a relatively predictable schedule. However, some payers delay reimbursement as long as possible. When patients are responsible for all or part of the payment, further delays may ensue. Providers must be diligent in following up and seeking payment for services so that cash is received as timely as possible.

## ACCOUNTING CONCEPTS

There are many branches of accounting and their uses depend on the needs of the organization. For example:

- **Financial accounting** is the process of measuring, recording, reporting, and analyzing financial data based on accepted principles. Financial accounting helps users compare organizational results from one year to the next or between organizations.
- Management accounting is the process of measuring future estimates of financial results against actual performance. Management accounting is used to help control financial activity.
- Cost accounting is the measurement of the inputs into a final product. Cost accounting helps organizations determine the price of a product.

Other branches of accounting pertain to specialties, such as auditing, taxes, forensics, and government accounting.

## Financial Accounting

Measurement of financial data in the United States is based on the US dollar. Recording of data is performed at the transaction level: when a purchase is made or anticipated. Some organizations use the *cash basis* of accounting, recording transactions only when they are completed, that is, when cash has changed hands. Thus the purchase of supplies is recorded when the supplies are actually paid for; salaries are recorded when the employees are paid. Cash basis accounting is appropriate for individuals and some small businesses. The cash basis of accounting poses some difficulties for large organizations, because purchases are rarely paid for on receipt and income may be earned long before it is received. Therefore most large organizations use the accrual basis of accounting: recognizing additions of money when it is earned and subtractions of money when expenses are incurred, regardless of when the funds enter or leave the bank accounts.

Traditionally, the point of accrual accounting is to match expenses incurred to the same time period in which the associated revenue was earned. When revenue exceeds expenses, the organization has generated a profit. When expenses exceed revenue, the organization has generated a loss. In a health care organization, revenue is generated primarily from providing services to patients. So, if a hospital earned $200,000 in revenue in June from treating clinic patients, the $190,000 in supplies, pharmaceuticals, utilities, salaries, and other expenses used to treat those patients would be recognized in June. A cash basis hospital would not recognize the revenue until it was received or the expenses until they were paid. This timing difference would make it difficult to figure out whether the hospital was profitable in a particular period of time, so most organizations use the accrual basis to account for transactions. Regardless of the method of accounting, an organization's transactions are periodically summarized into financial statements: balance sheet, income statement, and statement of changes in financial position.

The balance sheet is a snapshot of the organization's financial status at a point in time: what it owns (assets), what it owes (liabilities), and what it is worth (assets minus liabilities). There are two main categories of assets: short-term and long-term. Short term assets include cash, inventory, and accounts receivable. Long-term assets are buildings, equipment, furniture, and other items that are used for more than one FY. Such long-term assets are also called fixed assets and are typically categorized as property, plant, and equipment. Similarly, liabilities are categorized as short-term (e.g., accounts payable, short-term borrowings called notes) and long-term (e.g., mortgages). The difference between assets and liabilities is called equity (in a for-profit organization) or fund balance (in a not-for-profit organization). Fig. 6.7 shows a simple example of a set of financial statements.

Revenue is income that is earned by the activities or investments of the organization. It comes from providing services (in our case, to patients) and from interest and dividends from investments. Expenses are the costs incurred by the organization in the process of earning income. Expenses are expenditures related to earning revenue. Expenses include salaries and benefits, utilities, mortgage payments, and supplies. An income statement is a summary of revenue and expense activity over a period.

If assets minus liabilities equal equity, then what does equity represent? Equity, or fund balance, is literally the arithmetic difference between total assets and total liabilities. The representation of changes in equity is found in the income statement. If revenue exceeds expenses, then equity increases. If expenses exceed revenue, then equity decreases. This change is expressed in the statement of changes in financial position.

While HIM professionals are not expected to be accountants, it is very useful to understand the language of accounting and financial management and how revenue cycle activities impact the organization as a whole. The point of RCM is to ensure efficient and effective cash flow related to patient service revenue. This means that the revenue is accurately stated on the income statement and cash is received on a timely basis.

## Management Accounting: Budgets

Management accounting adds an analytical layer to the financial accounting data: what did the organization expect to happen and why? For example, if the hospital clinic was expected to earn $250,000 but it only earned $200,000, a management report would show the $50,000 difference. The development of the organization's expectations of financial performance takes place in the budget process.

Budgets, like financial statements, are based on an FY, which may or may not be the same as a CY. For example, FYs may start on July 1 and end on June 30 or may start on October 1 and end on September 30. The federal government uses an October 1 to September 30 FY, which is why IPPS rules, ICD-10-CM/PCS, and MS-DRG code changes are effective on October 1.

Budgets are a tool for facilities to plan for the cash needs of the organization. In order to pay all of its bills, the amount of cash coming in to the organization must exceed the amount going out. Cash coming in is the result of collecting earned income (e.g., patient service revenue), and cash going out is the result of paying obligations (e.g., expenses). Remember that on the accrual basis of financial accounting, we recognize revenue when it is earned and expenses when they are incurred. However, we might receive the cash a month (or more) after the revenue is earned and similarly may pay the bill in a different period than that in which the expense was incurred. The financial activity of cash coming in and cash going out is called cash flow. The process of projecting when cash will be received and what cash is needed to pay bills is the cash budget. The cash budget can be any useful period of time but is generally expressed as a monthly report. If cash coming in is expected to exceed cash going out, then there may be an opportunity for a short-term investment to earn interest on the excess cash. If cash going out is expected to exceed cash coming in, then there may be a need for a short-term loan to cover the difference. Again, while HIM professionals are not expected to work with the organization's cash budget, understanding what it means gives purpose to what we are expected to do, which is to minimize the DNFB dollars.

## DIAMONTE COMMUNITY HOSPITAL

### Balance Sheets
*(in thousands)*

| | December 31 | |
| --- | --- | --- |
| | **2019** | **2018** |
| **Assets** | | |
| Current assets: | | |
| Cash and cash equivalents | $ 32,000 | $ 35,000 |
| Patient receivables, net of discounts and allowances | 51,500 | 48,100 |
| Inventory | 7,000 | 6,500 |
| Total current assets | 90,500 | 89,600 |
| | | |
| Long-term assets: | | |
| Net property and equipment | 2,15,000 | 2,00,000 |
| Long-term investments | 1,25,000 | 1,30,000 |
| Total long-term assets | 3,40,000 | 3,30,000 |
| | | |
| **Liabilities and net assets** | | |
| | | |
| Current liabilities | | |
| Accounts payable | 30,000 | 23,000 |
| Accrued expenses | 20,000 | 8,500 |
| Other current liabilities | 2,000 | 2,500 |
| Total current liabilities | 52,000 | 34,000 |
| | | |
| Long-term liabilities: | | |
| Long-term debt and capital lease obligations | 1,60,000 | 1,50,000 |
| Other long-term liabilities | 25,000 | 20,000 |
| Total long-term liabilities | 1,85,000 | 1,70,000 |
| | | |
| Total liabilities | 2,37,000 | 2,04,000 |
| | | |
| Net assets (*Fund Balance, Equity*): | | |
| Unrestricted | 1,94,261 | 1,85,000 |
| Restricted | 976 | 976 |
| Total net assets | 1,95,237 | 1,85,976 |
| | | |
| Total liabilities and net assets | $ 4,32,237 | $ 3,89,976 |

### Statement of Operations
*(in thousands)*

| | December 31 | |
| --- | --- | --- |
| | **2019** | **2018** |
| Unrestricted revenue and other support | | |
| Net patient service revenue | 3,76,716 | 3,60,000 |
| Provision for bad debts | (4,683) | −3,000 |
| Net patient service revenue less provision for bad debts | 3,72,033 | 3,57,000 |
| | | |
| Other operating revenues | 7,608 | 9,000 |
| Gifts, bequests, and contributions | 3,620 | 3,000 |
| Total unrestricted revenue and other support | 3,83,261 | 3,69,000 |
| | | |
| Operating expenses: | | |
| Salaries and wages | 1,66,000 | 1,60,000 |
| Employee benefits | 60,000 | 58,000 |
| Contract services | 75,000 | 70,000 |
| Depreciation and amortization | 24,000 | 24,000 |
| Professional fees | 16,000 | 14,000 |
| Other | 13,000 | 12,000 |
| Supplies | 9,000 | 10,000 |
| Utilities | 4,000 | 4,000 |
| Interest | 4,000 | 4,000 |
| Insurance | 3,000 | 3,000 |
| Total operating expenses | 3,74,000 | 3,59,000 |
| | | |
| Operating income | $ 9,261 | $ 10,000 |

### Statement of Changes in Net Assets
*(in thousands)*

| | December 31 | | |
| --- | --- | --- | --- |
| | **Unrestricted** | **Restricted** | Total |
| Net assets, December 31, 2017 | 1,75,000 | 976 | 1,75,976 |
| Operating income | 10,000 | | 10,000 |
| Net assets, December 31, 2018 | 1,85,000 | 976 | 1,85,976 |
| Operating income | 9,261 | | 9,261 |
| Net assets, December 31, 2019 | 1,94,261 | 976 | 1,95,237 |

• **Fig. 6.7** Sample financial statements.

## Strategic Budget

Each year, the organization conducts an overall budget process to set its financial expectations for the FY. This process begins with the Board of Directors/Trustees.

The organization's Board of Directors/Trustees first develops a strategic budget, which gives managers guidelines about the organization's expectations and estimations of revenue and expenses. For example, the organization may be planning for an overall 3% increase in expenses and an overall 2% increase in revenue. Because a health care organization's revenue is earned primarily from delivering patient services, revenue is estimated by projecting patient volume and case mix. Factors that go into estimating patient volume include historical experience, the competition in the marketplace, and any planned expansions or contractions of the organization's services. The Board of Directors/Trustees communicates the strategic budget through administration to the department managers for their guidance in preparing the capital and operating budgets.

## Capital Budget

Capital budget expenditures are large purchases that support the organization's ability to generate revenue. There are two main financial accounting considerations in determining whether a purchase is a capital expenditure: useful life and cost. Fixed assets, such as computer systems, large furniture purchases, and diagnostic radiology equipment are examples of capital expenditures. Bulk purchases of small items, such as catheters and CDs, even if large dollars, are not capital items because the items themselves will not be used over a long period of time.

Each facility defines what constitutes a capital expense. For example, some facilities may require that any single item over $1000 be reviewed as a potential capital expenditure, while others may define this as $5000 or more. Expensive pieces of technology such as copy machines are fixed assets, unless the organization chooses to lease such items rather than purchase them.

### Requests and the Payback Period

During the capital budgeting process, department managers submit requests for new fixed assets, such as furniture, shelving and storage units, and technology. Although capital budget requests are submitted annually, projections for capital purchases may be required years in advance of the actual purchase. Capital budget requests are evaluated and approved based on the organization's available resources and strategic goals.

HIM department directors must think carefully about what they will need in the future in terms of new equipment and/or technology. While a purchase may seem logical to the manager and staff of the department, its value to the organization may not be clear to administration. Since HIM is competing with other departments, including clinical areas, for capital dollars, the value of the new asset to the organization will be an important factor in whether the capital budget request is granted. For example, the value of a new scanner may be found in faster turnaround to upload patient data to the EHR, reduction in staffing required to operate it, or significant reduction in maintenance costs over time.

When a capital equipment request is submitted, justification for the expense is required (Fig. 6.8). Financial justifications can be required in the form of a **payback period**, which determines how long it will take to recover the expense of the equipment. To calculate the payback period, the numerator is the total cost of the equipment and the denominator is the estimated cash inflow resulting from use of the new equipment:

$$\text{Payback period} = \frac{\text{Cost of equipment}}{\text{Estimated cash inflow}}$$

For example, a department might consider buying a new scanner to digitize health records. The model that best meets its needs has a sticker price of $12,000. But with this new technology, the department gets higher-quality scans and fewer rescans, amounting to monthly savings of $500, or annual savings estimated at $6000. The payback period would therefore be calculated as:

$$\text{Payback period} = \frac{\$12,000}{\$6000} = \frac{2}{1} = 2 \text{ years}$$

If the expected life of the equipment is 5 years, then a shorter payback period, such as 1–2 years, is likely preferred. Depending on the circumstances, that payback period may be too long. If the facility requires a 1-year payback period, then the HIM manager may need to look to other ways to meet this goal, such as a less expensive piece of equipment or a lease plan, rather than purchase.

### Return on Investment

Another way to look at the value of capital equipment purchases is **return on investment (ROI)**, which represents how much of the equipment cost is recovered per year. ROI is calculated with the average annual savings as the numerator over the purchase price, multiplied by 100 to get a percentage:

$$\text{Return on investment} = \frac{\text{Average annual savings}}{\text{Purchase price}} \times 100$$

Essentially, the ROI tells us how quickly the equipment pays itself off. Returning to the example of the scanner, we estimated this new equipment would save $500 per month, or $6000 annually:

$$\frac{\$6000}{\$12,000} \times 100 = 50\% \text{ return on investments}$$

In other words, 50% of the scanner is paid off after 1 year, and 100% after 2 years. If the facility has a required minimum ROI, such as 35%, then the new scanner would be considered

## CITYWIDE SURGI-CENTER
## CAPITAL EQUIPMENT REQUEST FORM

| BUDGET YEAR: | DATE: | | | | |
|---|---|---|---|---|---|
| BUDGET DESCRIPTION: | REQUESTED BY: | | | | |
| DEPARTMENT NAME: | Replacement | Yes ☐ | | No ☐ | |
| ACCOUNT / CENTER: | | | | | |
| CER AMOUNT: | New Item | Yes ☐ | | No ☐ | |
| DESCRIPTION OF NEED: | | | | | |
| | Revenue Stream | Yes ☐ | | No ☐ | |

**CAPITAL EQUIPMENT DESCRIPTION AND JUSTIFICATION**
List all other associated costs such as additional staffing, maintenance agreements, supplies, etc.



**EFFECT ON OPERATIONS**
List quality benefits, operational efficiencies, productivity improvements, other rationale



**COMPLETE THIS SECTION FOR ALL EQUIPMENT REQUESTS**

| Quantity | Vendor | Model Number |
|---|---|---|
| | | |
| | | |
| | | |

**SIGNATURE APPROVALS**

Director: _____    Date: _____

Administrator: _____    Date: _____

**FINANCE SCREENING AND PURCHASE AUTHORIZATION**

| PROJECT CATEGORY | Budget Amount | CER Amount | |
|---|---|---|---|
| Professional Fees | | | Date: _____ |
| Staff Salaries | | | ☐ Approved |
| Fringe Benefits | | | ☐ Approved with Modification |
| Supplies | | | ☐ Disapproved |
| Computer Support Services | | | |
| Training | | | Comments: |
| Installation | | | |
| Maintenance | | | |
| Depreciation | | | |
| Trade In (Amount) | | | |
| TOTAL PROJECT COST | $       - | $       - | |

**REVIEW AND APPROVAL**

| DIRECTOR OF PURCHASING | Date | CHIEF FINANCIAL OFFICER | Date |
|---|---|---|---|
| | | | |
| CHIEF OPERATING OFFICER | Date | FINANCE - RELEASE OF FUNDS | Date |
| | | | |

• **Fig. 6.8** Capital expenditure approval form. (From Abdelhak, M, Hanken, MA: Health information: management of a strategic resource, ed 5, St. Louis, 2015, Elsevier.)

a good investment. After 100% ROI, the organization makes a profit on its investment; it continues to save money each month but has already paid for the piece of equipment.

Obtaining equipment takes planning, and options for payment should be considered with the facility CFO. If new technology is constantly being introduced, then purchasing an expensive piece of equipment may not be the best answer. The department may want to rent for a year and then purchase the newer technology. In addition, even if the department purchases the scanner outright, it may choose to *amortize* the cost of the capital equipment over several years to represent the actual projected life of the equipment. **Amortization** finances the purchase with a fixed payment schedule of principal and interest over the life of a loan. This would also show as a monthly fixed cost rather than a one-time capital expense on your budget report.

This monthly cost is also known as depreciation expense, which is a common practice in accrual-based accounting. Very few material items *appreciate* (gain value), but most do, indeed, **depreciate** (lose value) as they age. Straight-line depreciation is calculated by devaluing the initial cost by the number of years that the item is projected to be used. For example, a high-capacity printer that costs $2500 and has an expected use of 5 years will depreciate $500 each year ($2500÷5 years=$500). The first year, it is worth $2500; the second year, $2000; by the third year, it is valued at $1500, the fourth $1000, and the fifth $500. After the fifth year, the printer's expected useful life has expired.

## Operational Budget

**Operational budgets** include department-level projected revenue and routine expenditures, such as supplies, utilities, and service contracts. They also plan for payroll, contractors, office supplies, and travel to conferences. Some of these expenditures would be **fixed expenses**, such as the price of equipment rental (assuming this is a flat rate and not based on amount of usage). In the preparation of a budget, the fixed costs are the easiest to fill in since they are based on a contracted amount between the vendor and the facility. The main characteristic of fixed expenses is that they do not change with the volume of activity. **Variable expenses** can change depending on the level of activity or volume. Variable expenses are estimated based on the prior year activity levels, along with any expected changes for the coming year. For example, if the capital budget includes the implementation of an EHR, postage and supply expenses would probably decrease as release of information requests would increasingly be fulfilled electronically. The HIM manager would have to take that change into consideration when preparing the postage and supply portion of the budget. To illustrate the difference between fixed and variable expenses, consider a department that uses an outside vendor for release of information. If the vendor charges a flat fee for performing the service, that is a fixed expense. If the facility performs all release of information functions in house, then the postage and supply expenses vary depending on the number of requests processed. Another example of capital purchases affecting the operating budget is supplemental or ongoing equipment training subsequent to the installation of a piece of equipment. Paid training can become costly, but additional training of personnel subsequent to a "go live" is essential to a successful outcome. In addition, service contracts to update and maintain the equipment and/or technology must also be considered. These may not be optional and can be costly. The HIM department is not typically a revenue-generating department; however, some HIM departments may offer transcription or coding services to area physicians or other facilities for a fee, in which case this limited revenue stream would be projected and reported. Otherwise, the budget concerns of the HIM director revolve around expenses.

The payroll portion of an operating budget is usually the largest expense. In addition to salaries and wages, the budget will include fringe benefit expenses of roughly 30% of payroll. If the employer provides raises at the same time for all employees, then payroll projections for all increases can be made in the operating budget beginning in the same month.

For example, the organization requires that the average raise for the department's employees must be no more than 2%. The adjustment in salary begins on January 1 for all affected employees. To budget, then, salaries would be estimated as an overall increase of 2%. Salaries that change mid-year (due to employee hiring anniversary being in the middle of the year) must be pro-rated-assigned salary budget dollars at the prior year rate until the anniversary, then at the new rate after the anniversary.

Say an employee earns $24,000 per year and is getting a 2% raise on their anniversary, which is July 1. The HIM director would adjust the budget for this payroll increase for half of the year at $24,000 ($2000 per month) and half of the year at $24,480 ($2040 per month), as seen here:

|  | January through June | | July through December | Total Salary Budgeted |
|---|---|---|---|---|
| Salary | $2000 × 6 | + | $2040 × 6 | = $24,240 |
| Calculation | $12,000 | | $12,240 | |

If a facility begins providing a new service, such as heart catheterizations, the HIM department should consider additional transcription and coding services at a minimum. It will need additional staff until its current staff is able to keep up with the volume of new cases and acquire the new skills needed to properly complete reports and provide codes for these services. Rather than hiring additional staff in this situation, many HIM directors would pay the existing staff overtime or hire an outsourcing company to assist temporarily with the extra work. Using current employees may be optimal since they will be more familiar with the physicians and work types. However, too much overtime can lead to errors and exhaustion, so these factors must be weighed in this decision. An outsourcing company should be able to quickly get up to speed with the demands and provide the extra resources needed. However, these resources can be more expensive than overtime expenses.

Conversely, sometimes there are declines in patient volume, and health care facilities are required to cut staff or hours. Ideally this is done by *attrition*, which means that employees who leave are not replaced. However, sometimes hours must be cut to avoid letting staff go. In this case, an HIM department director may be asked to cut hourly employees to a 32-hour work week from a 40-hour work week. Some jobs may be eliminated altogether. These are difficult decisions that must be undertaken with a great deal of research and forethought. It is important to remember the time and effort the facility has invested in the training of these highly skilled workers (Davis and Doyle, 2016).

## Variance

After the operational budget is created and approved, the department director reports on *variances* from the budget, usually on a monthly basis. A **variance** is the difference between what was budgeted and what was actually received or spent. A positive or favorable variance means that the department either earned more or spent less than was predicted. Conversely, a negative or unfavorable variance means that the department either earned less or spent more than was predicted. Negative variances in revenue can be offset by positive variances in expenses. For example, a decline in census affects revenue negatively; however, fewer resources would be consumed by patient care activities, resulting in a decline in variable expenses. Fig. 6.9 displays

| HIM Department Budget—July (month 7 of Fiscal Year) | | | | | |
|---|---|---|---|---|---|
| | Budget | YTD-Budget | Actual | YTD-Actual | Variance |
| Revenue: | | | | | |
| Expenses: | | | | | |
| Salaries | $12,000 | $84,000 | $11,458 | $82,880 | ($1120) or 1.3% |
| Supplies | $250 | $1750 | $308 | $1800 | $50 or −2.9% |
| Maintenance contract | | | | | |
| Copy machine | $500 | $3500 | $500 | $3500 | 0% |

• **Fig. 6.9** A sample budget.

## ❖ COMPETENCY CHECK-IN 6.5

### Accounting Concepts

#### Competency Assessment

1. What is the difference between financial accounting and management accounting?
2. How does cost accounting support the financial goals of the organization?
3. What are the two bases of accounting for transactions? What are the advantages and disadvantages of each?
4. Explain the difference between the operational budget and the capital budget, giving examples of the types of expenses in each.
5. If an HIM department considers purchasing a high-volume/high-speed scanner for $18,000 that would save the department $500 a month, what is the ROI after 1 year?
6. What is the payback period for a piece of equipment that costs $6000 and saves $250 per month?
7. Using straight-line depreciation, how much would an $11,800 piece of equipment depreciate each year on a 4-year depreciation schedule?
8. The HIM department pays $18 per box for a firm to remove, shred, and recycle its paper waste securely. In May the cost per box will increase to $20 per box. Is shredding a fixed cost or a variable cost?
9. Including benefits, you pay exempt employee Sally $6550 a month. Is Sally's salary fixed or variable?
10. The HIM department is allowed $300 per month for supplies. At the end of the third quarter, the department had spent $3000 on supplies. This means that the HIM department is:
    a. under budget YTD by $300
    b. over budget YTD by $300
    c. exactly as it should be on budget for supplies
    d. over budget $250

limited budget items for the HIM department during the month of July. An actual budget report would include many more line items or expenses. The "Budget" column displays the amount allocated for the corresponding expense. The "Actual" column displays the amount of money spent during the month of July. Notice that this information, budget and actual, is also displayed for year-to-date (YTD) expenses. The YTD information allows the manager to determine whether the budget is being met for the year. This is helpful because sometimes 1 month's expenses will be more or less than the actual budget, and knowing the YTD expenses helps the manager determine whether they will meet the budget for the entire year. The last column displays the difference, or the actual amount, that the department is over or under budget.

For example, in a small facility, if an employee has an unexpected illness or injury that causes them to be absent for a week, the unexpected cost of overtime may cause the payroll portion of the budget to show negative variance. Similarly, if the employee's work is being covered by a temporary or contract worker, the contractor expenses may be over budget for the period.

The presence of a positive or negative variance may need to be justified to administration, depending on the size and nature of the variance. So, a negative or unfavorable variance in payroll or contractor expenses is easily explained by the unexpected absence of the regular employee. Remember that the regular employee is likely still being paid at their regular rate in this example, assuming that there is sick time or personal time off accumulated.

## Chapter Summary

One of the key uses for coded data is reimbursement. Medicare PPSs arose out of cost-control measures and are based on code systems originally designed for other purposes. Inpatient hospitals are reimbursed using Medicare Severity Diagnosis-Related Groups (MS-DRGs). Medicare outpatient services are reimbursed under APCs. Additional PPSs include the IPF PPS, IRF PPS, LTCH-PPS, HH PPS, SNF PPS, and RUGs.

Billing in a hospital is generally the responsibility of the patient accounts department. Charges are posted to the patient's account on the basis of data maintained in the facility's Chargemaster, or CDM. Hospital-based services are submitted for payment using a Uniform Bill, currently UB-04. Outpatient services are billed using the CMS-1500 form. Because of the importance of the coded data in

correct billing and collections, health information professionals must maintain a strong working relationship with the patient accounts professionals.

All HIM professionals must understand basic accounting, as well as the planning and monitoring of budgets. Capital budget expenditures are large purchases of assets. Examples include computers and technology, furniture, and equipment. The operational budget consists of routine expenditures, such as supplies, utilities, payroll, vendors, travel, and service contracts. Requests for capital budget expenses are based on the payback period and the ROI of the purchase. After the operational budget is created and approved, managers report on variances from the budget, usually on a monthly basis.

## Competency Milestones

### CAHIIM Competency
*IV.3. Summarize regulatory requirements and reimbursement methodologies. (2)*

### Rationale
HIM professionals are employed in all areas that contribute to the revenue cycle.

### Competency Assessment
1. Each type of reimbursement has unique characteristics and a different approach to risk. Compare and contrast the four reimbursement methodologies discussed, identifying the financial risk to the parties involved. What incentives do physicians have to operate under each of the four methods of reimbursement discussed?
2. Discuss the impact of the PPS on the coding function.
3. Discuss the significance of a hospital's CMI and reasons that it should be monitored.
4. List three PPSs, and describe how reimbursement is obtained in each.
5. Provide an example of how incorrect inpatient coding would financially affect a hospital.
6. What are the major differences between MS-DRGs and APCs?

### CAHIIM Competency
*IV.3. **RM** Evaluate compliance with regulatory requirements and reimbursement methodologies. (5)*

### Rationale

An important career path for HIM professionals is in the revenue cycle—from coding to management; success in these roles depends on a thorough understanding of the data flow that drives reimbursement.

### Case Study

*You are a Patient Financial Services supervisor at a small Community Hospital. One of your staff has come to you with a problem. Normally, it takes the laboratory director a few days to review the codes, make any necessary revisions or corrections, and clear the claims, but your staff person noticed that they were suddenly being cleared very quickly. Curious, your staff person looked at a few claims and noticed that the laboratory was changing the diagnosis codes to other codes in order to bypass the medical necessity edit, regardless of whether the codes were correct, and then process the claims through the scrubber. You call over to the laboratory and find out that the laboratory's director has been on disability leave for a month, leaving a laboratory supervisor in charge of handling claims that have failed the scrubber's edits.*

1. Evaluate the scenario and describe the potential problems that are occurring.
2. What compliance issues are potentially at issue?
3. What are your (and the hospital's) next steps?

**CAHIIM Competency**

*IV.2. Describe components of revenue cycle management and clinical documentation improvement. (2)*

### Rationale

HIM professionals can be employed in all areas that contribute to the revenue cycle.

### Competency Assessment

1. When or where does the revenue cycle process begin?
2. What department/staff functions impact the data transmitted in the 837I?
3. What impact does clinical documentation improvement have on the revenue cycle process?
4. What management tool is used to track unbilled accounts?
5. What steps might someone take to use the tool described in Question 4?
6. In an ambulatory setting, an encounter form is often used for charge capture. Name three items that would be on an encounter form.

**CAHIIM Competency**

*IV.2. **RM** Evaluate revenue cycle processes. (5)*

### Rationale

HIM professionals can be employed in all areas that contribute to the revenue cycle.

### Competency Assessment

1. For the vaccination charge to appear on a patient's bill, how does the charge get to the patient's account?
2. What impact does the Chargemaster have on the revenue cycle?
3. The PFS department is backlogged processing failed claims due to a high number of errors in the patient's insurance identification. What is the most likely cause of the errors and what should PFS do about it?

### Case Study

*You are the coding manager in a small community hospital. Bill hold is 3 days, which accounts for 75% of the $8 million DNFB target. The clean claim rate averages 90%. Until recently, you have had no problem keeping the average DNFB under the target. However, over the past month, the DNFB has risen to $10 million. In discussions with the HIM department director, you determine the following:*

i. There have been only 3 sick days among the coders in the past month—all in the first week.
ii. The analysts are a day behind due to an analyst being on vacation.
iii. The interface between the transcription system and the EHR was down off and on for the past 2 weeks.
iv. PFS went live with a new claim review system at the beginning of this month. The conversion went smoothly; however, there were multiple staff who had not been trained by go-live, which delayed the handling of failed claims. PFS is beginning to catch up this week.

1. Evaluate each of these known issues and their possible impact on the DNFB. Include in your evaluation which of these issues is most problematic and what needs to be addressed in order to correct it.

## CAHIIM Competency
*VI.5. Utilize financial management processes. (3)*

### Rationale
HIM professionals are not expected to be accountants; however, a basic understanding of accounting terminology assists in budget preparation and the appreciation of the role of RCM in the financial health of the organization.

### Competency Assessment
1. You have completed the purchase of two replacement scanners for your department, which were approved from your capital budget request. The equipment is supposed to be delivered in March, but there has been a delay and it will not be delivered until June. What is the impact of the delay from a financial perspective?
2. You are the Director of HIM in a small Community Hospital. One of the clinical departments has noticed that there are two patients with the same name being treated in their area on different days and their charges were placed on the wrong accounts. The department is asking you what to do about it. Their position is that it is not a problem since the treatment they were having had the same dollar amount on the charges. What should be done?
3. This is your first year as Department Director and you are preparing your department budget for next year. You notice that last year's budget had a constant dollar amount for outsourced coding contractors, who are used on an as-needed basis. Is this the best way to budget for this expense? How would you characterize this expense in accounting terms? What should be taken into consideration in budgeting for these coding contractors?
4. Using straight-line depreciation, how much would an $11,800 piece of equipment depreciate each year on a 4-year depreciation schedule?
5. You sent out five requests for proposals (RFPs) to compare costs and benefits of a new patient check-in kiosk. You only received two of the RFPs back. Vendor A gives you a cost of $13,800. The cost savings per month for this first proposal is projected at $375. The second proposal from Vendor B is at a cost of $7100, but the software is not as sophisticated. Vendor B's kiosk would have a cost savings per month of $150. Which payback period is quicker?
6. You realize the department will need a new scanner in 3 years, so you anticipate the purchase price of a scanner in 3 years based on quotes from three of your sales representatives. As time passes, you realize this may need to be adjusted on budgetary restrictions or new technology, but you are comfortable budgeting $8400 and prepare a justification report to go along with the capital budget request. The hospital is asking for a 35% ROI in the first year for a purchase; otherwise, you will need to consider renting or leasing. Given the following information, which option should you choose?

| | Vendor A | Vendor B | Vendor C |
|---|---|---|---|
| Price | $7900 | $8400 | $6500 |
| Savings per month | $225 | $275 | $180 |

7. Community Hospital defines capital budget items as all items costing more than $10,000 that have a useful life of more than 2 years. Which HIM department expenses should be submitted under the capital budget?
   a. New paper shredder costing $3000 with a useful life of 5 years
   b. A 3-year supply of copy machine toner costing $6000
   c. New file cabinets and office furniture for the coding section costing $15,000
8. Cindy's salary (including benefits) is $31,200, and she received a score of 3 on her performance review, meaning her work "Meets Expectations." She will receive a 1% raise in May. Omar makes the same amount per year, but his score of 1, "Meets and Frequently Exceeds Expectations," will earn him a 5% raise. What is the payroll budget for these two employees for May?
9. Examine the following annual budget variance report and double-check the calculations. If available, use an Excel spreadsheet and embedded formulas for calculations. The "Budget" and "Actual" columns are correct, but are there any errors in the $Var or %Var columns? What possible explanations are there for why the variances exist? (Speculate what you would need to know in order to confirm your possible explanations?) Based on this report, how would you change the budget for next year?

| Item | Budget | Actual | $Var | %Var |
|---|---|---|---|---|
| Payroll | $1,560,000 | $1,555,555 | $4555 | 0.28% |
| Outsourcing | $5000 | $10,750 | ($5750) | 115% |
| Supplies | $3500 | $3000 | $500 | 12.4% |
| AHIMA dues and credentials | $2220 | $2405 | ($85) | (8.3%) |
| Equipment depreciation | $3750 | $3750 | 0 | 100 |

| Item | Budget | Actual | $Var | %Var |
|------|--------|--------|------|------|
| Equipment lease | $7200 | $6000 | $1200 | 0.16% |
| Equipment rental | $700 | $1400 | $700 | (100%) |

## Ethics Challenge

*VI.7. Assess ethical standards of practice (5)*

1. You are working in the patient financial services department and are responsible for resolving claims that have failed the initial scrub. The hospital's policy is to transmit to the payer daily 100% of all available claims. It has been challenging but possible to meet that goal until recently. You have noticed an increasing number of outpatient claims that are failing for physician NPI (national provider identification) numbers. You can see the physicians in the record and can look up their NPI. It usually takes a day to get the record corrected by going through patient access. You are not sure why it takes so long, since it only takes you a few minutes. There are more than usual today, so you decide to fix them and transmit the claims now. You will let patient access know tomorrow. Ethical or not?

## Critical Thinking Questions

1. HIM departments are frequently under intense pressure to code medical records as soon as possible after patient discharge so that the hospital may be reimbursed. Pressure may come from patient accounts department staff members, who may not completely understand the myriad reasons that all medical records cannot be accurately coded or even coded at all immediately after discharge. If you were the coding supervisor at a hospital, how would you describe the reasons for delays in coding with patient accounts department staff members? How would you discuss the DNFB (discharged, no final bill) and coding requirements under HIPAA with patient accounts staff members in a collaborative, rather than adversarial, way? Can you identify ways in which patient accounts staff members might help HIM employees decrease delays?
2. You are the manager of patient registration at a community hospital. When registering patients, your staff are required to obtain insurance information. The largest employer in your town has recently changed its employee benefit plan from an indemnity plan to a managed care plan. As manager of patient registration, you must educate your staff as to the differences in registering patients in a managed care plan versus an indemnity plan. For example, what will be your process for obtaining copays? How will your staff handle cash or checks? How will you ensure that cash or check copays are correctly credited to each patient's account? What will you instruct your staff to do if a patient with managed care insurance comes to the hospital for admission but the physician is not a participant in the patient's managed care plan?
3. In 2010 the federal government mandated that every person must have health insurance, and that all health insurance plans must meet MEC standards. Using the Internet, look up the standards for MEC. What services must qualified health plans cover? Why do you think legislators had to require plans to cover certain services? What is the current status of this requirement?

## Professional Profile

### Practice Manager

My name is Sherri, and I am the practice manager for a group partnership of six physicians who specialize in internal medicine, Ridgewood Medical Associates. I use my expertise in physician billing and contract negotiations to ensure that Ridgewood Medical Associates receives the appropriate payments and reimbursement from our patients and insurers after services are rendered.

I began my career in health care by taking a coding certificate course at my local community college. Our coursework included coding all types of patient records and outpatient encounters, and I realized that I preferred outpatient coding. After I completed the course, I sat for the American Health Information Management Association (AHIMA) Certified Coding Specialist-Physician-based (CCS-P) exam, passed it, and earned my credential as a CCS-P. I was fortunate to find a position working for a physician billing company.

As a physician biller, I applied my knowledge of HCPCS/CPT-4 and ICD-9-CM coding, adding the correct codes to billing claims so that physicians could be reimbursed for services rendered. After a few years as a physician biller, I was ready for new challenges to further my career. I applied for the position of practice manager for Ridgewood Medical Associates and was hired.

To perform my job well, I must manage and oversee the many daily tasks and functions of a busy medical practice. First, I must make sure that every new and existing patient is registered in our patient billing system with the correct information according to insurance type. Because we accept all types of patient insurance and also accept self-pay patients, we need to know who must pay a deductible, who must pay a copay, and who will pay out-of-pocket fees. We store this information and patient demographic details electronically, and we anticipate adding clinical information as we move toward adopting an electronic health record (EHR). Our goal is to become a paperless office within 5 years. I keep abreast of the latest information concerning the EHR through my professional association, AHIMA. I am also a member of the Medical Group Management Association (see http://www.mgms.com/).

Patients who are in managed care plans may require a referral from one of our physicians to see a specialist. It is my job to see that the referral process does not inconvenience either our patients or our physicians. To accomplish this goal, I need to know which managed care plans require a referral and for which specialties. I access referral forms from each managed care plan's website and download them from my computer. These referral forms are made accessible to our physicians at all times; they can either retrieve the forms online or use one of the hard copies that are readily available in patient treatment areas. If our physician orders a referral to a different specialist outside our group practice, I assist our patient by making the appointment and ensuring that our referral form and any necessary medical records are forwarded to the specialist in time for the appointment.

I supervise our billing staff and perform periodic audits of the codes submitted to insurers on claims submissions. We must submit accurate claims, including codes, to insurers to be properly reimbursed and also to avoid claim rejections. We submit most of our claims electronically. As a CCS-P, I stay abreast of any code changes or changes in claim submission requirements. I must also periodically remind our physicians to provide our billing staff with documentation that is complete and legible.

I also supervise our accounting staff. I receive detailed monthly reports that include an analysis of each insurer's payments to us. If I see that our expenses to treat a certain insurer's patients are not covered under the reimbursement we receive, I will negotiate with that insurer for a higher reimbursement to be applied for the next contract period. I must be able to review each insurer's contract and understand contract language so that I go into negotiations well prepared.

As a practice manager, I am involved in every nonclinical aspect of Ridgewood Medical Associates. I look forward to going to work each day because of the variety of functions that I oversee, and I also feel that I am helping our patients. The physicians value my work because I minimize the time that they must spend filling out paperwork and worrying about reimbursement. When I perform my job well, I enable our physicians to devote their time and clinical expertise to our patients.

### Career Tip

The level of skill needed to manage a physician group practice depends on the size and scope of the practice. A bachelor's degree in a health care–related field, such as HIM, is a good start. Experience in a physician's office setting is helpful, particularly demonstrating progressive increase in responsibility. For very large practices, a master's degree may be required.

### Patient Care Perspective

#### Maria

Recently, I received an explanation of benefits from our insurance company that denied payment for my radiology test because the insurance company had not given authorization for the test that the hospital had coded. I did not know what that meant, so I called Sherri in the doctor's office to help me make sense of it. She was able to coordinate a conversation with the hospital's preregistration department and the insurance company, and they solved the problem together.

### Patient Care Perspective

#### Dr. Lewis

The hospital uses codes for data analysis and billing purposes, and so do I. Recently, I sent my patient Isabel to the hospital for a blood test. I was surprised to get a call from patient registration that I had used an invalid code on the request (script). So, I called Sherri right away to help me find the right code. Without the right code to explain the medical necessity of the test, Isabel's insurance would not have paid for the test. Isabel was very happy to get that problem resolved on the spot.

## Works Cited

Centers for Medicare and Medicaid Services: *Three day payment window*. https://www.cms.gov/Medicare/Medicare-Fee-for-Service-Payment/AcuteInpatientPPS/Three_Day_Payment_Window.html. Accessed May 23, 2022.

Department of Health and Human Services, Indian Health Service: *Justification for estimates of appropriation committees*, Rockville, MD, 2019, Indian Health Service. https://www.ihs.gov/budgetformulation/includes/themes/responsive2017/display_objects/documents/FY2019CongressionalJustification.pdf. Retrieved January 2, 2019.

Health Information Policy Council: *1984, Revision of the uniform hospital discharge data set, Fed Regist* 50:31038–31040, 1985.

Liberty Healthshare: *How it works*, 2018. Retrieved from Liberty Healthshare. www.libertyhealthshare.org. https://www.liberty-healthshare.org/how-it-works. Accessed May 05, 2022.

United States Census Bureau. Health Insurance Coverage in the United States: 2020. https://www.census.gov/library/publications/2021/demo/p60-274.html. September 14, 2021. Accessed January 30, 2023.

## Further Reading

American Hospital Association, National Uniform Billing Committee: *About the NUBC*. https://www.nubc.org/about-nubc. Updated 2022. Accessed May 19, 2022.

Centers for Medicare & Medicaid Services: *Outlier payments*. Retrieved from CMS.gov: Centers for Medicare & Medicaid Services. https://www.cms.gov/Medicare/Medicare-Fee-for-Service-Payment/AcuteInpatientPPS/outlier.html. Updated December 1, 2021. Accessed May 19, 2022.

Centers for Medicare & Medicaid Services: *Minimum essential coverage*. Retrieved from CMS.gov: Centers for Medicare & Medicaid Services. https://www.cms.gov/CCIIO/Programs-and-Initiatives/Health-Insurance-Market-Reforms/minimum-essential-coverage.html. Updated September 27, 2021 Accessed May 19, 2022

Centers for Medicare & Medicaid Services: *Prospective payment systems—general information*. From CMS.gov: Centers for Medicare & Medicaid Services. https://www.cms.gov/medicare/medicare-fee-for-service-payment/prospmedicarefeesvcpmtgen. Updated November 15, 2022 Accessed January 30, 2023.

Centers for Medicare and Medicaid Services: *Acute care hospital inpatient prospective payment system*, February 2022. c. https://www.cms.gov/Outreach-and-Education/Medicare-Learning-Network-MLN/MLNProducts/html/medicare-payment-systems.html#Acute. Accessed May 23, 2022.

Cunningham RM: *The Blues: a history of the Blue Cross and Blue Shield System*, Dekalb, 1997, Northern Illinois University Press.

Davis NA, Doyle BM: *Revenue cycle management best practices*, 2nd ed. Chicago, IL, 2016, AHIMA Press.

Health Systems International: *Diagnosis related groups definitions manual*. 6th revision, Number 89-009 Rev. 00, New Haven, CT, 1989.

Kaiser Family Foundation (KFF): *Health insurance coverage of the total population*. 2021. https://www.kff.org/other/state-indicator/total-population/?currentTimeframe=0&sortModel=%7B%22colId%22:%22Location%22,%22sort%22:%22asc%22%7D. Accessed May 23, 2022.

# 7

# Statistics and Data Analytics

**NADINIA DAVIS**

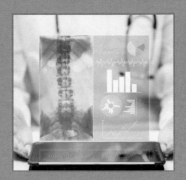

## CHAPTER OUTLINE

**Disciplines**
- Statistics
- Data Analytics in Health Care
- Health Informatics
- Health Information Management Role in Analysis

**Data Sources and Data Retrieval**
- Primary and Secondary Data
- Value of a Database
- Data Retrieval

**Types of Data**
- Nominal Data
- Ordinal Data
- Interval Data
- Ratio Data

**Common Statistical Analyses**
- Measures of Central Tendency
- Measures of Frequency
- Frequency Distribution
- Percentages, Decimals, Rates, and Ratios

**Measures of Variance**
- Normal Curve
- Skewedness
- Standard Deviation

**Routine Institutional Statistics**
- Admissions
- Discharges
- Length of Stay
- Average Length of Stay
- Transfers
- Census
- Days of Service
- Bed Occupancy Rate
- Hospital Rates and Percentages

**Research**
- What Is Research?
- Qualitative Versus Quantitative
- Research Design
- Institutional Review Board

**Reporting of Data**
- Reporting to Individual Departments
- Indices
- Reporting to Outside Agencies
- Specialized Data Collection Systems

**Presentation**
- Tables
- Pivot Tables
- Line Graph
- Bar Graph
- Histogram
- Pie Chart
- Dashboard

**Chapter Summary**

**Competency Milestones**

**Ethics Challenge**

**Critical Thinking**

**The Role of Health Information Management Professionals in the Workplace**
- Professional Profile: Clinical Data Analyst
- Patient Care Perspective

**Works Cited**

## CHAPTER OBJECTIVES

*By the end of this chapter, the student should be able to:*

1. Differentiate the disciplines of statistics, data analytics, health informatics, and decision support and discuss the health information management professional's role in these fields.
2. Differentiate primary and secondary data and use data collected in the facility to support organizational objectives.
3. Differentiate nominal, ordinal, interval, and ratio level data.
4. Calculate statistics used in health care, including measures of central tendency, measures of frequency, and measures of variance.
5. Utilize and compute routine institutional health care statistics.
6. Discuss research methodologies and how they are used in health care.
7. Understand the generation of reports within the facility and the reporting of data to outside agencies.
8. Explain the criteria for creating a report from a database.
9. Apply data visualization tools, present data graphically, and identify trends.

## VOCABULARY

accounting of disclosures
aggregate data
applied research
arithmetic mean
attribution
average length of stay (ALOS)
bar graph
basic research
bed control
bed count
census
central limit theorem
class intervals
clinical outcome analysis
cognitive definition
data analytics
discrete data
frequency distribution
geometric mean
health informatics
histogram
hypothesis
incidence
index
inpatient service day (IPSD)
Institutional Review Board (IRB)
interval data
key performance indicator (KPI)
length of stay
line graph
median

mixed method research
mode
morbidity
mortality
nominal data
normal curve
occupancy
operational definition
ordinal data
outlier
percentage
pie chart
population
prevalence
primary data
qualitative research
quantitative research
query
random selection
rate
ratio data
redact
registry
report
sample
secondary data
skewed
standard deviation
statistics
trend
vital statistics

### CAHIIM COMPETENCY DOMAINS

I.6.   Describe components of data dictionaries and data sets. (2)
III.1.  Apply health informatics concepts to the management of health information. (3)
III.3.  Calculate statistics for health care operations. (3)
III.4.  Report health care data through graphical representations. (3)
III.5.  Describe research methodologies used in health care. (2)
III.6.  Describe the concepts of managing data. (3)
III.6.  **DM** Manage data within a database system. (5)

In earlier chapters the collection of health data for documentation in the health record was discussed. Health data are stored in a physical location or database to facilitate retrieval for future use. Organizing specific data elements for each patient allows reporting of health information as it is mandated by law, accreditation, or policy or as needed by authorized users. Remember the difference between data and information: The data collected during patient care become health information only after careful organization and compilation. Data are raw elements. Information results from the interpretation of those data. This chapter focuses on the methods and tools used to compile and organize data to create information.

In the previous chapters the collection of health data was discussed in the context of providing proper patient care and following health care regulation and professional guidelines. This chapter focuses on the analysis and reporting of that data for a variety of uses. Basic analytical and reporting strategies are explored.

## Disciplines

To analyze data and report our findings, we need to utilize a branch of mathematics called statistics. We also may have occasion to apply the skills of data analytics and informatics as we gain proficiency in handling data.

### Statistics

According to the American Statistical Association (2019), "**Statistics** is the scientific application of mathematical principles to the collection, analysis, and presentation of numerical data." We already know that we are focused on health data and that health data needs to be collected in an organized manner so that we can retrieve it when it is needed. In our discussion of how a database is created for an electronic health record (EHR) (see Chapter 2), we learned that data elements to be collected are clearly defined in a data dictionary and stored in related tables. A key component in using statistics is understanding the data, so we have accomplished that in the previous chapters.

You already know (from Chapter 1) a useful statistical formula: **average length of stay (ALOS)**. ALOS is calculated by taking the total discharge days and dividing it by the number of discharges in the period. ALOS is one of the mathematical ways that we can turn data into information.

### Data Analytics in Health Care

Taking our need for information one step further, we can apply our understanding of data to a broader view of not only the data itself but also what the data can tell us about the organization as a whole and the behavior of its various components. To do this, we use **data analytics**, the process of extracting information from raw data to reveal trends and optimize organizational efficiency. So, instead of just calculating the ALOS or the average cost of treating a patient with a particular disease, we can retrieve all the charges for all of the patients and use that data to show how physicians compare to each other with respect to the cost of care and LOS. We can also use it to evaluate clinical outcomes that result from various treatment protocols. While we are still using statistical concepts, the goal of data analytics is to identify strengths, weaknesses, efficiencies, and inefficiencies in process.

Data analytics is extremely useful for decision support. In an EHR, clinical decision support can assist physicians and other providers with diagnosis, evidence-based treatment options, and pharmaceutical dosing data. For administrators, decision support comes by way of measurements of the success of the organization toward meeting its objectives. Data analysts compile data into information that quantify how well a function is being performed, or how well the organization is achieving its goals. Specifically, administrators obtain timely feedback through **key performance indicators (KPIs)**—predetermined values that tell a story about a function or an organization. Monitoring these day-to-day measurements helps administrators track progress toward organizational objectives, detect problems in efficiency and workflow, and find areas for improvement. For example, we already know how to calculate two important statistical measurements that are often used as KPIs: case mix index (CMI) and ALOS. We know mathematically that CMI tells us the average weight of the cases we have treated, from which we can estimate reimbursement. We know that ALOS is a measure of the resources that we have used to treat patients: beds, staff, and meals, for example. Statistically, the only thing the two measurements have in common is the number of discharges in the period. However, analytically, if CMI measures potential revenue and ALOS measures some of the related expenses, we would expect that they would rise and fall together, if we are being efficient. Higher weighted Medicare Severity Diagnosis–Related Groups (MS-DRGs) reflect more complicated cases and that causes CMI to increase. More complicated cases have higher expected LOS, so the ALOS should rise as well. Therefore, if CMI decreases and ALOS increases, our analysis is that we need to investigate a potential coding or utilization problem. See the Dashboard section for a discussion of how KPIs are monitored.

### Health Informatics

The power of statistics, data analytics, and technology come together in informatics. There are many definitions of informatics, but they all focus on the use of technology. **Health informatics**, also called biomedical informatics, "applies principles of computer and information science to the advancement of life sciences research, health professions education, public health, and patient care. This multidisciplinary and integrative field focuses on health information technologies (HIT), and involves the computer, cognitive, and social sciences" (American Medical Informatics Association [AMIA], 2011). For example, data analytics allows us to identify physicians who, compared to their peers, tend to use more resources and have longer LOS. Informaticists would design applications to collect, retrieve, and analyze this data efficiently, preferably real-time so that interventions with those physicians can be made on a timely basis.

Informatics supports a variety of applications, particularly decision-support systems. A clinical decision-support system (CDSS) delivers on-demand or just-in-time pertinent information to the user. For example, a physician types a dose of 500 mg of a drug for a pediatric patient and a knowledge-based system pops up a red flag telling the physician that this is a lethal dose at that patient's weight. A knowledge-based system can assist the physician to develop a diagnosis based on subjective and objective data it receives. You can see a rudimentary version of this in WebMD at https://symptoms.webmd.com. Nonknowledge-based systems are more useful in retrospect, as they can search for patterns in the existing data, learn from those patterns, and make predictions. So, a knowledge-based CDSS can assist at the point of care to diagnose and treat congestive heart failure (CHF), whereas a nonknowledge-based CDSS can point the physician at a patient who is at risk for developing CHF.

## Health Information Management Role in Analysis

Data analytics and informatics are certainly viable career paths for health information management (HIM) professionals who enjoy working with data and solving problems with data. Even for those for whom statistics, analytics, and informatics are not a chosen career path, the ability to use statistics and basic data analysis is useful for administrative support activities. HIM professionals understand the data, including the optimum source of data and the meaning of coded data. Therefore HIM professionals are uniquely positioned to help answer questions that require retrieval and reporting of collected data. For example, an administrator might want to know what percentage of bariatric surgeries in the hospital are gastric sleeves compared to other procedures. An HIM professional knows which ICD-10-PCS codes represent bariatric procedures and can quickly produce an index of these procedures, sorted by method, and either report the numbers or display the results graphically. This chapter focuses on the skills needed to answer these and other related questions.

is accomplished through the consistent use of forms and data screens to ensure timely, accurate, and valid data, as discussed in the previous chapters. When one is using the data, it is important to understand the source of the data, including the most appropriate source for the purpose.

## Primary and Secondary Data

Primary data come from original sources. They are used in direct patient care, such as patient health records. These data are collected or generated by clinicians while they are treating a patient. The clinician is the original recorder/reporter of the data: the firsthand account of the patient's treatment. Examples of primary data are the history given by the patient to the nurse (Fig. 7.1) and the patient's blood pressure or temperature reading as recorded by the nurse. These data elements are documented in the patient's health record in a format that helps transform the raw data into usable information. Because the data are from the original patient record, they are considered primary data.

Primary data are used when the identity of the patient is relevant to the user or the events recorded in the record are the focus of the review. For example, a physician who wants data for continuing patient care would be interested only in the patient-identifiable data from that specific patient's record. A nurse manager looking for documentation of compliance with protocols would probably need to review primary data.

Another example of primary data is the responses of the patient experience survey. This data is collected from each patient to determine his or her satisfaction with the services rendered.

Secondary data draw on the preexisting primary data for a different purpose. Abstracted data (data selected and reported from the health record) are secondary data and can be sorted and made available in a variety of formats. The compilation of health data for groups of patients is called aggregate data. For example, if we examine our patient

**COMPETENCY CHECK-IN 7.1**

### Disciplines

#### Competency Assessment
1. Define data analytics.
2. What is the difference between data analytics and health informatics?
3. What is a key performance indicator (KPI)?
4. How do KPIs aid administrators in decision support?

## Data Sources and Data Retrieval

To be analyzed in a meaningful way, the data must first be collected appropriately. Appropriate collection of data

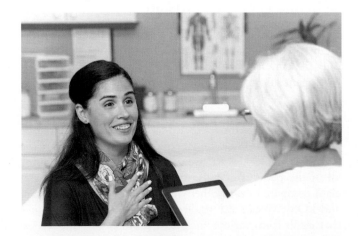

• **Fig. 7.1** Primary data are collected when the nurse talks to the patient to obtain her health history. (Copyright fstop123/iStockphoto.com)

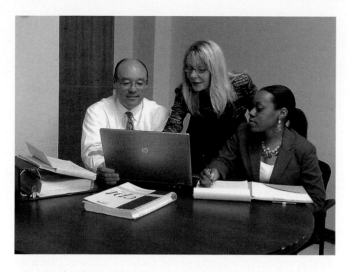

• **Fig. 7.2** As the health information management clerk reviews a health record and enters coded data into the abstract, she is creating secondary data.

records and make a list of patients who had pneumonia, this list is secondary data, aggregated from the primary data. A list of discharges sorted by physician is a physician index. The physician index is aggregated secondary data.

Scholarly articles are secondary sources. Government census data and publicly available mortality data are examples of secondary health data.

Secondary data are used when the identity of the patient is not integral to answering the question at hand. Secondary data may be patient identifiable, if that is appropriate, or may be **redacted** (removed or blocked). A hospital administrator may want to know how many cases of a particular surgical type were performed during a period of time. Although the primary data would be used to produce the abstracted report, the patient-identifying information would not be relevant—it would be omitted from the report. If the report generated from the computer system contains patient-identifiable data, such as name, such data would be redacted from the report before the report was transmitted to the administrator (Fig. 7.2).

Hospital administrators and managers use both primary and secondary data. It is used for monitoring, tracking, and forecasting hospital and departmental activities, for example. Physicians may use such data for tracking volume and outcomes. Questions such as "How many?," "How often?," and "How well?" may be answered through analysis of the appropriate data.

For example, a physician might want a list of patients that he or she treated for a specific diagnosis or with a specified procedure or to answer the questions "Which of my patients had a principal diagnosis of diabetes mellitus?" or "On which of my patients did I perform surgery?" In these cases, the identity of the patients is relevant to the physician, and primary data would be accessed to provide the data. The report itself, however, is secondary data. The report might contain only a list of the patients and perhaps the relevant identification numbers. The report gives no insight into other issues that might be relevant to the cases.

Using secondary data can be problematic. The data were collected for a specific purpose, such as to create a physician-specific list. Even a database of Uniform Hospital discharge data set (UHDDS) data contains only the data that were collected and reported according to UHDDS specifications. If you were studying Medicare patients who underwent hip replacements, you could search the UHDDS data for how many of those patients had a particular diagnosis, but you would not be able to tell whether those patients had an advance directive. You would know whether the patient went home or to another facility, but you would not know to which facility. Even more problematic is secondary data that do not identify the patient. Consider a review of summary data about deaths in your state. You query the database and determine that there were two patients under the age of 16 who died of AIDS-related complications last year. In a de-identified database, there may be no way to learn anything more about those deaths, if that were of interest to your review, because the etiology of infectious diseases was not a data element collected for that database. So, when using secondary sources for answering specific questions, care must be taken to learn exactly what data is available, how it was collected, and for what purpose it was collected. That will inform the user as to the usefulness of the data for their analysis.

Another issue that arises in the use of secondary data, particularly if the data are only partially de-identified, is whether the data can be used ethically. Data collected about humans are protected under a variety of statutes, regulations, and professional ethics rules and may not be usable for another purpose. As we will discuss later in the chapter, there are protocols that must be observed when using patient data. There are large amounts of de-identified data freely available on the internet that may be analyzed. However, as mentioned, care must be taken to understand the data before using it.

## Value of a Database

Because each data element is defined before it is collected, the patient database is a useful source of data for analysis. For example, attending physician is one of the data elements collected. One can collect this data element in the admission record by entering the identification number for the physician who matches the description of the attending physician (see Table 4.1). This data is collected per the specifications in the facility's data dictionary (see Chapter 2) and is reported on the Uniform Bill (UB-04) for each patient discharged. The collection of this data element on all patients in the database using specific, defined criteria makes it possible to **query**, or ask, the database for information specific to the attending physician. For example, facilities should review a representative sample of records on all physicians on the medical staff at the facility when conducting studies of documentation and quality. To do so, the user must be able to run a **report** that lists records for each physician. The ability to query the database on the attending physician data element is therefore quite useful. In addition to documentation and quality studies, such a report might also be part of a review of physician practice patterns, including patient volume.

Obviously, the value in a database is reliant on efficient construction of the data tables, as illustrated in Chapter 2. In addition to ensuring that data are clearly and unambiguously defined in the data dictionary, care must be taken to ensure that the data are not duplicated, that is, collected in two places with the potential of collecting it differently. This typically happens when there are multiple points of service using different systems that must share data in batches as opposed to real-time. For example, the transmission of transcription reports from an independent transcription system requires that the dictator of the report identify the patient in a way that permits matching of the report with the document management system at the facility. The XL7 interchange will match the patient if the physician has correctly relayed the patient name or medical record number (MRN). If there is no match, the report will be stored in a file of failed matches until a human can make the connection.

This issue of potential duplication arises again during the creation of a new form. As discussed in Chapter 2, the development of a paper form for use during downtime or for point-of-care printing for patient signature is the purview of the HIM Committee or its Forms subcommittee. Any new data collection that will have an associated computer screen component must consider the data that is already collected and available for use. So, a new clinical form would never capture the patient's name, for example, because the form should be populated with the existing data.

Database management is a discipline most closely associated with an information systems background. However, due to HIM professionals' intimate knowledge of the data, how it is collected, and how it is stored, database management is a strong potential career path for HIM.

As noted previously, some data are required by the federal government and other payers. However, some data elements are collected only as specified by the facility. These types of data must be collected in the way in which they will be useful in the future. For example, in some cases, the type and frequency of consulting services, such as cardiology and infectious disease, may influence the patient's outcomes and LOS. To collect this type of data (if not already captured), as each patient record is abstracted, the HIM professional identifies consulting services and enters the corresponding physician identifiers into the abstract. Later, the user can access that information in the database in the way that he or she prefers. For example, the user might look at consulting services associated with a specific diagnosis or procedure or with a particular attending physician. Examples of additional data that might be captured are type of anesthesia, length of surgery, and consent details.

An example of other data that may be collected is advance directive acknowledgments. Facilities can include fields containing Yes or No to capture whether a patient has signed the advance directive acknowledgment statement or whether the patient has signed an Advance Beneficiary Notice (ABN), accepting responsibility for charges not payable by Medicare. Copies of the documents themselves would be on file, but their presence is not retrievable as a data field unless specifically captured. This Yes/No field is an example of a **discrete data** point: a named and identifiable piece of data that can be queried and reported in a meaningful way. ICD-10-CM/ICD-10-PCS codes and MRN are also examples of discrete data.

Certain services provided to patients and supplies used to treat patients are not separately payable. However, hospital administration may wish to track such services and items for staff productivity or inventory control purposes. One way to do this is to enter charges to the patient's account that have no dollar amount associated with them. These data, then, would also be available for analysis by authorized users.

The point here is that to analyze data, the data have to be there in the first place and have to be collected in a consistent, organized fashion. We discussed data collection in Chapters 2 and 3, so at this point, you can visualize the examples herein and follow the logic of how to answer specific questions. If you are unsure, you may wish to review those chapters briefly to refresh your memory.

Some examples of routine inquiries of the patient database are as follows:
- List of patients for a physician (Fig. 7.3), often used for recredentialing or audits.
- List of patients by diagnosis, MS-DRG, or procedure (Fig. 7.4), used for a variety of analyses and audits.
- List of patients by patient financial class (Fig. 7.5), for contract negotiations and denials analysis.
- List of patients by age (Fig. 7.6), for review of utilization, staffing, and clinical competence.

Secondary data sources are only as useful as the source of the data from which they are derived and the skill of the individual querying the data. If patient access routinely records incorrect race/ethnicity data by guessing rather than asking the patient, then aggregate reports of race/ethnicity will not be useful. Similarly, a report on all obstetrical cases is incomplete if the preparer only includes deliveries. As a user, it can be difficult to know whether a report is accurate and complete.

One way to double-check is to compare the report to known data from another source. For example, if you are given a report that is supposed to contain all of the patients who were discharged in the month of March, you can compare the total number of patients on the report with the official number of discharges in March that is available from another source, such as a hospital statistical report.

Consider a question asking for a list of all patients with an asthma diagnosis during a specific period. You look at the report and see that all of the patients on the list had a principal diagnosis of asthma. But that was not the question. To list ALL of the asthma patients, the secondary diagnoses have to be considered.

**Diamonte Hospital**
**Discharges by Physician**
**Discharge Date 02/19/20XX**
**Attending Physician:**  Li, Xiaobo

page 1
printed 02/20/20XX

| Admission | Discharge | LOS | Disch Disp | DOB | Age | Gender | Financial Class | Account | Pt Last Name | Pt First Name |
|---|---|---|---|---|---|---|---|---|---|---|
| 02/16/20XX | 02/19/20XX | 3 | 1 | 02/03/1944 | 76 | F | M | 203673 | Anderson | Judith |
| 02/11/20XX | 02/19/20XX | 8 | 3 | 01/03/1943 | 77 | M | C | 203489 | King | Robert |
| 02/18/20XX | 02/19/20XX | 1 | 1 | 09/10/1937 | 82 | M | C | 203741 | Hill | Paul |

• **Fig. 7.3** List of patients by physician from a query to the abstract database.

**Diamonte Hospital**
**Disease Index**
**Discharge Date**
From 02/13/20XX through 02/20/20XX

page 1
printed 02/20/20XX

**Diagnoses**

| Z38.00 | Single liveborn, born in hospital, delivered without mention of Cesarean section |
|---|---|
| Z38.01 | Single liveborn, born in hospital, delivered by Cesarean section |
| Z38.30 | Twin birth, mate liveborn, born in hospital, delivered without mention of Cesarean section |
| Z38.31 | Twin birth, mate liveborn, born in hospital, delivered by Cesarean section |

| Principal Diagnosis | Secondary Diagnoses | | Principal Procedure | Secondary Procedure | Patient Last Name | Patient First Name | Admission | Discharge | LOS | Gender | MS-DRG | MR# |
|---|---|---|---|---|---|---|---|---|---|---|---|---|
| Z38.00 | Z23 | | 3E0134Z | | Johnson | Emma | 02/11/20XX | 02/13/20XX | 2 | F | 795 | 203290 |
| Z38.00 | Z23 | | 3E0134Z | | Williams | Mason | 02/11/20XX | 02/13/20XX | 2 | M | 795 | 203300 |
| Z38.00 | Z23 | | 3E0134Z | | Jones | Sophia | 02/12/20XX | 02/14/20XX | 2 | F | 795 | 203311 |
| Z38.00 | Z23 | | 3E0134Z | | Miller | Noah | 02/12/20XX | 02/14/20XX | 2 | M | 795 | 203314 |
| Z38.00 | Z23 | | 3E0134Z | | Rodriguez | Jackson | 02/13/20XX | 02/15/20XX | 2 | M | 795 | 203331 |
| Z38.00 | Z23 | | 3E0134Z | | Wilson | Ava | 02/13/20XX | 02/15/20XX | 2 | F | 795 | 203332 |
| Z38.00 | Z23 | | 3E0134Z | | Anderson | Ella | 02/14/20XX | 02/15/20XX | 1 | F | 795 | 203360 |
| Z38.00 | Z23 | | 3E0134Z | | Taylor | Ryan | 02/14/20XX | 02/16/20XX | 2 | M | 795 | 203365 |
| Z38.00 | Z23 | | 3E0134Z | | Hernandez | Michael | 02/15/20XX | 02/17/20XX | 2 | M | 795 | 203383 |
| Z38.00 | Z23 | | 3E0134Z | | Moore | Choe | 02/15/20XX | 02/20/20XX | 5 | F | 795 | 203396 |
| Z38.00 | P83.5 | Z23 | 3E0134Z | | Scott | Ethan | 02/17/20XX | 02/19/20XX | 2 | M | 794 | 203703 |
| Z38.00 | Z23 | | 3E0134Z | | Thompson | Sophia | 02/16/20XX | 02/18/20XX | 2 | F | 795 | 203437 |
| Z38.00 | Z23 | | 3E0134Z | | White | Wesley | 02/16/20XX | 02/18/20XX | 2 | M | 795 | 203440 |
| Z38.01 | Z23 | | 0VTTXZZ | 3E0134Z | Allen | Jayden | 02/15/20XX | 02/19/20XX | 4 | M | 795 | 203630 |
| Z38.01 | Z23 | | 3E0134Z | | Smith | Ethan | 02/11/20XX | 02/14/20XX | 3 | M | 795 | 203289 |
| Z38.01 | Z23 | | 3E0134Z | | Brown | Olivia | 02/12/20XX | 02/15/20XX | 3 | F | 795 | 203309 |
| Z38.01 | Z23 | | 3E0134Z | | Davis | Jacob | 02/13/20XX | 02/16/20XX | 3 | M | 795 | 203323 |
| Z38.01 | Z23 | | 3E0134Z | | Garcia | Aiden | 02/13/20XX | 02/17/20XX | 4 | M | 795 | 203327 |
| Z38.01 | Z23 | | 3E0134Z | | Martinez | Isabella | 02/14/20XX | 02/17/20XX | 3 | F | 795 | 203333 |
| Z38.01 | Z23 | | 3E0134Z | | Thomas | Lily | 02/15/20XX | 02/19/20XX | 4 | F | 795 | 203372 |
| Z38.01 | Z23 | | 3E0134Z | | Martin | Owen | 02/16/20XX | 02/19/20XX | 3 | M | 795 | 203416 |
| Z38.01 | Z23 | | 3E0134Z | | Jackson | Charlotte | 02/16/20XX | 02/20/20XX | 4 | F | 795 | 203431 |

• **Fig. 7.4** List of patients by diagnosis.

**Diamonte Hospital**
**Discharge Detail by Financial Class**
**Discharge Date 02/19/20XX**

Financial Class   B   Blue Cross/Blue Shield
                        C   Medicaid
                        G   Managed Care
                        M   Medicare
                        S   Self-Pay

| Financial Class | Admission | Discharge | LOS | Disch Disp | DOB | Age | Gender | MS-DRG | Account |
|---|---|---|---|---|---|---|---|---|---|
| B | 02/15/20XX | 02/19/20XX | 4 | 1 | 02/15/2024 | 0 | M | 795 | 203630 |
| B | 02/17/20XX | 02/19/20XX | 2 | 1 | 12/03/1970 | 49 | M | 153 | 203700 |
| B | 02/16/20XX | 02/19/20XX | 3 | 1 | 02/03/1952 | 68 | F | 069 | 203673 |
| B | 02/13/20XX | 02/19/20XX | 6 | 1 | 08/21/1960 | 59 | F | 330 | 203505 |
| B | 02/17/20XX | 02/19/20XX | 2 | 1 | 05/08/1973 | 46 | F | 743 | 203698 |
| B | 02/16/20XX | 02/19/20XX | 3 | 1 | 03/28/1967 | 52 | F | 378 | 203659 |
| C | 02/16/20XX | 02/19/20XX | 3 | 1 | 07/13/1962 | 57 | M | 379 | 203677 |
| C | 02/11/20XX | 02/19/20XX | 8 | 3 | 01/03/1951 | 69 | M | 885 | 203489 |
| C | 02/18/20XX | 02/19/20XX | 1 | 1 | 12/31/1982 | 37 | F | 770 | 203778 |
| C | 02/13/20XX | 02/19/20XX | 6 | 1 | 01/15/1975 | 53 | F | 745 | 203546 |
| G | 02/17/20XX | 02/19/20XX | 2 | 1 | 03/11/1979 | 40 | F | 775 | 203688 |
| M | 02/15/20XX | 02/19/20XX | 4 | 1 | 06/21/1941 | 78 | M | 864 | 203621 |
| M | 02/13/20XX | 02/19/20XX | 6 | 1 | 12/24/1935 | 84 | M | 378 | 203508 |
| M | 02/18/20XX | 02/19/20XX | 1 | 3 | 02/23/1944 | 75 | F | 809 | 203787 |
| M | 02/16/20XX | 02/19/20XX | 3 | 1 | 06/30/1936 | 83 | M | 195 | 203684 |
| M | 02/19/20XX | 02/19/20XX | 0 | 1 | 11/04/1925 | 94 | F | 313 | 203793 |
| M | 02/18/20XX | 02/19/20XX | 1 | 1 | 11/06/1983 | 36 | F | 885 | 203754 |
| M | 02/11/20XX | 02/19/20XX | 8 | 3 | 04/07/1933 | 86 | F | 179 | 203493 |
| M | 02/18/20XX | 02/19/20XX | 1 | 1 | 09/10/1945 | 74 | M | 244 | 203741 |
| M | 02/11/20XX | 02/19/20XX | 8 | 3 | 08/19/1918 | 101 | F | 945 | 203496 |
| M | 02/14/20XX | 02/19/20XX | 5 | 1 | 08/09/1953 | 66 | M | 189 | 203601 |
| M | 02/12/20XX | 02/19/20XX | 7 | 1 | 11/30/1924 | 95 | F | 242 | 203503 |
| M | 02/13/20XX | 02/19/20XX | 6 | 3 | 08/30/1918 | 101 | M | 280 | 203583 |
| M | 02/13/20XX | 02/19/20XX | 6 | 3 | 01/26/1950 | 70 | F | 640 | 203561 |
| M | 02/16/20XX | 02/19/20XX | 3 | 1 | 12/27/1924 | 95 | F | 379 | 203644 |
| M | 02/13/20XX | 02/19/20XX | 6 | 3 | 03/23/1943 | 76 | F | 871 | 203559 |
| M | 02/15/20XX | 02/19/20XX | 4 | 3 | 09/02/1921 | 98 | M | 872 | 203623 |
| M | 02/13/20XX | 02/19/20XX | 6 | 3 | 12/12/1933 | 86 | M | 872 | 203592 |
| M | 02/14/20XX | 02/19/20XX | 5 | 3 | 11/14/1937 | 82 | F | 256 | 203613 |
| S | 02/15/20XX | 02/19/20XX | 4 | 1 | 07/30/1988 | 31 | F | 766 | 203614 |
| S | 02/17/20XX | 02/19/20XX | 2 | 1 | 02/17/2024 | 0 | M | 794 | 203703 |

**SUMMARY BY FINANCIAL CLASS**

| | | # of Pts | LOS | ALOS | |
|---|---|---|---|---|---|
| B | Blue Cross/Blue Shield | 6 | 20 | 3.33 | |
| C | Medicaid | 4 | 18 | 4.50 | |
| G | Managed Care | 1 | 2 | 2.00 | |
| M | Medicare | 18 | 80 | 4.44 | |
| S | Self-Pay | 2 | 6 | 3.00 | |

• **Fig. 7.5** List of patients by financial class.

**Diamonte Hospital**
**Discharge Detail by Age**
**Discharge Date** 02/19/20XX

| Newborn | 0–30 days | Newborn |
|---|---|---|
| Pediatric | 31–364 days | Infant |
| | 1 year–16 years | Pediatric |
| Adults | 17–30 | |
| | 31–45 | |
| | 46–60 | |
| | 61–75 | |
| | over 75 | |

| Attending Physician Last Name | Attending Physician First Name | Admission | Discharge | Age | Gender | MS-DRG | PDx | Dx2 | Dx3 | PPx | Px2 | Px3 | Account | Pt Last Name | Pt First Name |
|---|---|---|---|---|---|---|---|---|---|---|---|---|---|---|---|
| **Newborn** | | | | | | | | | | | | | | | |
| Nelson | Kathleen | 02/17/20XX | 02/19/20XX | 0 | M | 794 | Z3800 | P835 | Z23 | 3E0134Z | | | 203703 | Scott | Ethan |
| Carter | Brent | 02/15/20XX | 02/19/20XX | 0 | M | 795 | Z3801 | Z23 | | 0VTTXZZ | 3E0134Z | | 203630 | Allen | Jayden |
| **Summary Newborns** | **Number of Patients** 2 | **Total Days** 6 | **ALOS** 3.00 | | | | | | | | | | | | |
| **Adults 31–45** | | | | | | | | | | | | | | | |
| Beard | Kristy | 02/15/20XX | 02/19/20XX | 31 | F | 766 | 0654 | O334xx0 | Z370 | 10D00Z1 | | | 203614 | Allen | Jessica |
| Hernandez | Antonio | 02/18/20XX | 02/19/20XX | 36 | F | 885 | F329 | R4585 | J45909 | | | | 203754 | Robinson | Jennifer |
| Perez | Catherine | 02/18/20XX | 02/19/20XX | 37 | F | 770 | O034 | | | 10D17ZZ | 10A07ZX | | 203778 | Martinez | Luz |
| Marks | Stacey | 02/17/20XX | 02/19/20XX | 40 | F | 775 | O702 | Z370 | | 0DQP0ZZ | 1097ZC | | 203688 | Scott | Donna |
| Shah | Lori | 02/13/20XX | 02/19/20XX | 45 | F | 745 | N898 | D500 | | 0UDB7ZZ | 30233N1 | 05HY33Z | 203546 | Thompson | Karen |
| **Summary Adults 31–45** | **Number of Patients** 5 | **Total Days** 14 | **ALOS** 2.80 | | | | | | | | | | | | |
| **Adults 46–60** | | | | | | | | | | | | | | | |
| Robert | Craig | 02/17/20XX | 02/19/20XX | 46 | F | 743 | D259 | D279 | N736 | 05HY33Z | 0UT00ZZ | 0DNW0ZZ | 203698 | Martin | Linda |
| Edwards | Gabriel | 02/17/20XX | 02/19/20XX | 49 | M | 153 | J101 | Z21 | F17200 | | | | 203700 | Hernandez | John |
| Thomas | Wendy | 02/16/20XX | 02/19/20XX | 52 | F | 378 | K921 | N390 | K862 | 0DJ08ZZ | | | 203659 | Harris | Susan |
| Donozo | Luis | 02/16/20XX | 02/19/20XX | 57 | M | 379 | K264 | R42 | I498 | 0DB68ZX | | 30233N1 | 203677 | Lopez | William |
| Marks | Stacey | 02/13/20XX | 02/19/20XX | 59 | F | 330 | K5660 | N321 | J9571 | 0DTN0ZZ | 0DQB0ZZ | 0DNW0ZZ | 203505 | Jackson | Carol |
| **Summary Adults 46–60** | **Number of Patients** 5 | **Total Days** 16 | **ALOS** 3.20 | | | | | | | | | | | | |

**Diamonte Hospital**
**Discharge Detail by Age**
**Discharge Date** 02/19/20XX

| | | Admission | Discharge | Age | Gender | MS-DRG | PDx | Dx2 | Dx3 | PPx | Px2 | Px3 | Account | Pt Last Name | Pt First Name |
|---|---|---|---|---|---|---|---|---|---|---|---|---|---|---|---|
| **Adults 61–75** | | | | | | | | | | | | | | | |
| Morgan | Randy | 02/14/20XX | 02/19/20XX | 66 | M | 189 | J960 | J441 | F10980 | HZ2ZZZZ | | | 203601 | Wright | John |
| Li | Xiaobo | 02/16/20XX | 02/19/20XX | 68 | F | 069 | G459 | I480 | I69998 | | | | 203673 | Anderson | Judith |
| Li | Xiaobo | 02/11/20XX | 02/19/20XX | 69 | M | 885 | F323 | G20 | I8390 | | | | 203489 | King | Robert |
| Phillips | Todd | 02/13/20XX | 02/19/20XX | 70 | F | 640 | E8352 | N179 | E232 | | | | 203561 | Taylor | Patricia |
| Li | Xiaobo | 02/18/20XX | 02/19/20XX | 74 | M | 244 | I441 | I452 | | Q2H63JZ | 0JH606Z | | 203741 | Hill | Paul |
| Campbell | Jeremiah | 02/18/20XX | 02/19/20XX | 75 | F | 809 | D590 | I425 | E119 | 30233N1 | | | 203787 | Moore | Barbara |
| **Summary Adults 61–75** | **Number of Patients** 6 | **Total Days** 24 | **ALOS** 4.00 | | | | | | | | | | | | |
| **Adults over 76** | | | | | | | | | | | | | | | |
| Stewart | Dennis | 02/13/20XX | 02/19/20XX | 76 | F | 871 | H7290 | N179 | J441 | | | | 203559 | Miller | Frances |
| Baker | Sandra | 02/15/20XX | 02/19/20XX | 78 | M | 864 | R509 | D469 | M069 | 30233N1 | | | 203621 | Young | Richard |
| Turner | Derrick | 02/14/20XX | 02/19/20XX | 82 | F | 256 | E1159 | I96 | E1042 | 0Y6P0Z0 | | | 203613 | Wilson | Virginia |
| Edwards | Gabriel | 02/16/20XX | 02/19/20XX | 83 | M | 195 | J189 | J449 | E119 | | | | 203684 | Clark | Thomas |
| Beard | Kristy | 02/13/20XX | 02/19/20XX | 84 | M | 378 | K2901 | D62 | I425 | 0W3P8ZZ | 30233N1 | | 203508 | Hall | Frank |
| Kabob | Elias | 02/11/20XX | 02/19/20XX | 86 | F | 179 | B59 | I509 | I10 | | | | 203493 | Brown | Mildred |
| Turner | Derrick | 02/13/20XX | 02/19/20XX | 86 | M | 872 | H61009 | J90 | T8584xA | | | | 203592 | Walker | Joseph |
| Gonzalez | Jacqueline | 02/19/20XX | 02/19/20XX | 94 | F | 313 | R0789 | I10 | K219 | | | | 203793 | Jones | Ruth |
| Rigger | Marcus | 02/16/20XX | 02/19/20XX | 95 | F | 379 | K921 | I129 | E119 | 0DJD8ZZ | | | 203644 | Williams | Margaret |
| Parker | Philip | 02/12/20XX | 02/19/20XX | 95 | F | 242 | I495 | N179 | E871 | 0JH606Z | 02H63JZ | | 203503 | Johnson | Dorothy |
| Stewart | Frank | 02/15/20XX | 02/19/20XX | 98 | M | 872 | H902 | I481 | A419 | | | | 203623 | Lee | James |
| Parker | Philip | 02/13/20XX | 02/19/20XX | 101 | M | 280 | I214 | J189 | I959 | 30233N1 | | 02HK3JZ | 203583 | Lewis | William |
| Mitchell | Frank | 02/11/20XX | 02/19/20XX | 101 | F | 945 | Z5189 | B370 | I509 | F07G7ZZ | F08Z1ZZ | | 203496 | Smith | Helen |
| **Summary Adults over 75** | **Number of Patients** 13 | **Total Days** 66 | **ALOS** 5.08 | | | | | | | | | | | | |

| Summary | | Number of Patients | Total Days | ALOS |
|---|---|---|---|---|
| Newborn | 0–30 days | 2 | 6 | 3.00 |
| Adults and Children | | | | |
| Pediatric | 31–364 days | | | |
| | 1 year–16 years | | | |
| Adults | 17–30 | | | |
| | 31–45 | 5 | 14 | 2.80 |
| | 46–60 | 5 | 16 | 3.20 |
| | 61–75 | 6 | 24 | 4.00 |
| | over 75 | 13 | 66 | 5.08 |
| | Total | 29 | 120 | 4.14 |

• **Fig. 7.6** List of patients by age group.

|  | A | B | C | D | E | F |
|---|---|---|---|---|---|---|
| 1 |  |  |  |  |  |  |
| 2 | MS-DRG | 291 - 293 |  |  |  |  |
| 3 | Discharges 02/01/20XX - 02/20/20XX |  |  |  |  |  |
| 4 |  |  |  |  |  |  |
| 5 |  |  |  |  |  |  |
| 6 |  |  |  |  |  |  |
| 7 | MR# | Patient | D/C Date | LOS | Physician | MS-DRG |
| 8 |  |  |  |  |  |  |
| 9 | 056023 | Austin, Dallas | 02/27/20XX | 5 | Angel, M. | 291 |
| 10 | 197808 | Bixby, Helena | 02/12/20XX | 3 | Kabob, L. | 292 |
| 11 | 945780 | China, Dollie | 02/14/20XX | 6 | Chow, A | 291 |
| 12 | 348477 | Combeaus, Plato | 02/02/20XX | 4 | Thomas, B. | 293 |
| 13 | 403385 | Dimaro, Cheri | 02/28/20XX | 5 | Angel, M. | 293 |
| 14 | 471416 | Dondi, Mac | 02/04/20XX | 3 | Thomas, B. | 293 |
| 15 | 362156 | Foster, Dan | 02/22/20XX | 4 | Chow, A. | 291 |
| 16 | 483443 | Lates, Ricky | 02/10/20XX | 6 | Kabob, L. | 292 |
| 17 | 483441 | Smeadow, Shane | 02/01/20XX | 5 | Thomas, B. | 292 |
| 18 | 201801 | Titan, Tami | 02/14/20XX | 4 | Thomas, B. | 293 |

• **Fig. 7.7** List of patients with congestive heart failure shows aggregate data retrieval.

## Data Retrieval

Once a database exists, the data can be used for analysis or comparison. When health information is needed for utilization review (UR), quality assurance, PI, routine compilation, or patient care, the HIM department is asked to retrieve relevant data. With the right instructions on the type of information needed and its intended use, HIM personnel can provide high-quality health information on both individual patients and groups of patients.

### Aggregate Data

**Aggregate data** are a group of like data elements compiled to provide information about a group. For example, a collection of the **length of stay (LOS)** data, the duration of an inpatient visit measured in whole days, for all patients with the diagnosis of CHF would be aggregate data, as shown in the report in Fig. 7.7. Further review of the report shows that the LOS data element for each patient has been retrieved. This report can be analyzed to determine the ALOS and the most common LOS. Sorting by any single data element for each of these patients produces a meaningful list of aggregate data.

Requests for data come into the HIM department frequently. Most of these requests are routine and can be satisfied quickly. Others are more complex and may require some analysis. In either case, the HIM professional needs to record the request in detail, partly to evaluate whether the request can be granted and partly to clarify the exact requirements of the requester. The following details are helpful: the name and contact phone number of the person making the request, the date of the request as well as the date parameters for the information requested, the specific information requested, and the reason for the request. This information helps the person querying the database ensure that the most appropriate information is retrieved from the database and provides an audit trail for **accounting of disclosures**. The facility should have an administrative policy regarding who may obtain data and for what purposes. For example, Dr. Braun may request data on her own patients but not on the patients of Dr. Wong. Residents may need to collect data on their own patients for educational purposes; however, a study involving other patients would require either faculty or possibly **Institutional Review Board (IRB)** approval. The IRB is a committee that is charged with ensuring that research conducted within the facility or by its employees and associates conforms to all applicable rules and regulations. The IRB is chiefly concerned with ethical issues, such as confidentiality and protection of the research subjects. However, other factors like the qualifications of the researchers to conduct a proposed project are also considered.

Data requests should be formatted to ensure clarity and reduce the potential for error. Fig. 7.8 illustrates a sample data request form. Note that the parameters for the report include the time period, the specific data elements requested, and the desired format of the output. In many cases the output format is determined by the system when predesigned reports are used. If it is possible to remove unnecessary data elements prior to delivering the report to the requester, such removal should be done. For example, if patient identity is not required, then patient name and account references should be removed from the report. Most systems provide for custom report design, which may or may not be the responsibility of the HIM department. The ability to identify and extract data from a database is a useful skill that renders the user a more valuable member of the organization. Combined with an HIM professional's knowledge of the underlying data, particularly code sets, this is a desirable skill in his or her practice.

**Hospital name** _____

**Request for data**   Date requested _____   Date needed _____

**Requestor**

      Name _____

      Title _____

      Department _____

This data will be used for: _____

**Data specifications**

      Time period _____

      Patient type (check box)

        □ Inpatient

        □ Outpatient

        □ Both

      Additional parameters (Check all that apply.  If ALL are required, state ALL.)

        □ MS-DRG (specify) _____

        □ Diagnosis (specify) _____

        □ Procedure

           ○ ICD (specify) _____

           ○ CPT (specify) _____

        □ Physician

           ○ Attending (specify) _____

           ○ Surgeon (specify) _____

           ○ Consulting (specify) _____

        □ Other (specify) _____

**Output**

      Data Fields (List all required fields on the report) _____

      _____

      _____

      Media

        □ Word

        □ Excel

        □ Paper

**Delivery (Specify email address or location)** _____

• **Fig. 7.8**   A data request form.

## Populations and Samples

The first step to retrieving appropriate useful information is to identify the population of interest. In health care a **population** can be defined as a group of people identified by a particular characteristic or group of characteristics, such as race, age, gender, diagnosis, procedure, service, or financial class. From hospital data, one can also identify patients by date of admission, date of discharge, charge code, payer, or virtually any data element that is resident in the database. The population, then, consists of all patients with the characteristic under consideration. For example, say we are doing a coding audit and want to review records coded in the first 3 months of the year. Our population would be *all inpatients discharged between January 1, 20XX, and March 31, 20XX.*

The next step is to narrow the data request, if desired. Although some users may want to review all of the patients

in the population, rarely will the user need all of the available data. Therefore the output of the data retrieval must be specified. In many systems, there are preprogrammed ("canned") reports that contain standard output that users would typically need: diagnoses, procedures, admission and discharge dates, gender, age, financial class, MRN, patient account number, and patient name. Customized reports may also be available. For a customized report, it is important to be very specific as to the output desired. The user will get only what the user has specified. Therefore, if the attending physician's name is required, the user must ask for the attending physician's name to be included in the report. A common reason to request data is for surgical case review or UR. For these studies, the population of patients may be based on a diagnosis or the operation that was performed and includes the period under study.

Sometimes, the population is too large to be analyzed. This might happen if the group is too large, such as all of

| TABLE 7.1 | Common Sampling Methods |
|-----------|--------------------------|
| Random | Selection is based on a list of random numbers. Items are sorted and numbered. The sample selection is made by matching the random number to the item number. If the items are unique, such as physician ID numbers, the random numbers can be matched to the items themselves. Selection can also be done with the use of computer software. |
| Systematic | Selection is made by choosing every nth item. Items are sorted in some logical order (e.g., by account number or discharge date). If there are 100 items and 20 need to be reviewed, then select every fifth item, beginning with one of the first five on the list. The first item might be selected randomly by choosing the number out of a hat or asking someone to pick a number between one and five. |
| Stratified | Before sample selection, the items are divided into segments to make sure that the segments are included in the analysis. For example, one might stratify cases by coder for a coding audit, by medical specialty for a documentation quality audit, or by month of discharge for ongoing record review. Once segmented, the individual items may be selected either randomly or systematically. |

the residents of Wyoming, or if the analysis is too time consuming, such as reviewing the coding of all inpatient records in a year. It is usually too expensive for auditors to review a population of 100% of the charts in a month, for example. If the population is too large to review completely, then the analyst will take a sample (subset) of the population. A **sample** is a small representation of the entire population. For example, if there are 1000 discharges in a month, the analyst may review 50 of the records.

For the analyst to make assumptions about the population using only a sample, the analyst must use a *random selection* of cases. In **random selection**, all cases have an equal chance of being selected and the cases are selected in no particular order or pattern. To select a random sample of 50 of the 1000 discharges, the analyst lists the discharges and numbers them (1–1000). A list of random numbers is selected, and each discharge that corresponds to a random number is selected for the sample. Other methods of sample selection may be used, depending on the needs of the analyst. The most common methods are described in Table 7.1.

### Optimal Source of Data

The next matter to discuss with regard to data retrieval is how to ascertain the optimal source of the data. In a well-constructed database, with unique data dictionary definitions, the computer program will have stored the data in only one place. Therefore the data will always be recorded at the best time by the best person, as defined in the data dictionary. For instance, the data dictionary probably specifies that the data element for a patient's name—and most other demographic data—will be recorded by the patient registration department when the patient arrives at the facility. Once the patient's name is recorded at registration, it is available in the system to populate electronic forms for all users. The name is not entered again and again by each user. Similarly, a nurse enters nursing assessments and notes—they are not entered by HIM personnel. The final diagnosis and procedure codes are stored in the system on abstraction and not a second time. For retrieval of a population report of all the patients with a principal diagnosis of pneumonia, there is only one database where the patient's diagnosis is

recorded: in the abstract. Thus writing a query or searching the database requires the user to understand the location of the data.

However, in a paper record or a record with scanned documents, understanding the optimal source of data becomes critical. In many paper environments the same information is recorded multiple times. The patient's admitting diagnosis, for example, is recorded by the admitting clerk; it is recorded on the nursing assessment by the nurse; and it is recorded on the admitting notes by the physician. What is the optimal, most reliable place to determine the patient's admitting diagnosis? It depends on the reason for the review. If one wants to learn why the patient thought he or she was admitted, the initial nursing assessment is probably the most important place to look, because nurses use that question to assess patient education needs. However, if one wants to know the physician's clinical reason for admitting the patient, the physician admitting note or the H&P are better places to look.

Another example of how important it is to identify the optimal source of data is during a survey by The Joint Commission (TJC). TJC surveyors may ask to review specific records (e.g., records of patients who were restrained). This information is not coded, either as a diagnosis or a procedure. From the HIM perspective, several different data elements in the database can indicate that a patient may have been restrained. In an electronic system a special data field can be added to indicate (Yes or No) whether a patient was restrained. If a special data field does not exist, other information in the abstract may help identify patients who were restrained. For example, a certain diagnosis indicates that a patient may have required restraints (e.g., organic brain syndrome or delirium). Optimally, there are appropriate and timely orders, nursing notes describing the application, duration, and monitoring of the restraints, and a restraints log maintained on the nursing unit; still, the surveyors may want to obtain corroborating evidence or to search for missing documentation.

Trying to find the optimal source of data requires knowing the database and knowing how to query it and relate the data elements, as well as a bit of detective work. Sometimes,

Report #1

| | A | B | C | D | E | F | G | H | I |
|---|---|---|---|---|---|---|---|---|---|
| 1 | | | | | | | | | |
| 2 | | FY 20XX | | | | | | | |
| 3 | | Final | | | | | | | |
| 4 | | Rule | FY 20XX | | | | | | |
| 5 | | Post- | Final Rule | | | | | | |
| 6 | | Acute | Special | | | | | Geometric | Arithmetic |
| 7 | MS-DRG | DRG | Pay DRG | MDC | TYPE | MS-DRG Title | Weights | mean LOS | mean LOS |
| 8 | 291 | Yes | No | 05 | MED | HEART FAILURE & SHOCK W MCC | 1.5010 | 4.7 | 6.1 |
| 9 | 292 | Yes | No | 05 | MED | HEART FAILURE & SHOCK W CC | 1.0214 | 3.9 | 4.7 |
| 10 | 293 | Yes | No | 05 | MED | HEART FAILURE & SHOCK W/O CC/MCC | 0.6756 | 2.7 | 3.2 |

Report #2

| | A | B | C | D | E | F | G | H |
|---|---|---|---|---|---|---|---|---|
| 11 | MS-DRG  291 - 293 | | | | | | | |
| 12 | Discharges 02/01/20XX - 02/29/20XX | | | | | | | |
| 13 | | | | | | | | |
| 14 | MR# | Patient | D/C Date | LOS | Physician | MS-DRG | MS-DRG Description | |
| 15 | | | | | | | | |
| 16 | 056023 | Austin, Dallas | 02/27/20XX | 5 | Angel, M. | 291 | HEART FAILURE AND SHOCK W MCC ◄ | =VLOOKUP(F16,$A$8:$F$10,6,FALSE) |
| 17 | 197808 | Bixby, Helena | 02/12/20XX | 3 | Kabob, L. | 292 | HEART FAILURE AND SHOCK W CC | |
| 18 | 945780 | China, Dollie | 02/14/20XX | 6 | Chow, A | 291 | HEART FAILURE AND SHOCK W MCC | |
| 19 | 348477 | Combeaus, Plato | 02/02/20XX | 4 | Thomas, B. | 293 | HEART FAILURE AND SHOCK W/O CC/MCC | |
| 20 | 403385 | Dimaro, Cheri | 02/28/20XX | 5 | Angel, M. | 293 | HEART FAILURE AND SHOCK W/O CC/MCC | |
| 21 | 471416 | Dondi, Mac | 02/04/20XX | 3 | Thomas, B. | 293 | HEART FAILURE AND SHOCK W/O CC/MCC | |
| 22 | 362156 | Foster, Dan | 02/22/20XX | 4 | Chow, A. | 291 | HEART FAILURE AND SHOCK W MCC | |
| 23 | 483443 | Lates, Ricky | 02/10/20XX | 6 | Kabob, L. | 292 | HEART FAILURE AND SHOCK W CC | |
| 24 | 483441 | Smeadow, Shane | 02/01/20XX | 5 | Thomas, B. | 292 | HEART FAILURE AND SHOCK W CC | |
| 25 | 201801 | Titan, Tami | 02/14/20XX | 4 | Thomas, B. | 293 | HEART FAILURE AND SHOCK W/O CC/MCC | |

• **Fig. 7.9** The combination of two reports using the VLOOKUP function in Microsoft Excel. This example assumes that the two "reports" are on the same worksheet.

one has to begin with known data and work backward. For instance, if the chief financial officer wants to know how many fertility treatments were performed in the facility, the user would have to know the procedure codes for fertility treatments to query the system for all of those procedures. The result should be a list of patients, their health record numbers, and the fertility procedures performed. Another requester may want a list of cases for MS-DRG 312 (Syncope and Collapse) and the total charges for each case. The HIM professional might have two preprogrammed reports: one that contains the MS-DRG but not the total charges and another that contains the total charges but not the MS-DRG. If the requester wants both, the professional has to look for a common field—usually the patient account number—and combine the two reports to get what the requester wants. One common task of this nature is the insertion of an MS-DRG description into a report that contains only the MS-DRG itself. Fig. 7.9 illustrates the latter example in which the VLOOKUP function in Excel is used.

## Types of Data

At this point, we need to take our discussion of health data in a mathematical direction. We understand the collection and storage of the data, but now we need to apply that understanding to the statistical analysis of the data. All of

**COMPETENCY CHECK-IN 7.2**

### Consent

#### Competency Assessment

1. What are primary data? Give an example.
2. What are aggregate data? Give an example.
3. What are secondary data? Give an example.
4. Define aggregate data.
5. What is the difference between a population and a sample?
6. What is the best source of the following data:
   a. medications given to a patient
   b. patient's current address
   c. principal diagnosis

the examples given here involve simple arithmetic, but they help the user answer important questions about the data. You may find it helpful to use a calculator or spreadsheet program to follow along and reproduce the example figures.

Once patient data have been collected and stored in a database, reports can be run and the data can be analyzed, interpreted, or presented with various tools. *Interpretation* is an explanation of the data within the context from which it was extracted. The exercises in this chapter contain sets of data that can be used to practice with the calculations

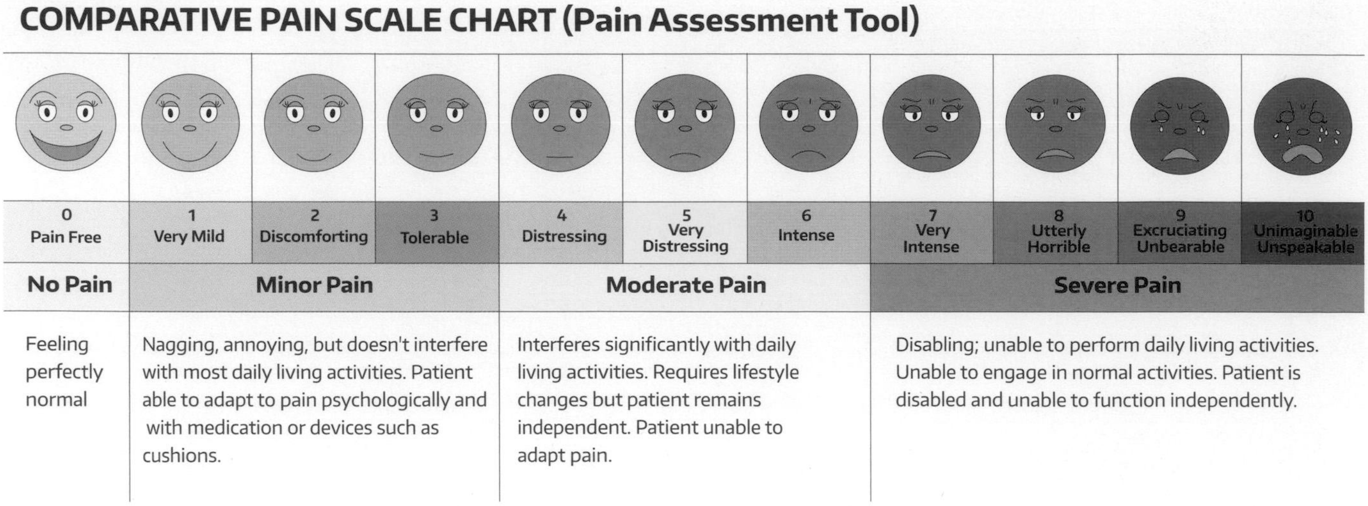

## COMPARATIVE PAIN SCALE CHART (Pain Assessment Tool)

| 0<br>Pain Free | 1<br>Very Mild | 2<br>Discomforting | 3<br>Tolerable | 4<br>Distressing | 5<br>Very<br>Distressing | 6<br>Intense | 7<br>Very<br>Intense | 8<br>Utterly<br>Horrible | 9<br>Excruciating<br>Unbearable | 10<br>Unimaginable<br>Unspeakable |
|---|---|---|---|---|---|---|---|---|---|---|
| **No Pain** | **Minor Pain** | | | **Moderate Pain** | | | **Severe Pain** | | | |
| Feeling perfectly normal | Nagging, annoying, but doesn't interfere with most daily living activities. Patient able to adapt to pain psychologically and with medication or devices such as cushions. | | | Interferes significantly with daily living activities. Requires lifestyle changes but patient remains independent. Patient unable to adapt pain. | | | Disabling; unable to perform daily living activities. Unable to engage in normal activities. Patient is disabled and unable to function independently. | | | |

• **Fig. 7.10** The numbers on a pain scale are ordinal data, where 0 represents no pain at all, and 10 is the most pain possible.

discussed later. Keep in mind that the purpose of the calculations is to derive meaning from the data, in other words, to answer a specific question. Therefore the appropriate calculation must be selected that will provide the desired answer. We will start here by classifying the data that we have collected. Data are classified by their nature and the extent to which they have an actual numeric value.

### Nominal Data

Gender is an example of **nominal data**. Nominal data are categorical because they give a name to each potential observation. The name describes the data. We typically name the categories of gender: Male, Female, Unknown, and Other. An emerging category of data is gender identity. While gender could be defined for data collection purposes as the gender assigned at birth, gender identity arises from the individual's perspective. So, an example of the categories of gender identity beyond male and female could include *gender neutral*. An individual may have been assigned male at birth but identified as female and vice versa. Medicare requires collection of gender as Male, Female, Unknown, and Other. Gender identity is relevant for patient care and inclusion purposes. For data analysis purposes, it is important to understand how gender data is being collected and to ensure that it is being collected consistently. While gender data have a finite number of categories, patient name—another nominal data example—has a seemingly infinite number of categories. Other examples of nominal data in health care are MRN, payer name, race and ethnicity, and marital status. Nominal data have no numerical value, but these can be counted. We can count the number of males at the facility and perform calculations on the sum. We can count the number of females, compare the total to the number of males, and provide a gender profile of the patients who received services. We can count patients by their names. Counting the number of patient records including

Marys or Roberts may not be useful; however, matching two Marys to help determine whether there is a duplicate medical record is extremely useful. Further, nominal data have no logical order. Males are not "better" or "greater" than females. Similarly, Marys are not better or greater than Roberts. Thus there is no sense of order or other empiric value to one category of numeric data over another. That is, there is no arithmetic or sequential relationship between the observations. So, we can count and match categorical data, but they have no inherent numeric or relative value that would give us a sense of hierarchy or worth.

### Ordinal Data

Another type of categorical data is **ordinal data**. Like numeric data, ordinal data consist of descriptive categories. However, unlike numeric data, ordinal data have an inherent hierarchy. An example of ordinal data is the data element *quality* with categories *good*, *better*, and *best*. These categories are descriptive, and they have no numeric value; however, they do have hierarchy or relative value. Although the value of *better* is greater than *good*, there is no measurable distance between *good* and *better* or between *better* and *best*. Another example of ordinal data is a pain scale. A pain scale enables a patient to communicate with the clinician by assigning a number (or happy/sad face) to the patient's subjective level of pain (Fig. 7.10). The depiction of the categories on a line, in order, is called a rating scale. A rating scale is commonly called a Likert scale, named after psychologist Rensis Likert, who developed it.

In the pain scale, while it is obvious that severe pain is worse than mild pain, there is no standard amount of pain that distinguishes level 2 from level 3 or level 5 from level 6, and so on. Further, the numbers assigned to the levels of pain are strictly for naming the levels. There is no relationship between them such that level 6 is three times level 2. Thus ordinal data are descriptive, have ordered categories

**Question**: *How satisfied were you with the overall patient registration experience?*

|  | Number of Responses | Percentage of Responses |
|---|---|---|
| Very satisfied | 150 | 50 |
| Satisfied | 60 | 20 |
| Neither satisfied nor dissatisfied | 15 | 5 |
| Dissatisfied | 30 | 10 |
| Very dissatisfied | 45 | 15 |

In this example, we counted the responses to the question by category, then calculated the percentage of each response.

that have a hierarchy, but there is no fixed measurable value among categories and no inherent numeric value associated with those categories. As with nominal data, we can count the frequency of the categories. Once we have counted the frequency, we can perform some additional analysis, such as the percentage of each category. See Box 7.1. In this example, we might say that 70% (50% + 20%) of patients were either Satisfied or Extremely Satisfied with the overall patient registration experience.

## Interval Data

Nominal data and ordinal data are categorical. They can be counted, but they have no inherent numeric value. Continuous data, on the other hand, are numeric and can take on an infinite array of values. **Interval data** are numeric and ordered and have an infinite array of values. Unlike ordinal data, which have order but no measurable intervals, the distances among levels of interval data are measurable and fixed. Temperature is a classic example of interval data. The distance between 23 and 33°F is the same as that between 55 and 65°F. However, despite their measurable numeric value, there is no true mathematic relationship between the values. So, 25°F is 2°F higher than 23°F. However, 40°F is not twice as warm as 20°F. This absence of a mathematic relationship is because there is no absolute zero. A measurement of zero, in mathematics, is the absence of value. So, for temperature to have an absolute zero, there would have to be a value of no measurable temperature—an absence of temperature. Instead, on a thermometer, zero is just the temperature in the exact middle between −2°F and 2°F.

Because the relationship between temperatures is consistent, we can attribute value to the temperatures themselves. One of the most common ways of analyzing and expressing the interpretation of these integer data is through graphing (see Fig. 2.3).

## Ratio Data

Our final category of data is **ratio data**: true numeric data. Time, weight, dollars, and distance are all ratio data. Ratio data are measurable by some defined standard. They have order and equal space between the levels of measurement. Most important, ratio data have an absolute zero that indicates the absence of value. Therefore mathematic relationships are possible. For example, zero time means that no time has passed or been spent, such as "I spent zero time working on my homework this weekend."

Since it is possible to have spent no time at all on your homework, 4 hours is twice as much time as 2 hours. One hundred dollars is half as many dollars as $200, and so on. We can perform addition, subtraction, multiplication, and division on the numeric values that measure ratio data.

## Common Statistical Analyses

There are a number of common statistical analyses that are performed to understand data. In general, these analyses are performed on ratio data: continuous, numerical values that can have an absolute zero. Some analyses also have limited application to other types of data. We will identify the types of data that can be analyzed with each method subsequently.

## Measures of Central Tendency

One of the most common analyses performed on numeric data is the average. The term *average* generally refers to the arithmetic mean. Average answers the question, "What does the typical case look like?" The requester may ask the following:

- What are the average total charges for patients in this DRG?

**Report of CABG Patients**
02/01/20XX–02/29/20XX

| MR # | Patient | D/C Date | LOS | Physician | Age |
|------|---------|----------|-----|-----------|-----|
| 560230 | Bianco, Helena | 02/07/20XX | 7 | Angelo, R. | 50 |
| 978081 | Chowski, Shane | 02/10/20XX | 8 | Kobob, L. | 53 |
| 045780 | Gombeaux, Glenn | 02/04/20XX | 12 | Chi, A. | 53 |
| 748473 | Phoster, Dodi | 02/12/20XX | 14 | Houmas, C. | 56 |
| 005338 | Sondi, Mac | 02/08/20XX | 8 | Angelo, R. | 59 |
| 671414 | Stephens, Henri | 02/14/20XX | 9 | Houmas, C. | 61 |
| 062150 | White, Jean | 02/20/20XX | 8 | Chi, A. | 62 |

• **Fig. 7.11** A list of patients who underwent a *CABG* procedure can provide data to find the mean age of this group: add all the ages in column 6 and divide by 7; the result, the mean age of this group, is 56 years. *CABG*, Coronary artery bypass graft.

## NOTE

Calculations often result in more decimal places than are necessary or appropriate. For example, the average of 3, 5, 8, and 11 is 6.75: two decimal places more than the source numbers. Sometimes, this many more decimal places is appropriate, such as in calculations of ALOS. At other times, the additional decimal places reflect more detail than is needed.

To reduce the number of decimal places, one can truncate the number. To do so, just remove the unwanted digits. To truncate 6.75 to one decimal place leaves 6.7. However, truncating does not always result in appropriate accuracy. For statistical purposes, we round the numbers.

To round a number, identify the digit immediately to the right of the desired place. In this example, 5 is immediately to the right of 7. To round digits that are 5, 6, 7, 8, or 9, add 1 to the digit on the left. In our example, 6.75 rounds to 6.8. If we wanted only a whole number, 6.75 rounds to 7. This is called *rounding up* because the resulting rounded number is numerically higher than the original number.

To round digits that are 0, 1, 2, 3, or 4, merely truncate. The number 5.34 rounds to 5.3 or 5. This is called *rounding down* because the resulting rounded number is numerically lower than the original number.

|  | A | B | C | D | E |
|---|---|---|---|---|---|
| 1 |  |  |  |  |  |
| 2 | **Calculation of the Mean** |  |  |  |  |
| 3 |  |  |  |  |  |
| 4 |  | 50 |  |  |  |
| 5 |  | 53 |  |  |  |
| 6 |  | 53 |  |  |  |
| 7 |  | 56 | ← | Median |  |
| 8 |  | 59 |  |  |  |
| 9 |  | 61 |  |  |  |
| 10 |  | 62 |  |  |  |
| 11 | Total | 394 | =SUM(B4:B10) |  |  |
| 12 | Total divided by 7 | 56 | =B11/7 |  |  |
| 13 |  | ↑ |  |  |  |
| 14 | Same result: | | =AVERAGE(B4:B10) |  |  |
| 15 |  |  |  |  |  |

• **Fig. 7.12** Using the AVERAGE function in Microsoft Excel.

* What was the ALOS for inpatients last month?
* What is the most common LOS for patients with this diagnosis?

### Arithmetic Mean

The **arithmetic mean** describes what is commonly called the *average of a group of numbers*. Add the sum of the group of numbers, and divide the sum by the number of items in the group. The mean is used to compute a wide variety of averages: LOS, cost per case, or patient age. The question may be, "What is the average age of patients receiving a coronary artery bypass graft (CABG)?" To answer the question, calculate the arithmetic mean. Add the sum of the ages of the group of patients and then divide by the total number of patients in the group. Fig. 7.11 provides a list of seven patients who had a CABG. To find the average age, add all of the ages (50, 53, 53, 56, 59, 61, 62 = 394) and then divide by 7 (394/7 = 56.29, which rounds to 56). The average, or arithmetic mean, age of patients in this group is 56 years. Calculate this easily in Excel using the AVERAGE formula: = AVERAGE(cell range). Fig. 7.12 provides an illustration.

The arithmetic mean is a useful and widely understood measure. It can be calculated meaningfully for ratio data (average age) and interval data (average temperature). It also has limited application in understanding ordinal data. For example, consider the following responses to a presentation: Meeting Evaluation Statistical Uses of Nominal Data Presenter #1 Attendee Responses.

| ◢ | A | B | C | D | E | F |
|---|---|---|---|---|---|---|
| 1 | | | | | | |
| 2 | **Calculation of the Mean with Outlier** | | | | | |
| 3 | | | | | | |
| 4 | | 20 | | | | |
| 5 | | 53 | | | | |
| 6 | | 53 | | | | |
| 7 | | 56 | ← | Median | | |
| 8 | | 59 | | | | |
| 9 | | 61 | | | | |
| 10 | | 62 | | | | |
| 11 | Total | 364 | =SUM(B4:B10) | | | |
| 12 | Total divided by 7 | 52 | =B11/7 | | | |
| 13 | | ↑ | | | | |
| 14 | Same result: | | =AVERAGE(B4:B10) | | | |
| 15 | | | | | | |
| 16 | The outlier (20) drags the arithmetic mean to a value that does not represent the population. | | | | | |
| 17 | | | | | | |
| 18 | | | | | | |

• **Fig. 7.13** Calculation of the mean with outlier.

| Number of Responses | Satisfaction |
|---|---|
| 15 | Very satisfied |
| 12 | Satisfied |
| 10 | Neutral |
| 6 | Dissatisfied |
| 2 | Very dissatisfied |
| 45 | Total responses |

We know that, as categorical data, we cannot perform arithmetic on the "satisfied" responses. We could, however, assign the numbers 1–5 to the descriptions and use those numbers to calculate the "average" response. This assigns a value or "weight" to the responses that is not inherent in the data but provides us with an artificial way to standardize the analysis of the responses.

$5 \times 15 = 75$
$4 \times 12 = 48$
$3 \times 10 = 30$
$2 \times 6 = 12$
$1 \times 2 = 2$
Total score: $75 + 48 + 30 + 12 + 2 = 167$
Average response: $167 \div 45 = 3.71$

The average response of 3.71 has no numerical significance other than to represent that the responses indicate that attendees tended to be satisfied with the presentation. However, as organizers of the presentation, we might develop a guideline that we would not invite speakers again who scored less than an average of 3.5 in the evaluations.

The arithmetic mean is sensitive to **outliers**: values that are very different from most of the other values in the sample or population. Going back to the example in Fig. 7.11, assume that the youngest patient undergoing a CABG procedure was 20 years of age (rather than 50 years of age; Fig. 7.13). In this case the average is 52 years of age. There are no patients younger than 53 years of age in the group, except for the patient who is 20 years of age. Therefore the average of 52 years of age gives an incorrect impression of the patients undergoing CABG procedures. One way to help the user of the information to understand the underlying data is to calculate the median and report it along with the mean.

## Median

The **median** describes the midpoint of the data. The median is often used to help describe groups of data that contain values that are significantly different from the rest of the group. Unlike the mean, which is a formula calculation, the median describes the value in a particular location on a list.

To determine the median, arrange the data in numeric order from lowest to highest and then count toward the midpoint to obtain the median. Using the same group of data from Fig. 7.11, first arrange the data in order: 50, 53, 53, 56, 59, 61, and 62. Because there are seven numbers, it is easy to determine the midpoint. Which number is halfway between 1 and 7? The answer is 4. Thus beginning with the first patient's age (50), count to the fourth patient's age (56). The median age in this group of patients is 56 (the age of the patient in the middle of the list). In this group of patients, the mean and the median are the same. This means that the data are equally distributed on the two sides of the mean and of the median: half of the observations are lower, and half of them are higher. If there is an even number of observations, take the middle two and average them to determine the median. For example, the median of the series 50, 53, 56, and 58 is 54.5: $(53 + 56) \div 2$.

In the example in Fig. 7.13, the mean is 52; however, the median is 56. Without looking at the data, you can tell that the data are unequally distributed around the mean because the middle observation is higher than the mean. In a small example such as this, these values hold no great significance. However, in a set of 300 observations, the data may be so unequally distributed that the mean must be adjusted to describe the data in a meaningful way. Because it is not a calculation, the median can be determined from most data that can be expressed numerically. However, it does not make sense for nominal data because there is no inherent order to nominal data.

### Adjusted Mean

One way to adjust the mean is to remove the highest and lowest observations. In a set of observations containing outliers (values that are very different from the rest of the observation values), this adjustment disregards the outliers and focuses on the observations that are most representative of the group under study. Try this with Fig. 7.13 as an example. Remove observations 20 and 62. This results in a mean of 56 and a median of 56. When this group is being reported, the source of the calculations must be stated so that the user knows what was done with the data to make them meaningful. In a larger group of observations, removing the highest and lowest observations may have no impact if there are multiple outliers. In that case, remove a percentage of the highest and lowest observations. Up to 5% of the highest and 5% of the lowest is generally acceptable. In the absence of policies or conventions, it is up to the presenter (the analyzer of the data) to determine what percentage should be adjusted. However, a clear explanation of the adjustment must accompany the report. It may be useful to provide the report both with and without the adjustment so that the user can see exactly what impact the adjustment had on the reported data. Compare the two reports in Fig. 7.14. Elimination of the three highest and lowest lengths of stay results in a mean and a distribution that more accurately reflect the most common observations. The adjusted mean can be used to analyze interval and ratio data. Unlike the arithmetic mean, it has no real application for ordinal data, because there are inherently no outliers in ordinal data.

### Geometric Mean

The problem with adjusting the mean is that valid cases are omitted from the report. This is problematic when all cases must be taken into consideration. The existence of outliers may be an important factor in the analysis, in which case they should not be ignored. If there are significant numbers of observations to be considered (usually more than 20), the geometric mean may provide a more useful expression of the average than the arithmetic mean. CMS uses geometric mean LOS (GMLOS or GLOS) to describe the expected LOS of patients in individual MS-DRGs. The ALOS and GLOS are both listed, illustrating the impact of outliers in the population on the ALOS.

The **geometric mean** is calculated by multiplying the values times each other and then taking the *n*th root of the product. This calculation is best performed with more powerful statistical software than the Microsoft Excel program provides. However, Fig. 7.15 gives a small example. Note that the arithmetic mean (12.09, which rounds to 12) in this example is not representative of the values in the group. The outliers 64 and 25 distort the arithmetic mean. The median is more representative of the group. The geometric mean (6.84, which rounds to 7) is more representative of the group than the arithmetic mean. The geometric mean is used primarily for ratio data and can be used for interval data. Since there are no outliers in categorical data, it has no relevance to ordinal data. As with the arithmetic mean, it is not used for nominal data.

### Mode

**Mode** describes the number that occurs most often in a group of data. The mode is helpful in the study of the most common observation or observations. It answers questions such as "What is the most common LOS for normal newborns?" Unlike the mean and the median, which have a single value, there can be multiple modes in a group of data. In the list of CABG patients in Fig. 7.11, the mode is 53. All of the other ages are observed only once. In a large group of observations, a mode with many observations may indicate a strong preference or tendency of the group. Because the mode is not a numeric calculation, it is possible that the group will have no mode. The lack of a mode is not inherently important. The mode can be expressed for any data type as it is a measure of frequency rather than any numerical value. We include it in this section because it is often referred to in association with the median and the arithmetic mean. (See the **Normal Curve** section.)

## Measures of Frequency

Measures of frequency are useful in looking at utilization. For example, when examining registration patterns in the patient access area, we may ask the question: "When is the department busiest?" The answer would help with assigning the appropriate number of staff during various times of the day or days of the week. To answer the question, we would count the number of patients registering during each hour of the day. There are a number of ways to express the answer, starting with a frequency distribution.

## Frequency Distribution

A **frequency distribution** answers questions such as "How many patients from each age category were admitted last month?" A frequency distribution is a way of organizing data into mutually exclusive **class intervals** (groups, categories, or tiers that are meaningful to the user). In Fig. 7.11, all of the patients are in their 50s and 60s: two class intervals that might be useful in identifying at-risk patients.

| | A | B | C | D | E | F | G | H | I | J | K |
|---|---|---|---|---|---|---|---|---|---|---|---|
| 1 | | | | | | | | | | | |
| 2 | **REPORTING ADJUSTED MEANS** | | | | | | | | | | |
| 3 | | | | | | | | | | | |
| 4 | **DATA:** | | | | | | | | | | |
| 5 | **Length of stay of 250 patients discharged in March 20XX** | | | | | | | | | | |
| 6 | | | | | | | | | | | |
| 7 | 1 | 2 | 3 | 3 | 3 | 4 | 4 | 5 | 5 | 6 | |
| 8 | 1 | 2 | 3 | 3 | 3 | 4 | 4 | 5 | 5 | 6 | |
| 9 | 1 | 2 | 3 | 3 | 4 | 4 | 4 | 5 | 5 | 6 | |
| 10 | 1 | 2 | 3 | 3 | 4 | 4 | 4 | 5 | 5 | 6 | |
| 11 | 1 | 2 | 3 | 3 | 4 | 4 | 4 | 5 | 5 | 6 | |
| 12 | 1 | 2 | 3 | 3 | 4 | 4 | 4 | 5 | 5 | 6 | |
| 13 | 1 | 2 | 3 | 3 | 4 | 4 | 4 | 5 | 5 | 6 | |
| 14 | 1 | 2 | 3 | 3 | 4 | 4 | 4 | 5 | 5 | 6 | |
| 15 | 1 | 2 | 3 | 3 | 4 | 4 | 4 | 5 | 5 | 6 | |
| 16 | 1 | 2 | 3 | 3 | 4 | 4 | 4 | 5 | 5 | 7 | |
| 17 | 1 | 2 | 3 | 3 | 4 | 4 | 4 | 5 | 5 | 7 | |
| 18 | 1 | 2 | 3 | 3 | 4 | 4 | 4 | 5 | 5 | 7 | |
| 19 | 1 | 2 | 3 | 3 | 4 | 4 | 4 | 5 | 5 | 7 | |
| 20 | 1 | 2 | 3 | 3 | 4 | 4 | 4 | 5 | 5 | 7 | |
| 21 | 1 | 2 | 3 | 3 | 4 | 4 | 4 | 5 | 5 | 7 | |
| 22 | 1 | 2 | 3 | 3 | 4 | 4 | 4 | 5 | 5 | 7 | |
| 23 | 1 | 2 | 3 | 3 | 4 | 4 | 4 | 5 | 5 | 7 | |
| 24 | 1 | 2 | 3 | 3 | 4 | 4 | 5 | 5 | 5 | 7 | |
| 25 | 1 | 2 | 3 | 3 | 4 | 4 | 5 | 5 | 5 | 7 | |
| 26 | 1 | 2 | 3 | 3 | 4 | 4 | 5 | 5 | 6 | 8 | |
| 27 | 1 | 3 | 3 | 3 | 4 | 4 | 5 | 5 | 6 | 8 | |
| 28 | 1 | 3 | 3 | 3 | 4 | 4 | 5 | 5 | 6 | 8 | |
| 29 | 1 | 3 | 3 | 3 | 4 | 4 | 5 | 5 | 6 | 10 | |
| 30 | 1 | 3 | 3 | 3 | 4 | 4 | 5 | 5 | 6 | 125 | |
| 31 | 1 | 3 | 3 | 3 | 4 | 4 | 5 | 5 | 6 | 250 | |
| 32 | | | | | | | | | | | |
| 33 | Mean = Total of all LOS / Number of patients | | | | | | | | | | |
| 34 | =SUM(A7:J31)/250 | | | | | | | | | | |
| 35 | OR | | | | | | | | | | |
| 36 | =AVERAGE(A7:J31) | | | | | | | | | | |
| 37 | Mean = 5.3 | | | | | | | | | | |
| 38 | | | | | | | | | | | |
| 39 | Median = average of 125th and 126th value | | | | | | | | | | |
| 40 | =(E31+F7)/2 | | | | | | | | | | |
| 41 | OR | | | | | | | | | | |
| 42 | =MEDIAN(A7:J31) | | | | | | | | | | |
| 43 | Median = 4 | | | | | | | | | | |
| 44 | | | | | | | | | | | |
| 45 | | | | | | | | | | | |

To illustrate the calculation of the mean using a weighted frequency distribution, the FREQUENCY formula is used below. This is a three-step process.

1. List the categories in numerical order. In this case, all LOS values are listed.
2. Enter the frequency formula in the first Number of Patients cell (in this example, corresponding to the value 1).
3. Highlight the Number of Patients cells, including the one below the last LOS listed. Press F2, followed by Ctrl/Shift/Enter.

| FREQUENCY: | | | |
|---|---|---|---|
| LOS | Number of Patients | Total LOS | |
| 1 | 25 | 25 | |
| 2 | 20 | 40 | |
| 3 | 57 | 171 | |
| 4 | 65 | 260 | |
| 5 | 52 | 260 | |
| 6 | 15 | 90 | |
| 7 | 10 | 70 | |
| 8 | 3 | 24 | |
| 9 | 0 | 0 | |
| 10 | 1 | 10 | |
| 125 | 1 | 125 | |
| 250 | 1 | 250 | |
| | 0 | | |
| | 250 | 1325 | 5.3 |
| Mean = Total LOS / Total Number of Patients | | | |

Because there are 2 extreme outliers (1 patient with an LOS of 125 days and another with an LOS of 250 days), the mean can be adjusted to remove the top and bottom 1%–2% of the cases. See how the mean approaches the median (4) below when the top and bottom 2 cases are removed.

| FREQUENCY: | | | |
|---|---|---|---|
| LOS | Number of Patients | Total LOS | |
| 1 | 23 | 23 | |
| 2 | 20 | 40 | |
| 3 | 57 | 171 | |
| 4 | 65 | 260 | |
| 5 | 52 | 260 | |
| 6 | 15 | 90 | |
| 7 | 10 | 70 | |
| 8 | 3 | 24 | |
| 9 | 0 | 0 | |
| 10 | 1 | 10 | |
| 125 | 0 | 0 | |
| 250 | 0 | 0 | |
| | 0 | | |
| | 246 | 948 | 3.9 |
| Mean = Total LOS / Total Number of Patients | | | |

While 5.3 is the actual mean, it is sometimes useful to calculate an adjusted mean and present BOTH means to illustrate the impact of extreme outliers on the group. One would not report ONLY the adjusted mean, because that would be misleading.

• **Fig. 7.14** Reporting adjusted means data: LOS of 253 patients discharged in March 20XX. *LOS*, Length of stay.

| | A | B | C |
|---|---|---|---|
| 1 | | | |
| 2 | **Calculation of the geometric mean** | | |
| 3 | | | |
| 4 | Discharges 02-09-20XX | | |
| 5 | Length of Stay | | |
| 6 | 25 | | |
| 7 | 64 | | |
| 8 | 5 | | |
| 9 | 5 | | |
| 10 | 4 | | |
| 11 | 5 | | |
| 12 | 8 | | |
| 13 | 6 | | |
| 14 | 4 | | |
| 15 | 5 | | |
| 16 | 2 | | |
| 17 | | | |
| 18 | 12.09 | =AVERAGE(A3:A13) | |
| 19 | 5 | =MEDIAN(A3:A13) | |
| 20 | 6.84 | =GEOMEAN(A3:A13) | |
| 21 | | | |

• **Fig. 7.15** Calculation of the geometric mean.

Five patients are in their 50s; two are in their 60s. This gives us a frequency distribution as follows:

| Age | Number of Patients |
|---|---|
| 50–59 | 5 |
| 60–69 | 2 |

To construct a frequency distribution, organize the data into mutually exclusive equal groups or class intervals (so that no observation can belong to more than one group). All of the observations fit into one of the two groups. Notice that in this example, only two groups are necessary. But the example data could also have been grouped as follows:

| Age | Number of Patients |
|---|---|
| 50–54 | 3 |
| 55–59 | 2 |
| 60–64 | 2 |
| 65–69 | 0 |

❖ **COMPETENCY CHECK-IN 7.4**

**Measures of Central Tendency**

**Competency Assessment**

| Age | LOS | Age | LOS | Age | LOS | Age | LOS |
|---|---|---|---|---|---|---|---|
| 20 | 3 | 34 | 1 | 49 | 1 | 71 | 6 |
| 21 | 2 | 36 | 1 | 50 | 3 | 72 | 6 |
| 21 | 4 | 36 | 2 | 51 | 2 | 73 | 5 |
| 22 | 2 | 38 | 5 | 52 | 4 | 75 | 2 |
| 22 | 2 | 39 | 2 | 55 | 1 | 75 | 3 |
| 23 | 2 | 40 | 2 | 55 | 6 | 76 | 1 |
| 25 | 1 | 40 | 6 | 57 | 1 | 76 | 7 |
| 25 | 3 | 42 | 11 | 60 | 3 | 80 | 2 |
| 25 | 4 | 43 | 2 | 61 | 1 | 80 | 5 |
| 25 | 8 | 44 | 5 | 62 | 1 | 80 | 11 |
| 26 | 2 | 46 | 2 | 62 | 2 | 82 | 2 |
| 27 | 1 | 46 | 5 | 62 | 4 | 83 | 5 |
| 28 | 2 | 47 | 7 | 66 | 3 | 83 | 7 |
| 29 | 3 | 47 | 3 | 66 | 4 | 84 | 14 |
| 33 | 4 | 48 | 3 | 66 | 5 | 85 | 2 |
| 33 | 11 | 48 | 1 | 69 | 4 | 87 | 1 |

Calculate:
1. Mean age
2. Mean LOS
3. Median age
4. Mode of the LOS

**Case Study**

*Over 12 months, an acute care facility compiled a report of the number of patients transferred by month to a neighboring skilled nursing facility*

| J | F | M | A | M | J | J | A | S | O | N | D |
|---|---|---|---|---|---|---|---|---|---|---|---|
| 13 | 4 | 10 | 10 | 11 | 6 | 10 | 12 | 34 | 8 | 9 | 5 |

1. What is the mean number of patients transferred per month?
2. What is the median?
3. What is the mode?
4. Which outliers would you remove to calculate the adjusted mean? What is your calculation?

This second grouping conveys the same data. The second grouping is more informative because it shows that the values are spread fairly evenly across the first three groups; however, there are no patients older than 65 years. Age is one of the criteria for Medicare eligibility. Therefore, if the potential third-party payer is of interest in this set of patients, Medicare is less likely than other payers. Note that the groups have an equal number of possible values. Each group has five consecutive observation values. A frequency distribution should have the lowest number of groups or categories that can present the data informatively. When the number of groups or categories is too large, it is difficult for the user to digest the information. Because it is grouped by counting, a frequency distribution can technically be created for any type of data. For nominal and ordinal data, the class is not an interval but rather the named categories.

## Percentages, Decimals, Rates, and Ratios

There are several common arithmetic ways to compare the relationship between two numeric values. For example, we might want to compare the number of men in the facility to the number of women. The question is "What is the relationship of male to female patients in the period?" The total number of patients in the period is 750, of which 500 are women and 250 are men.

*Ratios* show the two numbers as a fraction, typically reduced to its lowest common denominator. In this example, the ratio of women to men is 500/250, which can be expressed as 2/1 or 2:1. This gives the user a sense of the magnitude of the difference, but it is difficult to work with such a ratio or to compare it with another time period. For example, if the ratio in January is 500/250 and the ratio in February is 489:217, how do they compare?

To make the ratio easier to use, the ratio is converted to a decimal. 500 divided by 250 is 2.0; 489 divided by 217 is 2.25. Thus the ratio of women to men increased from January to February by 0.25.

Often, the actual number of observations is confusing to the user. In that case, it is useful to also provide the **percentage** of observations. Presentation of the percentage standardizes the data so that unlike groups can be compared. To calculate a percentage, divide the number of observations in the category by the total number of observations, and multiply by 100. In the previous example, the ratio in January was 2.0; the ratio in February was 2.25. The number of women in this case is 200% of the number of men in January, and 225% in February. Perhaps a more useful way to look at it is to express the numbers of women and men as percentages of the total number of patients and observe the changes in both figures.

| | January | | February | | |
|---|---|---|---|---|---|
| | Number | Percent | Number | Percent | Change in % |
| Women | 500 | 66.7 | 489 | 69.3 | 2.6 |
| Men | 250 | 33.3 | 217 | 30.7 | −2.6 |
| Total | 750 | | 706 | | |

**TABLE 7.2 Comparing Payer Mix**

| Payer | Hospital A | Hospital B |
|---|---|---|
| **Number of Discharges** | | |
| Medicare | 5000 | 13,229 |
| Medicaid | 2300 | 6032 |
| Blue Cross/Blue Shield | 1500 | 3975 |
| Commercial carriers | 950 | 2453 |
| Charity care | 500 | 1423 |
| Self-pay | 125 | 367 |
| Other payers | 90 | 325 |
| Total discharges | 10,465 | 27,804 |
| **Percentage of Discharges** | | |
| Medicare | 47.8 | 47.6 |
| Medicaid | 22 | 21.7 |
| Blue Cross/Blue Shield | 14.3 | 14.3 |
| Commercial carriers | 9.1 | 8.8 |
| Charity care | 4.8 | 5.1 |
| Self-pay | 1.2 | 1.3 |
| Other payers | 0.9 | 1.2 |
| Total discharges | 100 | 100 |

In Fig. 7.11 as an example, the percentages in each group are as follows:

| Age | Number of Patients | Calculation | Percentage |
|---|---|---|---|
| 50–54 | 3 | $3/7 \times 100 =$ | 42.86 |
| 55–59 | 2 | $2/7 \times 100 =$ | 28.57 |
| 60–64 | 2 | $2/7 \times 100 =$ | 28.57 |
| 65–69 | 0 | $0/7 \times 100 =$ | 0.00 |
| Total | 7 | – | 100.00 |

Percentages help the user compare observations in different time periods and when the group under study varies in size from the group to which it is being compared. For example, Table 7.2 compares the number of Medicare patients in Hospital A with the number in Hospital B. The actual numbers of patients are not comparable; however, the percentages show that the hospitals are very similar in the mix of payers.

Percentages are commonly used and can be applied to any type of data or frequency distribution. One of the most common errors in calculating percentage is to forget to multiply by 100. To check your work, always add up the percentages in your table to ensure that the total is 100%. That ensures that you have included all of the data you are analyzing and that you have probably calculated all of the percentages correctly.

Rates are comparisons of two numbers that are measured with *different* units of measurement, calculated as a numerator divided by a denominator. For example, the facility could compare the dollars in DRG reimbursement for each DRG, the unit would be *dollars per case*. The HIM department wants to know how many charts can be coded in a day, creating a rate of charts per day. Note that this is different than ratios that are expressed as simply one number compared to another, because in ratios the units of measure are the same.

Rates are common in health statistics and data analytics, both at the facility level and when looking at nationwide public health data. Because there is often an element of time involved, a facility frequently uses rates in its KPIs. For any given month or year, it might examine birth rates, death rates, rates of infection, and rates the physicians consulted with one another—just to name a few. Later in this chapter, we discuss the kinds of rates used for benchmarking.

### COMPETENCY CHECK-IN 7.5
**Measures of Frequency**

**Competency Assessment**

1. How do percentages facilitate data analysis?
2. What is a frequency distribution?
3. While looking at the salaries of hospitalists in the facility, you find a range from a low of $75,000 to a high of $150,000. How many categories would you have if you broke them into intervals of $5000?
4. If there are 1000 discharges in a month and the hospital treats patients of all ages, what is the most useful class interval to show the distribution of patients by age?
5. There were 400 Medicare patients last month out of a total of 945 discharges. Express the frequency of Medicare patients as a ratio, decimal, and percentage of total discharges.
6. Your department has budgeted for 2 sets of references for every 5 coders. Recently, a reorganization moved all of the coding to your hospital and now there are 25 coders. How many sets of references will you need?
7. Prepare a frequency distribution from the data set for patient ages in Competency Check-In 7.4.

## Measures of Variance

The difference between a benchmark or goal and the actual result or observation is a *variance*. If a facility expected 1000 admissions in May and there were 1200, then there is a variance of 200 admissions. The variance could be expressed as a number (200) or as a percentage (20%). Managers review and analyze these arithmetic variances to monitor results and take corrective action when results do not meet expectations. One routine review and analysis is financial:

how much did the department spend on supplies compared with the amount that was budgeted (predicted and authorized in advance)?

Comparing one value against another is a simple arithmetic calculation; however, it is limited in application. Certainly, one could list all the variances noted during the year and look at the trend (how the variances behave over time). If the variance in the cost of supplies is 20% over budget every month, some review of the budget preparation and the use of supplies should take place to determine the problem and develop a solution. Similarly, if bed occupancy is rising every month, administration will investigate whether the trend is seasonal or otherwise temporary versus a permanent change. Greater insight into the behavior of the observed values can be obtained by looking at the distribution of the values and their relationship to the arithmetic mean.

### Normal Curve

The distribution of values in multiple samples may be very different from one group of observations to the next. So the observations of patient ages during 1 week may be very different from the observations of patient ages during another week. Neither group of observations may be truly representative of the distribution of ages in the entire patient population. However, if one takes the arithmetic mean of each of those groups and displays the frequency distribution of those means, that frequency distribution approaches symmetry. A picture of such a distribution is called a normal curve. In a normal curve the observations are evenly distributed about the mean. The mean, median, and mode are equal. Note that the organization of the data is a frequency distribution of the values. This assumption of symmetry in the distribution of the means is called the central limit theorem. A set of observations that approaches a normal curve is illustrated in Fig. 7.16.

### Skewedness

Frequency distributions that are not symmetric are skewed. This skewedness might occur when a very small sample is taken and the observations do not truly reflect the population as a whole. For example, a review of coding using a sample of five cases out of 1000 may not yield results that are typical of the population. Nevertheless, a skewed distribution may truly represent the population. One would expect the ages of Medicare patients to be skewed, for example, since there are many more Medicare patients over the age of 65 than under.

### Standard Deviation

Another commonly used measure of variance is the standard deviation. The standard deviation describes how closely the observations are distributed around the mean. The higher the standard deviation, the more loosely the observations are distributed. Fig. 7.17 illustrates that 68.2% of observations fall within one standard deviation of the

| | A | B | C | D | E | F | G | H | I | J | K |
|---|---|---|---|---|---|---|---|---|---|---|---|
| 1 | | | | | | | | | | | |
| 2 | | | | | | | | | | | |
| 3 | | | | | | | | | | | |
| 4 | DATA: | | | | | | | | | | |
| 5 | Length of stay of 250 patients discharged in April 20XX | | | | | | | | | | |
| 6 | | | | | | | | | | | |
| 7 | 1 | 2 | 3 | 3 | 3 | 4 | 4 | 5 | 5 | 6 | |
| 8 | 1 | 2 | 3 | 3 | 3 | 4 | 4 | 5 | 5 | 6 | |
| 9 | 1 | 2 | 3 | 3 | 4 | 4 | 4 | 5 | 5 | 6 | |
| 10 | 1 | 2 | 3 | 3 | 4 | 4 | 4 | 5 | 5 | 6 | |
| 11 | 1 | 3 | 3 | 3 | 4 | 4 | 4 | 5 | 5 | 6 | |
| 12 | 1 | 3 | 3 | 3 | 4 | 4 | 4 | 5 | 5 | 6 | |
| 13 | 1 | 3 | 3 | 4 | 4 | 4 | 4 | 5 | 5 | 6 | |
| 14 | 1 | 3 | 3 | 4 | 4 | 4 | 4 | 5 | 5 | 6 | |
| 15 | 1 | 3 | 3 | 4 | 4 | 4 | 4 | 5 | 5 | 6 | |
| 16 | 2 | 3 | 3 | 4 | 4 | 4 | 4 | 5 | 5 | 6 | |
| 17 | 2 | 3 | 3 | 4 | 4 | 4 | 5 | 5 | 5 | 6 | |
| 18 | 2 | 3 | 3 | 4 | 4 | 4 | 5 | 5 | 5 | 6 | |
| 19 | 2 | 3 | 3 | 4 | 4 | 4 | 5 | 5 | 5 | 7 | |
| 20 | 2 | 3 | 3 | 4 | 4 | 4 | 5 | 5 | 5 | 7 | |
| 21 | 2 | 3 | 3 | 4 | 4 | 4 | 5 | 5 | 5 | 7 | |
| 22 | 2 | 3 | 3 | 4 | 4 | 4 | 5 | 5 | 5 | 7 | |
| 23 | 2 | 3 | 3 | 4 | 4 | 4 | 5 | 5 | 6 | 7 | |
| 24 | 2 | 3 | 3 | 4 | 4 | 4 | 5 | 5 | 6 | 7 | |
| 25 | 2 | 3 | 3 | 4 | 4 | 4 | 5 | 5 | 6 | 8 | |
| 26 | 2 | 3 | 3 | 4 | 4 | 4 | 5 | 5 | 6 | 8 | |
| 27 | 2 | 3 | 3 | 4 | 4 | 4 | 5 | 5 | 6 | 8 | |
| 28 | 2 | 3 | 3 | 4 | 4 | 4 | 5 | 5 | 6 | 8 | |
| 29 | 2 | 3 | 3 | 4 | 4 | 4 | 5 | 5 | 6 | 10 | |
| 30 | 2 | 3 | 3 | 4 | 4 | 4 | 5 | 5 | 6 | 12 | |
| 31 | 2 | 3 | 3 | 4 | 4 | 4 | 5 | 5 | 6 | 15 | |
| 32 | | | | | | | | | | | |
| 33 | Mean = Total of all LOS / Number of patients | | | | | | | | | | |
| 34 | =SUM(A7:J31)/250 | | | | | | | | | | |
| 35 | OR | | | | | | | | | | |
| 36 | =AVERAGE(A7:J31) | | | | | | | | | | |
| 37 | Mean = 4.144 | | | | | | | | | | |
| 38 | | | | | | | | | | | |
| 39 | | | | | | | | | | | |
| 40 | =STDEVP(A7:J31) | | | | | | | | | | |
| 41 | Standard Deviation = 1.66 | | | | | | | | | | |
| 42 | | | | | | | | | | | |
| 43 | | | | | | | | | | | |
| 44 | | | | | | | | | | | |
| 45 | | | | | | | | | | | |

| LOS | Frequency | % of Total Patients |
|---|---|---|
| 1 | 9 | 3.6% |
| 2 | 20 | 8.0% |
| 3 | 54 | 21.6% |
| 4 | 77 | 30.8% |
| 5 | 56 | 22.4% |
| 6 | 21 | 8.4% |
| 7 | 6 | 2.4% |
| 8 | 4 | 1.6% |
| 9 | 0 | 0.0% |
| 10 | 1 | 0.4% |
| 12 | 1 | 0.4% |
| 15 | 1 | 0.4% |
| | 0 | |
| TOTAL Patients | 250 | |

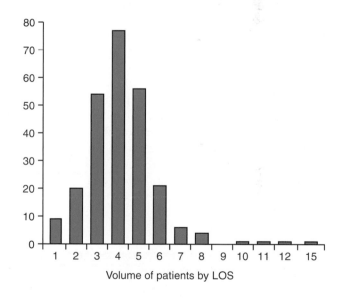

Volume of patients by LOS

• **Fig. 7.16** The frequency distribution of these observations approaches a normal curve. *LOS,* Length of stay.

mean, an additional 27.2% (total 95.4%) falls within two standard deviations of the mean, and an additional 4.2% (total 99.6%) falls within three standard deviations of the mean. Note in Fig. 7.17 that the standard deviation is represented by the symbol $\sigma$ (lowercase Greek sigma).

The standard deviation can be used to illustrate the extent to which an observation is different from the mean. This is useful for analyzing both clinical and financial data. For example, the ALOS of patients of a particular physician is 7 days, compared with the mean of 4 days for similar patients,

• **Fig. 7.17** Diagram of standard deviation.

varying greatly from the mean. It is not enough to say that the physician's patients on average stay 3 days longer than other patients, because there may be many physicians whose patients also stay 7 days. However, if the standard deviation of ALOS for these patients is 0.5, then an ALOS of 7 days is more than 3 standard deviations from the mean of 4 ($4 + 0.5\sigma + 0.5\sigma + 0.5\sigma = 5.5$): higher than 99.6% of all of the other physicians. The ALOS for these patients is tightly grouped from 2.5 to 5.5 days. In another example, if the total charges for a patient in MS-DRG 292 (Heart Failure and Shock with CC) are $65,000 and the mean for all patients in MS-DRG 292 is $50,000 with a standard deviation of $10,000, then the charges of $65,000 are only $1.5\sigma$ from the mean. In this case, 99.6% of the cases had total charges ranging from $20,000 to $80,000, a very loose distribution around the mean.

To calculate the standard deviation of a set of values, it is easiest to use a spreadsheet program. In Excel, for example, the formula for a sample standard deviation is =stdev([range of values]), as illustrated in Fig. 7.16.

## Routine Institutional Statistics

As discussed in Chapter 1, there are a number of ways to describe and distinguish among health care facilities. Analysis, interpretation, and presentation of data provide statistics that further identify a facility and its activities. Fig. 7.18 contains a list of important statistics for Community Hospital for the year 20XX.

## Admissions

Health care organizations always maintain statistics on the number of patients who are admitted to the facility. Review Fig. 7.18 to identify the number of patients admitted to Community Hospital during 20XX: 14,400 adults and children. The number of adults and children (14,400) does not include the number of newborn (NB) patients admitted (960). Unless otherwise specified, statistics for NBs are recorded separately from those of adults and children because the NBs are admitted to the facility for the purpose of being born. Even though an NB may be ill, that is not the

---

**◆ COMPETENCY CHECK-IN 7.6**

**Measures of Variance**

**Competency Assessment**

1. What is a normal curve?
2. What is the relationship between a normal curve and measures of central tendency?
3. What causes a frequency curve to skew?
4. What questions does standard deviation answer?
5. 50 patients were treated at the free clinic last week. Their ages are listed from youngest to oldest: 14, 15, 15, 15, 16, 16, 17, 17, 18, 18, 18, 18, 18, 18, 19, 19, 19, 19, 20, 20, 20, 21, 21, 21, 22, 22, 24, 24, 24, 25, 26, 26, 26, 27, 28, 30, 31, 32, 36, 40, 41, 41, 47, 52, 52, 59, 59, 60, 65, 72.
   a. Calculate the standard deviation.
   b. Calculate the arithmetic mean.
   c. Determine the median.
   d. What is the mode?
   e. Comment on the curve that represents this distribution.
   f. If this distribution represented the LOS of patients in a rehabilitation facility following a particular type of cerebrovascular accident with similar impairments, what questions would you have?

| ADMISSIONS | | |
|---|---|---|
| Adults & children | 14,400 | Total number of adults and children admitted during the year |
| Newborns | 960 | Total number of babies born in the hospital during the year |
| | | |
| **DISCHARGES (including deaths)** | | |
| Adults & children | 14,545 | Total number of adults and children discharged during the year |
| Newborns | 950 | Total number of newborns discharged during the year |
| | | |
| **INPATIENT SERVICE DAYS** | | Number of days of service rendered by the hospital |
| Adults & children | 75,696 | to adults and children |
| Newborns | 1993 | to newborns |
| | | |
| **TOTAL LENGTH OF STAY** | | Sum of all the individual lengths of stay of |
| Adults & children | 72,107 | all adults and children discharged during the year |
| Newborns | 1974 | all newborns discharged during the year |
| | | |
| **BED COUNT** | | |
| Adults & children | 220 | Number of beds staffed, equipped, and available |
| Bassinets | 20 | Number of bassinets staffed, equipped, and available |
| | | |
| **MORTALITY DATA** | | Deaths (these numbers are included in Discharges, above) |
| Total adults & children | | |
| Under 48 hours | 20 | Total adult and child deaths within 48 hours of admission |
| Over 48 hours | 138 | Total adult and child deaths 48 hours after admission |
| Total newborns | | |
| Under 48 hours | 3 | Total newborn deaths within 48 hours of admission |
| Over 48 hours | 2 | Total newborn deaths 48 hours after admission |
| Anesthesia deaths | 1 | Number of patients who died after receiving anesthesia |
| | | |
| **OPERATIONS** | | |
| Number of patients operated on | 1200 | Number of patients on whom operations were performed |
| Surgical operations performed | 1312 | Number of individual surgical procedures performed |
| Anesthesia administered | 1200 | Number of individual administrations of anesthesia |
| Postoperative infections | 30 | Number of patients who developed infections as a result of their surgical procedures |
| | | |
| **OTHER DATA** | | |
| Nosocomial infections | 231 | Number of patients who developed infections in the hospital |
| Cesarean sections | 303 | Number of deliveries performed by cesarean section |
| Deliveries | 1304 | Number of women who gave birth in the hospital |

• **Fig. 7.18** Community Hospital's 20XX year-end statistics.

reason for his or her admission. A birth is an admission, and a health record is created for each NB at birth.

## Discharges

Health care facilities also maintain statistics on the number of patients leaving the facility. The second item in Fig. 7.18 is discharges. Once again, the NBs are listed separately from the adults and children. Note that the discharges include deaths, because death is, effectively, a discharge. Because the number of deaths is important for statistical purposes, they are also listed. The usual way a patient is discharged is by discharge order from the physician. A transfer to a different facility is another discharge. Other ways include leaving against medical advice. Refer to Table 3.3 for a list of possible discharge dispositions. Discharge disposition is a discrete data point that can be queried for reporting purposes. It might answer these questions: How many patients with CHF were discharged to home? How many septicemia patients expired?

It should be noted that an individual who arrives at the facility already deceased (also known as *dead on arrival*, or *DOA*) is not counted as an admission and is therefore not a discharge. The DOA may, however, be included in certain autopsy rates, if the autopsy is performed by a hospital pathologist.

## Length of Stay

The time that a patient spends in a facility is called the *LOS*. LOS is the measurement, in whole days, of the time between admission and discharge. Fig. 7.19 illustrates

Length of Stay

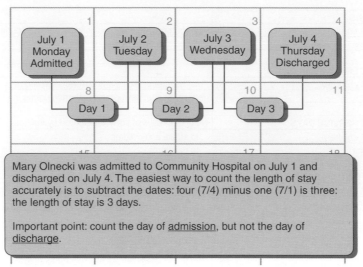

Mary Olnecki was admitted to Community Hospital on July 1 and discharged on July 4. The easiest way to count the length of stay accurately is to subtract the dates: four (7/4) minus one (7/1) is three: the length of stay is 3 days.

Important point: count the day of <u>admission</u>, but not the day of <u>discharge</u>.

• **Fig. 7.19** Calculation of length of stay within a calendar month.

how to calculate a patient's LOS. For example: A patient enters the facility on Monday, July 1, and is discharged on Thursday, July 4. The easiest way to calculate the LOS is to subtract the dates. Four minus one is three; therefore the LOS is 3 days.

It is important to note that when determining the LOS, one counts the day of admission but not the day of discharge. The times of admission and discharge are irrelevant to the calculation of inpatient LOS. In the previous example the patient is considered to have stayed in the hospital for 3 days: July 1, July 2, and July 3. On July 4, the patient is no longer there. This is a fairly easy calculation when the patient enters and leaves the facility during the same month because one can just subtract the dates of the month.

To calculate LOS if the patient enters and leaves the facility in different months, it is important to know how many days there are in a month. Four months have 30 days: April, June, September, and November. February has 28 days, except in leap years (every 4 years), when it has 29 days. All of the other months have 31 days.

If you have trouble remembering how many days there are in a particular month, try creating a mnemonic. Using the first letters of each of the 30-day months, create a silly sentence that will help you associate them. You will want to use April and June in the sentence, because there are other months that begin with those letters. For example: "April and June are Not Summer" or "April's Sister is Not June." As a child, you may have learned the jingle "Thirty days hath September, April, June, and November; all the rest have 31, except February alone, which has 28 in time, and each leap year 29."

So, if the patient enters the hospital in July and leaves in August, three calculations are required:

*Step 1:* Calculate how many days the patient was there in July.

*Step 2:* Calculate how many days the patient was there in August.

*Step 3:* Add the Step 1 and Step 2 results to obtain the total days.

Fig. 7.20 gives an example of this calculation. The patient is admitted on July 26 and discharged on August 6.

*Step 1:* The patient is in the hospital in July for 6 days. Remember to count the day of admission.

*Step 2:* The stay in August is only 5 days because the day of discharge does not count.

*Step 3:* Add the 6 days in July to the 5 days in August.

*Result:* The LOS for this patient is 11 days.

It is sometimes necessary to calculate LOS manually. In an electronic environment, however, a spreadsheet program can calculate this type of information for you. In a spreadsheet program, such as Excel, it is easy to subtract the two dates and format the result as a number. Fig. 7.21 shows the formula for subtracting two dates in Microsoft Excel.

## Average Length of Stay

LOS is very important in defining the type of facility and in analyzing its patient population. ALOS is the arithmetic mean of all the patients' LOSs within a certain period, calculated by adding up the LOSs for a group of patients and dividing by the number of patients in the group. Consider a list of patients in an acute care facility using patients who were discharged in July as an example:

| | |
|---|---|
| Patient A | 4 days |
| Patient B | 2 days |
| Patient C | 10 days |
| Patient D | 32 days |
| Patient E | 7 days |
| **Total** | **55 days** |

ALOS: 55 days ÷ 5 patients = 11 days

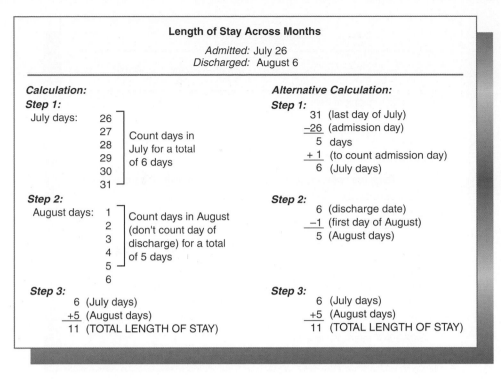

**Length of Stay Across Months**

*Admitted:* July 26
*Discharged:* August 6

**Calculation:**

**Step 1:**
July days: 26
27
28    Count days in
29    July for a total
30    of 6 days
31

**Step 2:**
August days: 1
2    Count days in August
3    (don't count day of
4    discharge) for a total
5    of 5 days
6

**Step 3:**
6 (July days)
+5 (August days)
11 (TOTAL LENGTH OF STAY)

**Alternative Calculation:**

**Step 1:**
31 (last day of July)
−26 (admission day)
5 days
+ 1 (to count admission day)
6 (July days)

**Step 2:**
6 (discharge date)
−1 (first day of August)
5 (August days)

**Step 3:**
6 (July days)
+5 (August days)
11 (TOTAL LENGTH OF STAY)

• **Fig. 7.20** Calculation of length of stay across calendar months.

|  | A | B | C | D |
|---|---|---|---|---|
| 1 |  |  |  |  |
| 2 |  | **Calculating Length of Stay Using Microsoft Excel** |  |  |
| 3 |  |  |  |  |
| 4 |  | Admission Date | 09/15/2020 |  |
| 5 |  |  |  |  |
| 6 |  | Discharge Date | 11/04/2020 |  |
| 7 |  |  |  |  |
| 8 |  | Length of Stay | 19/02/1900 |  |
| 9 |  |  |  |  |
| 10 |  | The formula in cell C8 is: | =C6-C4 |  |
| 11 |  |  |  |  |

|  | A | B | C | D |
|---|---|---|---|---|
| 1 | Admit | Discharge | LOS |  |
| 2 | 26-Jul | 6-Aug | 11 |  |
| 3 |  |  | =B2-A2 |  |
| 4 |  |  |  |  |

If you enter the formula without reformatting the cell, the result will be 2/19/1900. This is because Microsoft Excel stores dates as numbers with 1/1/1900 as the first date in the series. By subtracting two dates, the result cell (C8) carries forward the date format. In order to show the actual number of days, be sure to format the cell (in this case, C8) as a Number.

To double-check the results:

Count 16 days in September (30 minus 15, plus 1)

31 days in October

3 days in November

Total: 50

• **Fig. 7.21** Formula for subtracting two dates in Microsoft Excel to calculate length of stay (LOS).

**Intrahospital Transfers**

| | Unit A | Unit B | Total |
|---|---|---|---|
| 05/31/20XX midnight census | 3 | 2 | 5 |
| Transfers in | +1 | +2 | +3 |
| Transfers out | −2 | −1 | −3 |
| 06/01/20XX midnight census | 2 | 3 | 5 |

*Transfers between Units A and B have no impact on census*

Here is a table that reflects the same information:

| | Unit A | Unit B | Total |
|---|---|---|---|
| 06/01/20XX midnight census | 3 | 2 | 5 |
| Admissions | +2 | 0 | +2 |
| Discharges | −2 | −1 | −3 |
| 06/02/20XX midnight census | 3 | 1 | 4 |

• **Fig. 7.22** Intrahospital transfers.

As shown, the total LOS of all the patients combined is 55 days. Fifty-five days divided by 5 patients gives the average number of days, 11 days.

Usually, ALOS is calculated monthly or annually or in some relevant period. ALOS might also be calculated by medical specialty, and it can even be calculated in terms of a specific physician's practice. These calculations are useful in determining whether a physician or a particular medical specialty conforms to the average in a particular hospital or is higher or lower in terms of ALOS.

One of the characteristics of an acute care facility is that the ALOS of its patient population is less than 30 days. In reality, the ALOS of an acute care facility may be significantly less than that, depending on what type of patients it treats. For example, a community hospital with a large number of mothers and NBs, whose stay in the facility is generally 1–3 days, will tend to have a very low ALOS-perhaps only 4 or 5 days. On the other hand, a trauma center hospital with a large number of patients with serious trauma, burns, and transplants might have an ALOS closer to 12 or 13 days.

## Transfers

Patients can be transferred from one unit to another inside a facility, or they can be discharged and transferred to another facility. When a patient is transferred internally, there is no impact on the overall census or on the total admissions or discharges for the day. However, the transfer does affect the census on the nursing units from which the patient was transferred and to which the patient was transferred.

In the following example, two patients from Unit C were transferred: one to Unit A and one to Unit B. This did not affect the total number of patients in the hospital; it only affected the number of patients on the individual units.

| | **Patient Care Units** | | | |
|---|---|---|---|---|
| | Unit A | Unit B | Unit C | Unit D |
| Beginning | 4 | 6 | 8 | 18 |
| Admissions | +2 | +3 | +1 | +6 |
| Discharges | −1 | −2 | 0 | −3 |
| Unit transfers | +1 | +1 | −2 | 0 |
| Ending midnight census | 6 | 8 | 7 | 21 |

The transfer of a patient to another facility requires the transfer of sufficient information to support effective continuity of care. A special transfer form is used, and copies of all or part of the health record may accompany the patient. The receiving hospital (the hospital to which the patient is transferred) counts the patient as an admission. *Interhospital transfer* describes this movement of a patient from one facility to another. *Intrahospital transfer* reflects the movement of a patient between nursing units and therefore has no overall impact on the census. Fig. 7.22 shows the transfer of patients between two nursing units on May 31, 20XX.

## Census

The total number of patients in the hospital at any given time is called the census. The term **census** describes both the physical activity of counting (or confirming a computer-generated list of) the patients and the resultant total. Admissions increase the census; discharges decrease the census, as shown here:

| | Total |
|---|---|
| 06/01/20XX midnight census | 5 |
| Admissions | +2 |
| Discharges | −3 |
| 06/02/20XX midnight census | 4 |

For statistical purposes the census is taken at the same time every day, *usually* but not always at midnight, so that the facility can compare the census from day to day over time. This census number is also called the *midnight census*. For practical purposes a computer database allows the patient registration department to view the census at any time.

Because the number of discharges (decrease) was more than the number of admissions (increase), the inpatient census decreased.

Hospital administrators like to review the census by nursing unit, wing, or floor. This view enables administrators to identify underutilized areas for planning purposes. It also allows nursing managers to plan and control staffing. The impact of the two admissions and three discharges on the census taken between June 1 and June 2, 20XX, is detailed by nursing unit in the previous examples.

Historically, the admissions department used a chart to keep track of all of the rooms in the facility. The chart was called a bed board and provided a method for the facility to keep track of which patient rooms were vacant or occupied. If a room was occupied, the admissions clerk would put on the chart the name(s) of the patient(s) in that room and mark the room occupied. Today, this procedure has been automated; however, some hospitals have maintained the manual bed-board system as a backup. NB beds are called *bassinets* and are located in a part of the unit called the *nursery*.

The patient access (or registration) department is generally responsible for assigning a patient to a bed within a particular room. The function of assigning the bed is often called **bed control**. Manual tracking of patient admissions, discharges, and transfers between units can be very cumbersome and time consuming. Further, manual tracking systems are not available outside the bed control office. Therefore many facilities employ electronic bed control systems that can be accessed by nursing, housekeeping, and administration staff, as well as the bed control staff.

## Days of Service

A census does not measure all of the services provided by the hospital. What about the patient who is admitted at 10:40 a.m. and dies before midnight? That patient would not be present for the counting of the midnight census. The facility counts these patients in the service days for the facility

**TABLE 7.3 Number of Patients Who Received Services, Detailed by Patient**

| | Inpatients | Total |
|---|---|---|
| 06/01/20XX midnight census | M. Brown<br>S. Crevecoeur<br>F. Perez<br>P. Smith<br>R. Wooley | 5 |
| Admissions | C. Estevez<br>B. Mooney | 2 |
| Discharges | S. Crevecoeur<br>C. Estevez<br>B. Mooney | 3 |
| 06/02/20XX midnight census | M. Brown<br>F. Perez<br>P. Smith<br>R. Wooley | 4 |

called **inpatient service days (IPSDs)**. IPSDs are calculated by adding the admissions to the previous day's census, subtracting the discharges, and then adding the patients who were admitted and discharged on the same day.

In counting days of service, as in LOS, we count the day of admission but not the day of discharge. This makes sense because if the hospital counted the day of discharge as well, it would conceivably charge twice for the same bed on the same day. The same principle allows the facility to count 1 day of service for a patient who is admitted and discharged on the same day.

The previous census report does not indicate how many patients received services on June 2, 20XX. Table 7.3 shows the admission and discharge detailed by patient. The two patients who were admitted on June 2 were also discharged the same day. Table 7.4 analyzes the service days received by those patients. From this analysis, 6 days of service (IPSDs) were actually rendered by the hospital.

The census need not be analyzed patient by patient to calculate IPSDs. One can obtain the total number of patients admitted and discharged on the same day from census reports (Table 7.5). Once IPSDs have been calculated, the data can be added, averaged, graphed, and trended over time. The census is also a means to calculate occupancy, as mentioned, because it includes all patients who were admitted and discharged on the same day. Because the census counts only patients in beds at a point in time, calculating IPSDs is a better measure of the use of hospital facilities. Fig. 7.23 illustrates all the IPSD concepts discussed so far.

At the end of 2023, there were 325 patients in Community Hospital. At the end of 2024, the adults and children census was 180 (Fig. 7.24). There were 145 fewer adults and children in the hospital at the end of the year 2024 than there were at the beginning. How did that happen? Look at the admissions and discharges. There were more discharges than admissions during the year: 145, to be exact.

**TABLE 7.4　Analysis of Patients Who Received a Day of Service on June 2, 20XX**

| Inpatients | Analysis | 6/2 Day of Service |
|---|---|---|
| M. Brown | Inpatient on 6/1 and 6/2 | 1 |
| S. Crevecoeur | Discharged 6/2 | 0 |
| C. Estevez | Admitted and discharged 6/2 | 1 |
| B. Mooney | Admitted and discharged 6/2 | 1 |
| F. Perez | Inpatient on 6/1 and 6/2 | 1 |
| P. Smith | Inpatient on 6/1 and 6/2 | 1 |
| R. Wooley | Inpatient on 6/1 and 6/2 | 1 |
| Total days of service | | 6 |

**TABLE 7.5　Inpatient Service Days Calculated From Census**

| | Total |
|---|---|
| 06/01/20XX midnight census | 5 |
| Admissions | +2 |
| Discharges | −3 |
| 06/02/20XX midnight census | 4 |
| Patients admitted and discharged on 6/2 | +2 |
| 06/02/20XX inpatient service days | 6 |

Understanding the relationship among the statistics helps us to use these data effectively. For example, Fig. 7.18 shows that 14,545 adults and children were discharged in a single year. The total LOS for all of those patients combined was 72,107 days. Therefore the ALOS for adults and children in this year was 4.96 days (72,107 ÷ 14,545 = 4.96).

All health care facilities keep track of their statistics according to the fiscal year, which is a 12-month reporting period. A facility's reporting period can be the calendar year (January 1 through December 31), or July 1 through June 30, or October 1 through September 30. The fiscal year is then broken up into smaller reporting periods to help administrators and other users of data to make the data more timely and useful. To understand this concept, think of how a year is organized into days, weeks, and months. Hospital statistics are calculated by the relevant fiscal period. In addition to days, weeks, and months, data can be grouped into months or quarters. Each quarter represents 3 months, or approximately one-fourth of the year. Fig. 7.24 shows a hospital's data organized into quarters.

## Bed Occupancy Rate

Occupancy refers to the number of inpatient beds used by patients in a particular period. It is typically expressed as a percentage. As noted previously, the use of beds is measured by IPSD. Thus, if a hospital has 150 licensed beds and the IPSD for yesterday was 75, then yesterday's occupancy was 50%: (75 ÷ 150) × 100. Calculating occupancy with IPSD takes into consideration patients who are admitted and discharged on the same day.

Occupancy over a period of more than 1 day is calculated by dividing the number of days that patients used beds (total IPSDs) by the number of beds available (bed count×the number of days in the period). Bed count is different from licensed beds. Licensed beds are the number of beds permitted for the hospital according to the hospital's license from the state. **Bed count** is the number of beds that are actually staffed and available for patients at any time. A hospital may be licensed for 250 beds but have only 200 of them staffed and set up. Although the licensed beds cannot change without permission from the state, the bed count may change frequently. So the denominator of the occupancy equation needs to take into consideration how many days the hospital maintained bed count at various levels.

## Hospital Rates and Percentages

There are many ways to look at hospital statistics. The general rule is to look at the number of times something occurred in comparison with (divided by) the number of times it could have occurred in a given time period. This basic calculation provides a rate of occurrence.

Multiplied by 100, the rate of occurrence is expressed as a percentage.

$$\frac{\text{Number of times something occurred in a time period}}{\text{Number of times it could have occurred in the same time period}} \times 100 = \text{Rate}$$

For example, it might be necessary to know the percentage of hospital patients who acquired nosocomial infections. Fig. 7.18 shows that there were 231 occurrences of nosocomial infections at Community Hospital in a given year. Because 15,495 (14,545 + 950) patients were treated (discharged), 15,495 is the number of possible occurrences of nosocomial infections. The percentage of nosocomial infections is 1.5%.

The key to understanding hospital rates and percentages is to understand the underlying data and how those data elements relate to one another. For example, to calculate the facility's gross autopsy rate, the number of times an inpatient autopsy occurred is the numerator. The number of times

**Census Statistics**

A&C = Adults and children
N/B = Newborn

NICU = Neonatal ICU
Adm. = Admissions

D/C = Discharges
IPSD = Inpatient service days

| | Adults & Children | | | Newborns | | |
| --- | --- | --- | --- | --- | --- | --- |
| | UNIT A | UNIT B | TOTAL A&C | N/B nursery | NICU | TOTAL N/B |
| 06/01/20XX midnight census | 15 | 17 | 32 | 3 | 1 | 4 |
| Admissions/births | +4 | +2 | +6 | 2 | 0 | 2 |
| Discharges/deaths | −5 | −4 | −9 | 0 | 0 | 0 |
| Transfers in | +2 | +1 | +3 | 0 | +1 | +1 |
| Transfers out | −1 | −2 | −3 | −1 | 0 | −1 |
| 06/02/20XX midnight census | 15 | 14 | 29 | 4 | 2 | 6 |
| Adm. & D/C 06/02/2016 | +2 | +1 | +3 | 0 | 0 | 0 |
| 06/02/20XX IPSD | 17 | 15 | 32 | 4 | 2 | 6 |

*Sometimes these reports are generated from the main system. If the report from the main system is not in the desired format, it can sometimes be downloaded to a computerized spreadsheet program for reformatting or alternative presentation, such as a graph. Any report that is prepared on a spreadsheet should be spot-checked for accuracy potential errors.*

• **Fig. 7.23**  Census statistics.

**The Fiscal Year**

| QUARTER | Month | # of Days | Admissions | Discharges | Census | |
| --- | --- | --- | --- | --- | --- | --- |
| | | | | | 325 | **12/31/2023** |
| I | January | 31 | 1125 | 1148 | 302 | |
| | February | 29 | 1543 | 1555 | 290 | |
| | March | 31 | 1445 | 1430 | 305 | |
| II | April | 30 | 1406 | 1398 | 313 | |
| | May | 31 | 1242 | 1247 | 308 | |
| | June | 30 | 1004 | 994 | 318 | |
| III | July | 31 | 1254 | 1248 | 324 | |
| | August | 31 | 1145 | 1148 | 321 | |
| | September | 30 | 1212 | 1224 | 309 | |
| IV | October | 31 | 1478 | 1502 | 285 | |
| | November | 30 | 1567 | 1598 | 254 | |
| | December | 31 | 1229 | 1303 | 180 | |
| Total | | **366** | **15,650** | **15,795** | | **12/31/2024** |

*2024 is a leap year. In nonleap years, February has 28 days, for a total of 365 days in the year.*

• **Fig. 7.24**  The fiscal year.

an autopsy *could* have occurred is the number of inpatients who died in the hospital. So, if six patients died in the hospital this month and there was one autopsy performed, the gross autopsy rate is one divided by six or 17%. Sometimes, patient deaths are the domain of law enforcement, such as a patient who dies due to a criminal act. These deaths are subtracted from the inpatient deaths in the denominator, because the patients' bodies were removed for autopsy by the coroner or medical examiner and therefore were not available for autopsy by the hospital. This adjustment results in the net autopsy rate. Autopsies can also be done on outpatients, such as patients who expire in the emergency department (ED). They are included in the hospital autopsy rate, which divides the total number of autopsies performed divided by all of the deaths of patients whose bodies were available for autopsy.

Some of the most common types of calculations are shown in Box 7.2.

Thus there are many ways to report data. The way in which they are reported depends on the needs of the user. It is important for the HIM professional to understand the needs of the user to help identify the data for meaningful reporting and presentation.

 **COMPETENCY CHECK-IN 7.7**

**Routine Institutional Statistics**

**Competency Assessment**

1. What is the formula for computing the ALOS?
2. Why are census data important? How is census calculated?
3. The following patients were discharged from pediatrics for the week 7/15/20XX to 7/20/20XX. What is the ALOS of these patients?

| Patient Name | Admission Date | Discharge Date |
| --- | --- | --- |
| Groot | 07/13/20XX | 07/15/20XX |
| Smith | 07/12/20XX | 07/15/20XX |
| Brown | 07/11/20XX | 07/16/20XX |
| Kowalski | 07/10/20XX | 07/20/20XX |
| Zhong | 07/09/20XX | 07/19/20XX |
| Frank | 06/29/20XX | 07/18/20XX |

## Research

Throughout our discussion of health data, we have focused on the underlying meaning and source of various data elements. We talked about patient identification data as a UHDDS requirement and that the data are collected at patient registration. Patient name, address, gender, and date of birth are examples of patient identification data. In defining fields such as patient address for a data dictionary, we discussed the size of the field, whether it was text or

---

**• BOX 7.2**     **Health Care Statistics Formulas.**

**Average Inpatient Service Days**

$$\frac{\text{Total IPSDs for a period (excluding newborns)}}{\text{Total number of days in the period}}$$

**Average Newborn Inpatient Service Days**

$$\frac{\text{Total newborn IPSDs for a period}}{\text{Total number of days in the period}}$$

**Average Length of Stay**

$$\frac{\text{Total LOS (discharge days)}}{\text{Total discharges (including deaths)}}$$

**Bed Occupancy Rate**

$$\frac{\text{Total IPSDs for a period}}{\text{Total bed count days in the period}} \times 100$$

(Calculated as bed count × number of days in the period.)

**Newborn Bassinet Occupancy Ratio Formula**

$$\frac{\text{Total newborn IPSDs for a period}}{\text{Total newborn bassinet count} \times \text{number of days in the period}} \times 100$$

**Gross Autopsy Rate**

$$\frac{\text{Total number of autopsies per formed on inpatients for a period}}{\text{Total number of inpatient deaths for this period}} \times 100$$

**Other Rate Formula**

$$\frac{\text{Number of times something occurred}}{\text{Number of times something could have occurred}} \times 100$$

numbers, and who could enter the data. To use data that have been collected—or to develop a way to collect data that we need—we have to understand the nature of the data. What we need to do with the data drives how we collect and measure that data. For example, a media reporter who wants to explore the impact of an event on witnesses would likely conduct interviews of those witnesses and publish or broadcast the interesting comments. A hospital administrator, who wants to know whether patients are happy with the facility's services, would not wander around the hospital interviewing random patients for this purpose. The media reporter only needs interesting bits for an article to convey a story. The hospital administrator needs an organized, systematic approach to collecting data so that the results can be used to determine how well the hospital is running. The media reporter needs some quick information gathering. The hospital administrator needs research.

## What Is Research?

An important use of health care data is research. Many health care organizations, particularly teaching hospitals, perform research projects—often focusing on clinical outcomes. Government agencies, such as the Centers for Disease Control and Prevention (CDC), perform data analysis for operational purposes, often using research techniques. Other agencies, such as the Agency for Health Research and Quality (AHRQ), focus primarily on research. The AHRQ, in particular, does research designed to understand and help improve health care in the United States. The World Health Organization also performs research but on a worldwide scale.

Thus what is research? Research is a systematic investigation to answer a question. The difference between research and simply looking up facts on the internet or interviewing a few bystanders (to answer a question) is that "systematic investigation" involves a specific discipline of activities. Beyond looking up facts, research develops new ideas and new facts from the investigation. These new ideas and facts arise from the testing of a **hypothesis**, which is the anticipated answer to the question. For example, we might ask the research question, "Do HIM professionals maintain a personal health record (PHR) at a higher rate than non-HIM professionals?" One way to answer the question is to test the hypothesis: "HIM professionals are more likely to maintain a PHR than non-HIM professionals." Notice that the research question is phrased as a query, whereas the hypothesis is phrased as a statement. This hypothesis has two variables: the dependent variable, which is "maintain a PHR," and the independent variable, "HIM professional" status. The independent variable is the presumed cause of the dependent variable's value. In other words, the researcher's best guess as to the eventual results of the study are that the independent variable has a predictable impact on the dependent variable. Here are two more hypothesis examples:

- *Practicing coding* increases the *accuracy rate* of the coder. In this example, the independent variable, practicing coding, is predicted to have a positive impact on the dependent variable, coding accuracy rate.
- *Timely postdischarge follow-up* by the primary care physician decreases the rate of *readmissions of patients* with serious chronic illnesses. In this example, the independent variable, timely postdischarge follow-up, is predicted to have a negative impact on the dependent variable, patient readmissions.

Whether research consists solely of a comprehensive literature review (metaanalysis) or an experiment in a chemistry lab, there should be a systematic approach driven by a well-crafted hypothesis.

There are two fundamental types of research: basic and applied. In **basic research** a study is done to answer a question just for the sake of answering it. Mapping neural pathways and answering the question, "How do nerves and muscles work to enable movement?" is interesting but has no immediate practical applications. Basic research expands our knowledge of a subject, adding to the list of facts on which future research and the search for additional knowledge can be based.

**Applied research**, conversely, is designed to solve an existing or anticipated problem. Thus, using the results of basic research on nerves, muscles, and movement, researchers can answer the question, "Can nerves be trained to communicate with mechanical devices?" If the answer is yes, then it is possible to manufacture artificial limbs that can be manipulated by the wearer using nerve impulses—a very real and practical problem for amputees. **Clinical outcome analysis** is a type of applied research. In clinical outcome analysis, patients are studied to determine the most efficient and effective way to achieve a positive outcome in the treatment or management of a disease or condition.

To conduct research, certain logical steps are followed:
1. Topic
   a. Select a topic.
   b. Conduct a literature review.
   c. Examine the existing body of knowledge for gaps.
2. Focus
   a. Conduct a focused literature review.
   b. Develop a research question.
   c. Develop one or more hypotheses from the research question.
   d. Define the variables in the hypothesis(es).
   e. Determine how to measure the variables.
3. Study
   a. Design the study.
   b. Obtain approval/funding.
   c. Conduct the study.
4. Analyze
   a. Analyze the results.
   b. Reach conclusions.
5. Generalize
   a. Apply conclusions to the existing body of knowledge.
   b. Circle back to original question.
   c. Continue to explore the topic or move on to a different topic.

The process of research is cyclical in that researchers will circle back to the original question and determine whether more work is needed in the focus area, a shift in focus is needed, or another topic needs to be explored (Fig. 7.25). Of course, discussing the process of research and how it is funded is the topic of many stand-alone textbooks. For our purposes, it is helpful to understand some of the disciplines of research so that we can be of more assistance when asked for data and so that our own investigations have more rigor. One of the ways in which we can be of assistance is in defining and measuring the variables when research or other internal studies call for health care data. Therefore we need to take a closer look at the data with which we are already quite familiar and examine them in a slightly different way.

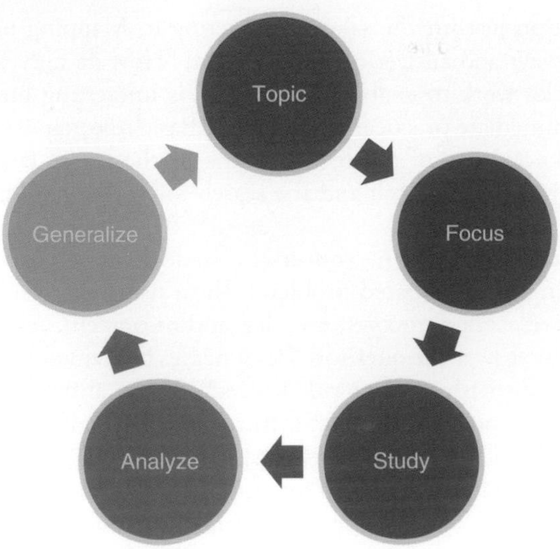

• **Fig. 7.25** The research process.

## Qualitative Versus Quantitative

In both basic and applied research, there are two approaches to data collection: quantitative and qualitative. As the name implies, quantitative data consist of data that are numeric or that can be collected using numeric representation. Counting the number of times an event occurs is a numeric activity—even if the underlying event is not. For example, gender is not numeric data—it is the description of whether an individual is male, female, or some other category. So, gender is a qualitative or categorical type of data. Interviews are qualitative data. The results of an interview are not numeric values but words. Words and other types of nonnumeric data are qualitative. Quantitative data are anything collected as a numeric value. Thus charges and DRG relative weights are numeric or quantitative data. Quantitative research relies on the ability to collect data that can be expressed numerically.

Qualitative research, in contrast, relies on observations that may have no numeric representation. For example, a study of children's behavior involves watching children in a particular setting and noting their behaviors. Since behavior is not inherently numeric, the data that are collected may be free text. Qualitative data, then, can be collected and categorized but may not be assigned any meaningful numeric value that can be analyzed.

When designing a study, a researcher may use both qualitative and quantitative methods: mixed method research. In the development of the actual study, the researcher may need to conduct open-ended interviews with colleagues and potential subjects to fully understand the topic and to develop the project more fully or to narrow down the topic. These qualitative data can be reviewed and analyzed to develop a quantitative study. For example, a researcher may want to study rates of record completion among physicians to determine why some physicians are very timely and others are not. To develop the study, the researcher may interview many physicians and many HIM professionals to identify the issues. From there, a quantitative study may be

designed in which the researcher collects data on completion rates and other identified record completion factors.

However, counting the number of males, females, or others who fall into those categories is a quantitative activity yielding a numeric value that can be used to analyze the gender mix of patients who received services at the health care facility. In this manner, qualitative data can be used to provide quantitative analysis. The extent to which we can use qualitative or categorical data for analysis depends on the nature of the underlying data.

## Research Design

Ultimately, when we are developing our hypotheses, we need to determine what types of data are represented by our variables and how we are going to measure them. The type of data we are trying to measure drives how we will collect it and how we will be able to analyze it. So, going back to our PHR example: "HIM professionals are more likely to maintain a PHR than non-HIM professionals."

Our dependent and independent variables are both nominal data. We will probably measure these by taking a survey of a group of individuals. All we will be able to do is count the responses. Once we count the responses, we can total them and create a table for analysis:

Employees of Community Hospital Who Maintain a PHR

Survey of 100 employees who attended a revenue cycle staff meeting

|  | Maintain PHR? | |
| --- | --- | --- |
|  | Yes | No |
| HIM professional | 25 | 10 |
| Non-HIM professional | 15 | 50 |

This example highlights several issues that arise when defining variables. The first is the specificity of the definition of the variables. For example, "What is a PHR?" Does everyone queried have the same understanding of what a PHR is? Does a copy of your latest blood work or active access to your primary care provider's (PCP's) portal count as a PHR? Further, "What is an HIM professional?" Is it a person with an HIM credential? Any credential? An HIM program student? We can't leave the answers to those questions for the survey participants. Their cognitive definition—what the participant thinks is the definition—may not match our operational definition—what we have determined are our criteria for defining the variable. So, we can't just ask, "Are you an HIM professional (yes or no) and do you maintain a PHR (yes or no)?" We will have to construct a survey that leaves no room for interpretation on the part of the person being surveyed. We might do that by asking whether a person has one or more of a specific list of credentials, what his or her job title is, and in what department he or she works. This would enable us to make the determination of the person's "HIM professional" status, based on our predetermined criteria. Further, since we think there may be other motivating factors in the maintenance of a PHR, we might ask a few more questions that elicit whether the person has a chronic illness. Fig. 7.26 is

## PERSONAL HEALTH RECORD SURVEY

*Please circle your response to each of the following questions. Unless stated otherwise, please circle only one response per question. Your responses are COMPLETELY confidential and anonymous.*

1. **What is your age?**

   A. Under 21
   B. 21–30
   C. 31–40
   D. 41–50
   E. 51–60
   F. 61–70
   G. Over 70

2. **What is the highest level of formal education that you have completed?**

   A. High school diploma or GED
   B. Associate's degree
   C. Bachelor's degree
   D. Master's degree
   E. Doctoral degree
   F. Other (please specify) _____

3. **What is your gender?**

   A. Female
   B. Male
   C. Other (please specify) _____

4. **Which of the following most closely describes your primary work setting?**

   A. Acute care facility
   B. Long term care facility
   C. Ambulatory care facility
   D. Other health care provider
   E. Third-party payer
   F. Pharmaceutical company
   G. Consulting firm
   H. Other (please specify)

5. **Do you participate in the health care decision-making process for any of the following? (check all that apply)**

   A. Child or children
   B. Spouse or significant other
   C. Parent or grandparent
   D. Other (please explain) _____
   E. None

1. **Do you have a chronic illness or disability?**
   A. Yes
   B. No

2. **Does anyone for whom you participate in the health care decision-making process have a chronic illness or disability?**
   A. Yes
   B. No
   C. I do not participate in the health care decision-making process for anyone but myself.

3. **Have you ever undergone a surgical procedure?**
   A. Yes
   B. No
   C. Not sure

4. **Has anyone for whom you participate in the health care decision-making process ever undergone a surgical procedure?**
   A. Yes
   B. No
   C. Not sure
   D. I do not participate in the health care decision-making process for anyone but myself.

**Continued on page 2**

• **Fig. 7.26** Example survey questions asking whether an individual maintains a personal health record. This is page 1 of the survey.

an example of a possible survey we might use. A survey is a type of measurement instrument that is used in descriptive research design.

The type of research design used will depend on the needs of the project and the extent to which the researcher can control the action of the variables. A chemist, for example, can control how much of a substance is introduced into a compound and measure the chemical reaction. On the other hand, a bariatric physician wanting to study different diet strategies in a patient population cannot control what patients do when they leave the office. Similarly, the chemist does not have to be concerned about the compound's feelings during a project. However, when working with humans, not only care for the subject's feelings but also informed consent to participate is necessary. Table 7.6 is a summary of the three types of designs we have discussed here.

## Institutional Review Board

Research involving human subjects requires review by an IRB. A university or teaching hospital may have its own IRB function; other organizations may rely on the services of an external board. The purpose of an IRB is to evaluate a research proposal to ensure that the research process is sound and that humans involved in the study will be treated with respect, their privacy protected, and their informed consent obtained. IRB approval is one aspect of a general concern for the ethical treatment of human subjects in research.

## Reporting of Data

Within a hospital's computer system, there are generally preprogrammed reports available to users. Who has access

5. Which of the following statements most closely reflects your understanding of a personal health record?
   A. I know what a personal health record is and can explain it to someone else.
   B. I know what a personal health record is, but I don't think I could explain it.
   C. I'm not sure how to define a personal health record.
   D. I do not know what a personal health record is.

6. Do you maintain a personal health record for yourself?
   A. Yes
   B. No
   C. Not sure

7. Do you maintain a personal health record for any or all of the individuals identified in question 9 (for whom you participate in the health care decision-making process)?
   A. Yes
   B. No
   C. Not sure

8. If you maintain a personal health record for yourself or anyone else, in what form(s) do you *receive* the data? (circle all that apply)
   A. Paper
   B. Electronically (portable storage, email, or portal access)
   C. I do not maintain a personal health record
   D. Other (please explain)

9. If you maintain a personal health record for yourself or anyone else, in what form(s) do you *retain* the data? (circle all that apply)
   A. Paper
   B. File on my computer
   C. Internet site
   D. I do not maintain a personal health record
   E. Other (please explain)

10. How many different primary care physicians have you seen in your lifetime?
    A. 0–2
    B. 3–4
    C. 5–6
    D. 7–8
    E. 9–10
    F. More than 10

11. Has a health care encounter ever been delayed due to lack of access to your health information (for you or for anyone for whom you participate in the health care decision-making process)?
    A. Yes
    B. No

12. Does your primary care physician have a full or partial electronic health record?
    A. Yes
    B. No
    C. Not sure

13. Does your current primary care physician offer a patient portal?
    A. Yes
    B. No
    C. Not sure

14. If the answer to Question 13 is Yes: do you log in and use the patient portal for access to your personal health records?
    A. Yes
    B. No
    C. Not sure

15. Do you have access to a personal computer? (circle all that apply)
    A. Yes—at home
    B. Yes—at work
    C. Yes—at school
    D. No—I have no access
    E. Other (please explain)

16. Do you have access to the Internet? (Circle all that apply)
    A. Yes—at home
    B. Yes—at work
    C. Yes—at school
    D. No—I have no access
    E. Other (please explain)

• **Fig. 7.26** *(Cont.)*

to which reports depends on the user's role in the organization. So, HIM staff might be able to run a detailed discharge register or a list of patients by diagnosis. A radiology department manager might have a report that details all of the radiology orders and the status of those orders. Typically, users have access to routine reports that they need to perform their job. However, as questions arise during the course of operations, the answers are not always available via these preprogrammed or routine reports.

## Reporting to Individual Departments

As we have discussed earlier in this chapter, the hospital's database, including the EHR, can be searched for specific data and customized reports prepared to answer almost any question. Some organizations have dedicated database analysts who spend their days answering questions via reports. In many cases, HIM professionals are needed to assist in the preparation of these customized or ad hoc reports because

## TABLE 7.6   Research Designs

| Design | Unique Characteristics | Example |
|---|---|---|
| Experimental | • Best for determining causality<br>• Researcher exerts control over the subject variables<br>• Subjects are randomly identified and assigned | Two equivalent groups are given a therapy; one group receives the test therapy, the control group receives either no therapy or the comparative therapy |
| Survey | Evaluates the existence of relationships but not necessarily causality<br>  • Used to explain what exists | Political polls, opinion surveys, customer satisfaction surveys |
| Metaanalysis | Solely literature review<br>  • Seeks to summarize and analyze the existing work in a particular area | A literature review of all published studies regarding the diagnosis of hypothyroidism |

## COMPETENCY CHECK-IN 7.8

### Research

**Competency Assessment**

1. A clinical department has received an unusual number of complaints from patients about their experience. Which of the following methods would yield the most detail regarding the patients' experiences?
   a. A survey with closed-ended questions
   b. Interviews with a sample of patients
   c. A double-blind placebo study
   d. Observation
2. You are asked to research the opinions of your staff. What is the first thing you need to know?
   a. What is the hypothesis?
   b. What data-gathering method will you use?
   c. What is the question to be answered?
   d. In what format should the report be presented?
3. You are considering taking a nutritional supplement and are reading some of the literature that is available about its usefulness. Which of the following is the most authoritative?
   a. A focus group of users
   b. A website blog with testimonials from users and physicians
   c. The manufacturer's website
   d. A double-blind placebo study conducted by a university
4. You are working with a team from Patient Access to improve the patient experience at registration. The discussion turns to wait times. Select an operational definition of wait time.
   a. The amount of time a patient has to wait
   b. The number of minutes and seconds a patient has to wait before being registered
   c. The difference between the time the patient is seen by the registrar and the time the patient arrived
   d. The difference in minutes and seconds between the time the patient begins the registration process, recorded by the registrar, and the time the patient arrived, recorded by the greeter
5. You want to conduct a research study to determine whether frequent, short yoga breaks during the work day will improve coding productivity. In framing your hypothesis, which represents a useful measurement of the independent variable?
   a. The coder's historical productivity
   b. The coder's productivity during the study
   c. The number and duration of yoga breaks
   d. The number and duration of breaks
6. You have been asked to query your staff to determine their satisfaction with a number of variables, such as break scheduling and collaboration between teams. What type of research design should you use?
   a. Survey
   b. Mixed method
   c. Experimental
   d. Metaanalysis

of our knowledge of the data and the way it is collected and stored.

Once a report has been run, further review of that report may be necessary to provide truly useful information for decision-making or interpretation. For example, refer to Fig. 7.7, which was used to illustrate patient LOS in the aggregate data explanation. That report could be useful in determining ALOS. Facilities typically review the ALOS for specific patient diagnoses. The facility's average is then compared with a national, corporate, or local average. This further analysis can determine whether a facility is within the expected LOS for that MS-DRG. The UR department analyzes patient LOS for each DRG and diagnosis. For an HIM professional to provide this information, he or she must run a report and then format it in an appropriate list or graph to represent the information for presentation.

Health data are used by various departments in the health care facility. The PI department uses the database to retrieve specific cases and review the documentation found in the health records to determine compliance with accreditation standards, perform PI studies, or study patient care outcomes. The finance department may use charge data to verify or prepare financial reports and budgets. Case management may perform retrospective reviews to investigate admission denials. Infection control needs to identify and analyze reportable infectious disease cases. The HIM department may help provide or analyze this data to these and other customers, both internal and external.

One important consideration in generating reports for other departments is whether the requesting user has the authority to view the requested data. For example, Dr. Brown may request a list of all of Dr. Garcia's patients. Assuming Dr. Brown is not a treating physician of Dr. Garcia's patients that would be an inappropriate request.

## Indices

An **index** is a list that identifies specific data items within a frame of reference. For example, the Master Patient Index (MPI) (see Chapter 2) is a list of all patients who have ever been admitted to the facility. The abstracting process has enabled facilities to create indices for diagnoses, procedures, physicians, admission date, and discharge date. For example, the attending physician is systematically identified on each patient record during the abstract process (attribution). A listing of patients by attending physician creates what is called the *physician index*. Additional indices can be created if the data are captured in the system. Referring physician, primary care physician, and consulting physician are typically captured, and each surgical procedure has a performing physician's name attached to it. Therefore reporting lists of visits by physician relationship is possible. The database can also provide information about any group of patients according to the instructions given by the person requesting the information to HIM personnel and further refined by HIM personnel queries to the database. As with any other data, the quality of the data capture dictates the completeness and accuracy of such reporting.

It should be noted that physician **attribution** is a matter of some importance to the physicians themselves. Increasingly, payers are reviewing facility and physician claims together and assessing whether the billing is consistent. As such, if a physician submits a claim as an attending physician, but the facility has a different physician listed as attending, then the payer may question either or both claims. Physician attribution is also an important issue for recredentialing. A physician may have a minimum volume requirement to maintain privileges at a particular facility.

Indices may also be generated on the basis of the principal diagnosis or the principal procedure. Although indices were a very important tool in the retrospective analysis of patient data before computerization, the automation of data collection and on-demand printing make the necessity for routinely maintaining physical copies obsolete. However, in the event of a system conversion (abandoning an old system for a new one) or an EHR implementation, care should be taken to preserve the historical data. Hospitals may be required by state regulation to retain the MPI permanently, and abstracted data may be attached logically during the conversion. Fig. 7.27 shows a diagnosis index of diagnosis code O80 for discharges in January 20XX in computerized format.

## Reporting to Outside Agencies

Various agencies associated with health care facilities routinely require information. Some states gather information from facilities to create a state health information network. The information in the database is shared (without patient identifiers) so that facilities can compare themselves with other facilities. Organ procurement agencies may request information on deaths for a certain period to assess the facility's compliance with state regulations for organ procurement.

Certain statistics must be reported to the CDC so that disease prevalence, incidence, **morbidity** (illness), and **mortality** (death) can be studied. **Prevalence** is the portion of the population that has a particular disease or condition. **Incidence** is how many new cases of a particular disease or condition have been identified in a particular period in comparison with the population as a whole.

Several issues arise in the reporting of data to outside organizations. Typically, reporting is accomplished via electronic data transfer. The receiving entity dictates the form and content of the data file. Matching of the data as collected with the required format must take place, usually with software customized for this purpose. During the development of a data transfer file, the completeness and accuracy of the data must be examined. For example, coding corrections to a failed claim in the billing system that are not also corrected in the patient's record will result in the same error appearing in the UHDDS reporting.

## Specialized Data Collection Systems

A **registry** is a collection of data specific to a disease, diagnosis, or procedure, the purpose of which is to study or

06/16/20XX

**Diagnosis Index          Discharges: 01/01/20XX – 01/31/20XX**

| Diagnosis Code | Description | Medical Record # | Admit Date | D/C Date | LOS | Physician |
|---|---|---|---|---|---|---|
| O80 | Encounter for full-term uncomplicated delivery | 010111 | 12/30/20XX | 01/01/20XX | 2 | Oscar, D. |
| | | 125544 | 12/31/20XX | 01/01/20XX | 1 | Jons, J. |
| | | 098805 | 01/02/20XX | 01/04/20XX | 2 | Vida, E. |
| | | 112096 | 01/05/20XX | 01/06/20XX | 1 | Oscar, D. |
| | | 113095 | 01/09/20XX | 01/12/20XX | 3 | Jons, J. |

• **Fig. 7.27** Diagnosis index shown in a computerized format.

improve patient care. Unlike an index, which lists all occurrences of a particular field, such as diagnosis or procedure, a registry is compiled of cases that conform to strict guidelines as defined by the registry (case finding) and the identification and reporting of very specific data related to the case. Common registries are the Tumor or Cancer Registry, Trauma Registry, AIDS Registry, Birth Defect Registry, and Implant Registry. The data are collected specific to the diagnosis, disease, or implant so that users can compare, analyze, or study the groups of patients. A registry is typically maintained by an agency external to the facility or provider and characteristically requires active follow-up of the reported cases.

## Tumor or Cancer Registry

The study of the causes and treatments of cancers is of importance to individuals and also as a public health issue. Many cancers, such as some types of lung cancers, are thought to be of environmental origin; others seem to have a genetic component. It is only by analyzing data collected from cancer patients that researchers can begin to identify the actual causes with the hope of finding preventive measures and effective treatments.

A cancer registry is a data system designed to capture specific facts about patients who have been diagnosed with cancer. Whenever a cancer is diagnosed, the hospital reports the case to the registry. Data are collected through the states electronically. Data collected include the type of cancer, whether it has metastasized, and what body systems are involved. Once a case has been identified, the patient is followed to determine the outcome of treatment. Registry data are centrally maintained by the National Program of

Cancer Registries (NPCR), which is administered by the CDC. Additional cancer data are collected through the National Cancer Institute's Surveillance, Epidemiology, and End Results (SEER) Program. Registry data are used to
- monitor cancer trends over time;
- show cancer patterns in various populations and identify high-risk groups;
- guide planning and evaluation of cancer control programs;
- help set priorities for allocating health resources; and
- advance clinical, epidemiologic, and health services research.

NPCR registry data about the incidence of cancer, combined with vital statistics data about mortality, provides valuable data for studying cancer over time (U.S. Department of Health and Human Services, Centers for Disease Control and Prevention, National Program of Cancer Registries [NPCR], 2015).

Detailed data collection includes demographic data (name, address, identification number) and clinical data (diagnoses, procedures, pathology). Pathology data include grading (classifying the growth of the tumor) and staging (describing whether the tumor has spread and how far). Many providers complete the basic registry reporting; however, a certified cancer registry also requires patient follow-up.

Individuals who specialize in collecting data for this registry may become Certified Tumor Registrars through the National Cancer Registry Association.

## Trauma Registry

Researchers can identify trauma (injury) victims by the ICD-10-CM codes associated with the external cause of morbidity and the injury itself. Because these codes are collected and reported on the UB-04 and through various data sets such as the UHDDS, they are available in the providers' and payers' databases and through state and federal databases. However, for study of the severity of the injury and the effectiveness of specific treatments, a trauma registry provides more data.

In 2006 the National Trauma Data Bank (2022) released "the National Trauma Data Standard (formerly National Trauma Registry) data dictionary, developed in collaboration with HRSA, state trauma managers, trauma registry vendors, and other stakeholders in the trauma community." Trauma registry data include traumatic injuries, such as head injuries and burns, of patients receiving care, as well as injury data related to patients who died before care could be rendered. The American Trauma Society offers a certification process for Certified Specialist Trauma Registry (https://www.amtrauma.org/page/CSTR).

### Other Registries

Birth defects and transplants are examples of other conditions for which registries may be maintained. Varying levels of detail are collected. Birth defects may not be detected at birth, and later reporting may be acceptable. Transplant registries match potential donors with recipients and follow those patients after the transplant.

### Vital Statistics

**Vital statistics** refers to the number of births, deaths, and marriages and to statistics on health and disease. In the health care facility, specific information regarding patient births and deaths is reported to the state's Department of Vital Statistics, also known as Vital Records. NBs must be registered with the Department of Vital Statistics within a specific time frame after birth. Within the health care facility, the HIM department is sometimes responsible for recording NBs' demographics, parents, and clinical information to submit to Vital Records.

Death certificates must also be submitted to the state's department of vital records after a patient's death. The death certificate records the patient's demographic information and the cause and place of death. In some states, this information is initiated by the nursing staff and completed by the funeral home; in others, the HIM staff may be required to participate in the submission of this information to the department of vital statistics.

Birth and death certificate data are increasingly collected electronically at the point of care. Paper submissions, where applicable, are collected at the point of care and submitted at the municipal level. The local registrar submits those data to the state, which in turn submits the data through the National Vital Statistics System to the National Center for Health Statistics (NCHS), a component of the CDC. Standards for data collection and reporting are developed by the NCHS. Appendix A contains the sample birth, death, and fetal death forms published in 1989. State forms vary depending on specific additional data the state wishes to collect (National Center for Health Statistics, 2018).

### COMPETENCY CHECK-IN 7.9
**Specialized Data Collection Systems**

**Competency Assessment**

1. What is a registry?
2. List and describe four registries.
3. List two departments within the health care facility that uses health databases. Why do they need the data?
4. What is an index? Give three examples.

## Presentation

After analysis and interpretation, the data can be presented as information. To present data in a meaningful yet simple manner, the analyst uses data visualization tools to illustrate the information. Although there are many tools, the most common are bar graph, pie chart, and line graph. In recent years, interactive tools, such as dashboards, have become common. Table 7.7 explains how these data visualization and presentation tools are used.

### Tables

A table is an organization of data into rows and columns. Each column and row contains a defined data element. Typically, the reporting of data from a database is initially presented in a table. For presentation purposes, rows and tables can be subdivided for clarity. For example, the presentation of the same data from two time periods may be displayed as two columns with one description and two subdescriptions. For small amounts of data, or summary data of a small number of categories, a table can be an easy, clear presentation. Fig. 7.28A illustrates a table in which the first column is the year, followed by a split column for the number of discharges: Hospital A and Hospital B. Each row contains the data for the corresponding year.

### Pivot Tables

For larger amounts of data, further analysis is generally necessary to provide information. One quick way to analyze data in a spreadsheet program, for example, is with a pivot table. Pivot tables rearrange the data from a large spreadsheet or database to summarize certain areas of interest. With a pivot table a user can use contiguous (adjacent) columns in a worksheet and summarize them in a meaningful way.

To prepare a pivot table, highlight adjacent columns of an Excel spreadsheet that has the data you want to analyze. From the Insert tab, select Pivot Table and choose New Worksheet to place the pivot table. In the pivot table worksheet, click and drag to select rows, columns, and data until the desired analysis is displayed. Additional configurations of the results can be achieved from the tool bar. Fig. 7.29 illustrates how a spreadsheet with over 1000 lines of data

**TABLE 7.7   Data Visualization and Presentation Tools and Their Uses**

| Presentation Tool | Construction | Purpose |
|---|---|---|
| Table | Column and rows. Construction depends on the items being compared. | Used to compare characteristics of items. Notice in this table that the items are listed in the first column and the two characteristics (construction and purpose) head the comparison columns. |
| Pivot Table | Select adjacent columns of an Excel spreadsheet. From the Insert tab, select Pivot Table. Choose New Worksheet. Click and drag to select rows, columns, and data until the desired analysis is displayed. Additional configurations of the results can be achieved from the tool bar. | With large amounts of data, it is not always easy to see relationships between the data elements. A pivot table allows the user to "play" with the data and explore possible relationships. Pivot tables are also a quick way to summarize multiple data elements without having to manipulate the original spreadsheet. |
| Bar graph | Bars are drawn to represent the frequency of items in the specified categories of a variable. One axis represents the category. The other axis represents the frequency. | Used to compare categories with each other, the same category in different time periods, or both. |
| Line graph | The horizontal (x) axis represents the observation. The vertical (y) axis represents the value of the observation. A point is made that corresponds to each observation, and a line is drawn to connect the points. | Used to represent data over a period of time; information is plotted along the x and y axes. Typically, time goes on the x axis and observation volume goes on the y axis. |
| Pie chart | In a circle the percentage of each category is represented by a wedge of the circle that corresponds to the percentage of the circle. Segments always represent 100% of the categories under review. | Used to compare categories with one another and in relation to the whole group. Percentages must add up to 100%. |
| Histogram | Like a bar graph except the sides of the bars are touching. Horizontally, each bar represents a class interval. Vertically, the height of the bar represents the frequency of the class interval. | Used to illustrate a frequency distribution in which the range of values is continuous. |
| Dashboard | Presents select statistics and graphical information for decision support and managerial control. May be interactive, static, or real-time. | Information is presented in logical spaces, often in color, and frequently with evaluative metrics. |

can be quickly analyzed to provide a meaningful summary of the data.

## Line Graph

A **line graph** is best used to present observations over time. The vertical axis represents the value or number of observations. The horizontal axis in a line graph represents the time periods. Fig. 7.28B provides an example of line graph construction. Note that the line graph is constructed by connecting the individual points that represent the observations.

Line graphs are also easy to read and interpret. Color presentation facilitates interpretation when multiple periods are superimposed on one another. For example, 3 years of data could be drawn on the same graph, with each year represented by a different color. In black-and-white presentation, the line for each year could be drawn with different patterns; however, that is not as clear as using color. A common use of line graphs is to depict this type of multiyear (or other time period) result. Fig. 7.28 shows Hospital A has an

increase or upward trend in discharges over the past 6 years; Hospital B has a downward trend.

Line graphs are also used to compare two variables. Fig. 7.30 shows a line graph that compares LOS with age. Each patient is represented on the horizontal axis. The patients are presented in order of age. In this example, there is no relationship between the two variables.

## Bar Graph

A **bar graph** is used to present the frequencies of observations within specific categories. Each bar can represent the number of observations in a particular category. Bar graphs are also used to represent frequencies or values attached to specific events or causes. Bar graphs can be drawn either vertically or horizontally. In a vertical graph the horizontal axis represents the categories, events, or causes. The vertical axis represents the value or number of observations, with the lowest value (often zero) at the bottom. Fig. 7.31 provides an example of bar graph construction using the data from Table 7.2. Note that the bars for each category are separate

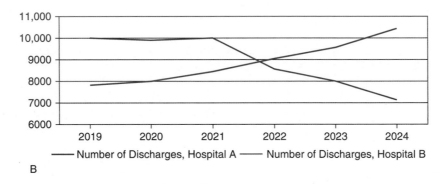

| | Number of discharges | |
|---|---|---|
| Year | Hospital A | Hospital B |
| 2019 | 7846 | 10,000 |
| 2020 | 7998 | 9887 |
| 2021 | 8432 | 9978 |
| 2022 | 9054 | 8553 |
| 2023 | 9578 | 7990 |
| 2024 | 10,456 | 7125 |

A

B

— Number of Discharges, Hospital A    — Number of Discharges, Hospital B

• **Fig. 7.28** Comparison of discharges between two hospitals, 2019–2024: (A) table and (B) line graph construction.

from one another but the bars for subcategories can be adjacent. The values on the vertical axis are expressed in equal increments. Note that Excel uses the term *column* for a vertical graph and *bar* for the horizontal graph.

Bar graphs are easy to read and interpret. Color presentation also helps the user, particularly when there are subcategories. Bar graphs can also be used to present a portion of the data to highlight a specific point, such as top 10 DRGs. Bar graphs are not particularly helpful when the data have a very wide range of values. For example, if one category has two occurrences and another has 30,000, the vertical axis might be difficult to draw in a meaningful way. Also, when there are many categories, including all of the appropriate descriptions can be difficult.

## Histogram

A **histogram** is a combination of a vertical bar graph whose sides are touching. Horizontally, each bar represents a class interval. Vertically, the height of the bar represents the frequency of the class interval. A line graph may be drawn to connect the midpoints of each class interval. Histograms are used only to draw frequency distributions of continuous data. Note that the bars are adjacent and we could add a line that approximates the curve created by the data (Fig. 7.32).

## Pie Chart

A **pie chart** is used to express the percentage of observations in each category of a variable. To use a pie chart, the analyst must convert the number of observations to a percentage. All of the observations (100%) must be included in the chart. Pie charts are drawn in a circle. Each "slice" of the circle or "pie" represents a category. The size of the slice corresponds to the percentage of observations. A complete circle is 360 degrees in circumference. To create an accurate drawing, multiply the percentages of observations by 360 to determine the number of degrees for the angle of the slice. To estimate the size of the slice, remember that a right angle is 90 degrees. Four 90-degree angles make a circle: 360 degrees. Therefore 25% of a circle is a quarter of the pie.

Pie charts have limited application and can be difficult to read if there are many categories. Because a pie chart represents 100% of the observations, all of the categories must be shown as a slice of the pie. If there are many small categories, it is sometimes useful to combine them in a meaningful way. However, pie charts can make a dramatic and easily understood statement. They are particularly useful when illustrating a variable with one or two dramatically large numbers of observations. Fig. 7.33 shows the

Showing four columns and twelve rows of a large Excel spreadsheet.

| MRN | DC Status | Sex | Attending |
|-----|-----------|-----|-----------|
| 50092976 | 3 | M | 35,679 |
| 50093391 | 2 | M | 37,549 |
| 50093513 | 1 | F | 38,124 |
| 50093707 | 3 | F | 37,549 |
| 50093701 | 1 | F | 32,546 |
| 50093801 | 1 | F | 33,675 |
| 50093971 | 1 | F | 32,546 |
| 50094435 | 1 | F | 45,324 |
| 50094446 | 1 | F | 64,352 |
| 50094136 | 1 | M | 37,549 |
| 50094167 | 1 | M | 32,546 |
| 50094165 | 3 | F | 37,549 |

**Question: what is the percentage of males and females in this period?**

To prepare this, we needed to change the value field setting from "sum" to "count," because we used MRN as the "data." Then we change the display to "percentage." No other data manipulation is required in order to answer the question.

| Row Labels | Count of MRN |
|------------|--------------|
| F | 58.43% |
| M | 41.57% |
| (blank) | 0.00% |
| Grand Total | 100.00% |

**Question: what is the frequency of patients NOT discharged to home?**

In this example, we used the DC Status as both the row and the data, again amending both the calculation to "count" and display of the data to "percentage." Patients discharged to home are DC Status 1; therefore the answer to the question is the sum of all of the other DC Status values or 26.64% (100% minus 73.36%).

| Row Labels | Count of DC Status |
|------------|--------------------|
| 1 | 73.36% |
| 2 | 2.84% |
| 3 | 15.28% |
| 6 | 2.01% |
| 7 | 1.35% |
| 20 | 2.62% |
| 50 | 0.26% |
| 51 | 0.13% |
| 62 | 0.35% |
| 63 | 0.22% |
| 64 | 0.26% |
| 65 | 1.31% |
| (blank) | 0.00% |
| Grand Total | 100.00% |

**Question: is there a possible relationship between discharge disposition and gender?**

To answer this question, we use Discharge Disposition as the rows and Gender as the Columns, again using "count" and "percentage" to get a quick look at any potential pattern. Taking a quick look at the numbers, there does not appear to be any significant difference in discharge disposition category between males and females.

| Count of DC Status | Column Labels | | |
|--------------------|------|------|-------------|
| Row Labels | F | M | Grand Total |
| 1 | 74.44% | 71.85% | 73.36% |
| 2 | 2.02% | 3.99% | 2.84% |
| 3 | 15.62% | 14.81% | 15.28% |
| 6 | 2.09% | 1.89% | 2.01% |
| 7 | 0.82% | 2.10% | 1.35% |
| 20 | 2.02% | 3.47% | 2.62% |
| 50 | 0.22% | 0.32% | 0.26% |
| 51 | 0.07% | 0.21% | 0.13% |
| 62 | 0.45% | 0.21% | 0.35% |
| 63 | 0.37% | 0.00% | 0.22% |
| 64 | 0.37% | 0.11% | 0.26% |
| 65 | 1.49% | 1.05% | 1.31% |
| (blank) | 0.00% | 0.00% | 0.00% |
| Grand Total | 100.00% | 1 | 100.00% |

• **Fig. 7.29** Pivot table example.

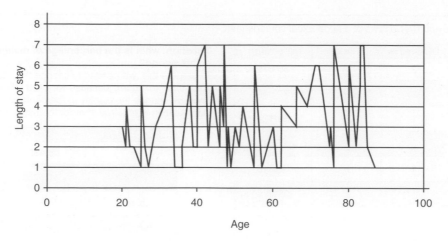

• **Fig. 7.30** Line graph comparing length of stay (in days) with patient age (in years).

Comparison of Hospital A and Hospital B by Payer

|  | Number of Discharges | |
| --- | --- | --- |
|  | Hospital A | Hospital B |
| Medicare | 5,000 | 13,229 |
| Medicaid | 2,300 | 6,032 |
| Blue Cross/Blue Shield | 1,500 | 3,975 |
| Commercial carriers | 950 | 2,453 |
| Charity care | 500 | 1,423 |
| Self-pay | 125 | 367 |
| Other payers | 90 | 325 |
| Total discharges | 10,465 | 27,804 |

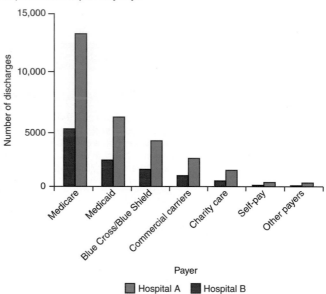

Comparison of Hospital A and Hospital B by Payer

|  | Percentage of Discharges | |
| --- | --- | --- |
| Payer | Hospital A | Hospital B |
| Medicare | 48% | 48% |
| Medicaid | 22% | 22% |
| Blue Cross/Blue Shield | 14% | 14% |
| Commercial carriers | 9% | 9% |
| Charity care | 5% | 5% |
| Self-pay | 1% | 1% |
| Other payers | 1% | 1% |
| Total | 100% | 100% |

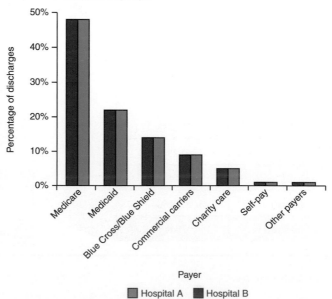

• **Fig. 7.31** Bar graph construction using data from Table 7.2 to compare Hospital A and Hospital B by payer.

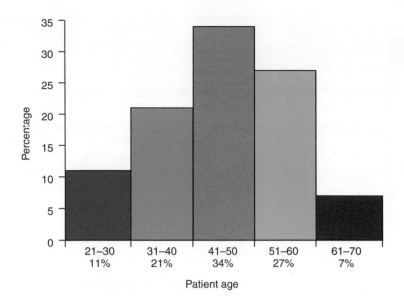

• **Fig. 7.32** Histogram.

|  | Hospital C | |
| --- | --- | --- |
| Payer | Discharges | % of Total |
| Medicare | 4500 | 43% |
| Medicaid | 2250 | 21% |
| Blue Cross/Blue Shield | 1625 | 15% |
| Commercial Carriers | 1100 | 10% |
| Uncompensated Care | 650 | 6% |
| Self-Pay | 250 | 2% |
| Other Payers | 180 | 2% |
| Total | 10,555 | 100% |

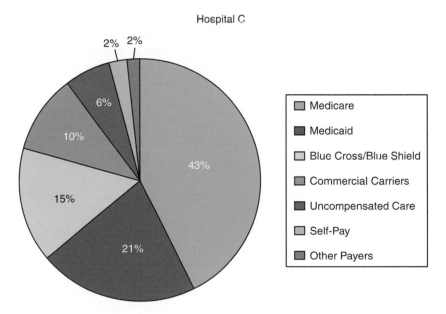

• **Fig. 7.33** Pie chart construction using payer mix data.

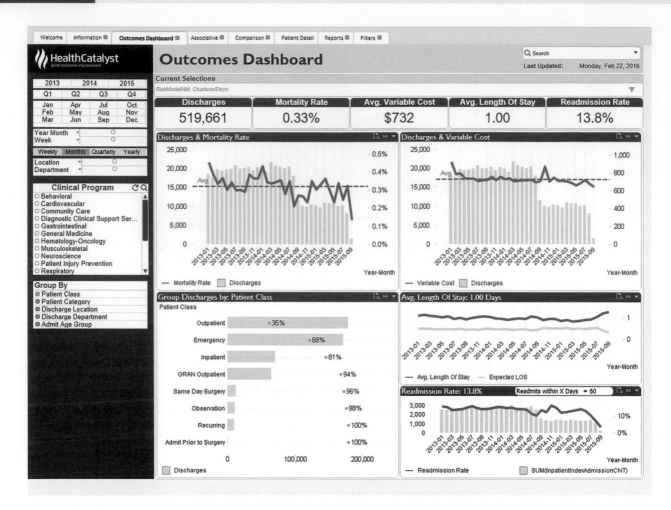

• **Fig. 7.34** Dashboards allow the visualization of the most important data on one screen. (Courtesy Health Catalyst, Inc., Salt Lake City, Utah.)

percentage of discharges, by payer, for Hospital C. Note that numerous payers who do not appear in the government and Blue Cross categories are combined together as "other payers."

Using a spreadsheet program, such as Microsoft Excel, to create graphs allows the user to experiment efficiently with the graph-making process and is best for professional-looking results.

## Dashboard

Every time you get in a car, you see a dashboard. Depending on the age of your car, it might tell you the following: current speed, distance traveled, time, average miles per gallon, current miles per gallon, and miles remaining on the current tank of gas. Imagine that same information on your computer screen when you log in every morning, only instead of automobile information it gives you current census, monthly discharges to date, month-to-date ALOS, month-to-date CMI, and today's Discharged, No Final Bill (DNFB). Increasingly, administrators and managers want real-time information that they can use to make decisions. These dashboards

of critical information (largely KPIs) can be collected and assembled manually to prepare a paper summary report, or the information can be gathered electronically and used to populate specific fields on a computer display (Fig. 7.34).

Typically, information on a dashboard is paired with a target or desired value for comparison. So, if it is desirable that DNFB be less than $8 million, then the current DNFB would display with that target. Depending on the number of information items needed, displays can be created that are colorful in a meaningful way—usually green, yellow, and red representing good, concerned, and bad, respectively.

Dashboards are useful not only at the administrative and managerial levels but also for supervision real-time. Workflow dashboards, such as for transcription and coding, can show—real-time—when a backlog is starting to happen so that the supervisor can take action to prevent it from getting worse. The number of dictations, by type (H&P, Operative Report, Progress Note, Discharge Summary), can show on a bar or speedometer, while the transcriptionist productivity can display by transcriptionist or work queue. An algorithm can be used to calculate the average transcription speed against the number of minutes of dictation pending to determine the estimated time to completion. If that estimated time approaches what is possible in the current staffing load, additional staff can be assigned to compensate. Obviously, this scenario is best applied to a 24-hour, 7-day-a-week operation for which on-call staff are available quickly.

Whether prepared manually or pushed electronically, dashboards can be a useful tool for decision support.

## Chapter Summary

Health information must be collected in a systematic, defined format. The database created by this systematic collection is then a source of information for departments within the organization and agencies external to the facility.

The data can be analyzed, interpreted, and presented to appropriate users through the use of statistical tools, including arithmetic mean, median, and mode, geometric mean, and standard deviation, as well as bar graphs, pie charts, and line graphs. The analysis of a facility's data is also referred to as the *facility's statistics*, which describes the services and activities of the facility. One important secondary use of health data is research. The research process identifies a topic, focuses on a question, conducts a study, analyzes the results, and determines what generalizations are possible from the results. To investigate a question, the researcher must identify and define the relevant variables. Depending on the nature of the variable (nominal data, ordinal data, integer data, or ratio data), the researcher will be able to analyze the data appropriately. Quantitative analysis is the easiest with variables that can be expressed numerically. Qualitative analysis relies on observations that are not inherently numerical.

An important use of health information databases is the identification of cases to report to registries, such as cancer registry and trauma registry.

## Competency Milestones

### CAHIIM Competency
*I.6. Describe components of data dictionaries and data sets. (2)*

#### Rationale
Understanding data elements and data requirements supports HIM professionals in their work with revenue cycle, database management, forms control, and release of information, for example. See also Competency Check-In 2.3: Data Collection and Storage.

#### Competency Assessment
1. What is the purpose of the unique field name in a data dictionary?
2. Compare and contrast data sets collected in a registry versus discharge data sets such as UHDDS.

### CAHIIM Competency
*III.1. Apply health informatics concepts to the management of health information. (3)*

#### Rationale
Although HIM professionals are not informaticists, the understanding of the underlying concepts supports the management of data quality and communication with information systems staff.

#### Competency Assessment
1. A CDSS is an example of
   a. A knowledge-based system
   b. A nonknowledge-based system
   c. A data dictionary
   d. A computerized physician order entry system
2. Patient access has been having trouble identifying Medicare patients who need to sign an ABN in case their laboratory test or procedure is not covered. They are considering having ALL Medicare patients sign the ABN; however, that is not necessary, nor is it appropriate. What informatics solution could support this function?

### CAHIIM Competency
*III.3. Calculate statistics for health care operations. (3)*

## Rationale

Analysis, interpretation, and presentation of data provide statistics that further identify a facility and its activities. HIM professionals are uniquely positioned to aid in answering questions that require retrieval and reporting of collected data.

## Case Study

Use the information in the table to answer the following questions.

First Quarter Data, Diamonte Hospital, 10/01/20XX–12/31/20XX.

| | | |
|---|---|---|
| Admissions | Adults and children | 9,218 |
| | Newborns | 290 |
| Discharges (including deaths) | Adults and children | 9,014 |
| | Newborns | 303 |
| Inpatient service days | Adults and children | 35,421 |
| | Newborns | 432 |
| Total lengths of stay | Adults and children | 32,542 |
| | Newborns | 608 |
| Bed count | Adults and children | 450 |
| | Newborns | 30 |
| Mortality data | Total adults and children: | |
| | <48 hours | 12 |
| | ≥48 hours | 132 |
| | Total newborns: | |
| | <48 hours | 2 |
| | ≥48 hours | 1 |
| | Anesthesia deaths | 1 |
| | Fetal deaths: | |
| | Early | 3 |
| | Intermediate and late | 9 |
| | Maternal deaths | 1 |
| | Postoperative deaths: | |
| | <10 days | 45 |
| | ≥10 days | 5 |
| | Removed by medical examiner | 7 |
| Operations | Number of patients operated on | 836 |
| | Surgical operations performed | 889 |
| | Anesthesia administered | 856 |
| | Postoperative infections | 12 |
| Miscellaneous | Cesarean sections | 69 |
| | Deliveries | 349 |
| | Nosocomial infections | 13 |
| | Autopsies | 6 |
| | Consultations | 2,756 |

1. What is the hospital's fiscal year?
2. Calculate to two decimal places:
   a. Average inpatient service days (adults)
   b. Average NB inpatient service days
   c. Average LOS
   d. Bed occupancy
   e. Consultation rate
   f. Nosocomial infection rate
   g. Hospital autopsy rate

CAHIIM Competency
*III.4. Report health care data through graphical representations. (3)*

## Rationale

After analysis and interpretation, the data can be presented as information. When information is requested, it is your job to present data in a meaningful and accessible manner. As we present the results of a data analysis, we need to consider the best way to make it informative to the target audience.

Trends are found in the presentation of data over time. Reporting data and identifying trends are tasks central to the healthy operation of any organization. Trend analysis helps the user identify whether performance is behaving in the desired way.

## Competency Assessment

1. What displays would you want on a dashboard if you were the Coding Supervisor?
2. Go to the CDC website at https://www.cdc.gov/injury/wisqars/fatal.html. Select Leading Causes of Death. Request a separate report for each of 2 or more years' causes of death in a category that interests you. You can download to Excel the results of each year's data. Prepare a 3-slide presentation explaining what the data represent. Include a title slide, a slide that explains what data you requested, and at least one slide with a graph that you created to explain or discuss the data you obtained.
3. Using the CABG report in Fig. 7.11 of the text, prepare a presentation for your instructor demonstrating the ALOS for the patients of each physician.
4. Health information professionals are commonly asked to analyze data for presentation. The presentation may be a simple table or report, or it may include graphs. Using the Internet, locate a database of patient information for query of a diagnosis-related group assigned by your instructor. Prepare a report with a graph for presentation to your instructor.

## Case Study

Your administration has noted an increase in injuries treated in the ED that were related to firearms and has asked you to look into trends in your geographical area. You do not have any current data, but you are able to review 3-year rates from the CDC at: https://www.cdc.gov/injury/wisqars/fatal.html. For deaths due to violence and firearms observe the trends associated with the following:

1. Five largest and smallest states.
2. Comparison of your state with your geographical region.
3. Comparison of your state with four other states of similar size.
4. Comment on your findings.

CAHIIM Competency
*III.5. Describe research methodologies used in health care. (2)*

## Rationale

Much of health care delivery is based on evidence-based practice. The evidence comes from a variety of sources, including research.

## Competency Assessment

1. You are searching for some evidence-based studies on the impact of clinical documentation improvement and come across a peer-reviewed journal article in which the authors collected data from numerous studies. What type of research is represented in the article?
   a. Survey
   b. Mixed method
   c. Experimental
   d. Metaanalysis
2. You are working with the coding staff to develop an operational definition of coding accuracy to study the impact of an upcoming implementation of an EHR in the ambulatory surgery department. Which should be included?
   a. The amount of time it takes to code a chart, measured in minutes.
   b. The number of correct codes assigned, divided by the total number of codes assigned.
   c. 100% minus the error rate on MS-DRG assignment.
   d. The number of correct codes assigned, divided by the total number of correct codes determined on audit.
3. You want to conduct a research study to determine whether frequent, short yoga breaks during the work day will improve coding productivity. In framing your hypothesis, which represents a useful baseline measurement of the dependent variable?
   a. The coder's historical productivity

b. The coder's productivity during the study

c. The number and duration of yoga breaks

d. The number and duration of breaks

4. The Zika virus is very rare in the United States. A group of researchers was able to collect demographic and clinical data from all 452 reported cases for their study. These researchers used a:

a. Convenience sample

b. Population

c. Stratified sample

d. Random sample

5. The HIM department does not have time to check the accuracy of all the coding, since the hospital averages over 1000 discharges every month. In fact, last year, the 281-bed facility had 14,182 discharges. Instead, they audit the coding of every third discharge. What is the population size for last year? What is the sample size?

6. Describe the type of study a physical therapist might conduct to determine whether the application of ice to an affected joint has an impact on posttherapy pain.

## CAHIIM Competency
*III.6. Describe the concepts of managing data. (3)*

### Rationale
Even if you are not working directly in data analytics or statistics, you will be supplying information to drive decision support. HIM professionals understand the data, including the optimum source of data and the meaning of coded data. Therefore HIM professionals are uniquely positioned to aid in answering questions that require retrieval and reporting of collected data.

### Competency Assessment
1. Why would the HIM department want to track data requests?
2. How does one determine the optimal source of data?
3. What is the optimal source for the following data in an inpatient record?
   a. Medications that the patient has already received.
   b. Possible diagnosis after 2 days in the hospital.
   c. Patient's temperature.
4. Your manager has asked you to use a publicly available Medicare database to compare the number of myocardial infarction patients who were admitted through the ED with your hospital's admission source for this type of patient. You know that the data she mentioned is compiled from UHDDS. What is your response?
5. How do facilities make discrete data available for query if it is not a data element required for collection by regulatory requirements, accreditation bodies, or payers?

### Case Study 1
Your administrator has asked for a summary of discharges by payer for commercial accounts for the month of March. You run a preprogrammed report that produces the following:

| March, 20XX | Discharges by Primary Payer |
|---|---|
| Blue Cross/Blue Shield | 350 |
| Medicare | 300 |
| Aetna | 250 |
| Cigna | 200 |
| Other commercial vendors | 80 |
| Medicaid | 75 |
| Worker's compensation | 10 |
| Total | 1265 |

1. How can you tell whether the report is complete?
2. Is any clarification of the request needed (from the administrator)?
3. Assuming you are satisfied with this report, what will you give the administrator?

## Case Study 2

*Refer to the Healthcare Cost and Utilization Project database HCUP.net:* https://healthdata.gov/dataset/hcupnet. *As you go through this assessment, pay attention to the explanatory notes on each page.*

1. Say your manager wanted you to query the HCUP database regarding a particular diagnosis for cases from 2016 through 2018. Could you do it?
2. Follow the query logic and select 2014 as your time period, inpatient as your population, and specify a search by diagnosis. Why can you not use ICD-10-CM codes to specify the diagnosis?
3. How many cases of uncomplicated benign prostatic hypertrophy (BPH) (ICD-9-CM code: 600) were there in 2014?
4. Does this represent all of the cases of BPH in the country during 2014?
5. Is HCUP a useful database? Why or why not?

## Case Study 3

1. You have been asked to find external data to help the hospital understand its case mix better. You turn to the National and State Summaries of Inpatient Charge Data, FY2016, Microsoft Excel version files that are available on the CMS Medicare Provider Utilization and Payment Data: Inpatient website at https://www.cms.gov/Research-Statistics-Data-and-Systems/Statistics-Trends-and-Reports/Medicare-Provider-Charge-Data/Inpatient.html. Of particular concern are these MS-DRGs, which are showing a high error rate on coding audits. Review the MedPAR file and comment on the comparison to your data. What other uses can you see for the MedPAR data?

| MS-DRG | Description | Weight | 12-month volume |
|---|---|---|---|
| 061 | ISCHEMIC STROKE, PRECEREBRAL OCCLUSION OR TRANSIENT ISCHEMIA W THROMBOLYTIC AGENT W MCC | 2.8477 | |
| 062 | ISCHEMIC STROKE, PRECEREBRAL OCCLUSION OR TRANSIENT ISCHEMIA W THROMBOLYTIC AGENT W CC | 1.9437 | |
| 063 | ISCHEMIC STROKE, PRECEREBRAL OCCLUSION OR TRANSIENT ISCHEMIA W THROMBOLYTIC AGENT W/O CC/MCC | 1.6280 | |
| 064 | INTRACRANIAL HEMORRHAGE OR CEREBRAL INFARCTION W MCC | 1.8692 | |
| 065 | INTRACRANIAL HEMORRHAGE OR CEREBRAL INFARCTION W CC OR TPA IN 24 HRS | 1.0315 | |
| 066 | INTRACRANIAL HEMORRHAGE OR CEREBRAL INFARCTION W/O CC/MCC | 0.7268 | |
| 067 | NONSPECIFIC CVA & PRECEREBRAL OCCLUSION W/O INFARCT W MCC | 1.5014 | |
| 068 | NONSPECIFIC CVA & PRECEREBRAL OCCLUSION W/O INFARCT W/O MCC | 0.8987 | |

### CAHIIM Competency

*III.6.* **DM** *Manage data within a database system. (5)*

### Rationale

Patient and performance data support the business of health care. As an HIM professional, you are a steward of the data that creates reports, which ultimately drive organizational strategy.

### Competency Assessment

1. What type of information could be obtained from indices?
2. What is the difference between a registry and an index?
3. List individual departments and outside agencies to which you might report information.
4. You have been asked to provide a report for administration summarizing the volume of cardiac catheterization and angioplasty procedures performed by several different practice groups of physicians. List the steps you will take to obtain the data. (See Optimal Source of Data earlier in the chapter to prepare the report.)

## Ethics Challenge

*VI.7. Assess ethical standards of practice. (5)*

1. You are the department manager in HIM. You have just received a request from a physician on staff who is doing a study for publication. The physician would like you to prepare a list of all patients in the past 2 years who underwent cardiac catheterization, from which he will be reviewing the patient records. He is doing a study on the correlation between clinical indicators, catheterization, and eventual angioplasty. According to the physician, the CEO of the hospital approved the request and will be sending you a memo. You run the list and give it to him. Ethical or not?

## Critical Thinking Questions

1. In Box 7.1, Example of Ordinal Data, 70% of patients were Satisfied or Extremely Satisfied with the overall Patient Registration experience. Does that seem like a good result? Is there room for improvement? What other questions would you like to ask? If you were the Manager of Patient Access, what action, if any, would you take after receiving this result?

## The Role of Health Information Management Professionals in the Workplace

### Professional Profile: Clinical Data Analyst

 My name is Maggie, and I am the clinical data analyst at Diamonte. I am responsible for overseeing the quality of the data contained in the health information management (HIM) database.

I am the contact person for all matters concerning the HIM database. In this role, I process all requests for reports from the HIM database. When quality management, administration, physician, or case management staff members need information from our database, they come to me. I make sure I know the following:

- What information they want.
- Why they need it.
- The time frame for the information.
- When they need the report.

This information helps me run the correct report so that employees may use the information as necessary in their presentation, decision-making, or investigation. Sometimes, the users have a question, but they do not really know how to answer it.

I find this part of my job very rewarding. I enjoy receiving a request that people think is impossible because I know that our HIM database contains the information that they need. Providing those reports is really exciting.

### Career Tip

Many individuals working in decision-support roles over the years did not have an HIM or even a hospital background.

With the increasing availability of electronically collected data, a background in the sources of data, such as a degree in HIM or a clinical discipline, is extremely helpful. Database skills with queries, postquery data manipulation, and software tools for data analytics are essential. For anyone wishing to pursue an interest in this area, courses (including continuing education) in database management, queries, and software tools are helpful.

### Patient Care Perspective

### Dr. Lewis

Our group is considering adding another physician and we wanted to confirm the gap in the group. We think we need a pulmonologist, because our own records show a high level of referrals, but we do not have enough data to make that decision. I called Maggie at Diamonte and obtained a report on all patients admitted by physicians in our group, as well as our patients who were treated by hospitalists. I asked for a spreadsheet that listed each patient for the past 2 years, the first five diagnoses, the first five procedures, and the ID for the attending physician and the PCP of record. With those data, we were able to determine that we admit enough patients with respiratory problems; however, they were mostly covered by the hospitalists. So we are looking for a pulmonologist who is comfortable working with hospitalists.

## Works Cited

American Statistical Association: *What is statistics?*, 2019. https://www.amstat.org//asa/what-is-statistics.aspx. Retrieved January 6, 2019.

American Medical Informatics Association (AMIA): *Why informatics?*, 2011. https://amia.org/about-amia/why-informatics/informatics-research-and-practice. Retrieved May 25, 2022.

National Center for Health Statistics: *Surveys and data collection systems*, 2018. https://www.cdc.gov/nchs/surveys.htm#tabs-1-2. Accessed February 1, 2023. Last reviewed June 22, 2022.

National Trauma Data Bank: *Trauma program: National Trauma Data Bank*, 2022. https://www.facs.org/quality-programs/trauma/quality/national-trauma-data-bank/. Retrieved May 31, 2022. copyright 1996–2022.

U.S. Department of Health and Human Services, Centers for Disease Control and Prevention, National Program of Cancer Registries (NCRPs): *About the program*, 2015. http://www.cdc.gov/cancer/npcr/about.htm. Accessed May 31, 2022. Updated July 2018.

# 8

# Confidentiality and Compliance

LISA REILLY

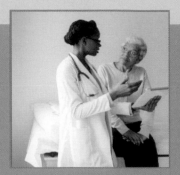

## CHAPTER OUTLINE

**Introduction**
 Compliance
 The Legal Health Record
**Legal and Legislative Landscape**
 Criminal Law
 Civil Law
 Litigation and the Judicial Process
**Consent**
 Informed Consent
 Admission
 Medical Procedures
**Privacy and Confidentiality**
 Scope
 Health Insurance Portability and Accountability Act
**Access**
 Continuing Patient Care
 Reimbursement
 Health Care Operations
 Litigation

 Public Health Activities
 Release of Information
 Record Retention
**Federal, Corporate, and Facility Compliance**
 Licensure and Certification
 Accreditation
**Risk Management**
 Disaster Planning
 Theft and Tampering
 Destruction of Health Information
**Chapter Summary**
**Competency Milestones**
**Ethics Challenge**
**Critical Thinking Question**
**The Role of Health Information Management Professionals in the Workplace**
 Professional Profile
 Patient Care Perspective
**Further Reading**

## CHAPTER OBJECTIVES

*By the end of this chapter, the student should be able to:*

1. Understand the legislative and legal landscape as it pertains to health care delivery and health care documentation and apply legal concepts and principles to the practice of health information management;
2. Comply with legal, ethical, and professional standards to protect patient privacy, especially regarding the provisions of the Health Insurance Portability and Accountability Act (HIPAA);

3. Adhere to policies and procedures surrounding access and disclosure of protected health information to patients and care providers;
4. Apply standards for accreditation, licensure, and/or certification; and
5. Promote risk management functions within the organization as they relate to compliance with accreditation and regulatory bodies.

# VOCABULARY

access
accounting of disclosures
accreditation
advance directive
amendment
American Recovery and Reinvestment Act (ARRA)
authorization
assault
battery
breach
business associates
business record rule
certification
competent
compliance
concurrent review
Conditions of Admission
confidential communication
confidentiality
consent
correspondence
court order
covered entities
custodian
defendant
designated record set
disclosure
discovery
emancipation
exception
Federal Drug and Alcohol Abuse Regulations
Health Information Technology for Economic and Clinical Health (HITECH) Act
Health Insurance Portability and Accountability Act (HIPAA)
hearsay rule
informed consent
jurisdiction
legal health record

liability
licensure
litigation
malpractice
minimum necessary
negligence
Notice of Privacy Practices
permitted disclosure
physician–patient privilege
plaintiff
potentially compensable events (PCEs)
power of attorney
preemption
privacy
privacy officer
prospective consent
protected health information (PHI)
release of information (ROI)
regulation
required disclosures
restriction
retention
retrospective consent
right to complain
right to revoke
risk management (RM)
security
statute
subpoena
subpoena ad testificandum
subpoena duces tecum
The Joint Commission (TJC)
tort
tracer methodology
use
verification
workers' compensation

## CAHIIM COMPETENCY DOMAINS

II.1. Apply privacy strategies to health information. (3)
II.3. Identify compliance requirements throughout the health information life cycle. (3)
V.1. Apply legal processes impacting health information. (3)
V.2. Demonstrate compliance with external forces. (3)
V.3. Identify the components of risk management related to health information management. (3)

## Introduction

Matters of law and accreditation underscore every aspect of the provision of health care. This chapter provides an overview of the US legal system and the laws that pertain to health care and health information management (HIM). We will also discuss the HIM activities that allow the facility to obtain and maintain accreditation. We will highlight confidentiality with an overview of the federal Health Insurance Portability and Accountability Act (HIPAA) Privacy Regulations as they pertain to patient rights, as well as uses and disclosures of health information. The importance of confidentiality, the rules critical to ensuring the confidentiality of a health record, and problems that can occur when requests for release of health information are received are also discussed. We will also discuss the standards needed to maintain accreditation, licensure, and certification, including those external forces requiring risk management (RM) processes.

## Compliance

**Compliance** means meeting standards. Within an organization, it also means the development, implementation, and enforcement of policies and procedures that ensure that standards are met. As a result of increasing pressure from the federal government, health care organizations have spent a great deal of time and effort in recent years demonstrating their commitment to data quality, particularly in terms of accurate billing. Some of this pressure comes from the Department of Health and Human Services (HHS) Office of the Inspector General, which has received increased funding for enforcing accurate billing through audits and penalties. In addition, the HIPAA legislation of 1996, the Balanced Budget Act of 1997, and the **HITECH** provisions in the **American Recovery and Reinvestment Act (ARRA)** legislation of 2009 increased the penalties for failure to comply with regulations. These officers can take this action if they find that their states' populations suffered because of a HIPAA violation. Compliance with the many and varied regulations governing health care has become a major focus of health care organizations and individual providers.

A compliance program is a facility-wide system of policies, procedures, and guidelines that help to ensure legal and ethical business practices. These policies, procedures, and guidelines should include, for example, ethics statements, strong leadership policies, commitment to compliance with regulations, and ways for employees to report unethical or noncompliant activities and behaviors. Part of a compliance effort is a coding compliance program. Such a program ensures accurate coding and billing through training, continuing education, quality assurance, and performance improvement (PI) activities.

## The Legal Health Record

Another challenge of health care organizations and individual providers, particularly in the context of an electronic health record (EHR), is the identification and maintenance of a **legal health record**, or the organization's officially declared business record of health care services a provider delivers to an individual. Exactly which sources, documents, and information comprise the legal health record varies depending on the needs of the organization. As we have discussed in previous chapters, there are multiple sources of patient data that constitute the health record, for example, paper forms, electronic form data entry, electronic data transfer, and scanned documents. There may also be audio files of provider dictation, digital images or video from imaging procedures, personal health record (PHR) data entered by the patient, and billing data. When considering the legal health record, the organization must decide what information to maintain for the longer term and, by extension, what information is released upon request. The challenge is not so much to understand all the sources, but to distinguish when the record is complete. By complete, we mean not just signed, dated, and timed but also containing all the necessary components in the appropriate location and on the proper medium.

To define what is a complete record, the organization must identify all the possible components of the record and where those components will be found in any given scenario. The health care organization must create a policy that defines the full legal heath record in a way that meets not only the record's primary purpose of clinical communication for the care of the patient but also the legal needs of the organization. For example, consider a patient who was admitted to the hospital from the emergency department (ED) and who had visited the ED 2 days previously for a related issue and had a diagnostic computed tomography scan as an outpatient at another facility in between, the report of which was scanned into the record. If the patient's record is requested to be used as evidence in court, what components, exactly, would be disclosed? The hospital must decide which of those components of the patient record constitute the legal record in the event that the record is used in a legal proceeding. In order to understand why that is important, we turn our attention to the legal system.

## Legal and Legislative Landscape

Laws are rules for conduct or behavior enforceable by a controlling authority, such as a government. In the United States, the authority to make laws comes from the US Constitution, the supreme law of the land, which establishes the power of the federal government. The Constitution also limits government power by recognizing the rights of states and individuals. No other laws from any level of government may contradict the laws of the Constitution, nor the rights it enumerates. The Constitution takes priority over any federal laws, state constitutions and statutes, and decisions of the courts. Each state has a Constitution containing the supreme law within the boundaries of each state but even they are subordinate to federal law and the US Constitution. States cannot pass statutes that conflict with the US Constitution because the Constitution's Supremacy Clause makes a conflicting law invalid through federal **preemption**.

A federal law passed by Congress is called an act. A **statute** is a law that has been passed by the legislative branch of government and signed by the executive branch. A **regulation** is a set of rules that enable the enforcement of compliance with a statute. Each state has licensure requirements for health care facilities. Generally, states also have regulations regarding medical records. Health care facilities must comply with these regulations to maintain their facility license. A facility must follow federal laws, federal regulations, state laws, and state regulations. So, a state statute would require a license to practice medicine; a state regulation is the set of rules that explains how to obtain a license, the requirements for licensure, what agency is responsible for enforcing compliance, and the penalties for practicing without a license.

Local governments and municipalities enact ordinances, their own laws or decrees, but these must not conflict with state or federal laws or statutes. As mentioned in Chapter 1, local governments typically impact the facility with respect to zoning ordinances and tax structures.

There are two areas of law: criminal law, which pertains to wrongs perpetrated against the government or the general public, and civil law, which involves disputes among individuals or organizations.

## Criminal Law

Criminal law concerns offenses against the laws of the government. When an individual commits a crime, he or she acts in violation of the law established by the government and therefore against the welfare of the public. Of course, crimes often do have a specific, individual victim. Murder, robbery, assault, and vandalism are examples of violations of criminal law. Charges of crimes are brought to the court by government officials, and punishments may include probation or prison time. In the health care industry, criminal violations usually involve charges of fraud, assault, or battery.

### Assault and Battery

The law treats a surgeon who operates without securing the patient's consent the same way it would if the physician attacked the patient with a scalpel. Battery is the crime of touching a person in a way that causes the individual harm or otherwise offends the individual. In health care, patients have a right to choose the treatments performed on them, therefore the physician's contact with the patient without consent is battery. Assault is the threat or intention of causing harm without physical contact. For example, a nursing facility aide who threatens to put a patient in restraints if the patient does not shower is committing an assault.

### Fraud

Health care fraud is committed when a provider, consumer (patient), or organization (such as an insurer or hospital) submits false or misleading information with the intent to somehow profit. There are several examples of health care fraud, which will be discussed further later, including:

- knowingly submitting false statements for payment;
- knowingly seeking and/or accepting payment for referrals of items or services ("kickbacks");
- billing for services that were not medically necessary;
- charging excessively for services or supplies;
- double-billing or filing duplicate claims for the same service; and
- misusing codes on a claim, such as upcoding, which is billing at a higher level than the actual service provided, or unbundling codes, where the service is billed in steps rather than as one total procedure.

Although it is more common for providers to commit health care fraud, patients may commit it by faking medical conditions in order to receive medications, falsifying medical claim information, or using someone else's insurance information to receive health care services.

Each state government and the federal government have laws against health care fraud. Regardless of the state law in place, federal health fraud law will apply in most situations, which usually applies when fraud is committed against any health care benefits program, such as Medicare and Medicaid. Health care fraud is punishable by fines and/or prison time, which may be at the minimum 5 years in federal prison, with fines ranging from $250,000 to more than $1 million, and even higher, depending upon the amount of money defrauded from the government. In addition to these penalties, health care providers who have been convicted of Medicare fraud or other felony fraud offenses may be excluded from federal health care programs. Exclusion prevents a person or entity from directly billing Medicare for any items or services. It can also limit a health care provider's ability to work for or contract with parties who receive funding through federal health care programs.

### Stark Law

The Stark Law is part of the Social Security Act and is commonly known as the "physician self-referral law." Providers are prohibited from making referrals for certain designated health services (DHS) payable by Medicare to any facility or health care business that the provider or an immediate family member either owns, has invested in, or receives payment from unless an exception applies. DHS include clinical laboratory; physical, occupational, or speech pathology; radiology; medical equipment and supplies; prosthetic devices; and prescription drugs.

The Stark Law was passed to control provider conflicts of interest and to prevent using patient referrals for the provider's personal financial gain. It was originally enacted to prevent providers from ordering unneeded clinical laboratory tests as a way of increasing profits but now covers an extensive list of testing and treatment facilities. However, providers can legally refer patients to testing facilities within a managed care organization.

### False Claims Act

The False Claims Act (FCA) allows for recovery of money from anyone who knowingly submits a fraudulent claim for reimbursement of services to the government. Health services administrators must be very careful when billing any governmental body, such as Medicare/Medicaid, for provider services, since the claim does not have to be entirely fraudulent to violate the FCA. Any false statement or document that supports a false claim can be considered breaking the FCA rules. If a provider or practice is convicted of submitting false claims, they can face fines of $5500–$11,000 plus three times the government's damages for each claim under issue. Any individual can be held responsible if he or she is convicted of acting willfully, recklessly, or with deliberate ignorance when creating false claims. Those found responsible may even face criminal charges in extreme cases.

### Sunshine Act

The Sunshine Act, or the Physician Payments Act, is designed to increase the transparency around the financial relationships between physicians, teaching hospitals, and manufacturers of pharmaceuticals, medical devices, and biologics. The law hopes to identify any questionable financial relationships between these parties and to help prevent inappropriate influence on research, education, and clinical decision-making.

Manufacturers must submit annual reports to the Centers for Medicare & Medicaid Services (CMS), which then itemizes the payments and transfers of value made to health care providers. There are some areas that are acceptable under the law and do not require reporting, such as:

- A sponsoring manufacturer can provide food or drink to a large group of conference attendees.
- Small payments of less than $10 do not need to be reported, except when the total annual value exceeds $100.
- Discounts and rebates for covered drugs or devices do not have to be reported.
- Manufacturers can donate supplies to patients who cannot afford them as long as the provider does not make money from the donation.
- Product samples, including coupons and vouchers, that can be given to patients do not have to be reported.
- Educational materials and items that directly benefit patients are excluded.
- Under certain circumstances, manufacturers can pay a provider for speaking at a continuing education program.

Once the manufacturer submits its annual report to CMS's Open Payments Program, which is the federal program that collects and compiles the data, the data are made available to physicians for review and to dispute any errors before the information is made public on the Open Payments website: https://openpaymentsdata.cms.gov/.

## Civil Law

Civil law addresses disputes among individuals and/or organizations. Rather than being prosecuted by the government, in a civil case, one party brings another party to court. **Litigation** is the process by which one party sues another in a court of law. Litigation often results when a patient has been injured, either accidentally or intentionally. Penalties for wrongdoing are usually in the form of financial compensation. The party requesting court intervention is the **plaintiff**. The party who must respond is the **defendant**. Sometimes, actions may be violations of both criminal and civil law. For example, a drunk driver swerves onto the sidewalk and hits a pedestrian, resulting in the victim's death. The government may prosecute the driver for driving while intoxicated and vehicular manslaughter, incurring fines and a prison sentence. The victim's family may also sue the drunk driver for damages

and wrongful death. The criminal offenses are crimes, while the wrongful acts of civil law are called **torts**.

Some types of litigation concern the delivery of patient care itself. A lawsuit may be filed when there is harm to the patient, even if the damage is unintentional. When a surgeon amputates the wrong foot, it is a clear example of harm or damage to the patient, although there are other cases. Invasion of privacy and **breach** of contract—especially when it concerns patient confidentiality—are common types of claims of which HIM professionals in particular must be aware. Many books are devoted solely to the complexities of health care and the law, but it is important to introduce several key concepts.

A legal **liability** is the responsibility for harm or damage caused by one's actions—or inactions. A physician who has amputated a patient's left foot instead of the right foot is probably liable for the harm caused to the patient. Employers are also liable for the actions of their employees and can be sued under the doctrine of vicarious liability (*respondeat superior*). However, many physicians are not employees of the hospital, and, as independent practitioners, vicarious liability historically excluded hospitals themselves from the actions of nonemployee physicians. This situation changed after the 1965 case, *Darling v. Charleston Community Memorial Hospital*. In *Darling*, a physician fitted a football player's broken leg with a cast that was too tight. Nurses employed by the hospital alerted the physician of the boy's worsening condition over the next several days, but the treating physician failed to take appropriate action, and eventually, the leg had to be amputated. The boy's parents sued the hospital, and the court found that the hospital failed to monitor the quality of care being delivered within. After the Charleston case, hospitals could be sued directly under "corporate negligence."

### *Unintentional Torts*

**Negligence** refers to a tort caused by carelessness or a lack of foresight. Negligence comes from a Latin word meaning "to neglect." A shopper slipped and fell at the grocery store. The supermarket may have been negligent if the floor had been recently mopped and it *neglected* to warn customers with "Caution-Wet Floor" signs. The type of tort this caused was not intentional, but reasonable care may have prevented the accident.

**Malpractice** revolves around the concept of negligence. When a patient seeks treatment from a physician, the physician and patient enter an agreement in which the physician is obligated to use his or her skills to treat the patient with care and at a standard of professional competence. Malpractice occurs when a health care provider incurs harm to a patient because of a failure to practice reasonable standards of care. Most instances of medical malpractice involve medical error, such as misdiagnosis of a patient's condition or a surgeon who inadvertently leaves an instrument inside a patient during an operation. Malpractice may also refer to intentional wrongdoing, although the majority of medical malpractice claims result from negligence on the part of the provider.

## Intentional Torts

Unlike unintentional torts, intentional torts are meant to harm an individual. Some criminal acts, such as fraud and assault and battery, are also intentional torts under civil law. Others bear special attention with respect to social media:

- Defamation—a false statement that harms another person's reputation, which is further classified as either:
  - Libel—false statements in print, text message or email, broadcast, or on social media
  - Slander—spoken false statements
- Invasion of privacy—publicly exposing a person's private affairs without consent

This chapter will discuss the legal aspects of privacy in detail later.

## Litigation and the Judicial Process

Most lawsuits based on injury require disclosure of medical records. The shopper slips on the newly mopped floor at the grocery store. A man sprains his back falling off a footbridge in the town park and sues the city. A pedestrian is hit by a car, breaks a leg, and sues the driver of the car. A physician amputates the wrong foot, and the patient sues the physician and the hospital. Each of these incidents will require medical records to both support the extent of the plaintiff's injuries and document that the plaintiff did not have the injuries before the accident.

The plaintiffs in these cases file a complaint with the court that states the issues, the reason they chose that particular court, and what outcome they desire. In the grocery store example, the plaintiff may file a complaint in a state court stating that the grocery store's floor was wet and posed a hazard, which was the cause of the accident. The complaint is filed in that court because the store is located in that state and the plaintiff lives in that state. The plaintiff wants the court to agree that the store was at fault and to order the store to pay for the plaintiff's medical care and loss of income. The steps in this type of litigation are listed and defined in Box 8.1.

---

**• BOX 8.1  Steps in Litigation**

1. Prelitigation medical review panel or tribunal (does not apply in all states for medical malpractice claims).
2. Filing of the lawsuit in the appropriate state or federal court
3. Discovery: Various techniques (e.g., depositions, interrogatories, requests for production of documents and things, admissions of fact, independent medical examinations) are used to discover pertinent information relating to the facts and issues of the case.
4. Pretrial settlement hearing.
5. Mediation before trial.
6. Trial by judge or jury.
7. Appeal of the decision or judgment.

From Aiken TD: *Legal and ethical issues in health occupations*, Philadelphia, PA, 2008, Saunders, p 221.

---

There are two steps in the aforementioned lawsuit in which health records may be required.

The first step is during the **discovery** process. During discovery, the lawyers may want a copy of the documentation of the plaintiff's treatment to verify the extent and timing of the injuries as well as the nature, extent, and cost of care. The record may be needed again in court during the trial if it is used as evidence. During both of these steps, a certified or notarized copy of the original record is usually required. **Certification** is the process whereby the official custodian of the medical records certifies that the copies are true and complete copies of the original records. The **custodian**, usually the HIM director, is the official keeper of the medical records and may be called to testify.

The certification and use of health records as evidence in court are based on the **business record rule**. The business record rule states that health records may be accepted as evidence in the following instances:

- They are kept in the normal course of business.
- They are recorded by individuals who are in a position to be knowledgeable of the events that are being recorded.
- They are documented contemporaneously with those events.

The business record rule is an exception to the **hearsay rule**, which prohibits secondhand accounts of events. If the hearsay rule were applied to health records, then a nurse's documentation of a patient's statements or a physician's subjective notes would not be admissible evidence (i.e., it would not be allowed to be presented in court) (28a U.S.C. § 803(6) 2015).

The choice of a court in which to file the complaint is primarily a matter of **jurisdiction**. Jurisdiction means that the court has authority over the issue, the person, or both. There are courts of limited jurisdiction, such as traffic court, which can only decide certain types of cases. Other courts have general jurisdiction, such as state courts, and they may decide a wide variety of cases. In general, these courts have jurisdiction over citizens of the states in which they operate. There are also federal courts, the jurisdiction of which extends to issues regarding federal statutes, regulations, and treaties; events that occur on federal land; and legal actions between citizens of different states.

### Subpoenas and Court Orders

There are several different avenues through which access to the record can be obtained during litigation. First, the patient can sign an **authorization**—a written direction to release the patient's information—directing the provider to release the information to either the patient's lawyer or the defendant's lawyer. It is presumed that when a patient institutes litigation and uses the medical condition as a foundation for the litigation, he or she is waiving the right to confidentiality.

Another avenue of approach is through the *subpoena* process. A **subpoena** is a direction from an officer of the court. The direction may be to testify (*subpoena ad testificandum*) or to provide documentation (*subpoena duces tecum*; Fig. 8.1). The HIM department may receive a subpoena from the patient's lawyer or from the defendant's lawyer. A subpoena is valid for access to health records only if the subpoena itself is valid and the court through which the subpoena is issued has jurisdiction over the party to whom the subpoena is addressed. Box 8.2 lists the common elements of a valid subpoena.

A **court order** is the direction of a judge who has decided that an order to produce the records is necessary. Again, the issue of jurisdiction arises. For example, if an older patient's children seek to declare the patient legally incompetent (unable to make decisions about his or her affairs), the judge may issue a court order to obtain the patient's health records. Box 8.3 gives the components of a valid court order authorizing disclosure.

AO 88 (rev. 07/10) Subpoena to appear and testify at a hearing or trial in a civil action

# UNITED STATES DISTRICT COURT

for the

_____

| | |
|---|---|
| *Plaintiff* | ) |
| *v.* | )    Civil Action No. |
| | ) |
| *Defendant* | ) |

## SUBPOENA TO APPEAR AND TESTIFY
## AT A HEARING OR TRIAL IN A CIVIL ACTION

**TO:**

    **YOU ARE COMMANDED** to appear in the United States district court at the time, date, and place set forth below to testify at a hearing or trial in this civil action. When you arrive, you must remain at the court until the judge or a court officer allows you to leave.

| Place: | Courtroom No.: |
|---|---|
| | Date and Time: |

    You must also bring with you the following documents, electronically stored information, or objects *(blank if not applicable):*

    The provisions of Fed. R. Civ. P. 45(c), relating to your protection as a person subject to a subpoena, and Fed. R. Civ. P. 45 (d) and (e), relating to your duty to respond to this subpoena and the potential consequences of not doing so, are attached.

Date: _____

     *CLERK OF COURT*

                              OR

_____      _____

  *Signature of Clerk or Deputy Clerk*               *Attorney's signature*

The name, address, e-mail, and telephone number of the attorney representing *(name of party)* _____
_____ , who issues or requests this subpoena, are:

• **Fig. 8.1** Sample *subpoena ad testificandum* to testify in a civil case.

## • BOX 8.2 Common Elements of a Valid Subpoena

- Name of the court and jurisdiction of the case
- Names of the plaintiffs and defendants involved in the case
- The docket number of the case, a numerical identifier
- Date, time, and place of the requested appearance
- Specific documents to be produced, if a subpoena duces tecum is involved
- Name and contact information of the attorney who requested the subpoena
- Signature, stamp, or seal of the official empowered to issue the subpoena
- Witness fees, where provided by law

## • BOX 8.3 Components of a Valid Court Order Authorizing Disclosure

- Name of the court issuing the order to disclose
- Names of the plaintiff and defendant of the case
- Docket number (identification number) of the case
- Specific components of the medical record to be disclosed
- Specific persons to whom the information is to be disclosed
- Any other limitations on disclosure, such as sealing the court proceeding from the public in order to protect the patient's privacy

## COMPETENCY CHECK-IN 8.1

### Legal and Legislative Landscape

#### Competency Assessment

1. What part of the US Constitution invalidates any local, state, or federal laws that conflict with the Constitution?
   a. The Preamble
   b. The Bill of Rights
   c. The Emoluments Clause
   d. The Supremacy Clause
2. Which type of subpoena asks for documents to be produced that pertain to a legal case?
   a. Subpoena duces tecum
   b. Subpoena ad litem
   c. Subpoena ad testificandum
   d. Subpoena respondeat superior
3. Posting a picture on social media of a patient's injuries would be which type of tort?
   a. Intentional tort
   b. Malpractice
   c. Negligence
   d. Unintentional tort
4. Which is the crime of touching a person in a way that causes the individual harm?
   a. Assault
   b. Battery
   c. Kickback
   d. Defamation
5. A podiatrist who regularly bills Medicare for detailed examinations even though he has only performed problem-focused exams is violating which law?
   a. False Claims Act
   b. Sunshine Act
   c. Stark Law
   d. The Health Insurance Portability and Accountability Act

## Consent

In health care, **Consent** refers to the patient's agreement to allow something to occur. Consents underlie virtually all of a patient's contacts with health care professionals. When a patient makes an appointment with a physician to get a flu shot, consent to have the shot is implied because the patient showed up for the appointment (although we typically do sign a consent form for a flu shot). Implied consent is generally only sufficient for simple treatments for which there is little or no risk or in emergency situations. Consider a patient who walks into the ED and loses consciousness during triage. By walking into the ED and participating in triage, the patient has implied consent to medical assistance.

Express consent involves a specific agreement by the patient to receive the shot, usually by signing a consent form or verbally stating that they consent. Informed consent is a requirement for more complicated treatments and procedures. **Informed consent**, which is a type of express consent, is the patient's signed agreement to a treatment following an explanation of the process, procedure, risks, or other activity to which the patient is consenting. Sufficient information must be provided to the patient so he or she can make an informed decision about the matter. Documentation of this informed consent is required before certain types of health care can be rendered, such as surgical procedures.

## Informed Consent

For a patient to give consent, the patient must be of legal age, competent, and provided with sufficient information to make a reasonable decision about the issue to which he or she is consenting. Only the provider may discuss the treatment, its risks, and alternatives, and only the patient or the patient's representative may sign the consent. It is the provider's responsibility to ensure the patient has a complete understanding of the plan for treatment. Without informed consent, a case could be made that the provider has committed the crime of battery.

*Legal age* generally refers to having achieved the statutory age, which is determined by state law. Statutory age is usually 18 years. There are some exceptions, such as emancipated minors and minors receiving psychiatric treatment, chemical dependency counseling, or prenatal care. State laws outline the conditions under which minors are given **emancipation** (i.e., consideration as an adult even though they are younger than the statutory age). A common reason for emancipation is marriage.

*Competency* is the patient's ability to make reasonable decisions. A patient is **competent** if a court has not declared the individual incompetent and the patient is capable of understanding the alternatives and consequences of his or her decision. A patient who has been declared incompetent by a court has a guardian who can consent on behalf of the patient. This guardian is given a health care **power of attorney**. In general, a patient is assumed to be competent unless there is evidence to the contrary. When a patient's competence is in doubt, the patient's physician and hospital attorney should be contacted for guidance.

Even in the presence of an informed consent, an implied consent can be given. For example, a patient signs an informed consent for the procedure, which includes the risk of excessive bleeding. During the procedure, to which the patient consented, the physician encounters excessive bleeding. The surgeon will take action to stop the bleeding under implied consent as this risk was explained to the patient, although the patient did not expressly consent to whatever the surgeon does to stop the bleeding. On the other hand, consider a patient who is undergoing an appendectomy, during which the surgeon unexpectedly observes extensive endometriosis or visible signs of cancer. Without an informed consent to proceed with investigation or excision, the surgeon will have to obtain informed consent, either from the patient or their designated medical representative, for further diagnostic or therapeutic procedures.

## Admission

For admission to a health care facility or a visit to a physician's office, the patient is asked to sign a document consenting to medical treatment. This type of consent is very general and covers routine procedures, such as physical examinations and medical therapies, nutrition counseling, and medication prescription. In an inpatient facility, this consent is usually called the **Conditions of Admission** (Fig. 8.2). The Conditions of Admission form generally also includes permission for the facility to use patient information for education, research, and reimbursement.

Under the Patient Self-Determination Act, all health care providers who receive Medicare or Medicaid funding are required to inform patients of their legal right to accept or refuse treatment and the right to formulate advance directives. An **advance directive** is defined as a written document such as a living will or durable power of attorney for health care.

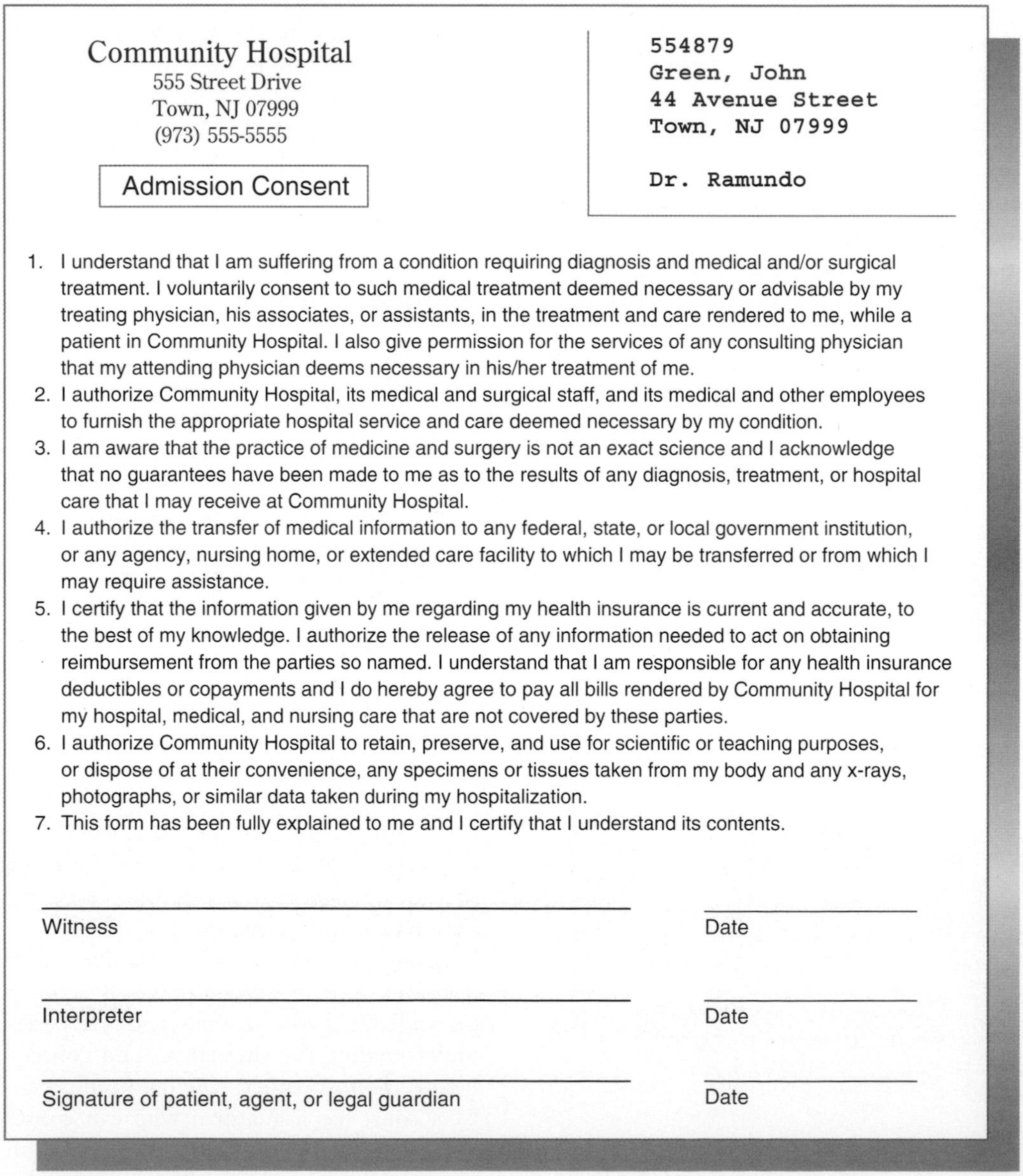

### Community Hospital
555 Street Drive
Town, NJ 07999
(973) 555-5555

| Admission Consent |

554879
Green, John
44 Avenue Street
Town, NJ 07999

Dr. Ramundo

1. I understand that I am suffering from a condition requiring diagnosis and medical and/or surgical treatment. I voluntarily consent to such medical treatment deemed necessary or advisable by my treating physician, his associates, or assistants, in the treatment and care rendered to me, while a patient in Community Hospital. I also give permission for the services of any consulting physician that my attending physician deems necessary in his/her treatment of me.
2. I authorize Community Hospital, its medical and surgical staff, and its medical and other employees to furnish the appropriate hospital service and care deemed necessary by my condition.
3. I am aware that the practice of medicine and surgery is not an exact science and I acknowledge that no guarantees have been made to me as to the results of any diagnosis, treatment, or hospital care that I may receive at Community Hospital.
4. I authorize the transfer of medical information to any federal, state, or local government institution, or any agency, nursing home, or extended care facility to which I may be transferred or from which I may require assistance.
5. I certify that the information given by me regarding my health insurance is current and accurate, to the best of my knowledge. I authorize the release of any information needed to act on obtaining reimbursement from the parties so named. I understand that I am responsible for any health insurance deductibles or copayments and I do hereby agree to pay all bills rendered by Community Hospital for my hospital, medical, and nursing care that are not covered by these parties.
6. I authorize Community Hospital to retain, preserve, and use for scientific or teaching purposes, or dispose of at their convenience, any specimens or tissues taken from my body and any x-rays, photographs, or similar data taken during my hospitalization.
7. This form has been fully explained to me and I certify that I understand its contents.

_____    _____
Witness                    Date

_____    _____
Interpreter                Date

_____    _____
Signature of patient, agent, or legal guardian    Date

• **Fig. 8.2** Sample of conditions of admission to a hospital.

AO 88 (rev. 07/10) Subpoena to appear and testify at a hearing or trial in a civil action (page 2)

Civil Action No.

*PROOF OF SERVICE*
*(This section should not be filed with the court unless required by Fed. R. Civ. P. 45.)*

This subpoena for *(name of individual and title, if any)* _____
was received by me on *(date)* _____.

☐ I served the subpoena by delivering a copy to the named person as follows: _____
_____
_____ on *(date)* _____ ; or

☐ I returned the subpoena unexecuted because: _____
_____

Unless the subpoena was issued on behalf of the United States, or one of its officers or agents, I have also tendered to the witness fees for one day's attendance, and the mileage allowed by law, in the amount of
$ _____.

My fees are $ _____ for travel and $ _____ for services, for a total of $ _____.

I declare under penalty of perjury that this information is true.

Date: _____

_____
*Server's signature*

_____
*Printed name and title*

_____
*Server's address*

Additional information regarding attempted service, etc.:

• **Fig. 8.2** cont'd

## Medical Procedures

The Conditions of Admission form includes only routine procedures and administrative issues. For invasive procedures, such as surgery, a specific consent is required. Anesthesia delivery and human immunodeficiency virus (HIV) testing are examples of other procedures that require specific consent. These consents are intended, in part, to document the extent to which procedures have been explained to patients, including the known risks of the procedures. Fig. 8.3 shows a consent for surgery form.

**Community Hospital**
555 Street Drive
Town, NJ 07999
(973) 555-5555

Consent to Operation
or Other Procedure(s)

554879
Green, John
44 Avenue Street
Town, NJ 07999

Dr. Ramundo

1. I understand that _____ is proposed to be
   performed by _____ and/or his/her associates
   and whomever may be designated as assistants.

2. I understand that the nature and purpose of the operation or procedure is to _____
   _____
   _____

3. I understand that possible alternative methods of treatment are _____
   _____
   _____

4. I understand that the risks and possible complications of this operation or procedure
   are _____
   _____

5. I am aware that the practice of medicine and surgery is not an exact science and I
   acknowledge that no guarantees have been made to me as to the result of this procedure.

6. I consent to the examination and disposition by hospital authorities of any tissue or parts
   which may be removed during the course of this operation or procedure.

7. I understand the nature of the proposed operation or procedure(s), the risks and possible
   complications involved, and the expected results, as described above, and hereby request
   that such operation or procedure(s) be performed.

8. I realize that an operation or procedure requires numerous assistants, technicians, nurses,
   and other personnel and I give my consent to care by such personnel before, during, and
   after the operation or procedure to be performed.

9. I also consent to videotaping or photographing of the operation or procedure for scientific
   or teaching purposes.

_____        _____
Witness (may not be a member of operating team)        Date

_____        _____
Interpreter        Date

_____        _____
Signature of patient, agent, or legal guardian        Date

I have discussed with the above patient the nature of the proposed operation or procedure(s),
the risks and possible complications involved, and the expected results, as described above.

_____
Signature of counseling physician

• **Fig. 8.3** Sample of consent for surgery.

❖ **COMPETENCY CHECK-IN 8.2**

**Consent**

**Competency Assessment**

1. Permission to perform a medical procedure generally requires the patient's _____.
2. A 16-year-old patient presents in the emergency room for treatment of stomach pain. She is conscious, alert, and oriented. Who is the appropriate individual to sign the consent for treatment?
3. Who is responsible for ensuring the patient understands the procedure, the alternatives, and its risks?
4. A patient who is incompetent has a guardian with _____ enabling the guardian to make health care decisions on the patient's behalf.

## Privacy and Confidentiality

Although the terms *privacy* and *confidentiality* are often used synonymously, they have different meanings. **Confidentiality** implies the use of discretion in the disclosure of information. In very simple terms, it is like keeping a secret. When a patient is receiving medical care, no matter what the facility, no matter who the provider, that information is confidential—it is secret. It cannot be released to a person who is not authorized to receive it. **Privacy** is the right of the individual to control access to that information. **Security** is the administrative, physical, and technological safeguards used to protect information.

The foundation for confidentiality is **physician–patient privilege**. This concept refers to the private nature of communication between the patient and his or her physician. To promote complete and honest communication between the physician and patient, the patient must know that any information relayed to the physician will be kept secret. Only the patient can waive the right to keep that communication confidential. Although the facility owns the physical or electronic record, the patient owns the information in the record. The concept of physician–patient privilege varies from state to state. This privilege generally prevents confidential communications between physicians and patients related to diagnosis and treatment from being disclosed in court without patient authorization or a court order to disclose.

### Scope

The scope of confidentiality is very broad. Health care professionals must not disclose any health information in any medium—whether written or spoken—that can be connected to the identity of the patient. There are some basic guidelines that a health care professional can follow when working in a health care facility. First, health care professionals should never discuss information about patients in a public place, such as the cafeteria, elevators, and hallways, because others may be able to hear their conversations.

If it becomes necessary to discuss a patient in a public place, the **minimum necessary** patient identifiers should be used, that is, the patient should be discussed only by diagnosis or in some manner that prevents others from being able to identify the patient. However, care should be taken even in this regard. For example, discussing a patient by room number can violate the patient's privacy if the conversation is overheard by someone who knows what room the patient is in (e.g., a family member). This may seem like common sense, but it is one of the most common violations of a patient's right to confidentiality. All employees must sign a confidentiality agreement when they are hired. Annual resigning of that document, along with in-service training in the necessity for understanding and complying with the facility's confidentiality policies and procedures, is recommended. Fig. 8.4 is a sample confidentiality agreement.

A second issue in confidentiality is the physical maintenance (security) of the patient's health record, as discussed in Chapter 4. Physical (paper) documents should be kept in a binder or folder at all times. Binders or folders containing a specific patient's documents should be identified only with the patient's name, medical record number (MRN), and room number (if applicable). No matter how the record is maintained, the outside of the folder or binder should not contain any diagnostic information or anything of significance that could be read by a casual passerby. In this way, the patient's health information is not connected to the patient's identity. On the nursing unit, only the bed number should be visible on the patient's binder. An important exception to this rule is a warning about allergies. Patient allergies should be clearly noted on the front of the binder. Employees are often tempted to mark the binder with clinically significant information, such as "HIV positive." Such sensitive information should not be visible. Some facilities place color-coded stickers or other symbols on the outside of the binder to circumvent this rule; however, these symbols should not be easily recognizable by the casual observer.

Confidentiality procedures extend to the hallways and to the patient's room itself. Even health care professionals do not have a right to access a patient's record unless they are actually working with the patient. The patient's actual diagnoses, procedures, and appointments should not be displayed where the casual observer can see them. This is a common failing in facilities where multiple individuals need to know the activities of a patient. For example, in an inpatient rehabilitation facility, patients do not generally remain in their rooms. They are transported to other parts of the facility for various therapies, or they may be taken out of the facility for a procedure. The temptation is to post the patient's schedule and other details in a common area where all health care providers can see it. To protect the patient's privacy, however, such postings should be confined to restricted areas.

### Technology

As discussed in Chapter 4, certain special considerations apply to electronics in the facility. Computer screens should be placed so that they are not in public view, and privacy screens should be placed on monitors that might be viewed by passersby. A health care professional accessing a patient's

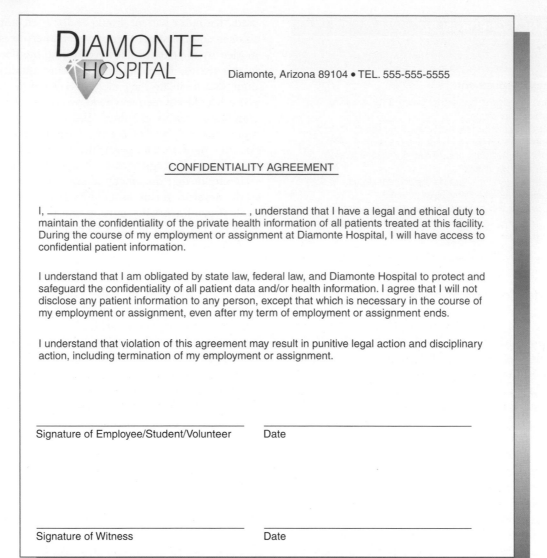

• **Fig. 8.4** Confidentiality agreement.

record at a computer terminal may be called away temporarily. It is very important for the person to log off or lock the computer before leaving so that patient information is not visible to anyone who is not authorized to view it. As an additional safeguard, computer systems should always provide an automatic log-off after a certain period of idle time. A typical screensaver is not sufficient for the purpose of protecting patient information.

Passwords must not be shared among caregivers, even for reasons of efficiency. Passwords must not be written near computers or anywhere that unauthorized users could obtain them. Passwords must be changed frequently, and best practice is for systems to force periodic change.

### Social Media
Every facility has policies for using electronic communications to protect itself and its employees from civil and criminal penalties. That policy covers the appropriate use of facility computers and may or may not address the use of mobile devices and home computers to discuss workplace

matters. Health care professionals face serious consequences for using social media inappropriately, even if they have the best interests of their patients in mind. For example, imagine a health care professional who has become very close to a child with cancer. She is so overjoyed when the doctor declares the child in remission that she posts a smiling picture of the patient on social media celebrating the patient's prognosis. While the health care professional intended nothing but good will toward the patient, this is a violation of the patient's privacy. Of course, negative sentiments are also violations of patient privacy as long as the patient can be identified. Even patient information that is deleted immediately is an infraction, since a screenshot of the material may have been saved or the content may still be retrievable from the social media site's servers. If the material is discoverable by a court of law, it is a breach of patient confidentiality, and therefore a violation of criminal and civil law, as well as facility policy and the standards of the profession. Box 8.4 contains guidelines for the use of social media.

# Health Insurance Portability and Accountability Act

Public Law 104-191 is the legal reference for the Health Insurance Portability and Accountability Act (HIPAA) of 1996, commonly known as HIPAA. Title II contains the Administrative Simplification Section. Within Title II are major categories dealing with health information: Electronic Transactions and Code Sets, Unique Identifiers, the Privacy Rule, and the Security Rule. The purpose of Title II is to improve the Medicare and Medicaid programs and to improve the efficiency and effectiveness of health information systems by establishing a common set of standards and requirements for handling electronic information. Health care delivery has changed significantly since HIPAA was enacted in 1996. The increased use of technology for the storage, sharing, and retrieval of health information raised new concerns about the confidentiality and use of health information. The HITECH Act provisions under ARRA, which President Obama signed into law in 2009, strengthened and revised the HIPAA Privacy and Security regulations.

The HIPAA Privacy Regulations address the use and disclosure of protected health information (PHI) in any format: verbal, written, or electronic. The HIPAA Security Regulations address administrative, physical, and technical safeguards to protect health information that is collected, maintained, used, or transmitted electronically. The Office for Civil Rights (OCR) is responsible for enforcement. Civil penalties can be imposed for noncompliance. Review HIPAA's Security Rule in Chapter 4. Review HIPAA's *transaction code sets* in Chapter 5.

Any organization that obtains and manages health information must comply with HIPAA Privacy and Security regulations. These groups are known as **covered entities** and include providers, health insurers, and health care clearinghouses. Business associates must also comply. **Business associates** are those contracted vendors that use confidential health information to perform a service on behalf of the covered entity. Typical business associates of the health information department are an outsourced medical transcription company, the release-of-information vendor, legal counsel representing the health care facility, reimbursement consultants, and the EHR vendor. Software vendors for scanning/indexing, practice management, and claims processing are other examples. They are not members of the facility's workforce, but they use or disclose health information to perform a function or activity on behalf of the health care facility. Fig. 8.5 illustrates the major sections of HIPAA.

Health information professionals play key roles in assisting health care facilities with HIPAA privacy compliance. The rule introduces the role of the **privacy officer**, the person appointed by the facility to handle privacy compliance. Facilities must also designate a professional to handle any complaints, although the privacy officer usually handles this role as well. Many health information professionals serve as privacy officers for their facilities. The American Health Information Management Association (AHIMA) offers a

---

**• BOX 8.4  The Health Care Professional's Guidelines for Using Social Media**

- Always recognize your legal and ethical responsibilities for patient privacy.
- Never take a picture of a patient or any part of a patient.
- Never share patient information or images unless you are required by law.
- Never post patient information that can be identified, even with the strictest privacy settings.
- Never post negative or disparaging comments about patients, coworkers, physicians, or managers, even if they are unidentifiable.
- Use the highest discretion when "friending" patients or former patients on social media. The lines of professional boundaries may become blurred.

From National Council of State Boards of Nursing, Inc. (NCSBN®): *A nurse's guide to the use of social media*, Chicago, IL, National Council of State Boards of Nursing, Inc. (NCSBN®), June 2018 https://www.ncsbn.org/NCSBN_SocialMedia.pdf. Retrieved January 29, 2019.

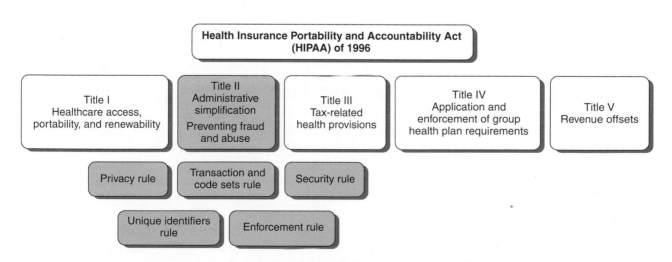

• **Fig. 8.5** The major sections of the Health Insurance Portability and Accountability Act of 1996 (HIPAA).

special credential: CHPS (Certified in Healthcare Privacy and Security).

## Protected Health Information

The Privacy Rule addresses the uses and disclosures of protected health information (PHI). PHI is individually identifiable health information that is transmitted or maintained in any form or medium by covered entities or their business associates. This includes oral, written, and electronic information. Some examples of identifiers are name, address, telephone number, fax number, email address, Social Security number, MRN, health plan number, account number, driver's license number, license plate number, URL, Internet service provider address, biometric identifiers (e.g., fingerprints), photos, and all relevant dates (e.g., dates of birth, admission, and discharge). These data items could identify the health information of a person, thereby violating his or her right to privacy.

## Uses and Disclosures

When a physician reviews a test result, it is a use of PHI. A disclosure occurs when PHI is given to someone. For example, an insurance company is given a copy of an ED record to verify that the patient's condition was indeed an emergency as defined in the patient's health insurance policy. This disclosure may be necessary to obtain reimbursement from the insurer.

PHI cannot be used or disclosed unless the Privacy Rule requires or permits it to be used or disclosed. There are two types of required disclosures: disclosures to the patient and disclosures to the Secretary of the HHS for compliance auditing purposes. There are also several permitted disclosures outlined in the Privacy Rule. All disclosures that are specifically authorized by the patient are permitted. Disclosures for treatment purposes, payment of the patient's bill, or health care operations are all permitted and do not need to be authorized by the patient. Some examples of health care operations that use PHI are RM, infection control, quality improvement, legal counsel, and case management. For example, an infection control nurse is allowed to review the medical records of a patient with an infectious disease without authorization in order to investigate the outbreak, keep statistics, and prevent the spread of a disease to other patients. The HITECH Act requires covered entities, when using or disclosing PHI or requesting PHI from another covered entity, to limit the information disclosed to a limited data set. If more information is needed, it must be the minimum necessary.

Uses and disclosures of PHI without patient authorization are also permitted for certain public priorities. Disclosures for research purposes are permitted under specific conditions. These are considered exceptions. Covered entities must comply with the conditions in the exceptions. Table 8.1 contains some examples of exceptions.

**TABLE 8.1  Exceptions for Using Protected Health Information Without Patient Consent**

| Exception | Example |
| --- | --- |
| As required by law | Transmission of discharge data to state repository |
| For public health activities | Reporting infectious diseases |
| About victims of abuse, neglect, or domestic violence | Reporting suspected abuse to appropriate local agencies |
| For health oversight activities | The hospital conducts outcomes analysis of its patient population |
| For judicial and administrative proceedings | The hospital receives a court order to release a patient's health record related to a trial |
| For law enforcement | Gunshot or knife wound |
| About decedents (to coroners, medical examiners, funeral directors) | A patient brought to the emergency department after being found unconscious in an abandoned vehicle. The patient dies within 3 hours of arriving in the emergency room. This case will likely be a coroner case. |
| To facilitate cadaver organ donation and transplants | The physician/surgeon for a patient who is the recipient of donor organs will likely require copies of the donor patient's health record |
| For certain research | Researchers conducting approved studies may be given access to patient information |
| To avert a serious threat to health or safety | A psychiatrist may warn a victim specifically threatened by a patient |
| For specialized government functions (e.g., military, veterans' groups, national security, protective services, State Department, correctional facilities) | A correctional facility may retain copies of records of patients treated at a local hospital |
| For workers' compensation (as authorized by law) | If an employee files a claim for workplace injury, the record will be used to substantiate the claim |

The HIPAA Privacy Regulations state that a covered entity may disclose PHI in the course of any judicial or administrative proceeding in response to the following:

- A court order, but only the PHI expressly authorized for release by the order.
- Subpoena duces tecum, provided that the covered entity:
  - receives a written statement and accompanying documents from the party seeking the information that reasonable efforts have been made to ensure that the individual who is the subject of the information has been notified of the request or that reasonable efforts have been made to secure a qualified protective order for the information.
  - makes reasonable efforts to limit the PHI used or disclosed to the minimum necessary to respond to the request.

The requirement to provide sufficient notice to the individual is met when a party provides a written statement and accompanying documentation that demonstrates the following:

- A good faith attempt was made to notify the individual.
- The notice included sufficient information to permit the individual to raise an objection with the court.
- The time for the individual to raise objections has lapsed, no objection was filed or objections have been resolved by the court, and the disclosure is consistent with the resolution.

A qualified protective order is an order of a court that prohibits the parties from using or disclosing the PHI for any purpose other than the litigation or proceeding for which such information was requested and requires the return to the covered entity or destruction of the PHI (including any copies) at the end of the litigation or proceeding.

### Notice of Privacy Practices

Covered entities are required to establish policies and procedures addressing HIPAA privacy issues. One of the most important policies is the Notice of Privacy Practices. This document summarizes the facility's privacy policies and explains how the facility may use or disclose patient health information. The notice must be written in clear, simple language and provide examples of uses and disclosures. Contact information, such as the telephone number, for the privacy officer/complaint designee, must be included in the notice. Facilities must also obtain a signed acknowledgment from the patient that the notice was received.

### Patient Rights

The Privacy Rule gives patients certain rights, including the right to receive a notice of the privacy practices. In some situations, patients may request a higher level of privacy. In this case, they have the right to ask for additional restrictions on the use of their PHI or additional limitations on the amount of PHI disclosed. For example, a patient may ask that the facility not allow her next-door neighbor, a nurse who would normally have access to the record for patient care, to have access to her PHI. Facility

administrators must decide whether they can comply with the patient's request. They do not have to honor such a request. For example, the facility may be small, with a limited nursing staff, and the next-door neighbor may need to be involved in the patient's care due to a staffing shortage. A common restriction (called an "opt-out" in HIPAA) is a patient's request to be removed from the patient directory. In other words, individuals calling the facility would not be told that the patient is there, and calls would not be forwarded to the patient. The patient may also ask for confidential communications. For example, the patient may ask that the bill be mailed to another address instead of the home address.

Patients have the right of access to their health information. Access refers to the ability to learn the contents of a health record by reading it or obtaining a copy. There are many reasons that patients would want access to their record. Many patients are now keeping their own PHRs. The purpose of a PHR is to document the patient's history and provide information for continuing patient care. AHIMA and the American Medical Association (AMA) are both encouraging patients to track their own health information. The patient is generally required to sign an authorization form or a request-for-access form to obtain or read copies of his or her health information.

The HIPAA Privacy Regulations require health care providers to define their designated record set to respond to an individual's right to request access, request amendment, and request restriction to his or her PHI. In contrast to the legal health record, the designated record set must include the patient's medical records, billing records, any information that includes PHI, and any other information with which a decision was made that affects the patient. Because it includes all PHI, the designated record set is a larger collection of information than the legal health record. Patients have full access to the designated record set. Access by others is discussed later in this chapter.

Patients may not always agree with the information in their medical record. The HIPAA privacy regulations give every patient the right to request an amendment of his or her health information. When a patient asks to amend health information, he or she should be given an amendment/correction request form to complete. It is generally given to the privacy officer for review and response to the patient within 60 days. If the facility cannot respond within 60 days, one 30-day extension is allowed. However, the patient must be informed in writing that there is a delay and given an expected date of response. The amendment can be denied if any of the following applies:

The information was not created by the facility.
The information is not part of the designated record set.
The information is not available for access.
The information is accurate and complete.

Usually, the privacy officer contacts the physician or health care professional whose documentation the patient is contesting. This professional reviews the request and decides whether to correct the information. If the professional stands by the information as being correct, the patient is notified that his or her request is denied because the information is accurate and complete. If the patient disagrees with the denial, he or she must be given the opportunity to provide a statement of disagreement. The patient may request that all future releases include a copy of the request for amendment, the facility's denial letter, and the disagreement statement.

Patients are also given the **right to revoke** authorization to disclose their PHI. For example, a patient may authorize his or her attorney to receive a copy of his or her medical record and later change attorneys. The patient would be allowed to revoke the original authorization to Attorney A and authorize a new disclosure to Attorney B.

Facilities are also required to give patients an **accounting of disclosures** on request (Fig. 8.6). This accounting is basically a list indicating who received information about the patient and when, why, and how the disclosure was made. Some disclosures do not require this accounting. Disclosures for treatment, payment, some health care operations, and patient-authorized disclosures do not require accounting. Most facilities track all disclosures, even those for which accounting is not required because thorough documentation is a good practice. HIPAA requires health care facilities to keep all documentation with regard to an accounting of

disclosures for 6 years. However, under the HITECH provisions of the ARRA, if a covered entity uses or maintains an EHR, the HIPAA exception for tracking and documenting disclosures for treatment, payment, and health care operations no longer applies if that disclosure is made through an EHR. In this situation, patients have the right to receive an accounting of disclosures made by the covered entity during the 3 years prior to the date on which the accounting is requested.

Finally, patients have a **right to complain**. They must be given the ability to discuss their concerns about privacy violations with a staff member and ultimately with the HHS. The Office of Civil Rights has been given HHS authority to investigate complaints, enforce the Privacy Rule, and impose penalties for HIPAA violations. Penalties may be civil or criminal and may involve fines and imprisonment depending on the circumstances.

### Breaches

Patients must be notified when there is a breach of PHI. This requirement applies to covered entities, business associates, PHR vendors, and companies that service PHRs. Notifications must be made without unreasonable delay and in no case later than 60 calendar days after the discovery of the breach. Covered entities are required to provide notice of a breach to individuals in writing, by first-class mail, sent

Patient Name: _____

Medical Record Number: _____

| Date Received | Name of Requestor | Address (if known) | Authorization or Written Request (Y/N) | Purpose | PHI Disclosed | Date Disclosed | Disclosed by | Amt. Billed | Amt. Received | Date. Received |
|---|---|---|---|---|---|---|---|---|---|---|
|  |  |  |  |  |  |  |  |  |  |  |
|  |  |  |  |  |  |  |  |  |  |  |
|  |  |  |  |  |  |  |  |  |  |  |

**Key:**
**Date received:** the date request is received to disclose or release information when applicable
**Name of requestor:** name of entity or person requesting information to be disclosed or released
**Address:** if known, the address of the entity or person requesting information be disclosed or released
**Authorization or written request (yes/no):** identify if there is a written request or authorization.
If not, indicate how request was received (for example, verbal)
**Purpose:** brief description of the purpose of the disclosure to reasonably inform the individual of the basis of the disclosure. If documented on authorization or written request, state "see authorization/written request"
**PHI disclosed:** brief description of the information disclosed/released
**Date disclosed:** date the information was released or disclosed
**Sent by:** staff member processing the request and disclosing the information
**Amount billed:** if applicable, the copy fee charged for records released
**Amount received:** copy fee received
**Date received:** date the fee was received

• **Fig. 8.6** An example of an accounting of disclosures.

to the last known address of the individual (or to the next of kin if the individual is deceased). In cases in which there is insufficient information to provide the written notice, a substitute form of notice must be provided. This could be a posting on the covered entity's website or in major print or broadcast media.

If the breach involves more than 500 patients, notification must also be made to prominent media outlets. Notice must also be provided to the Secretary of the DHHS at the same time notice is given to the patient. The Secretary publishes a list on the DHHS website of each covered entity involved in a breach of unsecured PHI involving more than 500 patients.

If a breach of unsecured PHI affects fewer than 500 individuals, a covered entity may choose to notify the Secretary at the time the breach is discovered, but it is required to make such notification within 60 days of the end of the calendar year in which the breach was discovered. The covered entity may report all of its breaches affecting fewer than 500 individuals on one date but must complete a separate notice for each breach incident.

Under the definition of *breach*, it is important to note that there are three exceptions: (1) any unintentional acquisition of, access to, or use of PHI by a workforce member; (2) any inadvertent disclosure by a person who is authorized to access PHI; and (3) a disclosure of PHI in which a covered entity and business associate has a good faith that an unauthorized person to whom the disclosure was made would not reasonably have been able to retain such information. For example, you are walking down the hall delivering records to the nursing units. You overhear the nursing staff discussing a patient. This would be considered an incidental disclosure and not a breach.

The following information must be provided in the breach notification:

- a brief description of what happened, including the date of the breach and the date of the discovery of the breach, if known;
- a description of the types of unsecured PHI that was involved in the breach (such as full name, Social Security number, date of birth, home address, and account number);
- the steps that individuals should take to protect themselves from potential harm resulting from the breach;
- a brief description of what the covered entity involved is doing to investigate the breach, mitigate losses, and protect against any further breaches; and
- contact procedures for individuals to ask questions or learn additional information, which must include a toll-free telephone number and an email, website, or postal address.

### Revisions to Health Insurance Portability and Accountability Act

As with many health care regulations, changes do occur from time to time as technology, public interest, and laws change. In 2018, due to continuity of care issues secondary to an

---

**◆ COMPETENCY CHECK-IN 8.3**

**Privacy and Confidentiality**

**Competency Assessment**

1. From the standpoint of patient care, why is it important for the patient to know the information he or she gives to a health care provider will be kept secret?
2. What are the differences among privacy, confidentiality, and security?
3. What is PHI?
4. What is a covered entity?
5. When a breach of the PHI of more than _____ patients occurs, covered entities must notify the media and the Secretary of the Department of Health and Human Services.
6. What document summarizes the facility's privacy policies and explains how patient information will be disclosed?
7. After seeing an embarrassing diagnosis in the health record, a patient files a(n) _____ form to have the information changed.

---

increase in opioid abuse and addiction, the OCR guidance regarding release of information (ROI) without patient consent in certain situations was changed. This underscores the need to stay abreast of legal and regulatory developments as they occur so that the hospital or other provider can prepare thorough analysis and revision, as needed, of policies, procedures, and training.

## Access

Despite the need for privacy, there are legitimate reasons for various parties to have access to a patient's PHI. These reasons include the following: treatment (continuing patient care), payment (reimbursement), and health care operations. In addition, the patient may wish to provide access to third parties, such as lawyers.

### Continuing Patient Care

Confidentiality presents some challenging issues for continuity of care. The attending physician and direct care providers involved with the patient should have full access to the patient's health information in order to treat the patient. However, what if physicians wish to review their neighbor's medical record? Should they be given access simply because they are physicians? No. The health care professional must have direct patient involvement or a specific "need to know" in order to obtain the patient's information. Any other access to a patient's record requires specific patient authorization. An example of inappropriate access is a facility employee looking at a family member's medical record without the patient's permission. This misuse of access would be a confidentiality violation. Electronic record systems should provide audit trails indicating who accessed what patient information so that compliance with confidentiality can be documented and violations identified.

It is important to convey to employees of the HIM department and the facility in general that inappropriate access to a record is illegal and will lead to disciplinary measures. The HIPAA Security Regulations discussed earlier in this chapter have a section dealing with workforce security and termination procedures if someone violates the rules. Dismissal of employees who inappropriately access health records is not excessively harsh; it is common.

Health care professionals outside the facility in which the patient was originally treated may also need certain health information. HIPAA's Privacy Regulations allow the use and disclosure of health information for continuing patient care, without specific patient authorization. However, it is common practice to ask for authorizations or at least written requests from outside health care providers because thorough documentation is required for accreditation and certification and as a record for accounting of disclosures.

## Reimbursement

Another reason to disclose health information is for reimbursement purposes. In the current health care environment, various payers may need to review the record. HIPAA's Privacy Regulations allow the use and disclosure of health information for payment purposes without authorization. However, it is common practice to have patients sign a **Conditions of Admission** (see Fig. 8.2) form on admission to a hospital; this form includes authorization for the release of health information to the party who is financially responsible. This type of authorization constitutes **prospective consent**. In other words, the patient is authorizing the ROI *before* that information has been generated.

Although this authorization is not required—because HIPAA allows release of health information for payment purposes without authorization—it is a common practice because it informs patients that their health information may be disclosed for the bill to be paid. In addition, the Notice of Privacy Practices informs the patient that his or her health information may be disclosed for reimbursement purposes.

In most other cases, such as third-party ROI for legal purposes, *retrospective consent* is necessary. **Retrospective consent** means that the patient authorizes the use or disclosure of health information *after* care has been rendered.

## Health Care Operations

HIPAA's Privacy Regulations also allow the use and disclosure of health information for health care operation purposes without authorization. Health care operations include functions such as RM, infection control, case management, and quality improvement. However, under the HITECH provisions of ARRA, the information disclosed should be a limited data set. If more information is needed, it must

be the minimum necessary. Under the minimum necessary standard, covered entities must make reasonable efforts to limit the patient-identifiable information they disclose to the least amount necessary.

### Internal Requests for Information

In everyday practice within a health care facility, there are numerous instances in which facility personnel routinely request health information. Some of these requests include utilization review, PI, and a variety of ongoing clinical reviews (e.g., surgical case review and infection control). These requests should be documented in writing both for internal control purposes (chart tracking) and to ensure that the request is valid.

The routine ROI for patient care should be handled with some caution. Even within a facility, many attempts are made to obtain information inappropriately. The culprits range from overly curious friends and family members who inquire about a patient's condition to unethical health care professionals who spy on one another. In the case of a physician's request, authorization is easily determined by checking the record to ensure that the physician requesting the chart is listed as an attending or consulting physician for that particular case. HIM departmental policies and procedures should be clear and specific regarding the internal ROI and should also include the steps to be taken when the legitimacy of the request is in question. Staff members should be allowed access to health information only on a need-to-know basis. In other words, what is the minimum amount of information necessary for the staff members to do their jobs?

### Sensitive Records

There are two major types of sensitive records: employee patients and legal files. Although there may be no statutory or regulatory requirement to handle these records differently from others, certain practical considerations apply. Maintaining the confidentiality of employee records is particularly difficult. In a small facility, a paper record can be maintained in a secure file. In the electronic environment, knowledge that an audit trail of access to the record will be monitored may serve as a deterrent to inappropriate access.

Facility policies and procedures should include specific language regarding the sensitivity of health information pertaining to fellow employees, including the nature and extent of disciplinary action in the event of violations. The confidentiality statement shown in Fig. 8.4 includes such language.

### Litigation

As mentioned earlier, nearly every lawsuit that involves injury requires the disclosure of the health record to either prove wrongdoing or mount a defense. The facility will receive requests for patient records via court order or subpoena. In general, the subpoena attaches urgency and deadlines to the request for information. However, patient authorization is required to release the records. A court order does not require patient authorization. Validating a subpoena or court order is necessary as some proceedings are discharged (settled or withdrawn) prior to the court date or other deadline. The nature of the case must also be noted. For example, a lawsuit may have been initiated by a defendant, who is requesting records of the plaintiff, who is the patient whose records are being requested. Contacting the patient and/or the plaintiff's lawyer is needed to ensure that they have been notified of the request.

Special attention should be paid to records that have been requested for litigation involving the facility, health care personnel, or a physician. In a paper-based environment, the HIM department obtains control of the record and copies it for review and circulation. The original is locked in a cabinet, so it cannot be altered. It may be viewed in the presence of an authorized individual. It is this original that may be requested by the court to be presented in evidence, although a certified copy is usually sufficient. In an EHR environment, all activity in the record must be tracked and audited to ensure that any amendments are duly noted. The EHR system will allow late posting of an entry to a record; however, the date of the entry will be logged, so there is no question of when the entry was actually made.

## Public Health Activities

Sometimes disclosures of PHI are necessary to ensure the health and safety of the general public. These are permitted disclosures in which authorization is not required as long as state law allows these exceptions (45 CFR 164.512(b)). In fact, many states require reporting of certain conditions of public health interest. Examples of mandatory reporting are occurrences of births and deaths. Some of these conditions include cancers, birth defects, and infectious diseases. Incidences of violence, such as gunshot wounds, knife injuries, or poisoning, are also required to be reported for compliance with the law. In these cases, patient consent is not required to file reports with the appropriate governmental agency, and timely disclosure is required under penalty of law. Suspected elder and child abuse is another instance in which reporting may occur without patient consent. Other examples are disclosures to coroners, law enforcement officials, and health licensing agencies, and for organ transplant activities, for certain research, for prevention of a bioterrorism event, and for other specific government functions and workers' compensation activities.

The federal government and the states monitor the incidence of certain diseases. Providers must report cases of certain sexually transmitted diseases, anthrax, rabies, meningitis, and cancer. Usually, the provider contacts the local or county authorities, who then report the incident to a state agency, who in turn reports the disease to the Centers for Disease Control and Prevention (CDC). This agency tracks diseases on a national scale. This information helps government officials develop health policy and contain outbreaks.

## Release of Information

In both paper-based and electronic environments, portions of the record must sometimes be disclosed. Duplication may be accomplished by photocopying the paper record, printing a copy from a computer or microfilm printer, or transmitting the information electronically, such as by faxing it from an electronic system. In practice, the duplicate is provided in paper format, regardless of how it is stored or maintained. The function of disclosing health information in the HIM department is often called **release of information (ROI)** or **correspondence**. This function is often outsourced (i.e., performed all or in part by outside contractors instead of facility personnel).

### Authorized Disclosures

The patient may authorize the release of his or her information to anyone. Remember that only the patient (or his or her personal representative) can waive the physician–patient privilege. Documentation of the patient's consent to release information is accomplished by completion of an authorization form. As with consents for medical procedures, the concept of informed consent applies. The patient must know in advance the nature and purpose of the consent for disclosure. Therefore consents for ROI should be retrospective. In other words, the patient cannot be fully informed about what is being released until after the information has been generated.

State laws and regulations vary regarding **retention**, but many facilities do destroy old records after the required retention period has passed, discussed later in this chapter. If a patient's appendectomy took place 30 years ago, the paper record may no longer exist. Therefore it is in the patient's best interests to maintain a personal file of health information.

The only legitimate reason to deny access to a patient is if the patient's health care provider decides that the information in the record would be harmful to the patient. This is an unusual circumstance that pertains primarily to behavioral health cases. If knowledge of the information in the record would be harmful to the patient, the provider must document reasons for the refusal of access. Health care providers must also follow a formal appeals process if access is denied. Fig. 8.7 illustrates the flow of the decision-making process with regard to access requests.

> ❖ **NOTE**
>
> A *personal representative* is an individual who is authorized to act on behalf of the patient. For example, a parent is generally a personal representative of his or her minor child. This title would also apply to a legal guardian or person acting *in loco parentis* of a minor child. In addition, if state law gives a person authority to act on behalf of a deceased individual (usually the executor, administrator, spouse, or next of kin), then that person would be considered a personal representative.

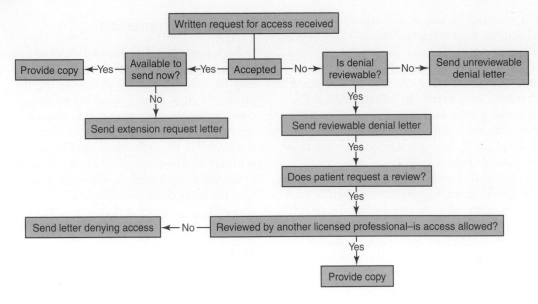

• **Fig. 8.7** The flow of the decision-making process with regard to access requests.

Technically, it is not necessary for a patient to complete a specific form to authorize the ROI. Each health care facility should have an access policy. A letter addressed to the facility should suffice if it contains all the elements of a valid authorization, but many facilities still require the use of a specific authorization form. HIPAA-compliant authorizations require the following core elements:
- *Identification of the party being asked to release the information:* The owner of the actual documents (i.e., the facility or health care provider who has custody of the documents) is named.
- *Patient name/identification:* The patient's name is the primary identifier. However, because many individuals have the same or similar names, additional identifiers, such as date of birth or Social Security number, should be documented. The MRN or account number is also very useful, if known.
- *Identification of the party to whom the information is to be released:* The person or class of persons to whom information is being released must be listed. This may be the name of a facility, a health care provider, or any other party. In other words, to whom does the patient want the information to be sent? It is also important to include the accurate address of this party.
- *Specific information to be released:* The authorization must include a description of the information to be used or disclosed that identifies the information in a specific and meaningful way.
- *Description of the purpose of the use or disclosure:* Common purposes for disclosure are for treatment purposes, legal reasons, application for disability benefits, application for life insurance, or simply "at the request of the individual."
- *Expiration date:* The authorization form must list an expiration date or expiration "event." For example, the patient may document an expiration event of "upon my death" or "specific date: 11/20/2019."

- *Signature of the patient or personal representative authorizing the disclosure:* If the personal representative of the patient signs the authorization, a description of such representative's authority to act for the individual must also be provided. For example, if a mother authorizes a disclosure on behalf of her minor child, she must sign and document the disclosure "as mother or parent." If a patient is deceased, the executor of the will provides such documentation as the patient's representative.
- *Date:* This is the date on which the patient makes the consent and signs the authorization documenting his or her consent.

In addition to the core elements, there are some required statements:
- *Patient's right to revoke the authorization*: The patient or authorized agent has the right to revoke the consent for ROI in writing at any time before the actual distribution of the information. This should be explicitly stated on the authorization form.
- *Redisclosure statement:* The information used or disclosed may be subject to redisclosure by the recipient and may no longer be protected.
- *Conditions of authorization:* Specifications as to whether the covered entity is permitted to condition treatment, payment, enrollment, or eligibility for benefits on the authorization.

When a patient visits the HIM department to obtain copies of his or her health record, the HIM professional must often help the patient complete the authorization form to ensure that it is properly filled out. Patients must always understand what they are signing.

### Defective Authorizations

An authorization is considered invalid if:
- Any of the core elements are missing.
- The expiration date or event has passed.

- It is filled out incorrectly.
- It is known that it was revoked.
- Any information in the authorization is known to be false.
- The authorization is not in plain language (i.e., in simple language that a person with a sixth-grade education would be able to understand).

Fig. 8.8 provides a checklist to ensure authorization validity.

## Special Consents

Special consents require consideration of federal law, state law, and federal and state rules and regulations. In general, health records containing chemical dependency information, HIV and acquired immunodeficiency virus information, behavioral health information, and adoption information are often addressed in state laws and regulations. As previously mentioned, the regulations that give the patient the highest level of protection should be followed. Most health care facilities have designed their authorization forms to be compliant with HIPAA and any state laws or regulations, but some facilities have a separate authorization form for special consents. In general, the authorization must specifically list the special nature of the

health information that is to be disclosed. Best practice is to notify the physician when a behavioral health patient requests a copy of their own records.

The *Code of Federal Regulations* (42 CFR Part 2), commonly referred to as the **Federal Drug and Alcohol Abuse Regulations**, outlines the requirements for disclosing chemical dependency information. In the absence of patient authorization, a subpoena for disclosure of chemical dependency information is not good enough—a court order is required.

## Preparing a Record for Release

There are several steps to take to properly release health care information. Each facility should have formal written policies and procedures regarding these steps. The specific policies and procedures vary among facilities; however, the issues can be discussed in general. Care should be taken to train and continually remind personnel of the confidential nature of health information.

### Validation and Tracking

After a request for information is received, the request should be recorded either in a manual log or in a computer database. The purpose of recording the request is so that

---

**AUTHORIZATION VALIDITY CHECKLIST:**

_____ Discloser (facility) name listed (e.g., Hospital Medical Center)

_____ Requestor name listed (e.g., attorney John Doe)

_____ Specific description of information to be disclosed (e.g., mammogram 03/01/20XX)

_____ Is the disclosure purpose listed or does it state something to the effect "at the request of the individual"? (e.g., to take to new physician)

_____ Is there an expiration date or event that has not passed? (e.g., an actual date or an event like "upon completion of this request" or "upon my death")

_____ Is it signed by the patient or by a personal representative with his or her authority documented? (e.g., parent of a minor)

_____ Is it dated? (e.g., must include the date the patient signed it)

_____ Is there a statement of the individual's right to revoke the authorization?

_____ Is this authorization still valid (i.e., has not been revoked?) (Check for revocation.)

_____ All of the information in the authorization appears to be true. (If you know that any information in the authorization is false, it will not be valid.)

_____ Is the authorization written in plain language? (i.e., a nonlawyer can understand it)

DECISION: _____ VALID or _____ INVALID

Employee _____   Date _____

• **Fig. 8.8** A sample checklist to help ensure that an authorization is valid. Individual states may require additional elements for valid authorization.

its status and disposition may be tracked. Many state regulations require that facilities fulfill such requests within a specific time frame. A correspondence-tracking log serves to document compliance and fulfill HIPAA's requirements regarding accounting of disclosures.

Every request should be fully read, and every accompanying authorization form should be analyzed to determine whether there is valid authorization. In addition, there should be verification that the patient indeed has consented. The signature of the patient should be validated in an appropriate manner. This may be as simple as comparing the signature on the authorization form with the signature on file in the health record. If such validation cannot be accomplished or is not clear, notarization of the signature or additional proof of identity may be required. It is also important to verify identity when a patient comes to the facility to obtain copies of records. Proof of identity should always be requested to verify that the person to whom records are disclosed is indeed the person who is authorized to receive them. Box 8.5 lists sample data elements contained in a typical correspondence-tracking log. Most logs today involve an electronic database.

### Retrieval

Retrieval of the patient's information is based on the specific information requested. It is very important to release only those portions of the record that are authorized for disclosure. Care should be taken to ensure that the information retrieved is complete. This verification may be complicated by the decentralization of paper-based records among facility clinics, across multiple systems, or by incomplete processing of the record. Incomplete records should not, as a general rule, be released unless the release is for treatment purposes and the facility is sending whatever is available. If

---

### • BOX 8.5 Correspondence-Tracking Log Data Elements

- Request ID number
- Date request received
- Patient name
- Medical record number/account number
- Admission date/discharge date
- Request type
- Requester name (including address or fax number)
- Information requested
- Purpose
- Information sent
- Date request canceled or returned (if applicable)
- Date information sent
- Basis for allowing disclosure (authorization, permitted use, etc.)
- Notes or comments
- Invoice number
- Invoice amount
- Employee name/initials of person who processed request

From Andress AA: *Saunders manual of medical office management*, Philadelphia, PA, 1996, Saunders, p 150.

---

an incomplete record is disclosed in response to a subpoena, the status of the record as incomplete should be clearly stated in the certification statement, affidavit, or cover sheet.

### Reproduction

Historically, photocopies or printed reproductions are made of the specific information requested. Every effort should be made to ensure the quality of the reproductions. When photocopying, personnel should compare the reproduction with the original to ensure completeness and clarity.

Increasingly, electronic media are requested. Patients may request records on CD, thumb drive, or electronic transmission. Unsecured email should not be used to transmit records. If the organization has a patient portal, the requested information may already be available for patient download. Alternatively, the record may be uploaded to the portal for the patient to access.

### Certification

When a copy of a record is required as evidence in a trial, a certified or notarized copy is usually acceptable in court. However, sometimes the original record is subpoenaed, and the custodian of the medical record accompanies the record to court. The custodian may be required to testify on the facility's procedures regarding development and retention of the record. When appearance by the custodian is required, a witness subpoena is usually issued in addition to the subpoena duces tecum for production of the record.

A certified copy contains a certification cover sheet signed by the custodian of the medical records, which states that the copy is a true and complete reproduction of the original record that is on file at the facility. The facility's policies and procedures should include the process by which verification of completeness can be obtained. With a paper record, completeness can be verified by numbering all the pages in the original record before it is copied. Every copy can then be verified as complete if they contain the same sequential numbering of the pages.

### Compensation

Most states permit facilities to charge a fee for providing copies of health records. Some states place a cap, or maximum, on the fees that may be charged. The fee covers the actual services performed: retrieval of the record (search fee), reproduction of the record, and delivery charges (postage). Therefore an important component of the ROI process is the preparation of the invoice. Some facilities may require that requesters pay the fee in advance, particularly for large records. As a professional courtesy, health care providers do not generally charge other health care providers for copies of records. In many cases, insurance companies and other payers have established set amounts that they will pay for copies of records. These fees may differ from the fees charged by the facility to other parties. HIPAA does not allow facilities to charge a retrieval or search fee to patients. Generally, the rate should be based on the actual cost to the facility of providing copies to the patient.

## Distribution

When a record is released, inclusion of a confidentiality notice is common practice. A typical notice might say, "This information is confidential and may not be used for other than the intended purpose and may not be rereleased." This is to remind the recipient that the information belongs to the patient—not the recipient. Table 8.2 lists the general steps in ROI.

The individual to whom the record is being released may arrive in person to pick up the record. Policies and procedures should define how the patient or individual's identity should be verified, and the individual picking up the record should sign a receipt. Usually, the copies are mailed. Care must be taken to ensure that the address is correct and legible on the envelope so that the record is not misdirected. Records may also be sent electronically, by fax machine, or via email. Extra care should be taken with electronic transmission of health information, as specifically addressed in the HIPAA Security Rule.

A cover sheet should accompany records sent by fax machine. The cover sheet should contain a confidentiality statement (Fig. 8.9). Internet transmission of confidential information is becoming more common, particularly in the physician's office setting. Consideration should be given to the transmission security and whether the recipient is able to handle the information confidentially. For example, many employers automatically monitor their employees' emails. Therefore sending medical information to a patient at his or her place of business may jeopardize confidentiality. The patient must be made aware of the issues before authorizing transmittal in this manner.

## Record Retention

The length of time a record is kept by a facility is the record retention schedule. Health records must be maintained by a facility to support patient care; meet legal and regulatory requirements; achieve accreditation; allow research, education, and reimbursement; and support facility administration.

The duration of **record** retention differs for the various types of records kept (e.g., laboratory data, radiology reports and films, fetal monitor strips, birth certificates, master patient indexes [MPIs]) and for different facilities and is defined by their respective accrediting agencies. Most states have laws mandating how long a facility must maintain health information. In the absence of state law, the facility must follow the federal requirements stipulated by the CMS, which is to save such records for 5 years. A facility should also consider extending retention time to allow for cases in which malpractice, patient age, or research activity requires review of the record.

The retention time for patient health records may be a specific number of years, or it can be counted from the date of the patient's last encounter. For example, assume that the retention schedule in a state is 10 years from the patient's last encounter and includes all previous records. Jane Ryan has an appendectomy at age 20 years, a broken ankle with repair at age 25 years, and treatment for a motor vehicle accident (MVA) at age 29 years, all at the same facility. Upon her admission for the ankle repair, the 10-year retention period for the appendectomy record starts over; it starts over again with the MVA admission. Jane's records are kept until a retention time of 10 years has lapsed from her last visit (when she is 39 years old, assuming no more admissions). However, if the retention schedule in the state does not include previous visits, then the appendectomy record can be destroyed when the retention period expires (when she is 30 years old). Refer to Table 8.3 for the retention schedule for health information suggested by the AHIMA.

### Retention Policy

Each HIM department must have a policy explaining how the medical records within the facility are stored. The policy describes which health records are maintained in the department, how each type of record is organized, the storage medium used, and the length of time each record is to be retained. The retention policy is very important to a facility with many records that may be stored in different locations.

**TABLE 8.2  Steps in Release of Information**

| Procedure | Comments |
| --- | --- |
| 1. Log-in request | Log request into a computer tracking system or onto a paper form. |
| 2. Validate request | Check signature; review the request for completeness. Obtain missing information if possible. Verify the validity of the subpoena or court order. |
| 3. Obtain record | Retrieve the record from storage. Complete an incomplete record before releasing it. |
| 4. Copy record | Photocopy or print from computer system. Download the electronic version, if the record is to be sent electronically. Copy only the required sections as specified in the request. |
| 5. Quality check | Verify that the request is being fulfilled correctly. |
| 6. Prepare invoice | Calculate charges, and prepare an invoice. |
| 7. Distribute copy | Mail, transmit, upload, or hand the copy to the requestor. Obtain signed receipt if requested information is picked up in person. |

| DIAMONTE HOSPITAL<br>Diamonte, Arizona<br>Tel: 928-555-1234 | **Fax** |
|---|---|

| RECIPIENT | SENDER |
|---|---|
| TO: | FROM: |
| DEPARTMENT: | DEPARTMENT: |
| FAX: | NUMBER of pages, including cover: |
| TELEPHONE: | DATE: |

RE:

MESSAGE:

This facsimile message and the document(s) accompanying this telefax transmission may contain confidential information which is legally privileged and intended only for the use of the addressee named above. If the reader is not the intended recipient or the employee of the intended recipient, you are hereby notified that any dissemination, copying, or distribution of this communication is strictly prohibited. If you received this communication in error, please notify us immediately by telefax or telephone and return the original documents to us via the U.S. Postal Service at the above address. Thank you for your help.

• **Fig. 8.9** Sample confidentiality notice for faxed information. (From Andress AA: Saunders manual of medical office management, Philadelphia, PA, 1996, Saunders, p 150.)

The policy must state that a record is maintained on every patient registered to the facility; provide the retention schedule; indicate how the records are identified, organized, or filed; state their location; and document alternative locations or media, if necessary. Visit the Evolve site for this text to view information specific to the retention of paper-based records.

### *Facility Closure*

What happens when a facility, physician's office, or clinic closes its operation? Where do the records go? In the event of a facility's closing, the retention schedule remains in effect. The facility must investigate the applicable laws to determine the best method for retaining the records. If the facility or practice is purchased, the records are managed by the new owner. However, if the practice or facility closes, the records must be maintained for the duration of the retention schedule in an appropriate, secure, confidential location.

The facility must notify its patients when it is closing. There are several excellent methods of informing patients of closure. One method is to run an advertisement in the local newspaper explaining the closure and what will happen to the health records (Fig. 8.10). Another method is to notify

## TABLE 8.3  Retention Schedule of Health Care Records

| Type of Health Information | Retention Schedule |
|---|---|
| Acute care facility records | 10 years for adults<br>Age of majority +10 years for minors (or statute of limitations) |
| Birth, death, surgical procedure registers | Permanent |
| Radiographs | 5 years |
| Fetal monitor strips | Age of majority +10 years |
| Master patient index | Permanent |
| Diseases index | 10 years |
| Emergency department register/log | Permanent |
| Employee health records | 30 years |

Medicare Conditions of Participation (COP) require retention of records, films, and scans for at least 5 years. Each provider should develop a retention schedule for records in its facility.
Modified from AHIMA Practice Brief: *Retention of health information.* http://library.ahima.org/xpedio/groups/public/documents/ahima/bok1_049250.hcsp?dDocName(bok1_049250.

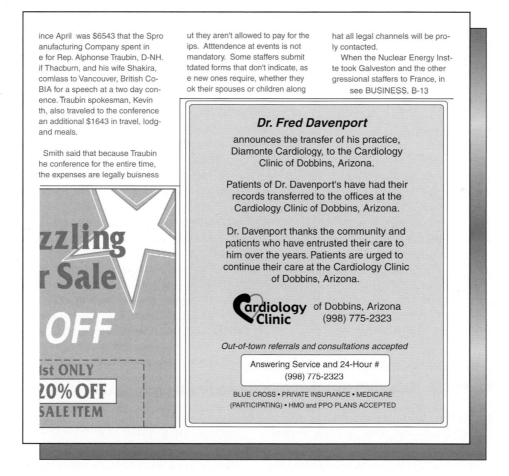

• **Fig. 8.10** Newspaper advertisement of facility closure.

patients of the closure through letters or notices mailed directly to the patients' homes. It is also important to post similar notices in and around the facility to notify patients of the closure. Because patient information is critical in the continuity of care, it is important to maintain patient access to the records even after the facility is closed. This goal may be accomplished by transferring the records to another local facility or physician's office, as appropriate.

**COMPETENCY CHECK-IN 8.4**

**Access**

**Competency Assessment**

1. How does a facility know which staff members accessed which patient records?
2. Even though, legally, the facility may disclose health information without patient authorization for reimbursement, it is common practice for Patient Access to have patients sign a _____ form authorizing the release of PHI to financially responsible parties.
3. A patient presents in the HIM department requesting a copy of the record for his recent appendectomy. Upon inquiry, the patient reveals that, in addition to wanting a record of the operation, he had an allergic reaction to the anesthesia and wants to keep a record of this event to avoid a similar problem in the future. What else should the patient be advised to request?
4. Discuss the steps to release patient information.

## Federal, Corporate, and Facility Compliance

An increasingly important responsibility of the HIM professional is that of ensuring compliance with the many statutes, regulations, and other rules imposed on the facility and the professionals who work there. There are many functions that require oversight. Some of these are specific to patient care or patient complaints. Other compliance functions focus on monitoring data quality of ensuring the completeness and timeliness of records. The following sections discuss the most common areas of concern to HIM professionals.

### Licensure and Certification

As discussed in Chapter 1, individual states license health care facilities for operation within that state. **Licensure** is the mandatory government approval required for performing specified activities. A state's licensure requirements, which can be found in the state's administrative code, may contain very specific provisions for the content and retention of specific clinical documentation. These provisions may take the form of a listing of elements to be maintained in a health record. They may also be included in statements about a facility's medical staff. The provisions for health records may be as detailed as specifying which documents should be included or which types of data should be collected. Whatever provisions are listed for a specific type of facility, HIM personnel must be aware of these rules and must ensure that any activities under their span of control are in compliance with those rules.

The first step in ensuring compliance with any rule is to review the rule and understand what it really means. Therefore every HIM professional should have access to a copy of the specific portions of the licensure regulations that apply to his or her activities. Although it is not necessary in terms of everyday practice for each person to have a copy of the document, it is certainly appropriate for such a document to be available to personnel in the facility.

In practice, each employee in the facility is responsible for a small portion of the compliance with the specific regulations. The responsibility for overall compliance with the particular regulations rests with the director of the particular department. In the case of the HIM department, the director typically is responsible for compliance. Regulations may also be identified in the medical staff bylaws, rules, and regulations or Hospital Policy and Procedures.

One of the best ways to teach HIM employees how to comply with various regulations is to ensure that there are written policies and procedures in the department that address these particular issues that are consistent with organizational policies and procedures. Employees should be trained with these issues in mind. It is also important to cross-reference the policies and procedures to the specific regulations for compliance. Chapter 9 discusses the development of policies and procedures in the HIM department.

HIM professionals often become involved in researching and interpreting regulations, and they assist in the development of policies and procedures to comply with those regulations. Frequently, HIM professionals aid in facility-wide compliance issues. This occurs because of the pervasive nature of the documentation that is handled after a patient's discharge. For example, if a regulation dictates that physician telephone orders be signed within a certain time frame after being ordered, HIM personnel are frequently involved in the development of the procedures and controls to ensure the monitoring of that activity because by analyzing the chart after the patient's discharge, they are in a position to note noncompliance with this regulation.

### Accreditation

State licensure of a facility is mandatory. Accreditation is optional. Remember that **accreditation** is the process by which independent organizations verify that a facility complies with standards of practice developed by that organization. There are accrediting bodies that deal with a specific type of health care facility, and there are accrediting bodies that deal with many different types of health care facilities across the continuum of care. **The Joint Commission (TJC)**, known primarily for accrediting acute care facilities, also accredits other facilities, such as rehabilitation, long-term care, and ambulatory care facilities. Because TJC is so important, it is used in this chapter to exemplify how accreditation works. The accreditation process is very similar, regardless of the accrediting body. Many health care payers mandate that an organization obtains accreditation in order to comply with their requirements for reimbursement. Currently, if a facility maintains TJC accreditation, it receives deemed status for its state and CMS survey requirements. Deemed status helps to reduce the administrative costs of health care.

TJC publishes its standards annually in several formats, including a *Comprehensive Guide* that pertains to each level of health care the commission accredits. The standards are updated annually to reflect changes in health care delivery, quality, organizational philosophy, evidence-based practices, and environment. To become accredited, a facility applies to the TJC, completes a detailed questionnaire, and undergoes an intensive site visit called a *survey*. TJC surveys facilities approximately every 3 years. Unannounced surveys or surveys focusing on previously identified problems may take place between formal surveys. Because TJC standards are modified frequently, reference to the most recent publications is essential to ensure compliance. See the TJC website for current publications and other information (http://www.jointcommission.org).

Ideally, a facility should be in continuous compliance with the standards; however, because the standards change annually, it may take facilities some time each year to adjust their operations accordingly. Many facilities spend a great deal of time preparing for a survey, ensuring that documentation and various procedures are in compliance. Although it is important to discuss the preparation for a TJC survey, it should be stated that if a facility is in continuous compliance with TJC standards, continually updates its procedures to ensure compliance, and structures its reporting to document that compliance, very little preparation is needed before a survey. Nevertheless, in reality, verifying TJC compliance is a time-consuming process, and facilities should scrutinize their compliance documentation and procedures on a periodic basis rather than a continual basis.

The preparation for a routine TJC survey frequently begins with the appointment of a TJC steering committee or task force. It is very important that the HIM department be represented on the steering committee. In some cases, the director of the HIM department chairs or cochairs that committee. Other members of the committee include a variety of department directors and managers. The director of nursing or his or her designee and a physician's representative are critical participants. There are a number of management-level staff members on the committee, and they divide the responsibilities for reviewing compliance among themselves.

Some of the activities of the TJC steering committee are to review current TJC standards and compare them with current policies and procedures, to ensure that the policies and procedures are updated, to conduct mock surveys, to prepare staff for the TJC visit, to review reports that will be required, and to assemble the large quantities of documentation required by the TJC surveyors. These activities are largely delegated to the appropriate department manager, but many employees become involved in preparing for the TJC survey. In corporate environments, a team from the home office usually conducts mock surveys in a facility before the actual TJC survey.

## Record Review

The quantitative and qualitative review functions performed by HIM professionals to ensure the quality of documentation in patient health records are also known as *record review*. The record review is required by TJC standards to be performed quarterly by a multidisciplinary team of health care professionals who are involved in patient care. HIM professionals read and understand TJC guidelines and then coordinate the review of the patient records at the facility and any follow-up required when deficiencies are noted. Typically, record reviews are retrospective. However, much of the record review that occurs during an actual survey is concurrent because of a methodology that TJC uses during the facility survey called *tracer methodology*.

## Tracer Methodology

TJC **tracer methodology** follows, or traces, a current patient's stay in the health care facility. At the beginning of TJC survey, the surveyors request a current patient census for the facility. From that census, the surveyors choose the charts that they will review during the survey. These charts are reviewed concurrently during the survey of those patients who are currently in the facility. From the review of these in-house charts, the surveyors determine which physicians they will review, which staff members they will interview, and which policies and procedures they will review. The goal is to evaluate how health care is being performed in "real time." In previous TJC surveys, the management team sat in a meeting and answered all of the surveyor's questions on policy and procedures, was able to choose (with some restrictions) the charts that the surveyors would review, and could sometimes even select the physicians who were involved. With the tracer methodology, the surveyors interview the staff members who are involved in patient care and ask them questions about policies and procedures. This is also how the surveyors determine which physicians will be reviewed in the credentialing portion of the survey and which employee files to review in human resources. This process shows whether all of the facility employees know the policies and procedures, rather than just the managers. In essence, the whole survey process revolves around the review of the concurrent health records of the facility during the survey. Therefore the **concurrent review** of health records is more important today than it was in previous years. The facility should have in place a process for regularly performing this type of record review before TJC survey takes place. In fact, to ensure continuous compliance with accreditation standards, it is wise for the PI team to have in place a process for performing frequent tracer surveys of patient care areas and support departments. Teams might walk through a nursing unit, for example, and use a checklist to indicate areas that are in compliance or that need attention. Issues such as environment of care, expired medications, and safety can be identified and resolved routinely. Tracer walkthroughs support compliance with not only accreditation standards but also RM.

### Value of Record Review

Qualitative analysis of health information serves several purposes. The most important reason to perform this review is to evaluate the quality of patient care. On review of a sample of patients with a diagnosis of pneumonia, for example, it may be found that a sputum culture was ordered in 50% of the cases. Additionally, the culture was obtained immediately after a diagnosis of pneumonia was suspected. The general treatment for pneumonia is to start the patient on some type of antibiotic. However, if the sputum culture reveals a Gram-negative specimen, normal antibiotics will not resolve the patient's pneumonia. The patient must be put on a more specific medicine. Early detection of the organism facilitates prompt medication and, ideally, a shorter period of recovery. The facility uses this information to educate the physicians and the clinical staff. The information shows the difference in patient outcome between those who received appropriate care and those who did not. The information can also show the effect of the treatment on the cost of health care or reimbursement.

These analyses—qualitative analysis and record review—are essential to the accreditation of the health care facility. Accreditation bodies expect facilities to continuously monitor and analyze their compliance with predetermined standards. The quarterly review of health information to determine this compliance can prevent a facility from failing an accreditation survey. If detected early, noncompliance with standards can be corrected before a survey.

### Record Review Team

It is important to formalize record review practices as a policy identifying who is responsible for performing the record reviews. Multidisciplinary or interdisciplinary teams are organized for this function. Health care professionals who document information in the patient health record meet at least quarterly to review records against the standards. Record review teams include physicians, nurses, physical therapists, occupational therapists, radiologists, laboratory workers, dietitians, case managers, and pharmacists. Members of the record review team are challenged to determine whether a record is in compliance with TJC standards. Record review requires team members to know where and by whom health information is documented. In the multidisciplinary team record review, health care professionals who document information in the health record learn the importance of the documentation. For example, a nurse reviewing records to measure compliance with patient education standards may realize that the documentation in the records does not support that patient

education is actually being accomplished. This problem may not have been identified and corrected without the record review.

The results of the record reviews must be communicated to the medical staff committee or a quality care review committee that understands the importance of health information and the effect it has on the quality of patient care and on facility accreditation.

## Risk Management

Risk management (RM) is the coordination of efforts within a facility to prevent and control **potentially compensable events (PCEs)**. A PCE is any event that could cause a financial loss or lead to litigation. RM is a TJC requirement and often one of the stipulations required by the insurance company that provides insurance coverage to the health care facility. Depending on the size and type of facility, the RM department may include an attorney who is an employee of the facility, or RM may simply be the responsibility of one of the leaders in the facility's administration. This department monitors PCEs, leads or is involved in the safety committee, and works to ensure a safe environment for patients and employees through training, education, and facility improvements.

The health record serves as evidence of patient-related events that occur within the facility. The patient health record includes documentation of the facts of an incident as they are related to the care of the patient. For example, if a patient falls out of bed during his or her stay in the health care facility, the documentation in the patient's record would indicate the time and date of the occurrence. It would also document the position of the patient's bed, use of side rails, and other pertinent information, such as the patient's diagnosis, medications administered, and instructions given to the patient before the incident.

The patient-centered documentation in the health record is different from the occurrence, or incident, report completed when there is an inadvertent occurrence (Fig. 8.11). An *incident report* is an administrative discovery tool used by the facility to obtain information about the incident. The

incident report is not a part of the patient's health record, and it is not mentioned in any documentation.

Incident reports should be completed immediately by the employee or employees most closely associated with the incident. The incident report is used to perform an investigation into the facts surrounding the incident. Facts discovered immediately after the incident can significantly affect

---

## Incident Report
### Do Not File in Medical Records

*Confidential and privileged health care quality improvement information prepared in anticipation of litigation*

Name: _____  Employee ☐  Patient ☐  Visitor ☐

Facility name: _____

Attending physician: _____

MR # _____  SS # _____

D.O.B. ___/___/___   Sex: M[ ]  F[ ]

Admission date: ___/___/___

Primary diagnosis: _____

Site (if applicable) _____

City _____

Facility ID# _____

State _____

Phone # _____

### SECTION I: General Information

**General Identification (circle one):**
001 Inpatient
002 Outpatient
003 Nonpatient
004 Equipment only

**Location (circle one):**
005 Bathroom/toilet
006 Beauty shop
007 Cafeteria/dining room
008 Corridor/hall
009 During transport
010 Emergency department
011 Exterior grounds
012 ICU/SCU/CCU
013 Labor/delivery/birthing
014 Nursery
015 Outpatient clinic
016 Patient room
017 Radiology
018 Recovery room
019 Recreation area
020 Rehab
021 Shower room
022 Surgical suite
023 Treatment/exam room

**Treatment Rendered (circle one):**
024 Emergency room
025 First aid
026 None
026 Transfer to other facility
027 X-ray

### SECTION II: Nature of Incident (Circle all that apply):

001 Adverse outcome after surgery or anesthetic
002 Anaphylactic shock
003 Anoxic event
004 Apgar score of 5 or less
005 Aspiration
006 Assault or altercation/combative event
007 Blood or IV variance

008 Blood/body fluid exposure
009 Code/arrest
010 Damage/loss of organ
011 Death
012 Dental-related complication
013 Dissatisfaction/noncompliance*
014 Equipment operation*
015 Fall with injury*
016 Fall without injury*

017 Handling of and/or exposure to hazardous waste
018 Informed consent issue
019 Injury to other
020 Injury to self
021 Loss of limb
022 Loss of vision
023 Medication variance*
024 Needle puncture/sharp injury

025 Paralysis
026 Patient-to-patient altercation
027 Perinatal complication*
028 Poisoning
029 Suspected nonstaff-to-patient abuse
030 Suspected staff-to-patient abuse
031 Thermal burn
032 Treatment/procedure issue
033 Ulcer: nosocomial stage III/IV

*\* Complete appropriate area in Section III*

### SECTION III: Type of Incident

**If death, circle all that apply:**
001 After medical equipment failure
002 After power equipment failure or damage
003 During surgery or postanesthesia
004 Within 24 hours of admission to facility
005 Within 1 week of fall in facility
006 Within 24 hours of medication error

**Blood/IV Variance Issues (circle all that apply):**
007 Additive
008 Administration consent
009 Contraindications/allergies
010 Equipment malfunction
011 Infusion rate
012 Labeling issue
013 Reaction
014 Solution/blood type
015 Transcription
016 Patient identification
017 Allergic/adverse reaction
018 Infiltration
019 Phlebitis

**Dissatisfaction/Noncompliance (circle all that apply):**
020 AMA
021 Elopement
022 Irate or angry (either family or patient)
023 Left without service
024 Noncompliant patient
025 Refused prescribed treatment

**Falls (circle all that apply):[†]**
001 Assisted fall
002 Found on floor
003 From bed
004 From chair
005 From commode/toilet
006 From exam table
007 From stretcher
008 From wheelchair
009 Patient states—unwitnessed
010 Unassisted fall
011 While ambulating
012 Witnessed fall

*† For any marks in this field, Section V must be completed*

**Medication Variance Issues (circle all that apply):**
013 Contraindication/allergies
014 Delay in dispensing
015 Incorrect dose
016 Expired drug
017 Medication identification
018 Narcotic log variance
019 Not ordered
020 Ordered, not given
021 Patient identification
022 Reaction
023 Route
024 Rx incorrectly dispensed
025 Time of dose
026 Transcription

• **Fig. 8.11** Incident report. *AMA*, (Patient left hospital) against medical advice; *CCU*, cardiac care unit; *ICU*, intensive care unit; *Rx*, medication (prescribed); *SCU*, surgical care unit.

the facility's ability to defend, comprehend, or determine the cause of the incident or the liability of the parties in an incident. Examples of inadvertent occurrences are listed in Box 8.6.

Occasionally, events are not recognized as incidents during the patient's stay. Review of documentation by HIM staff members may identify a PCE. As a result, health information is used in RM to gather facts surrounding an occurrence; support the claim should it require litigation; or provide information to prevent a future occurrence.

## Disaster Planning

In addition to complying with the Security Rule regarding e-PHI, organizations also have to plan for physical protection of nonelectronic PHI and the physical plant itself. Disaster planning is a method for planning and preparing to handle catastrophes and other emergencies that can adversely affect the normal performance of the health care environment. For example, a disaster can consist of a large number of patients requiring medical attention at the same time as a result of an explosion or a plane crash. In this situation, the increased number of patients needing treatment would necessitate implementation of a plan to handle their care and processing in a timely manner. All TJC-accredited facilities are required to maintain a disaster plan. Facilities must also educate HIM employees on the security procedures and make sure that they are prepared to follow procedure if a disaster occurs.

HIM practitioners must protect all health information, including records; diagnosis, procedure, and physician indices; the MPI; computerized health information databases; radiographic films; and admission, discharge, and transfer logs.

### Fire Damage

Providing protection from fire for the health information environment can prevent irreversible damage to the facility's health records. Some of the systems and barriers that can assist in the protection from fire are chemical systems, sprinkler systems, fire walls, fire compartments, and fire extinguishers.

Chemical systems deplete the oxygen from the air in an area where a fire exists. File rooms and computer facilities may be equipped with this type of system. The chemical system is designed to sense fire and release a chemical that removes oxygen from the air in the room. Removing the oxygen smothers the fire to prevent further damage to files or the facility.

Building structures such as fire walls or fire compartments are designed to contain a fire within a facility. Fire walls prevent a fire from moving in a parallel direction on a particular floor of the building. Health care facilities often feature double doors in the hallways, in which the doors are held open by magnets on each wall. When the fire alarm is triggered in a health care facility with fire walls, those double doors close to seal the fire and prevent it from spreading to other areas of the facility. A fire compartment is a structure in a building in which all sides of a room or area are protected by fire barriers. In other words, the walls, ceiling, and floor are all fire resistant. If a fire begins in a fire compartment, the compartment contains the fire; likewise, if the fire is outside the compartment, the contents within the compartment are protected from the fire. A fire compartment is the ideal solution to protect the permanent file area or a central computer system if a fire occurs in another part of the facility.

Sprinkler systems release water to extinguish fire when activated by heat or smoke. When a sprinkler system is used to safeguard files, it is important to have at least 18 in. of clearance between the top of the file space and the ceiling. Failure to keep these areas clear prevents the water sprinklers from extinguishing the fire at a lower level. In the event of a fire, sprinkler systems may extinguish the fire and cause minimal water damage to the facility's records.

All health care facilities are equipped with fire extinguishers. HIM employees must be familiar with the location of the nearest fire extinguisher. Employees must be able to operate the fire extinguishers in case of emergency. It is possible for a fire to begin in a very small trash can or near an electrical outlet. With use of a fire extinguisher, the fire can easily be controlled without activating a sprinkler system or chemical system.

### Water Damage

Water damage to health records, whether they are paper based or computerized, can occur because of flooding, storms, or fire control. A plan must be established to protect health information from water damage. For example, is the facility in an area where flooding is common? Some options for this scenario may be to relocate the file area to a higher floor of the facility, to elevate the file room a few feet, and to have an emergency plan that can be activated to move records on low shelves to a higher location in the facility if the need arises. Health records maintained in file cabinets or on shelves that are closed or covered must also be considered for protection from flooding. Although damage to contents of file cabinets from a sprinkler system is usually minimal, sprinkler systems do cause damage to contents of open shelving units. The HIM professional should evaluate the health record environment and the potential for flood or water damage and should remember to protect computer terminals and to have a plan in case of emergency.

On a positive note, there are processes to assist in the restoration of paper health records that are damaged by water. If paper records are soaked with water or other fluid, acting quickly can restore and protect the information. Once the paper records dry, the opportunity to salvage them may be lost. Wet paper records may be salvaged, but not those destroyed by fire. Meeting with disaster recovery companies before disaster strikes provides information for the department that might not have been considered otherwise. The companies can supply references to other facilities that have used their services. Proactive conversations can be very useful to the facility in a disaster because staff will know whom to contact, how long it will take for the records to arrive at the facility, and other helpful information to secure or preserve the health records.

## Theft and Tampering

The issues to consider when protecting health records from theft or tampering are the location of the health records, access to them, and security. Health information, both paper and electronic forms, must be protected from theft or tampering by parties both within and outside the facility. Within a facility, only authorized personnel should have access to patient health information, and they should have access only to the information that pertains to the completion of their job duties. Paper documents are secured by allowing release of an original record from the HIM department only if it is needed for the patient's treatment. The HIM department maintains appropriate measures to track the location of patient records. Other review of a patient's record must occur within the HIM department and is allowed only if the person reviewing the record is authorized to do so.

HIM professionals cannot follow every patient record checked out to every location in a facility. Therefore it is important to have policies and procedures in place to secure the information. This security may be achieved by (1) notifying others of the policies and procedures for security of information, (2) performing regular in-service training for facility employees to inform them of the rules governing health information, and (3) restricting the reasons for which a patient's health record is allowed to leave the department.

Additional security measures are as follows:

- After office hours, the HIM department should be closed and all access doors locked; only those people authorized to enter the department are allowed entrance. Anyone with a key to the area must be aware of all HIM policies and procedures regarding the appropriate use of health information.
- Areas may also be protected by a key code entry system. Access codes are assigned only to appropriate employees or physicians. After hours, an authorized physician can gain access to designated areas, such as the chart completion room, with this code.
- A swipe badge security feature allows entry to the HIM department only with the appropriate access card, which is assigned to authorized physicians or employees.
- Computer passwords assigned to authorized users allow the facility to limit and monitor the people who access health information.
- Biometric technology, such as fingerprinting and retinal scanning, is also a means of limiting access to health records. With this technology, the system scans a person's fingerprint or retina to evaluate his or her authority to enter an area or gain access to a system.
- Cameras are another security feature found in health care facilities. In areas where there is greater need for security, cameras monitored by the facility's security personnel guard against unauthorized entry.

For computerized health information, a facility must secure records when transferring files from one system to another within or outside of the facility. For example, upgrading software or changing computers may require patient health information to be transferred from one information system to another. Copying of records from one system to another is acceptable; however, the HIM department must supervise this type of data transfer. Additionally, the department must validate that patient information is not deleted in the transfer. Failure to maintain complete patient information may affect future patient care. Likewise, an incomplete medical record may not be admissible in court as evidence in the event of litigation. An index of the old system should be maintained to verify the accuracy of the new system.

Electronic health information must be protected. Equipment should be secure, and precautions should be taken to prevent others from accessing the system. It is also important to ensure that the facility can update current systems and still retrieve information from legacy systems.

## Destruction of Health Information

There are circumstances in which it is appropriate to destroy health information. For example, records (stored on paper, microfilm, or electronic formats) may be destroyed at the completion of the retention period or when paper-based records have been successfully transferred to another medium, such as scanned into the document management system. However, HIM employees must prevent negligent destruction. In a paper record environment, a common method of destroying health information is the shredding or incineration of the paper document. The destruction must occur in a confidential manner. It should be performed in the presence of a credentialed custodian of the HIM department or his or her delegate. Health information should never be left to be destroyed without the proper supervision. If a vendor is chosen for the destruction, the following questions should be answered: Do they use a third party for shredding? Is the third party compliant with HIPAA regulations? Is recycling an option? What is their procedure for destruction? How and when will written confirmation or a destruction certificate be obtained?

In the electronic record environment, destruction of health information may include entering a virus into the software system, destroying the equipment or software used to retrieve the health information, or otherwise removing the information from the system.

To prevent premature destruction of health information in the paper record environment, several measures must be taken. Employees should be aware of the appropriate content of the health record so that valuable patient information is not inadvertently thrown out. Likewise, the employees should be aware of the *record retention schedule* for all materials in the HIM department. If the facility has chosen to store records in an alternative format, the finished product—microfilm, optical disks, or EHR files—must be reviewed to ensure that all of the information is intact before the original paper record is destroyed.

In an electronic record environment, a backup file of all health information in all systems must be completed daily. The backup copy allows information to be restored up to the time that the backup was created. This procedure is usually performed daily in health care facilities. The backup file copies the information from the systems in the facility. If the system crashes the next day, at least the facility will have all of the information necessary to restore the system to the previous day's business.

Electronic health information should be kept in an environment that supports the use of computers. The HIM department must maintain the computerized equipment so that it is free from harm by temperature, water, and other environmental effects. These considerations also apply to microfilm and optical disk storage. Microfilm and optical disks can be damaged by intense heat. Computers are affected by temperatures as well. Water can damage a computer and cause loss of function and information. Falling objects can damage computer equipment and disks, and liquids spilled on keyboards or hard drives can impair or destroy a system.

### Restoration of Information Lost Inadvertently

What can be done when health records are lost or destroyed inadvertently? It is important to have a plan of action. In an electronic record system, daily backups of the information in the system should allow full recovery of all patient information (prior to backup). In the event of inadvertent destruction of paper records, the only information that can be reproduced is the duplicate paper documents maintained by allied health departments within the facility. For example, the laboratory and radiology departments usually maintain duplicate copies of reports, the transcription department or service may be able to recover transcription of any dictated reports, and in some instances the billing office may maintain a file including patient information. As a last resort, a facility may also find information in the attending physician's office. Often, the attending physician needs copies of patient information for follow-up care or to bill for services. Obtaining a copy of information sent to the physician can assist in the effort to recover this information.

**COMPETENCY CHECK-IN 8.6**

**Risk Management**

**Competency Assessment**

1. Define risk management.
2. Why does a health care organization need a formal risk management program?
3. How does risk management mitigate potentially compensable events?
4. Explain disaster planning and why it is important.
5. How is disaster planning and theft related to risk management?
6. Why would an organization destroy health information?

## Chapter Summary

At the foundation of HIM, we find the tenets of confidentiality, security, and privacy. In simple terms, health information is confidential. The patient–physician privilege ensures that information shared by patients with their physicians will be kept in confidence. Furthermore, release of this health information/record can only occur with the consent of the patient.

Informed consent underlies patient admission, treatment, and ROI. A valid consent for ROI comprises eight elements: identification of the party being asked to release the information, patient name/identification, identification of the party to whom the information is to be released, specific information to be released, description of the purpose of the use or disclosure, expiration date, signature of the patient or personal representative authorizing the disclosure, and date. However, in an emergency, records may be released without patient consent.

This chapter emphasizes the various legal and regulatory issues governing the development, retention, release, and use of health information. Other important issues include compliance with regulatory, accrediting, and professional standards. Health care facilities should make every effort to ensure continuous compliance with the standards imposed by authoritative bodies.

# Competency Milestones

*II.1. Apply privacy strategies to health information. (3)*

## Rationale
HIM professionals work at the intersection of patient privacy and information access. They have an ethical and legal obligation to maintain compliance while supporting quality patient care.

## Competency Assessment
1. What is the difference between privacy and confidentiality?
2. What is the legal foundation for confidentiality?
3. What is the function of the HIPAA Privacy Rule? What is required by the Security Rule?
4. What is an accounting of disclosure? What information is the health care facility required to release to the patient, and how long must this information be maintained?
5. What is the Notice of Privacy Practices? Find or create an example to be used by a health care facility.
6. What is a business associate?
7. A permission that is given after the event to which the permission applies is called _____.
8. What are the elements of a valid authorization for ROI?
9. Describe situations in which authorization is not necessary to release information.
10. Compare and contrast the procedures for preparing a record for release to the patient versus a certified copy for court.
11. List examples of occurrences for which reporting is mandatory in the interest of public health.

## Case Study
*A nurse aggregating information about cases of pneumonia at the facility left printouts of the progress notes for 40 different patients on his desk when he was called away urgently. When he came back 10 minutes later, the patient records were gone. Working with the privacy officer, the staff looked everywhere for the printouts. Three days later, they were found on a shelf near the nurse's desk, just above eye level.*
1. What is the facility required to do at this point?

*II.3. Identify compliance requirements throughout the health information life cycle. (3)*

## Rationale
Health information is gathered for patient care, reporting, reimbursement, and administrative reasons. Ensuring its integrity while it is useful and destroying it appropriately when it is not is an important HIM professional skill.

## Competency Assessment
1. Describe the health information life cycle.
2. Your facility is merging with another. The facilities are on different computer systems and will be retaining the data in your facility and creating an enterprise-wide MPI going forward. The implementation team has suggested that your MPI data generated in the past year should be uploaded to the new MPI. What is your response to that suggestion?
3. In the process of merging your facility with another, it was decided to migrate to a cloud-based storage strategy for archiving. While the storage capacity is virtually unlimited, administration wants to archive only what is necessary and asks for your recommendation. What is your response?

*V.1. Apply legal processes impacting health information. (3)*

## Rationale
Legal matters permeate the health care industry, both to protect the rights of patients and the rights of providers. As a keeper of documentation, you will be required to provide evidence on the side of both plaintiffs and defendants.

## Competency Assessment
1. What is the designated record set? Why is it important for a health care facility to identify the designated record set?
2. Create a policy to define a designated record set for an acute care hospital.
3. What is jurisdiction?

4. What is the hearsay rule? How does it affect cases involving health records?
5. What are the components of the business record rule?
6. What is the purpose of informed consent, and why is informed consent necessary?
7. Explain the difference between retrospective consent and prospective consent. Why is the difference important?
8. Over what events or circumstances does a federal court have jurisdiction?
9. Number the steps in a civil lawsuit in their correct order:
   __A. Appeal
   __B. Complaint
   __C. Discovery
   __D. Pretrial conference
   __E. Satisfying the judgment
   __F. Trial
10. The legal term for harm and damages suffered by an individual is _____.
11. How has the doctrine of corporate negligence affected hospitals?
12. Your ROI clerk is questioning a subpoena because the instructions do not seem "right." Upon review of the document, you agree that the language is not standard. The document came in the mail with a patient authorization attached. What should you do?

### CAHIIM Competency

*V.2. Demonstrate compliance with external forces. (3)*

### Rationale

As an HIM professional, you will frequently support the facility's accreditation and licensure with documentation.

### Competency Assessment

1. What is compliance? Why is it important?
2. Locate the licensure regulations for your state.
   a. What are the provisions for the content of a health record?
   b. What are the rules regarding the timeliness of completion of a record?
3. Describe the accreditation process.
4. Explain the role of HIM department in maintaining compliance with the rules and regulations for Medicare coding and billing.
5. What are the licensure requirements for an acute care hospital in your state?
6. Why must a court order for a patient record be validated?

### CAHIIM Competency

*V.3. Identify the components of risk management related to health information management (3).*

### Rationale

HIM works closely with RM on matters related to health information.

### Competency Assessment

1. One of your staff tripped and fell in your department. What should you do?
2. You have received a subpoena for records and notice that the case involves a patient suing a physician on staff at your hospital. What should you do?

## Ethics Challenge

*VI.7. Assess ethical standards of practice (5)*

You are the director of HIM in a small community hospital. One day, an employee in the incomplete file area comes to you with a coat. One of the physicians left it in the dictation room, but the employee does not know to whom it belongs. You decide to look in the pockets of the coat to see whether any identification is present. You find in one of the pockets a prescription bottle of Antabuse (disulfiram), a medication given to alcoholics to help them stop drinking. The patient named on the bottle is a physician at your facility. What should you do with this information? What are the confidentiality issues? Should you have handled this situation differently?

## Critical Thinking Question

1. An unconscious patient arrives via ambulance to the emergency room with multiple abdominal scars. Doctors need information about previous history to thoroughly consider the course of treatment. Records were requested from another hospital. What might the HIM-ROI clerk release in these circumstances?
2. In Chapter 2, we discussed health information exchanges (HIEs). What impact does an HIE have on patient access to their records? How does an HIE impact continuity of clinical care? What challenges exist in accessing records through an HIE?

## The Role of Health Information Management Professionals in the Workplace

### Professional Profile:

#### Customer Service Representative

 My name is Zak, and I am a customer service representative with a company that performs release of information (ROI) services for acute care facilities. The company and others like it were once referred to as *copy services* because our employees spent so much time making photocopies. Today we can assist patients with accessing their information via our hospital's patient portal. With the patient portal, patients have access to test results, doctor's appointments, and information related to their diagnosis/procedures, making it easier for patients to stay informed about their care.

I am a registered health information technician. While I was in school, I was hired by the copy service to work as a copy representative. At the facility where I was placed, health information management (HIM) department employees logged in the requests, validated the requests, and retrieved the records. Then I would copy the required sections, prepare an invoice, log the completion of the request, and send out the copies. Eventually, the facility turned over the entire function to me.

As a copy representative, I need to know the laws in my state governing the ROI as well as the hospital's policies and procedures. I need to know the contents of the record, how to retrieve it, and how to ensure that the record is complete. In addition, I had to learn the copy service's computer logging and invoicing system. Most importantly, I'm required to maintain a professional attitude at all times and employ good communication skills to ensure a cordial and professional relationship with my clients.

After I graduated from my health information technology program, I was promoted to customer service representative. Now I am responsible for training new employees, scheduling and managing their assignments, solving problems that arise, and occasionally substituting for someone who is ill or on vacation. Sometimes, I accompany the marketing manager when she makes presentations to potential new clients. I like to travel to different hospitals and meet new people, and I enjoy the responsibilities, so I am very happy in this new position.

One thing is certain—the duties related to my job are constantly evolving, with legislative, regulatory, accreditation, and technology changes occurring on a regular basis. I am very excited about the future of HIM—being able to facilitate patient access to their PHI so that they can take an active role in their care and sharing patient information via health information exchanges (HIEs). These are very exciting times in our field.

#### Career Tip

Making copies of records for ROI is an example of an entry-level position in HIM. Although many clerical staff are trained on the job, extensive experience or HIM formal education is usually needed for supervisory roles. ROI vendors, to whom health care providers outsource all or part of this function, are a major employer of these workers.

### Patient Care Perspective

#### Maria

After my experience with Mom and not having immediate access to medical records, I decided to make a file of all of our family's important health care records. I found a good PHR website that lets me enter key data and upload documentation. I was not sure what documentation was really important, so I called Diamonte and spoke with Zak. He helped me understand what documentation was important for continuing medical care, and he helped me fill out the consent forms that were needed to get it. He was also able to give me the documentation electronically and share the information with me to set up my patient portal account so I can access future records! Now I am all organized. I was really surprised to find out how much was missing from my own early records and my husband's. We should have started this process sooner, but we will have it all going forward.

## Further Reading

American Health Information Management Association (AHIMA): Fundamentals of the legal health record and designated record set, *J AHIMA* 82(2), 2011. expanded online version. Retrieved from https://library.ahima.org/doc?oid=104008. March 7, 2022

McLendon K, Dinh RA: Notice of privacy practices (2013 update), October 2013. *AHIMA Practice Brief*. http://library.ahima.org/PB/NPP. Accessed March 7, 2022.

National Council of State Boards of Nursing, Inc. (NCSBN®): *A nurse's guide to the use of social media*, Chicago, IL, June 2018. National Council of State Boards of Nursing, Inc. (NCSBN®).https://www.ncsbn.org/NCSBN_SocialMedia.pdf. Retrieved March 7, 2022.

U.S. Department of Health and Human Services: *Summary of the HIPAA Privacy Rule*. *HHS*.gov: U.S. Department of Health and Human Services website, July 26, 2013. https://www.hhs.gov/hipaa/for-professionals/privacy/laws-regulations/index.html. Accessed March 7, 2022.

# 9

# Management and Leadership

## LISA REILLY

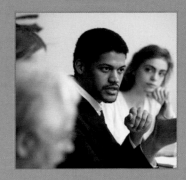

## CHAPTER OUTLINE

**Organizational Structure**
- Accountability
- Shared Governance
- Management Responsibilities
- Health Information Management Department Organization
- Health Information Management Department Workflow

**Strategic Planning**
- Mission, Vision, and Values
- Data and Information Governance
- Rolling Out the Strategic Plan

**Operational Planning**
- Goals and Objectives
- Policies and Procedures
- Customer Satisfaction

**Human Resources**
- Legal Aspects
- Job Analysis and Description
- Recruitment and Retention
- Performance Standards
- Workload
- Workflow and Process Monitors
- Employee Evaluations
- Organization-Wide Orientation
- Health Information Management Department Orientation
- Clinical Staff Orientation
- Discipline
- Outsourcing

**Communication**
- Oral Communication
- Communicating with Physicians
- Communicating with Outside Agencies or Parties
- Written Communication
- Meetings
- Work Teams

**Interpersonal Skills**
- Leadership
- Diversity

**Training and Development**
- Planning a Training Session
- Calendar of Education
- Evaluating the Training Program
- Educating the Public
- Continuing Education

**Chapter Summary**

**Competency Milestones**

**CAHIM Competency**

**Critical Thinking Questions**

**The Role of Health Information Management Professionals in the Workplace**
- Professional Profile: Health Information Management Director
- Professional Profile: Health Information Management Assistant Director
- Patient Care Perspective
- Patient Care Perspective

**Works cited**

**Further Reading**

## CHAPTER OBJECTIVES

*By the end of this chapter, the student should be able to:*

1. Describe the organizational and governance structures of health care organizations and health information management departments;
2. Articulate the process of strategic and operational planning;
3. Articulate the value of human resources and human resources processes to the work of the organization and the delivery of health care;
4. Practice professional oral and written communication in the workplace;
5. Identify leadership strategies and advocate for diversity in the workplace; and
6. Facilitate training and development for health care professionals.

## VOCABULARY

agenda
chain of command
continuing education (CE)
cross-training
cultural competence
diversity
dual governance
full-time equivalents (FTEs)
functional organization
goal
information governance
in-service
job analysis
job description
matrix reporting
memorandum (memo)
minutes
mission statement

objective
organization chart
orientation
outsource
per diem
performance improvement plan (PIP)
performance standards
policy
procedure
productivity
shared governance
span of control
unity of command
values statement
vision
workflow analysis
workflow

### CAHIIM COMPETENCY DOMAINS

I.6.   **DM** Evaluate data dictionaries and data sets for compliance with governance standards. (5)
VI.1.  Demonstrate fundamental leadership skills. (3)
VI.3.  Identify human resource strategies for organizational best practices. (3)
VI.6.  Examine behaviors that embrace cultural diversity. (4)
VI.7.  Assess ethical standards of practice. (5)
VI.9.  Identify processes of workforce training for health care organizations. (3)

In this chapter, human resources (HR), organization, planning, policy, procedures, equipment, and supplies are discussed in the context of their importance, relevance, or function in the health information management (HIM) department. Note that the general topics discussed apply to supervision and training in many areas. This chapter focuses on issues, tools, and techniques used to manage HIM employees who perform HIM department functions.

## Organizational Structure

One method used by health care facilities to describe the arrangement of departments and positions is the **organization chart**. The organization chart illustrates the relationships among departments, positions, and functions within the organization. The traditional structure of an organization chart resembles a pyramid, in which there are more departments and personnel at the bottom than at the top. An organization chart uses boxes and lines to represent departments and positions within the facility (Fig. 9.1). Each box indicates a department or position. The higher the box is located within the chart, the higher the authority and responsibility of the position or department that it represents. Boxes on the same level indicate similar levels of authority or responsibility. Lines connecting the boxes indicate relationships. Solid lines indicate a direct relationship. Broken lines indicate an indirect (or shared) relationship.

The lines in the organization chart illustrate the subordination of positions in the chain of command. The **chain of command** refers to the order in which decisions are made

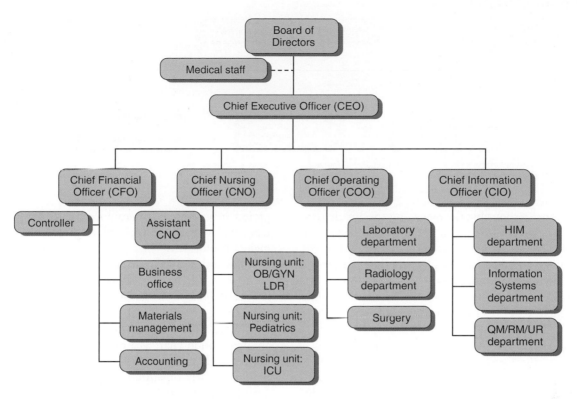

• **Fig. 9.1** Example organization chart for a small- to medium-sized acute care hospital. *HIM*, Health information management; *ICU*, intensive care unit; *LDR*, leader; *OB/GYN*, obstetrics/gynecology; *QM*, quality management; *RM*, risk management; *UR*, utilization review.

within the facility: the line of authority through which decisions are formally authorized. Therefore the organization chart also represents the reporting structure; it indicates which individuals manage or have authority over another employee or department. An employee should follow the chain of command for approval related to his or her job in the department, including discussion of disagreements with supervisors.

The traditional health care facility is composed of departments with specialized personnel or services; these are related to the health care professions discussed in Chapter 1. The chart in Fig. 9.1 is a useful reference when you are considering the organization chart of a medium-sized acute care facility. The box at the top of the chart represents the ultimate authority and responsibility within the organization. This authority is usually called the *Governing Body, Board of Directors (in a for-profit organization)*, or *Board of Trustees (generally not-for-profit)*. Every health care facility has this type of authority at the top of the organization.

There are typically 8–25 members on the Board, depending on the size of the facility. Members of the Board include the Chief Executive Officer (CEO), members of the medical staff, and members of the community. The Board meets regularly to review the business of the health care facility, set direction, and monitor progress. The Board has two distinct relationships, as shown in Fig. 9.1. One is their delegation of authority to the CEO for the daily operations of the facility. The other is the relationship with the facility's medical staff. These two lines of authority constitute **dual governance**, a shared organization structure consisting of

the administration, headed by the CEO, and the medical staff, headed by the Chief of Medical Staff.

The medical staff is organized as a membership group of physicians governed by the facility's medical staff bylaws, rules, and regulations. They admit patients to the health care facility and provide care during the patient stay. In addition, the medical staff has a responsibility to aid the administration in the longer term planning of the health care facility. An example of medical staff structure is shown in Fig. 9.2.

The CEO, under the Governing Board, is given the authority to oversee the daily management of the health care facility. The CEO must guide, motivate, and lead the organization, receiving direction from the Governing Board.

Below the CEO are several administrative positions. These positions have authority over specific departments within the organization. These administrators report to the CEO and are accountable for the operations of their departments. This level of the administration is also known as the chiefs, or the "C-Suite." The term C-Suite refers to the executive leadership of an organization and, if applicable, the area in the building in which their offices are located. Executive leadership titles common in health care are:
• Chief Executive Officer
• Chief Operations Officer
• Chief Medical Officer
• Chief Nursing Officer
• Chief Financial Officer
• Chief Information Officer

Assistant administrators and vice presidents report to these administrators.

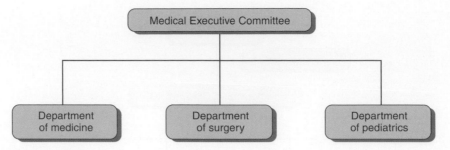

• **Fig. 9.2** Medical staff organization chart.

The personnel responsible for managing specific departments are known as directors, department heads, or managers. Below department directors are assistant directors, supervisors, and then staff employees. The managers of each department have authority over the supervisors within their departments, and finally, the staff employees within each department report to their respective supervisors.

## Accountability

The exact titles of administrative positions are less important than their chain of command and **span of control**, the number of employees or departments that report to one individual. In an organization chart, the number of positions or employees shown below the box for an administrator, manager, or supervisor indicates the span of control for that position. The span of control for one supervisor must be appropriate so that management is efficient and effective. Too many varied responsibilities or employees under one supervisor can lead to ineffective management. A large facility may require more managers than a small facility because of the number of employees needed to accomplish tasks or functions.

It is equally important that any individual employee reports to only one manager. This concept is called **unity of command**. If one employee has two supervisors, this can cause a dilemma as to which manager's authority is higher or which manager's rules and requests take precedence. If both managers have deadlines, which one must be met first? Who decides? If the employee has only one manager, the employee knows that he or she is accountable to that manager according to the role and responsibility of the position. This traditional arrangement is a **functional organization**. In HIM, that means that a staff person, such as a coder, reports to a supervisor who reports to an assistant director who reports to a director. The director usually reports to an administrator, such as the Chief Financial Officer.

An alternative to the functional organization is **matrix organization**. In a matrix organization, some staff may be grouped by product or service and generally have multiple reporting lines. In an increasingly challenging health care environment, it is not always possible or practical to maintain strict unity of command. Furthermore, with performance improvement (PI) and other quality efforts crossing all aspects of a facility, the functional responsibility for a

project may result in an employee, particularly a manager, reporting to multiple higher-level individuals, either formally or informally. This type of cross-departmental chain of command is called **matrix reporting**. In health care, this occurs most often when teams are created to solve a problem, work on a particular project, or oversee some aspect of monitoring organizational performance, Temporary teams to solve a problem or work on a project do not show up on an organization chart as a matrix. Similarly, standing committees such as Infection Control and Revenue Cycle are not true matrix organization. However, the assignment of a patient access registrar to a clinical department for a centrally organized patient access department could certainly be reflected on the organization chart as a straight line to patient access and a dotted line to the clinical supervisor or manager. One might be more likely to see matrix organization in a project-oriented organization such as a consulting firm or technology development company.

Matrix reporting is typically represented by broken or dotted lines on an organization chart, if the reporting line is permanent and inherent in the duties of the employee. Less formal matrix reporting that results from project work is not generally represented on the table of organization. Matrix reporting does not necessarily solve the problems of workload prioritization mentioned above. It does formalize the relationships, though, so that accountability is apparent to all. Clear communication, documentation of responsibilities, and measurable performance objectives are common ways to overcome dual reporting issues.

## Shared Governance

The concept of **shared governance** refers to the empowerment of all staff to be responsible for their particular areas. Instead of top-down direction from management to employees, employees are part of the team and participate in decision-making. Shared governance implies a decentralization of management to the point of service that defies traditional organizational chart description. Thus all participants in a process collaborate and build relationships that include the participation of all staff in an effective partnership. Staff determine what must be done, what goals to pursue, and how to do it. The goal of the partnership is to develop and maintain the best possible service, including patient outcomes. The standards set to measure success emphasize that all members of the team have equity or equal importance in the accomplishment of the goal. The price to be paid for that equality is to hold each team member accountable for his or her own performance. Therefore each team member has ownership of the process, as well as his or her individual role, and thus there are typically shared responsibilities for what might be normally considered supervisory or management activities such as scheduling (Guanci, 2018).

## Management Responsibilities

There are countless different managerial roles that are performed by individuals with a variety of titles. In general, a manager is responsible for one or more operational processes and has one or more individuals who report directly to them in order to perform the process. As a general rule, upper management refers to the vice president and C-Suite levels, middle management are directors and managers, and lower management are supervisory personnel. Managers plan, organize, lead, control, and direct to varying degrees depending on the needs of the organization and the specific role.

Managers are responsible for efficient and effective use of all the resources in an organization, including the people. They organize **workflow** (the order of tasks to complete a

process), establish policy and procedures, hire, and monitor employee productivity and performance. In this chapter we discuss many of the tools HIM managers employ to coordinate these functions. Please note that HIM departments differ among health care facilities. The methods and workflow that work in one department may not work efficiently in another department.

## Health Information Management Department Organization

Fig. 9.3 illustrates a table of organization within the HIM department. This is an organization chart for an HIM department with 35 employees. The box at the top of the chart represents the department director. The person in this position has the delegated authority from the administration of the facility to act as the custodian of health information. This position also has the responsibility and authority to manage the daily operations of the HIM department. This example department has 1 director, 1 assistant director, 3 supervisors, and 32 staff employees. Keep in mind that job titles for positions within the HIM department vary among facilities. The HIM department may also be called the *medical record department* or *health information services*. Names of HIM departments remain diverse across the country.

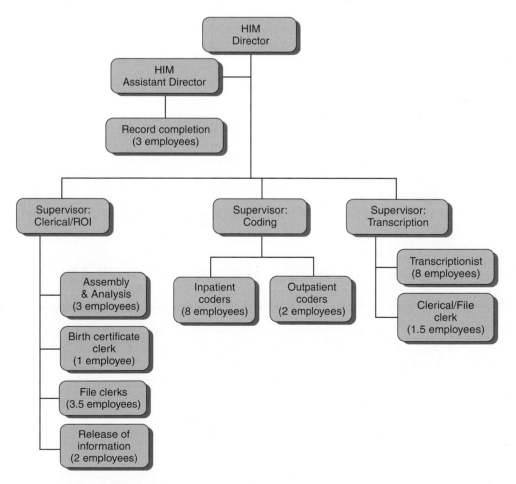

• **Fig. 9.3** Health information management department organization chart. *HIM*, Health information management; *ROI*, release of information.

The organization chart in Fig. 9.3 shows a department that is organized into three supervised sections of health information functions. Each supervisor is responsible for specific functions within the department. There is a supervisor for the assembly, scanning, analysis, release of information (ROI), and filing functions, also known as the *clerical*, or *ROI*, *supervisor*. Another supervisor, called the *coding supervisor*, oversees the coding and abstracting functions. The third supervisor, *the transcription supervisor*, is responsible for the transcription function.

Supervisors work at the staff level to ensure that the daily tasks in the HIM department are accomplished in a timely and accurate manner. Supervisors typically work in close proximity to or with the employees they supervise. They are on hand to handle in a timely manner issues, questions, and situations that arise. Responsibilities of the supervisor positions differ in each department, but they may include scheduling, hiring, training, monitoring, coaching, disciplining, and terminating staff. The supervisor is responsible for ensuring that staff employees are performing their functions efficiently and consistently with the policies of the department.

Within the HIM department, employees are further identified by the positions that they hold or job functions that they perform. HIM departments have clerical and technical staff positions (Table 9.1). The director of the HIM department in collaboration with the HR department typically determines the titles for employee positions. Some titles are generic (e.g., HIM Tech I), whereas other titles describe the employee's responsibilities (e.g., inpatient coder, outpatient coder, scanning technician, ROI clerk, and revenue cycle supervisor).

Clerical employees are responsible for the functions known as *scanning* (or assembly), indexing and data validity (analysis), and ROI. Technical employees perform functions such as coding, abstracting, and transcription (Table 9.1 describes possible job titles). Such positions are sometimes referred to as *HIM Tech II*. These staff employees typically report to the first or lowest level of management, either the HIM supervisor or a team leader. The titles, roles, and responsibilities of positions within the HIM department vary. Smaller facilities with few patient admissions have fewer positions as well as fewer levels of management. However, larger health care facilities have several employees performing one function, and they require more supervisors and levels of management to oversee daily functions.

## Health Information Management Department Workflow

The collection, organization, coding, abstracting, analysis, storage, and retrieval of patient health information are organized into a workflow within each health care organization to best suit that facility. Efficient workflow allows department employees to accomplish their functions in a timely, accurate, and complete manner. Although managers should continually look for ways to remove obstacles and streamline the workflow in their departments, **workflow analysis**, or a careful look at how work is performed, is especially crucial

| TABLE 9.1 | Staff Positions in the Health Information Management Department | | |
|---|---|---|---|
| **Position** | **Responsibility/Function** | **Hours** | **Status** |
| HIM Director | Daily management of the HIM department | Monday through Friday, 8:00 a.m.–4:30 p.m. | Full time |
| Supervisor | Clerical/ROI/filing | Monday through Friday, 7:00 a.m.–3:30 p.m. | Full time |
| Scanning Clerk | Assembly and analysis of all patient records | Sunday through Thursday, 6:30 a.m.–3 p.m. | Full time |
| Birth Certificate Clerk | Birth certificates Saturday assembly/analysis | Tuesday through Saturday, 8:00 a.m.–4:30 p.m. | Full time |
| HIM Tech I | File clerk | Monday through Friday, 5:00 p.m.–9:00 p.m. | Part time |
| Inpatient Coder | Inpatient coding | Monday through Friday, 8:30 a.m.–5:00 p.m. | Full time |
| Outpatient Coder | Outpatient coding | Monday through Thursday, 4:00 p.m.–9:00 p.m. | Part time |
| ROI Clerk | Release of information | Monday through Friday, 8:30 a.m.–5:00 p.m. | Full time |
| Revenue Cycle Manager | Daily management of revenue cycle activities, including quality of claims-related data | Monday through Friday, 7:30 a.m.–4:00 p.m. | Full time |
| Transcriptionist | General transcription and STAT requests | Saturday through Sunday, 8:00 a.m.–4:30 p.m. | Part time |

*HIM*, Health information management; *ROI*, release of information; *STAT*, immediate.

when a facility is implementing new software or anticipating changes, such as additional departmental responsibilities.

Because every HIM department is different, this section covers general workflow concepts such as the management and organization of HIM functions with only a few variations. Variations in the workflow among different facilities are necessary to accommodate the type, size, and structure of each health care facility.

As a refresher, let's look at the HIM workflow, as discussed in Chapter 4. As shown in Fig. 9.4, health records undergo several distinct processes that enable the current and future use of the data they contain:

*Collection*—the retrieval of any paper documentation related to the health record from the patient care unit for every patient treated by the facility;

*Organization*—the assembly of the record into a batch that enables scanning of the paper into the document management system associated with the electronic health record (EHR);

*Analysis*—the review of quantitative (and sometimes also the qualitative) health information to ensure timely, accurate, and complete records;

*Coding*—the assignment of alphanumeric or numeric codes to patient diagnoses and procedures for reimbursement and data retrieval;

*Abstracting*—the validation of certain data elements, such as discharge status, by either analysts or coders, to ensure the accuracy of the record;

*Transcription*—the method by which the physician's dictation is turned into a medical report;

*Record completion*—the processing of an incomplete record as more health data are entered from appropriate health care personnel;

*Storage*—the electronic or other method used to maintain records for future use; and

*Retrieval*—the function that locates a record for future use following patient care for placement in the patient's record.

Fig. 9.5 shows a typical HIM department layout and the locations where these actions might occur for the most efficient workflow. These HIM functions occur sequentially and are typically grouped into sections under a supervisor for efficient management (see Fig. 9.3).

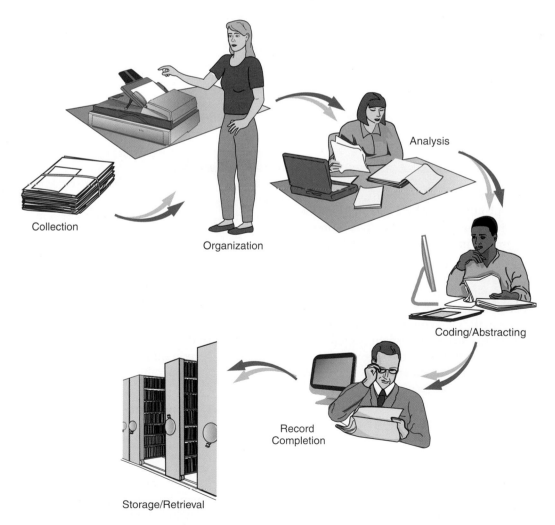

Collection

Organization

Analysis

Coding/Abstracting

Record Completion

Storage/Retrieval

• **Fig. 9.4** Retrospective processing of health information.

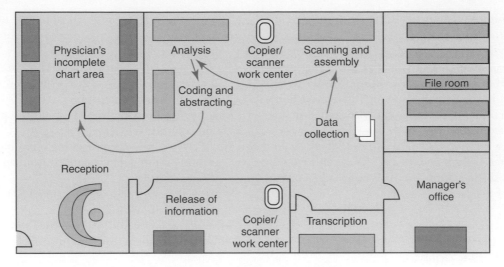

• **Fig. 9.5** The layout and workflow of a typical health information management department.

---

**COMPETENCY CHECK-IN 9.1**

**Organizational Structure**

**Competency Assessment**

1. The _____ is an illustration used to describe the relationships between departments, positions, and functions within an organization.
2. Judy, the physician record clerk in the HIM department, is responsible to Jovan, the supervisor, and Michelle, the director. This violates the _____ principle.
3. Janet is a supervisor responsible for eight coding employees. This statement represents Janet's _____.
4. In a dual governance organizational structure, the _____ heads the medical staff.
5. The order of tasks and functions in the department is called the _____.

---

## Strategic Planning

One of the key responsibilities of the Board of Directors/ Trustees is strategic planning. Strategic planning involves envisioning where the organization will be years from now and setting an organizational course to enable the vision. Strategic planning is an ongoing activity in which the Board reviews organizational outcomes on a regular basis to ensure that strategic goals are on track. The Board will also consider actual and anticipated changes in its community of interest, as well as competition in the marketplace. Strategic planning might involve evaluating whether a hospital should search for a partner organization with which to merge, in order to expand its current market share or enhance existing services. Strategic thinking takes into consideration the aging population of its geographic area or perhaps the influx of retirees in determining how it wants to position or develop its geriatric services. As the strategic plan is developed, the key strategies then become a map to how management will set its operational priorities in order to achieve the strategic goals. The alignment of operational priorities with the strategic plan is a key factor in whether the administration will approve a departmental plan or request for additional resources (see Management Accounting: Budgets in Chapter 6).

• **BOX 9.1    Corporate/Enterprise Strategic Plan Example**

Diamonte prioritizes:
- Patient-focused care in all we do, including price transparency
- Continuous improvement in outcomes through clinical excellence and patient engagement
- Community engagement and support for population health

In order to develop and steer a strategic vision, the Board needs to keep in mind the *mission, vision,* and *values* of the organization. An example strategic plan is shown in Box 9.1.

### Mission, Vision, and Values

A **mission statement** is a declaration of the organization's purpose. A mission statement provides a common purpose, which helps the organization unify, serving its community as a team with a specific direction. The mission statement for Diamonte Hospital (our hypothetical acute care facility) might be: *Diamonte Hospital provides high-quality health care through dedication to the community* *we serve and commitment to excellence.* The mission statement is important for the development of a *culture.* If the employees demonstrate the mission in their actions, it impacts how the organization functions. The development and periodic reevaluation of the mission statement is a strategic planning activity. Input from employees and other stakeholders is taken into consideration in revising the mission.

HIM departments, as well as other departments in the facility, also have a mission. The department mission should align with the mission for the entire facility. The following is the mission statement for the HIM Department of Diamonte Hospital: *The Health Information Management Department of Diamonte Hospital exists to provide timely, complete, accurate health information to authorized users in support of the delivery of high-quality health care to the community.* As with the mission statement for the organization, when the HIM employee actions reflect the HIM mission statement, their purpose is evident to the customers.

While the mission articulates the organization's purpose, a **vision** statement clearly states the organization's expected future. Although the mission is to provide high-quality patient care through dedication and excellence, the vision may be: *Diamonte Hospital will be the highest rated acute care facility in the state, recognized for its customer service, superlative outcomes, and desirable place of employment.* By definition, *vision* conveys an intelligent foresight: that "years down the road" image that the Board envisions. A vision for the HIM department might be: *To be the benchmark for excellence in customer service, compliance, and employee satisfaction,* which supports the organization's vision of being the leading provider in the community.

An organization's **values statement** reflects its commitment to its mission and vision. In general, values statements speak to the culture that the organization strives to achieve or maintain.

Diamonte Hospital Values are as follows:

*These values support our mission and inform our service to the community at every instance.*

*Treat everyone with respect and dignity: patients, their families, and our colleagues.*

*Honor our ethical responsibilities through compliance with our professional standards and exceeding expectations in our interactions with others.*

*Deliver outstanding care to our patients through clinical excellence in evidence-based practice with a judicious eye toward innovation.*

*Adhere to our culture of teamwork and collaboration throughout the organization.*

## Data and Information Governance

Strategies, goals, policies, and procedures that address data and information governance reflect the "tone at the top"—the priority placed by organizational leadership on protecting and managing these important resources. Without leadership priority and support, efforts to manage data and information will be fragmented and ineffective.

**Data governance** is, at the organizational level, the development, implementation, and monitoring of policies and procedures that ensure the quality of the data that are captured and the integrity of that data as they are stored and used across the multiple applications and systems within the organization. Thus the patient's demographic data are captured accurately at the point of registration, appear the same in all systems within the organization that use those data, and cannot be changed without changing them everywhere they appear. Why would it change? Think about billing. A patient submits his or her correct address at the time of service. However, when the organization tries to send the bill to the patient 2 months later, the patient has moved. Data governance policies and procedures are needed to guide patient financial services and patient access staff on how to deal with these new data.

Data governance affects all users in the organization who collect, use, or otherwise impact data. For much of this book, we have been discussing data quality. Data governance, then, creates the organizational structure and policies within which the departmental and functional areas can operate.

Traditionally, HIM professionals have played an important role in developing and maintaining the tools with which all areas collect and maintain data. By leading and participating on medical records committees, they helped develop the various forms on which data were collected and managed the postdischarge completion and retention of the data as paper medical records. In the electronic environment, that role changes as HIM professionals consider not just the data capture but also the access to the captured data and the extent to which individuals can view and amend the data. For example, patient registration staff often enter the admitting diagnosis as a component of the registration process. If, on discharge, the health information coder determines that a significant error has occurred in the capture of the admitting diagnosis (such as "abdominal actinomycosis" instead of "abdominal pain"), should the coder have the ability to make a correction to those data or should the error be referred back to patient access for correction?

The decision regarding what system access to grant is generally based on the role that the individual plays in the organization—typically as defined in the job description. Access to view a system component may be less risky than allowing the ability to enter or alter the data. So, to answer the coding question above, the organization has numerous choices: allow the coder to make the change, require that someone in patient registration make the change, or perhaps need that the change be made by a supervisor in either department. One consideration in choosing one or all of these options is the internal control of correction. If the coder fixes a registration error, there should be a process in place to ensure that registration is alerted so that the registrar can be educated not to make the same mistake again.

Health care providers must handle patient information very carefully. In an EHR environment, failure to have an organization-wide plan to handle information can result in regulatory and legal difficulties, hence the need for information governance. **Information governance** is, at the organizational level, the development, implementation, and monitoring of policies and procedures regarding the use of the organization's data as they are retrieved, analyzed, reported, and transmitted. Information governance is, by its very nature, a strategic responsibility of the governing body and administration rather than a task-oriented function. Organization leadership must understand the nature of, and make decisions about, the life cycle of the information it obtains and retains. This was a significantly simpler task in the days of paper records in which the location of the actual record was closely tracked and transmission of the data it contained was largely via photocopies and sometimes faxes. With the implementation of electronic data capture and the interfacing of multiple complex systems, the touch of a button can create a reportable privacy breach. Thus we can no longer regard privacy, security, and ROI as issues related solely to entities outside the organization. We must also have policies and procedures that address the use of information throughout the organization.

While data governance deals with the capture of data, information governance deals with its use. Think of it as data going into the system and information coming out. You can also think of it as information governance being an all-encompassing umbrella that includes data governance as a component. Either way, organizations must be proactive in ensuring that they control all aspects of the data that are being collected every day in ever-increasing volume.

As with data governance, HIM professionals have played an important role in managing the health information that is released from organizations. As the gatekeepers to the paper records, it was difficult to obtain access to data without our knowledge and cooperation. In the electronic environment, our role becomes not so much gatekeepers but leaders in the development and implementation of the policies and procedures that drive access. Previously we would have denied access to a record by an unauthorized person. Now we develop the policies to grant or deny access to specific parts of the record, define the type of access, and monitor the audit trails of such access to ensure compliance.

## Rolling Out the Strategic Plan

Strategic planning may incorporate feedback from patients, employees, and other stakeholders. However, once the plan is articulated, those goals must be operationalized throughout the organization. As illustrated above, the mission and vision of various departments should mirror that of the organization. So must the departmental goals and objectives mirror the strategic plan. As with the organization, the

department should have a long-term strategy that is driven by the organization's strategic objectives. In other words, if the organization is committed to quality, then the department's goals and objectives should address and support quality. If the organization has a strategic goal of achieving a paperless EHR system within 3 years, the HIM department should not have a strategic goal of obtaining more filing space, but rather of ensuring appropriate computer training for all staff. Similarly, if the organization has strategically decided to accelerate its use of outsourcing to improve workflow, the HIM department should not be asking for space for new employees, but rather should be investigating remote coding and other outsourcing options.

## Operational Planning

Planning is used by organizations to prepare for the future: expansion of the facility, providing new services that require knowledge of regulations and guidelines, and even conversion to an EHR. Some situations require more planning than others, and some plans are more formal and elaborate than others. Implementation of the strategic plan requires attention to the alignment of operations with the organization.

A plan is a guide that describes the way events are expected to take place in the department. For example, the workflow in a department is the result of a plan. Before employees begin performing the functions of assembly, analysis, and coding, HIM managers must plan to ensure optimal productivity.

The HIM department may also plan for changes or improvements. Managers can plan to implement a new procedure, for example, concurrent coding, purging of records, or scanning of paper files into digital images. We mentioned the strategic budget in Chapter 6. That budget is derived from Board-level planning and is passed down to the departments for their budgeting. Planning involves analyzing the current situation, determining the goal, and strategizing to accomplish goals.

## Goals and Objectives

Departments annually set goals to maintain existing levels of performance and to accomplish new or improved functions. **Goals** are statements that provide the department with direction or focus. Goals can reflect different time frames; they can be annual, short term, or long term. Examples of goals for an HIM department are listed in Table 9.2.

To reach a goal, the department sets objectives to direct how the goal will be achieved. **Objectives** specify what must be accomplished. The expectation is that when the action for each objective is implemented, the goal is attained. So, if your goal is to arrive at work on time (95% of the time), your objectives would include rising with the alarm at least 95% of the time and perhaps listening to the traffic report at least half an hour before leaving (at least 95% of the time) in order to plan an alternative route or leave early.

| TABLE 9.2 | Health Information Management Department's Goals and Objectives[a] | |
|---|---|---|
| **Goals** | **Objectives** | |
| 1. Maintain continuous compliance with The Joint Commission (TJC) accreditation standards for timely record completion | 1a The monthly number of delinquent health records will be less than 50% of the average monthly discharge (AMD) | |
| | 1b The number of delinquent history and physical records will not exceed 1% | |
| | 1c The number of delinquent operative reports will not exceed 1% | |
| 2. Transcription services will facilitate compliance with TJC requirement for timeliness of documentation regarding history and physical records, discharge summary records, consults, and operative reports | 2a History and physical records will be transcribed within 6 hours of dictation | |
| | 2b Consultation reports will be transcribed within 12 hours of dictation | |
| | 2c Operative reports will be transcribed within 12 hours of dictation | |
| | 2d Discharge summaries will be transcribed within 24 hours of dictation | |

[a]*Note*: These goals are, for example, only; they are not all inclusive.

If the goal is to pass the Registered Health Information Technician (RHIT) exam the first time, then an objective would be to engage in a pattern of study to support that goal. Importantly, objective statements are measurable so that it is easy to see if the action has been completed or not. Thus if the strategic plan of the organization is to reduce employee turnover by focusing on employee satisfaction, then a departmental goal would be to reduce employee turnover by a specified percentage and a measurable objective might be to conduct employee team meetings weekly to engage staff in collaboration. Table 9.2 also provides some examples of HIM department objectives.

## Policies and Procedures

The policies and procedures of a health care facility are documented so that the employees, customers, accreditation agencies, licensing bodies, regulatory agencies, and legal authorities can identify the philosophy and methods under which the facility operates.

A **policy** is a statement, in broad terms, of what the facility expects to happen on a routine basis. It is a general guideline. For example, a policy might require that bills be dropped within 3 business days of patient discharge. The **procedure** is the process of how the policy is carried out. For example, what specifically has to happen in order to drop a bill: chart completion, coding, and finalization of the abstract? Policies and procedures provide details about the following:

- How, when, and why are things done?
- Who performs which tasks, jobs, and functions?
- Who is responsible for an activity, an authorization, and so forth?
- Quality controls and audits.
- Historic, routine, and emergency situations.
- Volume and timing productivity expectations.

Fig. 9.6 shows an example of the policy: *A health record is maintained for every patient treated in this facility.*

The health care organization has policies and procedures that affect everyone in the facility. Each department in the health care facility should have specific policies and procedures that outline their processes, responsibilities, and services. All employees of the facility must have access to the policy and procedures manual (PPM). Today PPMs are often stored electronically so that all employees have easy access from any computer. The HIM department manual contains policies and procedures that relate specifically to health information. Fig. 9.7 contains a list of contents for an HIM department PPM.

Special consideration for a facility's policies in the digital environment includes securing access to prevent unauthorized people from making changes to policies. It is also important to have a paper copy of the policy statements in case the computer is inaccessible. Since corporate policies are typically authorized by the Board of Directors, an official, signed copy is likely kept in a central location and the organization's document management system.

The HIM department director is responsible for ensuring that the departmental policies and procedures are current. This is accomplished by making sure that policies exist for all necessary functions, responsibilities, and services under his or her control. All policies and procedures should be reviewed annually and as significant changes occur in procedures, regulations, or legislation. Review is as simple as reading through each policy and procedure to verify that the contents are accurate and then initialing and dating the review for authentication.

Inherent in the construction of policies and procedures is the need to ensure that they support corporate compliance with regulations and accreditation standards. For example, there must be a policy that states that records must be completed within the maximum number of days allowed by the accrediting organization (usually 30 days). Organizations that have taken the initiative to reduce the number of days allowed must reflect that tighter standard in all related policies. Similarly, coding quality is a matter

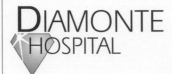

**Effective:**

**Approved:**

Rationale: TJC - IM.02.02.01 The hospital effectively manages the collection of health information; IM.04.01.01 The hospital maintains accurate health information; Standard IM.01.01.01 The hospital plans for managing information. CMS COP - §482.24(b) Standard: Form and Retention of Record: The hospital must maintain a medical record for each inpatient and outpatient. Medical records must be accurately written, promptly completed, properly filed and retained, and accessible. The hospital must use a system of author identification and record maintenance that ensures the integrity of the authentication and protects the security of all record entries.

**Policy:**

Each patient will be identified using a unique medical record number that will be used for all subsequent visits. A unique patient account number will be assigned for each visit. Patients may only have one medical record number.

**Procedure:**

1. Upon registration at Diamonte Hospital for any service, the registrar will search for previous visits to identify an existing medical record number.

2. At the point of registration, the registrar will query the patient for any previous visits or name change in order to ensure that a duplicate number is not assigned.

3. At the point of registration, the registrar will initiate a new visit and unique patient account number associated with the patient's medical record number.

4. If at any time a Diamonte team member becomes aware that a duplicate medical record number or a duplicate patient account number has been assigned, it is the responsibility of that team member to alert Patient Access and Health Information Management so that remediation can take place.

5. Once a week, Health Information Management will run the Duplicate MPI program to identify potential duplicate medical records and remediate any duplicates according to HIM Department Policy No. 8.04, MPI Maintenance.

6. Merging of medical record numbers will always flow from the incorrect duplicate back to the historical number. Variation from this procedure requires administrative approval.

• **Fig. 9.6** Policy and procedure for *MPI* integrity. *MPI*, Master patient index.

of accurate reimbursement, but it is also a regulatory issue in that routing coding errors that result in excessive reimbursement to the hospital may trigger a false claims audit. Therefore policies and procedures that support accurate coding—including supervision, queries, clinical documentation improvement, and routine and targeted audits—should be in place and enforced.

## Customer Satisfaction

Typically, when we think about customer satisfaction in health care, we think about patients. No doubt, patients are our customers in the HIM department, both as requesters and recipients of ROI, and as users of our accurately coded bills. However, the HIM department has many other customers, including the physicians who need to complete their records, the patient financial services department that needs our codes quickly, and the administrators who rely on our data. It behooves us to build into our policies and procedures how we expect to treat our customers, both internal and external. Since the HIM department is not routinely reflected in customer satisfaction surveys, some customized alternative to assess satisfaction may be required to obtain reliable data regarding our success in this area.

| Diamonte Health Information Management Department Policy and Procedure Manual | |
|---|---|
| **Table of Contents** | |
| **Section 1** | **Introduction** |
| 1.01 | Purpose |
| 1.02 | Responsibility for policy development, update, and approval |
| 1.03 | Distribution and access of policies |
| 1.04 | Diamonte mission statement |
| 1.05 | Diamonte organization chart |
| 1.06 | Health information management department mission statement and organization chart |
| **Section 2** | **General Department Policies** |
| 2.01 | Centralized health information management department |
| 2.02 | Scope of service |
| 2.03 | Hours of operation |
| 2.04 | Confidentiality, privacy, and data security considerations |
| 2.05 | Confidentiality statement |
| 2.06 | Department orientation |
| 2.07 | Training and education of department employees |
| 2.08 | Employee competency |
| 2.09 | General policies of the health information management department |
| 2.10 | Health information management department organization chart |
| **Section 3** | **The Health Record** |
| 3.01 | Creation and definition, unit medical record number assignment |
| 3.02 | Ownership of the health record |
| 3.03 | Guidelines for entries into the health record |
| 3.04 | Abbreviations list |
| 3.05 | Fax copies in the health record |
| 3.06 | Completion of discharge summaries |
| **Section 4** | **Assembly and Analysis** |
| 4.01 | Health record assembly and chart order |
| 4.02 | Retrospective record analysis |
| **Section 5** | **Storage, Access, and Security** |
| 5.01 | Health record storage system |
| 5.02 | Security of health information |
| 5.03 | Confidentiality and security of computerized information |
| 5.04 | Retention schedule for health records and related documents |
| 5.05 | Procedure to access health records |
| 5.06 | Health record locations |
| 5.07 | Removal of unprocessed health record components from the health information management department |
| 5.08 | Destruction of records |
| **Section 6** | **Record Completion** |
| 6.01 | Incomplete chart/record completion process |
| 6.02 | Notification of incomplete health records for physicians |
| 6.03 | Suspension process |
| **Section 7** | **Release of Information** |
| 7.01 | General policies for release of information |
| 7.02 | Consent for release of information |
| 7.03 | Notice of recipient of Information, disclosure laws |
| 7.04 | Patient's right to health information, copies of health records |
| 7.05 | Copy and retrieval fees |
| **Section 8** | **Quality of Health Information** |
| 8.01 | Monitoring and evaluation of quality in the health information management department |
| 8.02 | Record review process/clinical pertinence |
| 8.03 | Compliance with regulations and standards |
| 8.04 | MPI Maintenance |
| **Use of Contract Services or Agencies–Business Associate Agreements** | |
| **Job Descriptions** | |
| **Safety in the Health Information Management Department** | |
| Materials Safety Data Sheets (MSDS) | |

• **Fig. 9.7** Table of contents of a health information management department policy and procedures manual.

**Strategic and Organizational Planning**

**Competency Assessment**

1. For the 2021–22 fiscal year, the manager has set a _____ to implement a document imaging system.
2. To reach a desired goal, the department must establish _____, directions for achieving a goal.
3. The purpose of the organization documented in a formal statement is known as the _____.
4. Above and beyond the mission statement, a _____ sets a direction for the organization for the future.
5. The HIM director established the following: "The HIM department delinquency percentage will not exceed 50% of AMD by July 1." This is an example of a(n):
   a. plan
   b. goal
   c. objective
   d. mission
6. In addition, the director stated that the suspension procedure will be performed weekly (as approved in the bylaws). This is an example of a(n):
   a. plan
   b. goal
   c. objective
   d. mission
7. The following is a _____ of Diamonte Hospital, an equal opportunity employer: "All new hires will be drug tested."
8. A process that describes how to comply with a policy is a _____.
9. The policy and procedure manual does not need policies for compliance, since those mandates are already part of the compliance standards.
   a. True
   b. False
10. The HIM department is the only department in the organization that has a policy and procedure manual.
    a. True
    b. False
11. At a minimum, how often should the HIM department manager review and update the policy and procedures manual?
    a. Annually and as needed due to change
    b. Weekly as needed due to change
    c. Quarterly and as needed due to change
    d. Monthly and as needed due to change

## Human Resources

The HR department is responsible for the development and implementation of policies and procedures related to the people who work there. The size and complexity of the department depends on the number of employees in the organization and how some of the functions, such as hiring, are performed. HR ensures that the organization is in compliance with all laws and regulations governing employment.

## Legal Aspects

The impact of labor laws cannot be overemphasized in health care. While we tend to think of health care law in terms of the Health Insurance Portability and Accountability Act (HIPAA) and other patient-centered regulations, the body of law impacting HR is also extensive. It is extremely important that HIM managers and supervisors comply with appropriate and legal hiring practices. Over many years the United States has passed a number of laws pertaining to age, gender, race, religion, and disability that affect hiring practices, outlined in Table 9.3.

Employers are allowed to hold their employees to certain standards; for example, the law allows health care employers to perform a drug screen before making a job offer. An employee working under the influence of certain substances does not have the ability to provide high-quality health care and would expose the employer to liability. Department standards, however, must not contradict the law at any level—local, state, or federal.

### Labor/Employment Laws

The US Equal Opportunity Commission (EEOC) is the federal agency charged with enforcing these laws, which apply not only to discrimination in hiring and firing but also to fair compensation and harassment (EEOC, 2022).

Employers must be certain that their hiring practices do not discriminate among candidates. Additionally, employers must be sure that all employees are managed in an appropriate, law-abiding manner. The Americans with Disabilities Act (ADA), passed into law in 1990, makes it illegal for any employer to discriminate against a person, who is qualified to perform a job, on the basis of his or her disability. Under this legislation, as long as a disabled individual has the necessary background, experience, and skill set and is able to perform the "essential functions" of the job, he or she may not be discriminated against in any employment practice (Guerin, 2019). For this reason, HIM managers must be

TABLE 9.3 **Employment Laws**

| Law | Area of Concern |
|---|---|
| Age Discrimination in Employment Act (1967) | Protects employees between the ages of 40 and 70 years. |
| Americans with Disabilities Act (ADA) (1990) | Outlaws discrimination against disabled people and ensures reasonable accommodation for them in the workplace. |
| Title VII of the Civil Rights Act (1964) | Prohibits discrimination on the basis of race, color, religion, sex, or national origin and ensures equal employment opportunity. |
| The Pregnancy Discrimination Act (1978) | Amended to Title VII, this law makes it illegal to discriminate against a woman because of pregnancy, childbirth, or related medical complications. |
| Fair Labor Standards Act (1938) | Sets minimum wage, overtime pay, equal pay, child labor, and record-keeping requirements for employers (Equal Pay Amendment [1963] forbids sex discrimination in pay practices). |
| Family Medical Leave Act (1993) | Grants unpaid leave and provides job security to employees who must take time off for medical reasons for themselves or family members. |
| Equal Pay Act (EPA) (1963) | Men and women must make the same wage if they perform equal work in the same workplace. Retaliation against a person because the person complained or filed a charge about discrimination is also against the law. |
| Genetic Information Nondiscrimination Act (GINA) (2008) | Makes it illegal to discriminate against employees or applicants on the basis of genetic information, including genetic tests of an individual or his or her family, as well as any disease, disorder, or condition. |

Modified from U.S. Equal Employment Opportunity Commission: *Laws enforced by EEOC.* www.eeoc.gov/laws/statutes/index.cfm. Accessed February 8, 2019.

TABLE 9.4 **Employee Classifications**

| Classification | Common Terms | Description |
|---|---|---|
| Full time | FT | Employee who works 32–40 hours each week or 64–80 hours every 2 weeks, earning full benefits |
| Part time | PT | Employee who typically works less than the minimum full-time hours; frequently less than 20 hours each week, occasionally earning benefits at half of the full-time rate |
| Temporary | Pool, PRN, per diem | Employee scheduled to work as necessary because of an increased workload |

sure to consider this law when writing job descriptions and must include in the description the necessary physical requirements of the job. For example, if an essential function of a job is the ability to move freely throughout the hospital to pick up and deliver documents, this must be stated in the job requirements.

The Fair Labor Standards Act (FLSA) of 1938 addressed the issues of many workers' rights. In addition to the implementation of strict rules surrounding child labor, the FSLA set a national minimum wage, and it guaranteed overtime pay for some jobs. Although the provisions of the FLSA continue to cover most industries in the United States, some jobs are exempt from the rules regarding overtime. A position is generally exempt if the wages are high, wages are paid by a salary (not hourly), and there is some administrative or supervisory role. Specific salary limits and detailed criteria are available on the FLSA website. *Nonexempt* employees are paid according to the number of hours worked and, under the FLSA, must be paid overtime, usually for work beyond

40 hours in any given week, although some states set different guidelines. State guidelines that are different, such as overtime for over 46 hours a week, would only apply to jobs not covered by the FLSA (U.S. Department of Labor, 2022).

## Classification of Employees by Hours Worked

Employees may be classified according to hours worked (full time or part time [PT]) or by position—such as management or staff. Those in management or supervisory positions have responsibility for other employees. Staff employees are responsible for daily tasks and functions, and they report to a supervisor or manager.

As shown in Table 9.4, employee classifications by hours worked are full time, PT, and **per diem** (also known as temporary, PRN [as needed], extra help, or pool). The classification of employees by hours worked is up to the individual companies; there is no federal definition that requires a specific number of hours for such classification. However, there are hour-based rules that affect the employer's responsibility to offer health insurance benefits without incurring an employer-shared benefit payment under the Affordable Care Act (ACA). In general, an employer with over 50 full-time equivalents (FTEs) is required to offer a full-time employee (and the employee's dependents) health insurance benefits as offered by the organization, per minimum essential ACA standards (IRS 2022). Full-time status may be different for health insurance benefits than for other benefits. Full-time status also affects employees' benefits in terms of hours earned in paid time off (PTO), vacation, holiday benefits, and retirement options. For example, an employee who works 40 hours each week is considered a full-time employee, and he or she may earn a specified number of hours of vacation each pay period or year, depending on the organization. Additionally, the organization might match retirement benefits for the full-time employee at a rate higher than that for other classes of employees. It is important to note that the classification of an employee for benefits purposes is independent of the organization's definition of a full-time employee for staffing purposes.

Understanding the staffing complement requires the definition of a standard work week. For example, a company may define a standard work week as being 40 hours in 5 days. That means 8 working hours per day, not including breaks and lunch. If the employer allows two 15-minute breaks and 30 minutes for lunch, then a full-time employee who begins work at 8 a.m. will be expected to work until 5 p.m.: 8 working hours and 1 hour nonworking.

The staffing complement can be expressed not just by the number of employees but also by how many **full-time equivalents (FTEs)** are used. The FTE calculation enables managers to better understand their utilization of HR. FTEs are calculated as the total number of hours worked (allowed or budgeted), divided by the number of standard full-time hours per week (e.g., 40). The resulting number, which may include a fractional employee, helps account for the PT employees. For example: The HIM department is allowed 100 hours each work week for coding. How many FTEs equal 100 hours? The answer is 100 hours divided by 40 hours (per full-time employee) equals 2.5 FTEs; 2.5 FTEs are allowed in the coding department each week. We discuss FTEs in more detail later in the chapter.

A PT employee is one who typically works less than the standard full-time hours (frequently less than 20 hours) per week, thereby earning benefits at half the weekly rate of a full-time employee, if at all. For example, a permanent PT employee may earn 2 hours of vacation, sick leave, or PTO for every 20 hours of work. Temporary or per diem employees rarely earn any type of employee benefit. Per diem employees are scheduled to work as needed in the facility when the amount of work exceeds what the regular employees can accomplish. Temporary workers are commonly used to accommodate unusual work volume and fill in for vacationing staff when the work cannot be absorbed by the remaining staff.

Staffing complements are often described by the number of FTEs. For example, if the organization's normal work week is 40 hours, an employee working 20 hours is one half of an FTE. Similarly, two PT employees working 20 hours per week is equivalent to one employee working 40 hours per week, or one FTE. All of the regularly scheduled hours for the week are added and then divided by the full-time work week hours to arrive at the total number of FTEs for the department.

Example:

| | |
|---|---|
| Sue | 20 hours |
| James | 15 hours |
| Mary | 40 hours |
| Alison | 40 hours |
| *Total hours* | *115 hours* |

In this example, the department staff are scheduled to work 115 hours per week. The full-time work week is 40 hours. Therefore the employee complement is 2.875 FTEs (115 divided by 40).

Some people who work in the HIM department are employed by an agency or company that contractually agrees to perform certain job functions for the HIM department or health care facility. These workers are employed by the agency or company, and not the health care facility. A facility might choose to make this arrangement to acquire specialized help in a particular HIM function such as ROI, transcription, or coding. This type of contractual arrangement is also called **outsourcing**, whereby the work is performed by workers *other than those* employed by the facility. These categories are discussed in more detail later in the chapter.

## Job Analysis and Description

It is important to have the right employee performing the appropriate function at the right time in order to effectively manage the HIM department. **Job analysis** is the review of a specific function to determine all of the tasks or components from the job. When a job analysis is performed, the job tasks are reviewed to ensure that the process works efficiently.

Job analysis can be performed by a supervisor or manager working with the employee; together, they review and perform the employee's job function. As the supervisor works with the employee, he or she is able to determine the procedures performed by the employee. The supervisor must document the procedures as performed by the employee so that they can be reviewed in total. Following this observation, which can take a few hours or even an entire day, the evaluator or supervisor has actual information with which to develop a job description and performance standards. If you have involved the employee in a job analysis, the employee should review the job's functions and responsibilities when the job description is complete.

Another effective way to perform a job analysis is by asking the employee to explain how he or she performs the job. This method employs a data-collection device used by the employee to analyze his or her job. The form shown in Fig. 9.8 is an example of this sort of tool. The employee uses this form to communicate to the manager in detail what the job involves on a daily basis, using his or her own words.

The **job description** is a list of the employee's responsibilities. Each position in the department should have a job description. The job description communicates the expectations of the job to the employee. If an old job description needs to be updated, it is appropriate to give the employee a copy of the job description for review. Allow the employee to review the job description and ask him or her to identify how the job has changed. This involvement gives the

employee an opportunity to clearly communicate to the manager/supervisor how the job is currently being performed. Job descriptions should be reviewed annually by managers and employees. Employees sign the job description to acknowledge their awareness of their responsibilities and job function.

A job description contains several key elements that describe the job specifically. The job description has a heading that briefly describes the position. The heading should include the facility in which the position is located, the title of the position, the supervisor for the position, and the effective date of the job description (Fig. 9.9). The remainder of the job description includes information regarding

Employee: _Tim Tall_
Position: _file clerk_
Hours worked: _8:00AM–4:30PM_

Use this form to communicate your job duties or daily routine. Use the comments section to document any unusual occurrences.

| | Monday | Tuesday | Wednesday | Thursday | Friday |
|---|---|---|---|---|---|
| 7:30AM | | | | | |
| 8:00AM | Locate charts for coders | | | | |
| 8:30AM | | | | | |
| 9:00AM | | | | | |
| 9:30AM | | | | | |
| 10:00AM | | | | | |
| 10:30AM | Organize files | | | | |
| 11:00AM | File | | | | |
| 11:30AM | | | | | |
| 12:00noon | | | | | |
| 12:30PM | | | | | |
| 1:00PM | | | | | |
| 1:30PM | | | | | |
| 2:00PM | | | | | |
| 2:30PM | | | | | |
| 3:00PM | | | | | |
| 3:30PM | | | | | |
| 4:00PM | | | | | |
| 4:30PM | | | | | |
| 5:00PM | | | | | |

Comments: _Periodically answer phone calls and bring charts to the floor._

• **Fig. 9.8** Job analysis tool.

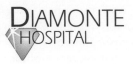

**JOB DESCRIPTION**

**Health Information Management Department**
**Position Title:** Birth Certificate Clerk

| | |
|---|---|
| **Position #:** 070530 | **Grade:** G2 |
| **Reports to:** HIM Manager | **Effective:** 01/15/20XX |

Position Description: Under the general supervision of the HIM Manager, the Birth Certificate Clerk completes a birth certificate, and supporting forms as necessary, for each baby born at Diamonte Hospital. The birth certificates are electronically submitted to the Office of Vital Records, and original certificates with signatures are mailed to the Office of Vital Records in a timely manner. The clerk must maintain a current knowledge of the rules regarding birth certificates. The Birth Certificate Clerk is a member of the Health Information Management department team and maintains knowledge of various other functions in the department to assist as necessary.

**Position Qualifications:**

*Education:*                                          High school diploma

*Licensure/Certification/Registration:* None necessary

*Experience:*                                        Excellent communication skills. Ability to type 30 WPM. Previous clerical experience preferred. Ability to function in busy office environment with multiple shifting and evolving priorities.

**Responsibilities:**

1. Monitors Labor and Delivery log and Admission reports to identify all patients requiring a birth certificate.

2. Collects birth certificate information from parent(s) and completes birth certificate accurately. Parent(s) review birth certificate to verify accuracy and sign in appropriate areas.

3. Maintains current knowledge of all birth certificate rules, regulations, and issues. Reviews and implements state laws governing completion of birth certificates.

4. Ensures completion of other forms relating to the birth as necessary (e.g., paternity, social security verification).

5. Maintains current and accurate birth certificate log.

6. Contacts any parents who have left the hospital prior to completion of the birth certificate. Processes new, delayed, or corrected birth certificates.

7. Obtains physician's signature on the birth certificate within 1 week of completion.

8. Submits electronic birth certificates immediately following completion, mailing completed original certificate within 15 days of completion.

9. Maintains electronic birth certificate software in working condition; performs backups regularly.

10. Follows established policies and procedures regarding confidentiality and security of health information, infection control, safety and security management, and emergency preparedness.

• **Fig. 9.9** Job description for an HIM department position. *HIM*, Health information management; *WPM*, words per minute.

hours worked, the purpose of the job, its responsibilities, and skills required. It also includes a description of the physical demands of the environment in which the work is performed and the basic physical requirements of the position. It is important to list only physical requirements that are essential to the performance of the job, in accordance with the stipulations of the ADA requirements. The job description also contains any numbers, grades, and classification (exempt or nonexempt) used by the HR department or the organization to describe that position.

## Recruitment and Retention

Certain jobs in the HIM departments are staffed by credentialed employees. For example, the director of the HIM department must hold a current RHIT (Registered Health Information Technician) or Registered Health Information Administrator (RHIA) credential. Coding positions may require the Certified Coding Specialist (CCS), Certified Coding Specialist-Physician (CCS-P), or Certified Coding Associate (CCA). At the very core, HIM-credentialed

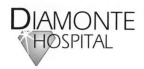

**JOB DESCRIPTION, continued**

**Health Information Management Department**
**Position Title:** Birth Certificate Clerk

| **Position #:** 070530 | **Grade:** G2 |
|---|---|
| **Reports to:** HIM Manager | **Effective:** 01/15/20XX |

11. Displays a positive and courteous manner toward patients, visitors, customers, and co-workers.

12. Follows all policies and procedures of the facility and HIM department.

13. Completes annual employee in-service and required department training.

**Physical Requirements:**

| | |
|---|---|
| ***Mental and emotional requirements:*** | Employee must be able to manage stress appropriately, work independently, handle multiple priorities. |
| ***Working conditions:*** | Employee spends approximately 90% of time inside the health care facility. The work area has adequate lighting, good ventilation, comfortable temperature. Employee work station provided with appropriate access to rest rooms and lunch and break areas. |
| ***Physical demands:*** | Employee is responsible for light work—lifting maximum of 20 lb, with frequent lifting or carrying of objects weighing up to 10 lb. Work positions include sitting 50%, standing 20%, walking 20%, lifting/carrying 10%. |

**Example only**

• **Fig. 9.9** *(Continued)*

employees must adhere to the American Health Information Management Association (AHIMA) code of ethics in handling HIM procedures and health information. Hiring credentialed employees is one way to ensure that the fundamental tenets of HIM are a part of the employees' background. It is important to note that the topics discussed may vary by state, region, and employee association. Department managers should be very careful to understand the labor rules and regulations associated with the employees in their department. When in doubt, one should consult the facility's HR department.

## The Hiring Process

Hiring of new employees is a key HR department activity. Department managers play varying roles in this activity, depending on the needs of the organization. There are multiple steps in the process, starting with the request to hire. Again, the complexity of the process varies among organizations and the absence of a particular step is not necessarily a problem.

Retention is the rate at which staffing of positions does not change over a time period. High turnover rate—the rates at which positions are replaced during a time period and can be a sign of widespread problems that need to be addressed. There are many reasons that employees leave an organization. A spouse moving and retirement are two reasons over which the organization has no control. Other reasons, however, are a matter of concern. As you may have gleaned from the discussion thus far, it can be costly and time consuming to hire and train a new employee. Common reasons for employee resignations are: career advancement, increase in pay, change in career, and dissatisfaction with their job or the company. Since individuals are motivated by different issues, keeping an eye on the trends for these reasons rather than focusing on individuals is a good way to identify systemic problems. The hiring process can be an excellent safeguard against high employee turnover. Finding a person with the right skill set who is also a good fit for the organization is key.

When a department manager identifies the need for a new employee, whether creating a new position or replacing departing staff, approval is needed. The hiring of a new employee is both an operational concern and a budgetary issue, so the justification for the position is formally made. The organization may have a specific form for this process and the manager may be required to specifically identify the benefits of filling the position and the problems that will occur if the position is not filled. Depending on the level of employee requested (staff, management, and executive), the approval may be required at several levels up to the CEO and Board of Directors/Trustees. Once approval is received, the recruiting process can begin.

Recruiting involves disseminating information about the position to likely candidates. This may include advertising, networking, and internal notices.

To locate potential candidates for a job, the organization must let others know that the position is open. An open position can be publicized in a number of ways, such as by placement of an advertisement on the organization's employment website, on popular recruiting websites, and in local newspapers, professional journals, and community and association newsletters.

The right advertisement should include all of the qualifications that a candidate should possess. The advertisement must specify how much education is required (e.g., college degree, high school degree, or equivalent) along with specific training or credentials (e.g., training in anatomy and physiology, medical terminology, or transcription). The advertisement should also specify (1) the amount of prior experience that a candidate should have, (2) whether the experience needed is specific to a job function or generally

related to the HIM field, and (3) the means by which candidates should apply for the position (e.g., by sending a résumé by fax or email or applying in person to the HR department) (Fig. 9.10). Other information about the position that may be included in the advertisement pertains to employment status: full time or PT, the hours worked per week, responsibilities, benefits, and pay scale. Interested candidates should follow the instructions in the advertisement to apply for the position.

One strategy for filling positions is to hire from within: identifying an employee of the organization who may be a good fit for a new position or even a promotion. Many

◆ **NOTE**

Many HIM positions are advertised by word of mouth. Participation in local HIM associations can put you in touch with large numbers of professionals who are potential candidates for open positions in the department. This activity is often called *networking*-getting to know other HIM professionals and sharing information, knowledge, and strategies as appropriate.

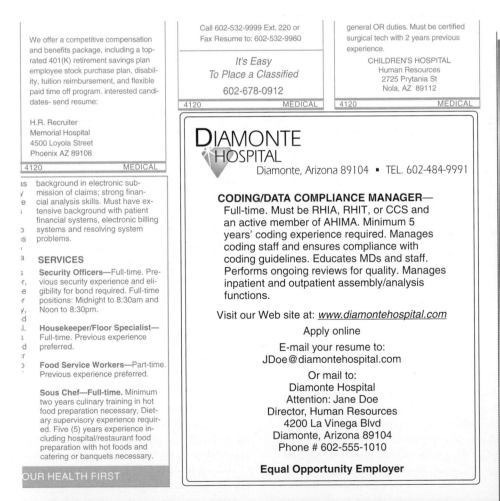

We offer a competitive compensation and benefits package, including a top-rated 401(K) retirement savings plan employee stock purchase plan, disability, tuition reimbursement, and flexible paid time off program. interested candidates- send resume:

H.R. Recruiter
Memorial Hospital
4500 Loyola Street
Phoenix AZ 89108

4120                                    MEDICAL

Call 602-532-9999 Ext. 220 or
Fax Resume to: 602-532-9980

*It's Easy*
*To Place a Classified*
602-678-0912

4120                              MEDICAL

general OR duties. Must be certified surgical tech with 2 years previous experience.

CHILDREN'S HOSPITAL
Human Resources
2725 Prytania St
Nola, AZ  89112

4120                              MEDICAL

ıs    background in electronic sub-
y     mission of claims; strong finan-
e     cial analysis skills. Must have ex-
;     tensive background with patient
      financial systems, electronic billing
ɔ     systems and resolving system
ıs    problems.

a     **SERVICES**

;     **Security Officers**—Full-time. Pre-
ır,   vious security experience and eli-
e     gibility for bond required. Full-time
ır    positions: Midnight to 8:30am and
y,    Noon to 8:30pm.
d
ıl.   **Housekeeper/Floor Specialist**—
;     Full-time. Previous experience
d     preferred.
ır
ɔ     **Food Service Workers**—Part-time.
.     Previous experience preferred.

      **Sous Chef—Full-time.** Minimum
      two years culinary training in hot
      food preparation necessary, Diet-
      ary supervisory experience requir-
      ed. Five (5) years experience in-
      cluding hospital/restaurant food
      preparation with hot foods and
      catering or banquets necessary.

OUR HEALTH FIRST

**D**IAMONTE
**H**OSPITAL
Diamonte, Arizona 89104  ▪  TEL. 602-484-9991

**CODING/DATA COMPLIANCE MANAGER**—
Full-time. Must be RHIA, RHIT, or CCS and an active member of AHIMA. Minimum 5 years' coding experience required. Manages coding staff and ensures compliance with coding guidelines. Educates MDs and staff. Performs ongoing reviews for quality. Manages inpatient and outpatient assembly/analysis functions.

Visit our Web site at: *www.diamontehospital.com*

Apply online

E-mail your resume to:
JDoe@diamontehospital.com

Or mail to:
Diamonte Hospital
Attention: Jane Doe
Director, Human Resources
4200 La Vinega Blvd
Diamonte, Arizona 89104
Phone # 602-555-1010

**Equal Opportunity Employer**

• **Fig. 9.10** Newspaper advertisement for health information management personnel. *AHIMA,* American Health Information Management Association; *CCS,* Certified Coding Specialist; *MDs,* medical doctors; *RHIA,* Registered Health Information Administrator; *RHIT,* Registered Health Information Technician.

organizations require the posting of a position internally for a specified period, such as 2 weeks, prior to advertising externally. This option promotes a positive environment in which good performance, productivity, and work ethic can result in advancement within the organization. Identification of a suitable internal candidate may halt further recruitment activities until the internal candidate is either hired or not.

External advertising for a position is typically controlled by the HR department to ensure that appropriate language is used, including the accurate description of the position and instructions for applying.

Screening of candidates may be performed by the HR department or delegated to the manager. If the HR department performs the screening, it will typically exclude any candidates whose résumé does not exactly conform to the stated requirements of the position in its official description that is on file in the HR department. So, if a position requires an RHIT credential, any candidate who does not list that credential will be rejected. The HIM department manager, on the other hand, may be more likely to consider a candidate who has significant related experience and is nearing graduation from an HIM program.

Typically, candidates must complete an application for employment to be considered for a position. Today most applications are completed on a website and submitted to the hiring authority electronically. All applicants must provide accurate and complete information on the application. Depending on the organization's policies and procedures, applications may be screened electronically or by a human HR person or department manager. Increasingly, electronic applications are the norm and candidates who do not exactly fit the criteria may be automatically rejected. This can be frustrating for both the applicants and the department manager. As a manager, it is important to ensure that the job requirements are accurately listed with HR before the position is posted. Qualifications include the type of education, training, and experience required to perform the job duties. Modification of an "RHIA or RHIT required" statement may include a phrase like "RHIT eligible" if the manager is willing to consider an HIM program graduate who has not passed the exam yet.

Those job applicants who are screened but not interviewed, at a minimum, should receive some correspondence letting them know how their applications will be handled. Again, the electronic application may result in an electronic rejection in the form of an email. Typically, these emails do not contain the rationale for rejection.

The manager uses the applications to determine which candidates meet the minimum qualifications for the job to receive an interview. An applicant should expect that inconsistent, vague, or incomplete information on any part of the application may require further explanation during the interview. Therefore, when reviewing applications, the hiring authority looks to see that each question on the application is answered. The candidate should not leave any spaces blank, even if he or she believes that the information is covered on the résumé and attached to the application.

Inconsistencies on an application are a warning to the manager that the candidate is not honest. Electronic applications must be completed carefully. Be sure to complete each portion or field in the application accurately. Read all of the instructions carefully before finishing the application and hitting the submit button. Electronic applications typically offer the opportunity to attach a copy of your résumé, letters of reference, and other transcripts, certificates, or supporting documents. It is a best practice to convert documents into a pdf file so that they can be opened by the hiring personnel for review so they can read the documents regardless of the software suite they use. However, some applications require all the information typed directly into the form.

References should be current and appropriate, because employers will check the references before making a final hiring decision. Best practice as an applicant is to confirm permission from the references used. Use of a reference without permission or without preauthorization after prolonged lack of contact may result in no response from the reference when they are contacted. It is also a good idea to let the references know who will be contacting them and what position is being sought. On a practical note, staying in touch with key references is an important networking activity that makes job searching a little less stressful.

## Interviewing

The interview is typically a face-to-face meeting between the applicant and the organization's representative. Each organization has a specific process for performing an interview. Sometimes, the applicant is interviewed over the phone or with the HR department before meeting with the HIM department manager. Other organizations perform a group interview, in which the applicant meets with several different members of the organization at the same time. For the applicant, the interview is an opportunity to learn about the organization and the responsibilities of the position. For the organization, the interview is a way to assess the candidate's qualifications for the position. Interviews may be very formal and structured, informal, or somewhere in between. The interviewer should plan ahead, determine an appropriate location, decide on the style, and write down the questions he or she wants to ask.

All interviews begin with a greeting between the candidate and the interviewer. Experienced interviewers can tell a lot about a candidate within these first few moments. Therefore the interviewer must be prepared and must pay close attention to the responses given by the interviewee.

During the interview in the HIM department, the manager describes the position to the candidate, explaining the expectations, requirements, environment, and philosophy of the organization or management style. The manager also asks questions to obtain further information about the candidate's qualifications. This exchange gives the candidate and the manager more information with which to develop an opinion about the candidate's suitability for the position. The interview is the opportunity to find out whether the candidate is appropriate for the job and a good fit for the department. Box 9.2 provides a list of the questions often asked during an interview. The same questions are used for each person interviewed for the position.

• BOX 9.2 **Interview Questions**

- Tell me a little bit about yourself.
- Describe your last job. What did you like or dislike about the job?
- What expectations do you have for your supervisor?
- Describe your relationship with your former supervisor.
- Explain a stressful situation and how you handled it.
- What is the one word that best describes you? Which of your strengths best suit you for this job?
- Which of your weaknesses may cause a problem for you in this job?
- Do you have any future education goals?
- Where do you see yourself in 5 or 10 years?
- Are you available to work weekends, evenings, or some holidays?

In the United States, a series of federal laws enacted since the 1960s govern job discrimination (Table 9.4). Known collectively as *Equal Employment Opportunity laws*, they prohibit employment discrimination based on age, gender, race, color, religious beliefs, nation of origin, disabilities, genetics, and plans to marry or have children. Interviewers must consider carefully whether their inquiry is relevant to the applicant's capacity to perform the job. Table 9.5 lists some questions that may be discriminatory. The goal of the interview is to determine the applicant's qualifications for the position. Interviewers must avoid any inquiry that may be discriminatory. Table 9.5 lists common examples, but it is not comprehensive. Consult the organization's HR department for guidance on the interview process. Fair employment practices are discussed in more detail later.

### Assessment

Although the questions asked in an interview are necessary and inform a manager about a candidate's ability and

TABLE 9.5    **Interview Guidelines**

| Category | May Ask | May be Discriminatory by Asking |
|---|---|---|
| Gender and family | Whether applicant has relatives who work for the health care facility | Gender of applicant<br>Number of children/childcare arrangements<br>Marital status/living situation<br>Spouse's name or occupation<br>Plans to have children<br>Any question that could determine gender or family status |
| Race | – | Applicant's race or color of skin, hair, or eyes<br>Request for a photo before hire |
| National origin or ancestry | Whether applicant can be legally employed in the United States<br>Ability to speak/write English (if job related)<br>Other languages spoken (if job related) | Nationality/ethnicity of name<br>Birthplace or birthplace of applicant's parents<br>Nationality<br>Nationality of spouse<br>Country of citizenship<br>Applicant's native language/English proficiency<br>Maiden name |
| Religion | – | Religious affiliation/church or services the applicant attends<br>Religious holidays observed |
| Age | Whether applicant is over age 18 years<br>Whether applicant is over age 21 years if job related | Date of birth<br>Date of graduation<br>Age<br>Length of time until applicant plans to retire |
| Disability | Whether applicant can perform the essential job-related functions | Any question about an applicant's mental or physical disability, including its nature or severity<br>Whether applicant has ever filed a workers' compensation claim<br>Current, recent, or past diseases, treatments, or surgeries |
| Other | Academic, vocational, or professional schooling<br>Training received in the military<br>Membership in any trade or professional association<br>Job references | Numbers and kinds of arrests<br>Height or weight<br>Veteran status, discharge status, branch of service |

*Note*: The physical requirements essential to the performance of the position are included in the job description. The Americans with Disabilities Act requires employers to make reasonable accommodations to qualified individuals with disabilities, unless those accommodations cause undue hardship to the employer. Refer to http://www.eeoc.gov/policy/docs/accommodation.html#reasonable for more information.

knowledge, it is often necessary to test the candidate's skills. The interviewer must determine whether the candidate is competent to perform the job. For example, if the manager wants to hire a skilled coder, he or she should give an assessment to each candidate that resembles actual coding work to determine whether the candidate is capable of performing the work required for this job. Health care workers are also required to pass a criminal background check and drug tests before being formally offered a position with the organization.

There are at least two different types of applicant assessments—one for skills and the other for aptitude. A skills assessment is designed to identify the applicant's ability to perform the job. The aptitude assessment evaluates the applicant's inclination, intelligence, or appropriateness for a position and the likelihood of his or her fitting into a particular organization or position. The assessment is typically a test given during the interview. Some tests are lengthy. Skills assessments should include activities that the applicant would encounter on the job; for instance, if the position is for outpatient coding, have the applicant code some of the emergency room or outpatient records. It is not a fair practice to assess an applicant with a test that is different from the actual work that he or she will be expected to perform.

HIM managers should always test the coding skills of an applicant for a coding position and test the keyboarding/typing and terminology skills for a transcription position. There are different screening practices for clerical positions, such as testing filing skills for a file clerk.

## Performance Standards

Managers can use the information they gathered in job analysis to set **performance standards**. Performance standards determine how much work should be accomplished within a specific time frame. Additionally, performance standards let the employee know that quality (percentage of accuracy) is required for this position. Supervisors can use these standards to evaluate employee performance.

Performance standards are drawn from the job description and job analysis. Table 9.6 provides examples of performance standards for various job descriptions for the HIM department birth certificate clerk. These performance standards establish a time frame in which the employee's work is to be completed and include a scale that explains how each score is achieved. The birth certificate clerk is responsible for completing a birth certificate for all newborn admissions according to the facility's policy and state law. Performance

**TABLE 9.6 Performance Standards[a]**

| Employee/Position | Standard | Performance Rating Scale |
|---|---|---|
| Coder | All health records will be coded within 48–72 hours of patient discharge | Exceeds expectations: 36 or more records coded daily<br>Meets expectations: 28–35 records coded daily<br>Does not meet expectations: Fewer than 28 records coded daily<br>*Supervisor uses daily productivity reports to average the coder's performance* |
| Coder | Health records will be assigned appropriate and accurate codes according to applicable coding guidelines | Exceeds expectations: 96%–100% of records reviewed coded appropriately and accurately<br>Meets expectations: 90%–95% of records reviewed coded appropriately and accurately<br>Does not meet expectations: Less than 90% of records reviewed coded appropriately and accurately<br>*Supervisor will review a representative sample of the coder's work to ensure appropriateness and accuracy of coding* |
| Assembly/analysis clerk | All patient health records will be assembled and analyzed within 24 hours of patient discharge | Exceeds expectations: 95%–100% of all records assembled and analyzed within 24 hours of patient discharge<br>Meets expectations: 85%–95% or all records assembled and analyzed within 24 hours of patient discharge<br>Does not meet expectations: Less than 85% of all records assembled and analyzed within 24 hours of patient discharge<br>*Supervisor will routinely assess and document the clerks' productivity to determine score* |
| File clerk | Accurate filing of all patient health records will be completed daily | Exceeds expectations: 100% of all health records filed accurately on a daily basis<br>Meets expectations: 96%–99% of all health records filed accurately on a daily basis<br>Does not meet expectations: Less than 96% of all health records filed accurately on a daily basis<br>*Supervisor will perform routine checks of filing area to determine accuracy; results will be documented to determine file clerk's score* |

[a]*Note:* These standards vary in each facility.

standards for this requirement might be stated as follows: "A birth certificate is completed on all newborn admissions according to facility policy and state law prior to the newborn's discharge. If at any time a birth certificate is not completed before the newborn is discharged, the employee has not met the standard, thereby affecting the employee's performance rating."

Employee performance affects the productivity of the entire department. Therefore the standards are developed specifically for each position to ensure that each employee's performance promotes effective and efficient progress in the HIM department.

## Workload

Each department must have a method for completing its workload. The amount of work in the HIM department is determined by the number of discharges, by the type (e.g., outpatient, inpatient, and rehab), and by length of stay (LOS). The number of patients discharged each day will be equal to the number of records that must be processed. The patient type (e.g., inpatient, outpatient, rehab, and psych) determines the extent of the processing. For instance, ambulatory/outpatient records are very brief and are relatively easy and thus quick to process. Ambulatory surgery records require less time to review than inpatient stays. Likewise, the LOS for patients who have been discharged affects the length of time that it will take to process (and code) the patients' charts. A patient with a long LOS may have generated more material to be scanned and the record itself will likely take longer to review and code.

Supervisors may use time studies to determine the appropriate number of employees for the workload. A time study can be accomplished by monitoring the employee(s) performing the function and the time that it takes to complete each task. This helps the supervisor identify how much work can be done by one employee in a specific period. It also determines the percentage of accuracy with which the work should be completed. If the supervisor is actually present while the employee performs the job, the employee may become nervous or irritated. Likewise, a supervisor does not want to waste valuable time watching employees work. Other methods exist to capture this information without physically watching employees. Employees can fill out forms to indicate their performance, productivity, and time (Fig. 9.11). In an electronic system or with document conversion, data may be available from the system through reporting.

The standards set for the department must comply with organizational, professional, licensing, and regulatory requirements. These standards determine when many of the functions must be performed (e.g., scanning/assembly and analysis within 24 hours of discharge and coding within 48 hours of discharge; Table 9.7). Some internal standards may lead the way for new processes, such as concurrent analysis or coding, to successfully accomplish department functions within the set time frame.

The standards, along with the amount and type of work, dictate the operating hours of the HIM department and the scheduling of the employee(s) work hours. Some departments in large health care facilities are open 24 hours a day, 7 days a week. Other departments have limited hours (Monday through Friday 7 a.m.–9 p.m. and PT on weekends) and use cross-trained staff (i.e., nursing) to cover emergency issues when the department is closed (see Table 9.1).

**Coder:** ____________________ **Month/year:** ____________________

| | M | Tu | W | Th | F | M | Tu | W | Th | F | M | Tu | W | Th | F | M | Tu | W | Th | F |
|---|---|---|---|---|---|---|---|---|---|---|---|---|---|---|---|---|---|---|---|---|
| Date | | | | | | | | | | | | | | | | | | | | |
| Inpatient | | | | | | | | | | | | | | | | | | | | |
| Medicare | | | | | | | | | | | | | | | | | | | | |
| Non-Medicare | | | | | | | | | | | | | | | | | | | | |
| Outpatient | | | | | | | | | | | | | | | | | | | | |
| Observation/surgeries | | | | | | | | | | | | | | | | | | | | |
| Diagnostics | | | | | | | | | | | | | | | | | | | | |
| Emergency department | | | | | | | | | | | | | | | | | | | | |
| | | | | | | | | | | | | | | | | | | | | |
| Hours worked | | | | | | | | | | | | | | | | | | | | |
| Physician contacts | | | | | | | | | | | | | | | | | | | | |
| Other (please comment below) | | | | | | | | | | | | | | | | | | | | |

Comments:

• **Fig. 9.11** Coding productivity sheet.

| TABLE 9.7 | Typical Health Information Management Department Standards[a] | |
|---|---|---|
| **Department's Function** | **Standard** | |
| Assembly and analysis scanning | Completed within 24 hours of patient discharge | |
| Coding and abstracting | Completed within 48–72 hours of patient discharge | |
| Record completion | Completed within 30 days of discharge | |
| Filing | Completed daily | |
| Release of information | Completed within 48–72 hours of receipt of an appropriate authorization or request for information | |
| Transcription: | | |
| History and physical | Transcribed within 4 hours of dictation | |
| Consults | Transcribed within 12 hours of dictation | |
| Operative reports | Transcribed within 6 hours of dictation | |
| Discharge summary | Transcribed within 24 hours of dictation | |

[a]*Note*: These standards are, for example, only; standards in health information management departments may vary.

Workload is also affected by the amount of computerization in the HIM department. In some instances, technology reduces the complexity of a function, making it easier to complete HIM processes in a timely manner, and at other times it increases the steps in the process to complete a function. For example, in a hybrid record, the time needed to process a record for scanning and indexing can add complexity to the process formerly called *assembly and analysis*. On the other hand, computer-assisted coding may reduce the amount of time it takes to code a record.

## Workflow and Process Monitors

Once workload measures have been established, it is important to ensure that processing is maintained at an appropriate level. For example, if the workload standard is 20 inpatient charts per day but the coder is processing only 15, it is important that this variance (the difference between expected and actual performance) be identified and remedied quickly. Similarly, if the expected discharges per week are 300 and they spike to 325, additional resources must be allocated to the various tasks.

In a paper-based environment, HIM department workflow was relatively easy to manage by walking around. The supervisor could see the pile of charts or stuffed shelves and instantly know the status of the workflow. In a largely electronic environment, computer-based workflow software can generate queues for distributing work automatically to employees based on predetermined algorithms. It can also develop reports to inform the supervisor of the progress in any given area. We thus become more reliant on the software to let us know when something has gone awry. Nevertheless, it still rests with the supervisor to take action when an anomaly is identified.

In order to effectively monitor workflow and process, key performance indicators should be established. The dollar value and number of records in the Discharged, No Final Bill (DNFB) report, for example, are key performance indicators as to the timeliness of the discharged record process—particularly the finalizing of charges and coding. While an appropriate expectation as to the size of the DNFB is generally communicated by administration, the HIM department should examine this report closely to ensure that there is not a lag in coding that is being masked by a low number of discharges. The DNFB should always be viewed in the context of the volume of discharges. Similarly, the number of requests for ROI and the number and age of outstanding requests should be monitored to ensure that productivity remains at an appropriate level.

In the event of variances in productivity, the supervisor may need to take action in the form of requesting additional staffing, calling up per diems, or even sending staff home. One of the major advantages of maintaining per diem staff is the flexibility of the organization to staff up or down in the face of volume increases or decreases. It is also extremely beneficial to cross-train staff to perform work other than their regularly assigned tasks. This helps with vacation and sick time coverage, as well as volume needs.

## Evaluating Productivity

**Productivity** is the amount of work produced by an employee in a given time frame. There are several ways to collect information on the employee's performance and productivity: manually, by observation, or by using computerized reports from computer applications. The goal is to have an objective tool that reflects the amount of work performed by the employee. Later, the accuracy and quality of the employee's work can be assessed by sample review of his or her work.

### Manual Productivity Reports

Manual productivity reports can be designed to obtain information about the employee's performance. Fig. 9.11 gives a sample form for collection of data on the productivity of a coding employee.

This form contains information to identify the employee, the time frame in which the information is collected, and specifics about the employee's job. Because the employee in our example is responsible for inpatient coding, the form shown in Fig. 9.11 collects information about the number of records coded each day. In addition, the form collects information about activities related to the employee's job, including conversations with physicians, problems with chart documentation, and other activities as they occur.

This form can be developed by reviewing the job description and creating categories for each responsibility. The employee uses the form to collect statistics regarding his or her job performance. The completed form is turned in to the supervisor. The supervisor is then able to review the employee's productivity against the job's performance standards. This information, collected on a regular basis, provides a picture of the employee's job performance for the entire review period, discussed later in the chapter. Routine collection of this information over time provides a larger picture of the employee's performance so that the evaluation is not skewed in one direction toward his or her performance over a limited time period.

### Computerized Productivity Reports

Some of the functions in the HIM department are performed in a computer system that produces a productivity report. The report is maintained by the computer system as the employee logs onto the system and completes job tasks. Some electronic reports not only tell the supervisor how much work is performed but also indicate the time frame in which the work was done. With regard to our coding example, coders are often expected to code a specific number of records within an hourly time frame (i.e., six to eight charts per hour). The software system used by the coders keeps track of productivity without additional effort from the coder. Fig. 9.12 illustrates this type of productivity report.

### *Productivity Calculations*

All staff are typically held to some sort of performance standard. In coding, for example, the number of charts completed per day is a common standard. In transcription, it might be the number of words, lines, or even characters. This sort of volume productivity standard can be common across all staff in the same role or may be scaled by the rank of the employee. For example, a beginning Coder I may

be expected to complete 8 inpatient charts per day, but a more experienced Coder II may be expected to complete 12. Volume productivity standards may also be tied to the type of work. So, a Coder I may be expected to complete 8 inpatient records or 20 ambulatory surgery or 80 emergency department (ED) records in a day.

Volume productivity is relatively easy to track, even manually. A transcriptionist listens to a digital recording of the physician's report. As she listens, she types. Every measurable unit of productivity (character, word, and line) is identified and tallied by the software. The sum of the productivity is used for employee evaluation and billing to the client. In coding, the employee can count how many charts are done in a day and report it manually. More usefully, the coding software can produce a report that shows what charts were completed by which coders. More sophisticated volume productivity calculations can be performed using such software by incorporating factors such as the patient LOS or type of procedure.

Quality is a component of productivity requirements. A coder making an error in the assignment of the principal diagnosis will likely affect reimbursement. A transcription error may affect patient care. A scanner who misses a page affects the user of the record. Therefore quality control standards are applied to the work and quality assurance activities ensure that the standards are being met. The calculation of a number that represents the quality of the work can be controversial. In transcription, the number of errors is calculated against the total amount of work. For example, 2 errors per 1000 words (2/1000 is the same as 0.2%). Unless the employer wants to rate errors by type (grammar, spelling, or the wrong body part), transcription error rates are relatively easy to calculate. Code errors are more difficult. An incorrect fifth digit on a secondary code describing a patient's inguinal hernia (i.e., recurrent or not) when the patient was admitted for a myocardial infarction is clearly not as problematic as assigning chest pain as the principal diagnosis on that record. Therefore coding errors are often categorized

| Coder | IP Total | IP Mcare | IP Non-Mcare | OP Total | ER | OP Refer | OBS | SDS |
|---|---|---|---|---|---|---|---|---|
| JBG | 22 | 20 | 2 | 40 | 0 | 40 | 0 | 0 |
| CRB | 15 | 15 | 0 | 55 | 48 | 0 | 7 | 0 |
| TLM | 30 | 25 | 5 | 12 | 0 | 0 | 0 | 12 |
| SNK | 32 | 20 | 12 | 5 | 0 | 0 | 0 | 5 |

**Coding Productivity Report** 02/20/20XX

• **Fig. 9.12** Productivity report of coders in a health information management department.

by severity when an audit is performed; for example, wrong principal diagnosis, wrong diagnosis-related group, wrong code, and missing code. Furthermore, the volume of errors is often expressed in multiple ways: number and percentage of records with errors and number and percentage of code errors among all codes assigned. Consider an audit of 20 records, each coded by Coder A and Coder B. Here are the results:

|  | Number of Records Reviewed | Records with Errors | Number of Codes Assigned | Code Errors |
|---|---|---|---|---|
| Coder A | 20 | 15 (75%) | 230 | 15 (7%) |
| Coder B | 20 | 5 (25%) | 100 | 15 (15%) |

In this simple example, it appears by the number of records with error that Coder A has a much higher error rate than Coder B. However, looking at the number of codes assigned, Coder A achieved a 93% accuracy rate based on the number of codes assigned. Coder B is at 85%. Depending on the type of error, the supervisor might recommend that Coder A slow down a bit, but Coder B would likely have to be monitored closely and possibly undergo some remedial training. So, it is confusing to say that coders are expected to achieve in excess of 95% accuracy without specifying the numerator and denominator of the calculation. This same quality issue arises in scanning.

## Employee Evaluations

Employee evaluations allow management to provide feedback to the employee on the basis of the employee's job performance. Feedback is an important aspect of a manager's communication with employees. The evaluation entails one-on-one communication from the manager about an employee's job performance. Performance standards, measures of productivity, and the job description are used as a rubric to perform the employee rating. This rating of the employee's performance is called an *evaluation*. Evaluations should be performed at the end of the probationary period and annually thereafter for each employee. Sometimes, the employee's annual evaluation is tied to a merit pay increase. The result of an evaluation can determine whether an employee receives a 1%, 2%, or 5% increase in pay, and occasionally it affects an employee's promotion. Fig. 9.13 illustrates a sample evaluation form.

The employee evaluation is not the first communication that the employee receives regarding his or her job performance. Each employee is given performance expectations and performance standards when he or she receives a copy of the job description. Routine communication between the employee and the supervisor should indicate whether the employee's performance is acceptable. The employee evaluation should not be the first occasion on which an employee learns that he or she is not meeting expectations. The manager or supervisor should regularly communicate with the

employees, especially when their performance is unacceptable. Poor communication by the management can negatively affect functions in the HIM department.

Routine feedback to employees about their job performance improves effectiveness if there is a problem and makes the employee performance evaluation go more smoothly because the necessary information has been gathered over the entire evaluation period (i.e., over the course of a year). If the manager does not gather information over the course of the entire evaluation period and waits instead until the evaluation is due to complete it, the manager may be able to recall only the most recent incidents. If these are not favorable, the manager may not consider the employee's positive performance during the entire evaluation period. In other words, employees should receive regular feedback, both positive and negative, from the supervisor. These conversations should be documented for future reference. Because employees have job descriptions and understand the productivity expectations, evaluations should not be a surprise to them.

The employee evaluation should be performed in person by the employee's direct supervisor. If at all possible, the employee should sit down with his or her manager to discuss the evaluation; this is an excellent opportunity for feedback and communication. The employee evaluation is the formal summary of the employee's performance (as required in the performance standards) for the evaluation period. It is documented and maintained in the HR department, and a copy is kept in the employee's file maintained by the HIM manager.

What occurs if the evaluation is not favorable? Is the employee immediately terminated for poor performance? Typically, an employee who has successfully completed a probationary period and later performs poorly is put on a **performance improvement plan (PIP)**. The PIP informs the employee of the poor performance and describes the consequences of not performing according to the acceptable standards. The standard disciplinary process requires counseling, a verbal warning, and then suspension. This can vary, depending on specific HR guidelines at the organizational level or union contracts. Regardless of the process, regular communication that includes both positive and negative feedback fosters an environment in which the results of an evaluation should not be a surprise to an employee.

## Organization-Wide Orientation

When an employee begins a job at a health care facility, it is very important for him or her to learn about the environment and the new job, so an orientation is essential. The purpose of **orientation** is to make the employee familiar with the surroundings. Some facilities hold organization-wide orientations weekly, which are followed by second orientations specific to an employee's job within the department, led by his or her direct supervisor.

Typically, before new employees report to their departments, they attend an organization-wide orientation in

## FY 20XX Employee Evaluation—Criteria-Based Appraisal

**Employee Name:** Erin Rene Ory            **Position:** Emergency Department Coder

**Supervisor:** Tami JoAnne Davi            **Date:** March 23, 20XX

Ratings scale to assess performance: **Exceeds (E = 3 points)**—consistently performs at a level over and above standards; **Satisfies (S = 2 points)**—consistently performs at the level defined by the standards; **Opportunity (O = 1 point)**—generally meets more standards in the function, but needs improvement; **Unsatisfactory (U = 0 points)**—Consistently performs at a level below the standards.

| Job Functions | % Weight | Rating | Score =: Weight × Rating |
|---|---|---|---|
| 1. **Job Function: Codes patient medical record information for diagnosis and procedures.**<br>• Assigns ICD-10-CM codes accurately in accordance with coding guidelines, CMS regulations, and hospital policies.<br>• Assigns CPT-4 codes accurately in accordance with coding guidelines, CMS regulations, and hospital policies.<br>• Assigns ED charges, as needed, in accordance with coding guidelines, CMS regulations, and hospital policies. | 40% | ☒ E (3)<br>☐ S (2)<br>☐ O (1)<br>☐ U (0) | 1.20 |
| 2. **Job Function: Maintains acceptable coding productivity for outpatient claims.**<br>• Codes, charges, and abstracts an average of at least 110 ED charts per day.<br>• Maintains a minimum 99% accuracy rate as determined by independent audit. | 30% | ☒ E (3)<br>☐ S (2)<br>☐ O (1)<br>☐ U (0) | 0.90 |
| 3. **Job Function: Employs full use of encoding software and abstracting system.**<br>• Uses the encoder to ensure proper coding and sequencing.<br>• Accurately abstracts all information in the abstracting system to reflect correct UB-04 data.<br>• Correctly refers to the computer system when necessary for lab results, transcription, and older claims information. | 15% | ☒ E (3)<br>☐ S (2)<br>☐ O (1)<br>☐ U (0) | 0.45 |
| 4. **Job Function: Performs other financial and compliance duties as necessary.**<br>• Assists patient financial services personnel with any claims issues to ensure that proper billing is facilitated.<br>• Works with the registration department to ensure data integrity on patient information.<br>• Complies with the standards set by department policy, CMS, and other regulatory agencies. | 5% | ☐ E (3)<br>☐ S (2)<br>☒ O (1)<br>☐ U (0) | 0.05 |
| 5. **Job Function: Continuing Education**<br>• Maintains credentials through ongoing education.<br>• If uncredentialed, seeks to obtain a coding credential, as appropriate.<br>• Attends mandatory educational sessions for coding information. | 10% | ☐ E (3)<br>☒ S (2)<br>☐ O (1)<br>☐ U (0) | 0.20 |
| | | **TOTAL** | **2.8**<br>Performance above standard |

• **Fig. 9.13** Sample evaluation form. *CMS,* Centers for Medicare and Medicaid Services; *CPT,* Current Procedural Technology; *ED,* emergency department; *ICD-10-CM,* International Classification of Diseases, Tenth Revision-Clinical Modification; *UB-04,* Uniform Bill.

which they learn about the organization and its mission statement, vision, and values. During the orientation, they have an opportunity to ask questions regarding employment. In most cases, an organization orientation includes the organization chart for the entire facility and the following topics:

• Personnel considerations
• Customer service expectations

- Quality
- Building safety and security
- Infection control
- Body mechanics
- Confidentiality
- HIPAA
- Information systems
- Tour of the facility
- Incident reporting
- Compliance
- Phone and email systems

This orientation should take place before employees begin their job activities; however, because these orientations are sometimes offered only once a month, employees may actually begin work before their organization orientation. It is important that all employees receive orientation, including those employees who work from home or remotely.

Each topic in the organization-wide orientation is typically presented by the employee within the organization who is the authority on that issue. For example, the safety topic is presented by the facility's security officer; body mechanics is presented by a physical therapist; infection control is presented by the infection control nurse; and confidentiality is presented by an HIM professional. An excellent way to keep track of the important orientation topics that must be covered with a new employee is to complete an orientation checklist (Fig. 9.14). The employee should initial and date each item as it is completed. This form is kept in the employee's file folder for future reference, as verification of the orientation.

**DIAMONTE HOSPITAL** Diamonte, Arizona 89104 • TEL. 602-484-9991

**EMPLOYEE ORIENTATION CHECKLIST**

Employee: _____ Date: _____
Position: _____ Supervisor: _____

The following items have been reviewed with the employee.
(The employee and supervisor should initial and date items as they are reviewed.)

| | Employee | Supervisor | Date |
|---|---|---|---|
| Employee identification card policy | | | |
| Explanation of payroll procedures, including time clock location | | | |
| Absence and tardiness policy | | | |
| Employee job description | | | |
| Employee performance standards | | | |
| Introduction to department employees and physical layout | | | |
| Review of department functions | | | |
| Review of functions involving related departments | | | |
| Departmental Policy and Procedure manual | | | |
| Review of specific job-related policies and procedures | | | |
| Dress code | | | |
| Performance improvement activities | | | |
| Security and confidentiality policies | | | |
| Review and sign confidentiality statement | | | |
| Safety policy, disaster plan, and safety manual | | | |
| Review of break schedule | | | |
| Location of restrooms and area to secure belongings | | | |
| Password assigned and related policies covered | | | |

Employee signature: _____ Date: _____
Supervisor: _____ Date: _____

*Example only. This list is not all-inclusive.*

• **Fig. 9.14** Employee orientation checklist.

## Personnel Considerations

Some of the first materials that employees receive during the orientation explain the benefits to which they are entitled as employees of the organization. During this part of the orientation, employees complete necessary forms for income tax purposes and learn about enrollment in other special savings plans, insurance, or retirement accounts. Because compensation for the job is important, orientation is an opportunity to ask about pay periods, proper completion of payroll forms, and use of the time clock. Employees are also informed of health care facility policies and procedures that affect their employment, and they must receive a copy of the employee handbook. Information in the employee handbook includes facility dress code, attendance policy, hours earned for vacation and sick leave (paid time off [PTO]/paid time sick [PTS]), grievance procedures, and holidays. New employees also acknowledge receipt and understanding of their ethical and HIPAA compliance responsibilities. This latter acknowledgment is required at hire as well as annually.

## Customer Service

By definition, a *customer* is one who receives goods or services from another. Each person who interacts with the HIM department, whether that person receives material or services, is a customer. Therefore fellow employees in another department in the hospital can be customers, as well as physicians, patients, and third-party payers. During the initial orientation, the new employee learns about the organization's expectations for customer service. It is an opportunity to inspire the use of positive techniques when interacting with all customers. Many organizations use a customer satisfaction survey to measure their service to customers. The results are used to improve the quality of customer service, and when the survey results are overwhelmingly favorable, the organization can use them in marketing efforts. Employees are encouraged to:

1. identify all of their customers by name,
2. greet each customer with a smile,
3. provide assistance or find someone who can assist the customer, and
4. follow up on a customer's request.

Employees may have an opportunity to participate in a role-playing exercise in which they learn how to deal with a disgruntled customer.

## Quality

Because of its importance, employees are informed about the expectations and methods that the organization uses to ensure quality. The orientation should introduce the employee to the PI method used by the organization. New employees learn that everyone in the facility is responsible for quality. As appropriate, employees are encouraged to identify and report opportunities to improve quality.

## Building Safety and Security

The health care environment should be safe for patients, visitors, and employees. Safety issues are covered in the organization orientation to make the employee aware of the policy and procedures for maintaining a secure environment and for handling situations in the event of an emergency (i.e., the disaster plan). Two commonly discussed topics are fire safety and response to code emergencies. A common fire response uses the acronym RACE—rescue, alarm, confine, and extinguish. Every employee learns to rescue patients, employees, or visitors from the area of the fire. He or she should go to the closest fire alarm and inform the operator of his or her name and the location and status of the fire. Then the employee should confine the fire by closing all doors in the area. If possible, he or she should extinguish the fire with a fire extinguisher or other appropriate device.

During a visit to a health care facility, you may have heard the operator announce a code over the intercom system. Common codes are "code blue" for cardiac arrest and "code red" for fire. These codes alert the employees to an emergency that is occurring in the facility (Table 9.8). These codes may also be announced as fictitious physician names (e.g., Dr. Red instead of "code red" or Dr. Strong for "security"). All employees must recognize the codes in the facility and know their roles in response to the emergency.

## Infection Control

By nature of the job environment, health care workers may be exposed to a number of infectious agents. For this reason, several significant issues are covered under the topic of infection control, including hepatitis, acquired immunodeficiency syndrome, and universal precautions for blood and body fluids. During this part of the orientation, new employees learn how to protect themselves and others from infection; the discussion provides information about how these infections are spread and then share procedures that help protect employees.

**TABLE 9.8**    **Sample Emergency Codes**

| Code | Emergency |
| --- | --- |
| Dr. Strong | Security requested in a specific area of the facility |
| Black | Bomb threat |
| Red | Fire |
| Orange | Radiation disaster |
| Pink | Infant abduction |
| Blue | Cardiac arrest |
| Yellow | External disaster |

In a discussion about universal precautions for blood and body fluids, employees are informed that one of the best and easiest methods to prevent the spread of infection is by washing their hands. Employees are encouraged to always wash their hands before and after having contact with a patient, eating, and using the restroom. Universal precautions also include wearing masks and gloves when interacting with potentially infectious material and properly discarding needles and other contaminated objects.

Because some blood-borne organisms can survive for days outside the body, health care workers are advised to exercise caution when handling items contaminated with body fluids. For example, a paper record contaminated with blood should be filed in a sealed plastic sheet protector.

### Confidentiality

Confidentiality has always been an important part of the new health care employee orientation. HIPAA legislation increased the need for organizations to ensure that all employees and contractors receive training regarding the confidentiality and security of health information. Typically, this topic is presented by an HIM professional. All employees must recognize the sensitivity of confidential information in a health care facility and the proper manner in which it should be handled. The confidentiality policy is reviewed, and all employees are asked to sign a confidentiality statement, as discussed in Chapter 8 (see Fig. 8.4). Additionally, all employees must be made aware of any applicable federal and state laws and organization policies regarding patient confidentiality and security. Security matters can include review of the information technology (IT) policy on password security and access to the organization's electronic health information. All employees will be asked to review the guidelines for security and to sign statements acknowledging their understanding and compliance.

### Information Systems

Many facilities require a training session before a new employee is given access to its computer systems, and The Joint Commission (TJC) requires that new employees complete this training within 7 days. During orientation, new employees receive their login or user names, even though access will be limited until training on the various computer systems is complete. They are also given information on rules for setting passwords and the frequency that passwords must be changed and learn about the use policies surrounding the facility's information systems. This information, along with training on the use of software applications, may be presented by an IT professional, although the use of computer-based learning modules for this procedure is common.

### Body Mechanics

All employees should maintain proper body mechanics, particularly while sitting at the workstation and when lifting, pushing, pulling, or transporting patients or equipment.

Employees can be injured if they use poor body mechanics, and injuries are very costly to the entire organization; injuries could lead to missed work, workers' compensation claims, and reduced productivity. The orientation may include demonstration of proper body mechanics for employees to use in their job duties.

## Health Information Management Department Orientation

After the organization-wide orientation, employees report to their supervisors in their assigned departments for orientations specific to their jobs. Each employee is given an opportunity to become acclimated to the work environment, meet the employees who are part of the work group or team, and learn what is expected by management.

During this orientation, a new employee in the HIM department is given a copy of the job description, performance standards, rules, and policies and procedures of the department. The employee becomes familiar with the physical layout of the HIM department and other related departments within the organization.

One way to orient new employees is to have them sit with coworkers in each section of the department so they become familiar with everyone's duties. This experience helps new employees understand the impact of their roles in the department.

Although the organization-wide orientation covers payroll issues (as discussed earlier), there may be specific policies within the department that are important for the employee to learn. HIM employees should know the hours and shifts that they are expected to work. HIM employees also need to understand which holidays they may be required to work and how to request time off.

Another topic discussed in the organization-wide orientation is security of health information. HIM employees are given a password with access to appropriate systems that they will use to perform their job duties. In the HIM department orientation the employee is reminded of the rules associated with the password; for instance, employees cannot share passwords with others, and when they leave a computer station, they must log out to prevent unauthorized access by someone who might try to access that computer after they walk away. Once their passwords are assigned, employees can begin training on the computer systems associated with their jobs.

Employees who change positions within an HIM department should undergo a formal orientation to their new duties and responsibilities.

Department managers must understand the proper way to request records from the HIM department. Managers often request records for a study or project in which they are involved or to obtain information for a meeting. They need to know how much notice the department needs to complete the request. Does the request need to be specific? Does the person requesting the information need to include the patient's name, medical record number, and discharge dates on the request form? While in the past most audits were conducted using paper abstraction forms and paper medical charts, with the increased use of EHRs, many audits are now conducted by accessing electronic health data. If your health care facility or practice uses EHRs, you may be able to get the system to generate a report with the data you need. Covering these policies in an orientation eliminates a great deal of confusion and stress in the future.

## Clinical Staff Orientation

HIM department employees are not the only members of the organization who require an orientation to the department. Clinical staff, physicians, and members of other departments should be familiar with the functions and services of the HIM department. Physicians require orientation to the HIM department because they will visit the department to complete their health records and perform research. Physician orientation can be by personal appointment or in the form of a letter (Fig. 9.15) introducing or explaining HIM department functions.

A general orientation explaining HIM department operations will help these members when they interact with the department. HIM customers need to know the requirements for requesting information or records and the procedures for completing or reviewing records.

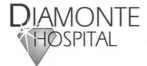

Diamonte, Arizona 89104 • TEL. 602-484-9991

November 30, 20XX

Eileen Dombrowski, MD
1101 Medical Center Blvd.
Diamonte, Arizona 89104

Dear Dr. Dombrowski,

On behalf of the Health Information Management department, welcome to Diamonte Hospital. I would like to introduce you to the HIM department staff and the services provided.

**Release of Information**
To obtain copies of health information for a patient under your care, please contact Shelly Pontiac, 565-1411. She will be happy to provide the appropriate forms and process your request.

**Coding**
Our coding department is supervised by Joanne Davis, CCS. If you have any questions regarding coding, please feel free to contact her.

**Request for an old chart for patient care**
The unit coordinator will typically request previous records for patients under your care by contacting the Health Information Management department at 565-1400. If you encounter difficulty retrieving a previous patient record, please feel free to contact John Brown, Supervisor.

**Medical record completion**
In keeping with our policy for timely completion of health records, we will e-mail weekly reminders to your office to notify you of any incomplete records. If you plan to come by our office to complete your records, please call in advance, 565-1455. We will be happy to pull your records and leave them in the physicians' lounge for 48 hours.

I look forward to working with you. If you need any further assistance, I can be reached at 565-1416.

Sincerely,

Michelle Parks, RHIA
Director, Health Information Management

• **Fig. 9.15** Orientation letter to physicians.

Physician orientation is an excellent opportunity to cover information relevant to completion of records, specifically the suspension policy. The suspension policy is typically found in the medical staff bylaws. But even if the orientation is no more than a simple letter of correspondence, it tells the physician how to avoid negative correspondence and unfortunate consequences as a result of delinquent records. Whatever format, the physician orientation should let the physician know whom to contact to gain access to incomplete records and how the HIM department can assist the physician in record completion.

## Discipline

When an employee is first hired, there is typically a period of probation. The probation period varies but is often the first 90 days of employment and may be extended, if company policy permits, in order to provide additional training and observation. During the probation period, employees are allowed ample time to learn their new tasks and responsibilities. At the end of this time, employees who are performing at an acceptable level are considered permanent. If at any time during this probation period the employer feels that an employee is not performing as expected, the employee can be released from the job.

The disciplinary process is defined in an organization's HR manual. In general, the process starts with a verbal warning and progresses through a written warning, retraining, reevaluation, and eventually termination.

## Outsourcing

It is increasingly common for HIM departments to outsource functions performed within the HIM department. To **outsource** means to hire a vendor or consultant from outside of the facility to perform the HIM function; another term for this practice is to *contract out* the function. For example, many facilities use contract coders when they have a backlog or need temporary help during an employee's vacation or sick leave. However, some facilities permanently outsource these functions-meaning that a facility signs a contract for a period with a company who will perform the function and bill the facility for the services. Another HIM function that is commonly outsourced is ROI. HIM departments use a contract service to perform this very important and specialized function on a full-time basis for a specific contract period. The advantage for the facility is the shift of employee management responsibility to the company/consultant. The facility must be careful to hire a reputable company/consultant and to monitor the outsourced work just as they would that of an onsite employee. Even though a contract exists, the facility remains responsible for the overall quality and integrity of the HIM department.

## COMPETENCY CHECK-IN 9.3
### Human Resources

#### Competency Assessment

1. The department within the health care organization responsible for employee management is:
   a. the HIM department
   b. HR
   c. materials management
   d. operations management
2. Which of the following Fair Employment Laws prohibits discrimination based on race, color, religion, or sex?
   a. Fair Labor Standards Act
   b. Civil Rights Act
   c. Americans with Disabilities Act
   d. Age Discrimination in Employment Act
3. Which of the following fair employment laws sets minimum wage, overtime pay, and equal pay?
   a. Fair Labor Standards Act
   b. Civil Rights Act
   c. Americans with Disabilities Act
   d. Age Discrimination in Employment Act
4. Which of the following Fair Employment Laws prohibits discrimination against handicapped people and ensures reasonable accommodation for them in the workplace?
   a. Fair Labor Standards Act
   b. Civil Rights Act
   c. Americans with Disabilities Act
   d. Age Discrimination in Employment Act
5. An employee who works 16–20 hours each week, occasionally earning partial benefits, is:
   a. FTE
   b. PRN
   c. part time
   d. LPN
6. A pool of employees used as needed when workload increases are:
   a. FTE
   b. part time
   c. PRN
   d. coders
7. A formal list of the employee's responsibilities associated with his or her job is called a(n) _____.
8. A(n) _____ involves the review of a function to determine all the tasks or components that make up an employee's job.
9. _____ are guidelines specifying the quantity and quality of work that must be done and in what timeframe.
10. One method of monitoring the amount of work an employee performs is:
    a. reviewing the organization chart
    b. reviewing the productivity report
    c. monitoring payroll
    d. limiting employee breaks
11. The _____ is an opportunity for management to provide feedback to the employee based on the employee's performance.
12. Identify some HIM functions that may be outsourced.
13. Which of the following organization-wide orientation topics should be presented by an HIM employee?
    a. Safety
    b. Infection control
    c. Personnel issues
    d. HIPAA, confidentiality, and security
14. What is the purpose of orientation?
15. Explain the importance of a job description.

# Communication

Employees in the HIM department communicate using written, verbal, physical, and electronic methods. The HIM department also communicates with other departments inside and outside the facility—clinicians and physicians, other health care facilities, insurance companies, attorneys, and patients. Communication should always be clear and appropriate regardless of the parties involved.

Communication requires two or more parties and the conveying of a message. First, the message must be transmitted from one party to another. The message can be written, verbal, or electronic or can be expressed by body language. The first party—called the sender—initiates the message. The second party—the receiver—is the recipient of the message. Regardless of the intention of the sender, it is the recipient's interpretation that matters: Was the message conveyed? Therefore every effort must be made to present a professional tone, eliminating slang, "text talk" and other colloquialisms from both spoken and written communication. With this understanding, consider typical communication within the HIM department.

## Oral Communication

Oral or *verbal* communication occurs among employees within the HIM department and throughout the organization. Communication may be verbal, written, or electronic and may involve job-related or personal subjects. Positive, appropriate communication among employees enhances productivity.

It is very important that communication about or to patients is kept confidential. Patient health information should be communicated in an appropriate method to employees on a need-to-know basis in accordance with HIPAA regulations and health care facility policy.

Communication between employees and their immediate supervisors is also important. Employees need to know how their performance is perceived by their supervisor (management). They also need to be informed of changes in their work, processes, and functions that affect the daily operations.

Occasionally, conflicts arise in the workplace between a supervisor and a staff member or among two or more coworkers. Conflict in the workplace can create a poor work environment and should be resolved. For example, when the conflict involves two or more employees, one effective method of addressing the conflict is to establish clear lines of communication between the employees involved. This is best done in a private setting. A supervisor may use the following procedure as one way of handling conflict:

1. Listen to each employee involved in the conflict to clearly understand each side of the conflict. Stay calm, and ensure that the other parties do as well. If the situation is tense, enlist the help of HR or another department supervisor/manager to witness and assist if necessary.

2. Ensure that each individual knows that his or her point of view is valuable. A resolution will be impossible if any one side feels he or she is misunderstood or misrepresented.

3. After hearing both sides, assess the best method of compromise. You may need the expertise of a HR manager to ensure that the best method is chosen.

## Communicating with Physicians

The HIM department communicates routinely with physicians regarding record completion, ROI, continuity of care, and documentation of health information for case management or reimbursement. Communication with a physician should be respectful. Consider the physician's time, and make your communication appropriate. To communicate record completion requirements, HIM employees use email and official mail, and for questions on health record documentation, they post notes on EHRs or attach paper memos to health record files, if appropriate. The message/communication must be meaningful, brief if possible, and, most important, clear.

## Communicating with Outside Agencies or Parties

HIM departments often communicate with agencies external to the organization. For example, the HIM department ROI employees receive requests from attorneys and third-party payers (insurance companies) for copies of health records. As discussed in Chapter 8, information should be released only according to applicable policy or state or federal law. As a part of the release process, the HIM/ROI employee may need to discuss with the requestor the circumstances, charges, or additional forms necessary to comply with the request. Communication should be clear, preferably in writing, and should provide information so that the recipient can reply as necessary. Many departments create form letters to handle this type of communication in a standard, law-abiding, and professional manner.

## Written Communication

Written communication provides documentation of the message intended for the recipient. Therefore written communication serves two purposes: It conveys a message and records it. A common form of written communication in a health care facility is the memorandum, better known as the *memo* (see later). Memos can be written on paper and delivered individually to each employee or communicated in electronic form via email.

### Electronic Communication

It is extremely common for health care facilities to use email for communication and notification. This method of communication allows the same message to be sent to

- Do not type an email message using all-capital letters. In the email context, all-capital letters are considered the equivalent of shouting. Use all-capital letters sparingly, only to emphasize a word.
- Be careful to read your email for grammar, spelling, punctuation, and tone.
- Tone is very important. Never send an email written in anger; save it as a draft and rewrite it later. Save the emoticons for friends and family.
- Avoid long messages. Keep the message brief and to the point. If someone sends you an email message that requires a response, be careful to reply to the sender as appropriate. Include the previous message so that the person knows why you are communicating a specific message. In a business email, end your message with your name, title, and business address, including phone numbers as appropriate. You want the person to be able to contact you appropriately.
- Email is not private. Be careful what you send via email. Messages can be read by others, misdirected, or forwarded. Send only what you feel comfortable expressing to the whole world.
- Use punctuation appropriately.
- Email is faster than conventional mail. However, the quicker arrival of email does not mean that the intended recipient will actually read the message any faster.

all employees instantly. Email systems provide a record of a communication sent, and an indication, using a read receipt function, that the receiving party has opened the email.

With the use of email, messages can be conveniently tracked for receipt, returned, forwarded, or saved. When sending an email, it is easy to send a copy to others (cc: carbon copy) in receipt of the message so that they have the information. Additionally, copies of emails can be sent to others in such a way that the intended original recipient does not know that others are included or copied in the message (bcc: blind carbon copy).

Because email is a form of written communication, appropriate grammar, punctuation, and etiquette must be used in creating it. Additionally, email is not a private method of sending communication; therefore health care facilities must use encryption to enhance the security of this communication and employees must comply with HIPAA guidelines for ROI by email. Box 9.3 contains guidelines for sending email.

## Memos

A **memorandum (memo)** is typed communication for informational purposes. A memo is used to provide clear, concise information about a new procedure, process, or policy to all those affected by it (Fig. 9.16). The memo is more formal than verbal communication. Memos can be addressed to a group or an individual but are not as formal as a letter addressed specifically to an employee.

Memos can also serve as proof of communication to an employee. When a memo is shared with employees in a department, it may be posted in a highly visible and frequented place (e.g., near the time clock or in the break room). At other times, memos are copied for each employee and handed to the employee personally by another staff member. Regardless of the means, the manager wants to be sure that the message is communicated. One easy method for obtaining confirmation of the employee's receipt of the memo is to have the employee initial a master copy of the memo. This system allows management to record employees' receipt of the memo.

## Meetings

Department meetings are another method of face-to-face communication. Department meetings should be held monthly or more often as the need arises. A good way to schedule the meetings is to set aside one day each month for the meeting. This routine helps employees and managers know when to expect the next department meeting so that scheduling conflicts do not arise. The department meeting is an opportunity for employees to come together to discuss, learn, communicate, and share information. The department meeting is an ideal forum for reviewing policies and procedures to ensure that everyone understands the appropriate course of action. Department meetings are an excellent opportunity for holding brief training, discussing productivity goals, planning for major workflow changes, and providing development opportunities, such as presentations.

In a small department, a single meeting may suffice to communicate necessary information to all employees. However, in a large department, more than one meeting is necessary during different shifts so that all employees can attend.

### Conducting and Documenting Meetings

To conduct an orderly meeting, teams and committees might adopt some form of Robert's Rules of Order. These rules explain how business is conducted during the meeting and include the making of motions, voting, and the preparation of formal resolutions. Robert's Rules explain how debate should proceed and how motions can be made to present new business, make amendments, or vote on issues at hand. Likewise, there is a formal method for keeping track of old business on the agenda until it is resolved to the satisfaction of the meeting members. These rules may be important for conducting business in board meetings and with large groups, such as corporate annual meetings and legislatures. For most meetings, however, just a few key rules can be sufficient. Meetings are formally called to order by the leader, a specific agenda is followed, individuals who wish to speak are called on, any voting takes place by a show of hands, and the meeting is concluded with adjournment.

**DIAMONTE HOSPITAL**    Diamonte, Arizona 89104 • TEL. 602-484-9991

**MEMO**

TO: Health Information Management Employees

FROM: Michelle Parks, RHIA
        Director, Health Information Management

DATE: May 8, 20XX

RE: Monthly Department Meeting

A Health Information Management department meeting will be held Wednesday, May 31, in the hospital auditorium at 2:00 p.m.

We will have a brief presentation by the Human Resources department followed by the regular monthly agenda. Please make necessary arrangements to attend this meeting.

Thank you.

• **Fig. 9.16** A memo.

## Agenda

Regardless of the style or purpose of meetings, an **agenda** is used to ensure that all of the necessary topics are covered. Although agendas vary, the example in Fig. 9.17 is typical for an HIM department. A meeting officially begins with the call to order, whereupon the events of the meeting begin to be recorded. *Minutes* from the previous meeting may be reviewed and approved, depending on the formality of the meeting. Next, old business (if any) from the previous meeting is discussed. Occasionally, topics discussed will require more than one meeting to be resolved. Some topics require further investigation and will be on a future agenda under old business until they are resolved, closed, or completed. The next part of the agenda is new business.

At this point in the meeting, new items are introduced for discussion or information. This is followed by items that are discussed each month, such as reports from sections within the department, quality management activities in or related to the department, safety issues, and special announcements from the administration or about the facility. It is usually during this last part of the meeting that comments and issues from attendees may be solicited.

## Minutes

Appropriate discussion and decisions from each meeting should be recorded for future reference in the **minutes**. When preparing the minutes, the agenda should be used as a guide. This ensures that the content or discussion surrounding

HIM Department

Monthly Department Meeting

Date: September 30, 20XX

Time:          2:00 a.m.–2:30 a.m.

Location: Conference Room B, First Floor

AGENDA

| TIME | TOPIC | | RESPONSIBLE |
|------|-------|---|-------------|
| 2:00 | I. | Call to Order | M Parks |
| 2:02 | II. | Review of Minutes | All |
| 2:05 | III. | Old Business | |
| | | Uniforms | S Gibbons |
| 2:10 | IV. | New Business | |
| | | Required Flu Shots<br>Handwashing protocols | S Gonzalez, RN<br>Infection Control |
| 2:20 | V. | Announcements | M Parks |
| 2:25 | VI. | Open Forum | All |
| 2:30 | VII. | Adjourn | M Parks |

• **Fig. 9.17** Agenda.

each topic presented at the meeting is recorded. Review the minutes shown in Fig. 9.18 and notice how the content of the topics discussed as recorded just as they were presented at the meeting. The preparer must be careful to include only pertinent meeting information and participants' comments without mention of the participants' names in the minutes; gossip, slang, and irrelevant comments by the participants should not be included in minutes.

The minutes should clearly document the events of the meeting as presented, discussed, and decided. The template provided in Fig. 9.18 is an example of how minutes can be organized; here the topics presented are documented in a table format. Under the column titled "Topic/Discussion," the general discussion or information provided for each topic is recorded. The decision or action of the meeting members is documented under "Recommendation/Action." The final

column, "Follow-up," identifies whether a topic has been closed (i.e., the business for that topic is concluded). Most importantly, topics that are not finalized should be recorded so they may be carried forward to the next meeting until the business is concluded.

All employees should attend the scheduled monthly HIM department meetings. When employees miss a meeting, they still need to hear the information. Therefore posting or copying minutes from the meeting serves as notification for these employees. Also, employees should initial the transmittal memo attached to the minutes of the meeting, indicating that they have read the minutes.

It is important to keep a precise record of supporting information used at each monthly meeting. These records will support any future business, discussion, and accreditation requirements. You can set up a file folder or a binder to

Health Information Management
Department Meeting
September 30, 20XX

Employees present: M. Parks, Director; R. Applegate, E. Baker, W. Coppola, X. Davidson, T. Edwards, S. Fernandez, S. Gibbons, D. Gentley, Y. Hernandez, R. Johnson, W. Johnson, T. Owens, I. Parks, S. Quigley, M. Rosen, F. Weatherly, T. Zapato, S. Zhen

Employees absent:

| Topic/Discussion | Recommendation/Action | Follow-up |
|---|---|---|
| I. Call to Order<br>The Health Information Management meeting was called to order by Michelle Parks at 2:00 p.m. | | |
| II. Review of Old Minutes<br>The minutes from the August Health Information Management department meeting were reviewed and approved as presented. | | |
| III. Old Business<br>**Uniforms**<br>Employees in the department are interested in adopting a uniform as the dress code. During the previous meeting it was decided that the employees would invite three uniform companies to present at the next meeting. M & R Uniforms, Acorn Uniforms, and B & B Direct presented uniforms, pricing, and payment options to the employees. | After review of the information presented by all uniform companies the employees voted for the uniform and options presented by B & B Direct. The uniform company will return in 2 weeks to take orders and the dress code will take effect in 2 months. | 11/20XX |
| IV. New Business<br>Samantha Gonzalez, RN, from Infection Control explained the hospital policy regarding flu shots. All employees are required to have evidence of flu vaccination and to display flag on their badge at all times on the premises.<br>As cold and flu season approaches, all employees are reminded to observe proper handwashing techniques. S. Gonzalez demonstrated. There is a video demonstration on the intranet under Infection Control tips. | Flu shots are free to employees. If the shot is obtained elsewhere, documentation must be provided to Employee Health before October 31.<br><br>HIM staff absent from this meeting must review the handwashing video, complete the quiz at the end, and submit a printout of the results to M. Parks by October 31 and complete the | All, by October 31<br><br><br>Absentees, by October 31 |
| V. Announcements<br>Safety Inservice 10/15–17<br>Flu Shots in employee health 10/8–10/15, 7 a.m.–7 p.m. | Informational | |
| VI. Open Forum<br>A coder asked whether the department would be offering Coding inservice in December for CPT code changes. | M. Parks stated that the hospital has contracted with a vendor for an online training. Information will be provided at the October department meeting. | Agenda item for October meeting. M. Parks. |
| VII. Adjourn<br>With no further business to discuss the meeting was adjourned at 2:30 p.m. Next meeting is October 28, 20XX. | | |

_____          _____
Michelle Parks, RHIA                                    Date

• **Fig. 9.18** Minutes of health information management department meeting.

organize each month's meeting information. Be sure to keep a copy of the agenda, the sign-in sheet, any attachments or handouts shared with the group, and the final draft of the minutes. The records from these meetings should be kept for at least 3 years, or longer if required by legal or regulatory bodies.

The HIM department meeting should be held in a location able to accommodate the number of the department's staff. In a small department the meeting may be held in the HIM office area. For a large department an alternative location may be necessary to accommodate all the employees. Management must make sure to consider the time of the meeting. If it is held during the normal hours of operation, more than one meeting may be necessary so that employees can rotate attendance in order to cover HIM responsibilities during the meeting. Otherwise, the manager should try to find a time when the office is not too busy. In order to cover the normal business, one employee may need to remain in the department to answer requests and handle business. Another way to handle this is to have someone from another department cover the functions briefly while the employees are at the meeting. Furthermore, it must be scheduled so that employees working from off-site locations can travel conveniently or so that remote access to the meeting can be arranged. There should be a sign-in sheet for all of the employees to record their attendance at the meeting.

## Work Teams

*Teamwork* is a familiar term. In the workplace, employees are often called upon to work together as a "team" to accomplish common goals. One example of a health care work team is the patient care team: the employees of the health care facility who work together to treat the patient. In the ED the team may include emergency medical technicians who transport the patient into the ED, the ED physician, nurses, radiology technicians, and phlebotomists. On the rehabilitation unit the team may consist of physical therapists, occupational therapists, nurses, and physicians.

These are not the only employees who have to work in teams to accomplish goals. For instance, in an HIM department the coding team may have a large number of charts that must be coded for final billing. (These charts and the dollar amount for each account are typically listed on an unbilled report.) Timely and accurate coding helps the health care facility receive the appropriate reimbursement for each patient case. A delay in coding will extend the amount of time it takes for the health care facility to send a bill to the payer, thus delaying payment to the facility. One single patient record can represent a large sum of reimbursement for the health care facility, and consequently, many charts can add up to a large sum of money. To reach the goal of coding all of the charts, the coding team and other HIM department employees must work together in an efficient manner to get the job done.

A likely game plan for addressing a long list of charts that need to be coded will involve a team meeting to discuss the goal, a review of the list of accounts that need to be coded, division of the tasks among the team members, and then action. In larger facilities, coders are often assigned to either inpatient or outpatient charts, but when the workload is exceptionally heavy, outpatient coders may be able to help with some of the less complicated inpatient charts. Other team members in the HIM department may be able to assist with physician communications, by researching questions, or even by looking up coding clinic guidelines.

### Roles and Functions

Every team or committee has a *leader*, generally called the *chairperson* of a committee. The leader runs the meetings and typically controls the development of the agenda for the meetings. In a committee, the leader is often a person in authority.

In meetings, the leader fosters a collaborative atmosphere. Meetings of individuals with disparate ideas and roles in the organization may result in contentious dialogue if ground rules and protocols are not clearly established. Furthermore, individuals with strong personalities may monopolize the conversation. The leader, then, must ensure that all voices are heard, generally by inviting silent members to speak. Therefore building a collegial team is very important to the success of the venture.

One barrier to collegiality that has arisen in recent years is the distraction of cell phones, tablets, and laptops which impair the ability of all members to participate. In the first meeting of the group, the members should mutually decide to what extent communication devices will be used or permitted. There are some individuals, such as physicians on call, who must leave their cell phones on and need to check them when they "ring." However, they can be kept on vibrate and glancing at the screen is usually not problematic. This mutual agreement can be a first step to developing a collegial atmosphere and fostering mutual respect.

A secretary or recorder should be designated to document the meetings of the team or committee. It is most efficient for this person to have no other official role during the meetings so that they can concentrate on the discussion. It may be helpful to audio record the meetings so that the secretary can take notes and also participate in the discussion more fully. Sometimes, the role of secretary or recorder is rotated among committee members when a volunteer to perform the task is not immediately identified.

An often-overlooked role on teams and committees is a *timekeeper*. The HR involved in teams and committees are organizational resources. There is a cost to participating, which should not be wasted through inefficiency. The agenda should clearly state the topics to be discussed and the time allocated to each topic. It is the leader's responsibility to keep to the agenda, but having a timekeeper to give friendly warnings helps the leader bring closure to a topic without drama. Further, the timekeeper can be an objective arbiter of time allotted to individuals so that a member who tends to talk too much can be reminded when their time has expired.

## Interpersonal Skills

The HIM department is responsible for supporting a variety of patient-centered activities, such as completing health records, ROI, and billing. As such, it cannot operate in a vacuum or silo. Significant interdepartmental relationships must be developed for the department to operate effectively. For example, the HIM department deals with physicians on a daily basis. Therefore relationships with the medical staff and the medical staff office personnel are critical to ensure success. Also, coding is a part of the revenue cycle. Other components of the revenue cycle include scheduling, patient access, patient financial services, and clinical charge capture. Thus relationships with all of these areas are important for effective revenue cycle management.

Because interdepartmental relationships are not necessarily reflected on an organizational chart, the parties to the relationship often have informal leadership. It is in these off-chart relationships that HIM professionals often have the opportunity to exert their leadership skills. The need arises here to inspire one's colleagues to collaborate in order to achieve the common goal of timely record completion, clean claims, or quality data.

## Leadership

Leadership inspires others—to accomplish, to perform, or to follow—in a similar manner or on a certain course to achieve common goals for the department or organization. Sometimes people use the terms *leadership* and *management* interchangeably. However, it is important to understand the difference. Management can be described as ensuring that the tasks, processes, or tools associated with the work are performed within established standards. A manager will make sure that all of the discharged records are analyzed, coded, and billed correctly and on a timely basis. A skilled leader provides support and encouragement for others to take on challenges and change with a positive, purposeful attitude. While we tend to think of managers as leaders, and they may very well be, there is not necessarily a direct correlation. Managers direct and control subordinates in order to get them to perform. Leaders inspire others to perform. Note that the organization chart defines the management relationships in an organization. Leadership—the ability to influence others to achieve a common purpose—can happen anywhere in an organization.

There are many styles of leadership, each with its own characteristics. Work in the department is affected by the HIM department director's leadership style. The three major categories of leadership are autocratic, democratic, and *laissez-faire*.

The *autocratic* leader controls everything. Employees function under strict control of this manager. All operations and decisions are overseen by this type of leader. Autocratic leaders are sometimes called *micromanagers* because they

---

❖ **COMPETENCY CHECK-IN 9.4**

**Communication**

**Competency Assessment**

1. A written/typed communication tool used to communicate or provide information to members of an organization is a
   _____.
2. _____ are used to record the events, topics, and discussions of a meeting.
3. An _____ is used to organize the topics to be discussed during a meeting.
4. The first item on the monthly HIM department meeting agenda is:
   a. call to order
   b. review of old business
   c. new business
   d. adjournment
5. What is the first step in conflict resolution?
   a. Listen to both sides
   b. Contact the HR department
   c. Affirm the value of each side's point of view
   d. Assess a compromise
6. Which is true of an email message?
   a. It is private and confidential
   b. The recipient will read the message faster than a letter
   c. Spelling and grammar are optional
   d. It should end with the sender's name, title, and business address

oversee even the smallest details of the department. The autocratic leader focuses on efficiency of decision-making. Dialogue tends to be one way.

The *democratic* leader allows all employees to provide input in decision-making or operations of the department. He or she seeks input and then typically makes decisions on the basis of this feedback. This style is considered most effective as it increases both productivity and morale.

The *laissez-faire* leader allows the employees to run the department and gets involved only when assistance is requested. This is a true "hands-off" manager. The *laissez-faire* style is effective when team members are very experienced and trustworthy.

Although thousands of books have been written about the qualities of effective leadership, here are a few points to consider.

- Leaders *delegate* for several reasons: to be more efficient handling duties or responsibilities, to empower others and allow them to own a responsibility in the organization, and to create partnerships or relationships between management and staff. Delegating can allow employees to share in the department's or organization's success!
- Leaders *lead* by example. In the workplace, people tend to gauge their behavior by the actions of those around them, but perhaps none more so than those of their supervisor. Exemplary behavior sets the tone, encouraging the best from the organization.
- Leaders *support* the staff by both praising in public and coaching in private.
- Leaders *identify and remove* obstacles that keep staff from doing their jobs; whether ensuring the right equipment, the right workload, or the right processes, leaders are supportive in a problem-solving role.
- Leaders *are accessible*, often by having a so-called open-door policy, which allows employees to enter the office anytime to share information and ask questions.
- Leaders *encourage* continuous improvement and provide an environment in which employees feel welcome to share their suggestions.
- Leaders *develop* the staff—an investment in an employee ensures performance, both in his or her current position and in his or her further career. Career counseling can inspire others to do their best, and advancement within the organization can create networks of individuals who have a common goal.

Because leadership can occur anywhere in the organization, HIM professionals can create opportunities through leadership, beginning by effectively managing themselves and demonstrating a commitment to the work and providing added value to the organization. Here are some examples.

- Focus continuing education (CE) on acquiring and enhancing relevant skills (such as public speaking or technical writing) and on broadening knowledge (such as financial accounting or data analytics).
- Maintain a positive attitude in establishing and maintaining intra- and interdepartmental relationships.

- Manage yourself by refraining from participating in gossip and other negative behaviors.
- Polish oral and communication skills.
- Learn the organization. Know your administrators and key management in addition to your own department colleagues.
- Network with your peers in other organizations. Stay in touch with classmates and individuals you meet at external meetings.
- Attend conferences for CE and to network.
- Volunteer with your local HIM organization to develop your leadership skills and gain insight into current issues in your area.
- Eliminate the phrase "that's not my job" from your vocabulary. Every moment you are at work, be aware of opportunities to assist someone else: a lost patient, a confused volunteer, or a harried coworker. Sometimes a kind word is all it takes.
- Exceed expectations in your own work.

## Diversity

Health care as an industry attracts workers and serves patients from a wide diversity of backgrounds. It is important that, within the organization, there is both an expectation and a corporate culture of professionalism when dealing with individuals from different backgrounds. This is so important that the AHIMA Code of Ethics includes this standard.

*XI. Respect the inherent dignity and worth of every person.*
*A health information management professional* **shall**:
  *11.1. Treat each person in a respectful fashion, being mindful of individual differences and cultural and ethnic diversity.*
  *11.2. Promote the value of self-determination for each individual.*
  *11.3. Value all kinds and classes of people equitably, deal effectively with all races, cultures, disabilities, ages and genders.*
  *11.4. Ensure all voices are listened to and respected.*

AHIMA Code of Ethics. Revised & adopted by AHIMA House of Delegates. http://bok.ahima.org/codeofethics#.XE7e_FxKhPY. Published October 2, 2011. Accessed January 28, 2019.

Professionalism in this area is not just a "tolerance" of others, but rather **cultural competence**. By cultural competence, we mean the ability to work with others and deliver care to patients in a way that meets their needs: culture, language, and customs, for example.

Since we have acknowledged the importance of teams in a health care organization, we must discuss diversity. In simplest terms, **diversity** refers to the differences that exist among or between team members. Those differences, which make a team diverse, can be any number of varied things such as age, race, position, length of service in the organization, education, and abilities or disabilities.

Can you think of other differences not listed here? Teamwork is inevitably affected by diversity, hopefully in a positive manner, but sometimes it represents obstacles for the team that have an impact on performance. Team members must be able to perform their duties in a way that is not disruptive.

Diversity training can be an effective way to educate team members so that they perform in a respectable manner. This training would include:

- identification of the many and varied ways that people are different;
- a global perspective of how many specific types of people there are in the world; for example, the percentage of people in the following categories: men/women, level of education, religious affiliation, financial class, languages, sexual preference, and so on;
- how these differences might influence a person's behavior (can be done with scenarios and using group activities);
- review of cultural assumptions, biases, and stereotypes related to the things that make people different;
- self-assessment of cultural diversity, personally and of others;
- best practices for handling situations related to diversity; and
- activities that ask each participant to draw an object or do something and then discuss how differently the task was done by the participants.

Diversity can be a very positive and necessary part of teamwork. However, it is important for team members to have an awareness of diversity so that diversity is not disruptive. Training and support for a diverse population are not only an ethical responsibility of all HIM professionals; there are laws and regulations that require this activity. For example, the ADA prohibits discrimination against individuals with disabilities and requires reasonable accommodations for employees faced with these challenges. Various governmental agencies support enforcement of this and other legal issues, including the Equal Employment Opportunity Commission (EEOC) and the Office for Civil Rights. Private organizations, such as the American Civil Liberties Union, also provide training and support for issues related to diversity.

In a 2005 article, Beach et al. describe evidence that cultural competence training improved not only the knowledge and attitudes of practitioners but also patient satisfaction. Training methods included discussions, case studies, interviews, and audiovisual presentations, for example. Although their literature review focused on clinical professionals, the results of the studies were generally consistent in that cultural competence training is beneficial to the clinician/patient relationship (Beach et al., 2005).

In 2008 TJC published a study that detailed four themes for the engagement of providers in diversity and cultural competence. The four themes are as follows:

- Theme 1: Building a Foundation. Establishing a foundation of policies and procedures that systemically support cultural competencies, a crucial component of meeting the needs of diverse patient populations.
- Theme 2: Collecting and Using Data to Improve Services. The collection and use of community- and patient-level data is essential to developing and improving services in health care, including services developed to meet the needs of diverse patient populations.
- Theme 3: Accommodating the Needs of Specific Populations. Accommodating the needs of specific populations includes practices aimed at providing safe, quality care and decreasing health disparities for particular populations in the service community.
- Theme 4: Establishing Internal and External Collaborations. Collaborative practices encompass those that bring together multiple departments, organizations, providers, and individuals to achieve objectives related to culturally and linguistically appropriate care (Wilson-Stronks et al., 2008).

Throughout the report, there is an emphasis on flexibility with respect to the environment of the health care organization and a specific identification of the communities being served.

In 2015 the American Hospital Association released *Equity of Care: A Toolkit for Eliminating Health Care Disparities*, which is both a compendium of resources and a call to action: improve the collection of accurate diversity data, increase cultural competence through training, and expand diversity within the executive and governance levels (Equity of Care Committee, American Hospital Association, 2015).

These examples serve to highlight the emphasis being placed on cultural competence throughout the health care industry. The CLAS consist of 15 action steps that organizations can take to "advance health equity, improve quality, and help eliminate health care disparities by providing a blueprint for individuals and health and health care organizations to implement culturally and linguistically appropriate services." The standards are reproduced in Box 9.4.

Several of the CLAS standards target the organization itself and would, if implemented, support the creation of a sustainable organizational culture of diversity and cultural competence. Basically, the organization should set the tone at the top, hire a diverse workforce that is on board with the concept, keep training the workforce to stay on top of it, tell everyone what you're doing, and keep improving.

Circling back to work teams, we can see that a strong organizational culture that embraces diversity and is culturally competent will yield a rewarding experience for all of the team members. Effective teams consist of skilled members who have respect for one another and confidence in their teammates. Other factors such as leadership, collaboration, communication, and cooperation support this teamwork.

> **• BOX 9.4    National Standards on Culturally and Linguistically Appropriate Services**
>
> Principal Standard:
> 1. Provide effective, equitable, understandable, and respectful quality care and services that are responsive to diverse cultural health beliefs and practices, preferred languages, health literacy, and other communication needs.
>
> Governance, Leadership, and Workforce:
> 2. Advance and sustain organizational governance and leadership that promotes CLAS and health equity through policy, practices, and allocated resources.
> 3. Recruit, promote, and support a culturally and linguistically diverse governance, leadership, and workforce that are responsive to the population in the service area.
> 4. Educate and train governance, leadership, and workforce in culturally and linguistically appropriate policies and practices on an ongoing basis.
>
> Communication and Language Assistance:
> 5. Offer language assistance to individuals who have limited English proficiency and/or other communication needs, at no cost to them, to facilitate timely access to all health care and services.
> 6. Inform all individuals of the availability of language assistance services clearly and in their preferred language, verbally and in writing.
> 7. Ensure the competence of individuals providing language assistance, recognizing that the use of untrained individuals and/or minors as interpreters should be avoided.
>
> 8. Provide easy-to-understand print and multimedia materials and signage in the languages commonly used by the populations in the service area.
>
> Engagement, Continuous Improvement, and Accountability:
> 9. Establish culturally and linguistically appropriate goals, policies, and management accountability, and infuse them throughout the organization's planning and operations.
> 10. Conduct ongoing assessments of the organization's CLAS-related activities and integrate CLAS-related measures into measurement and continuous quality-improvement activities.
> 11. Collect and maintain accurate and reliable demographic data to monitor and evaluate the impact of CLAS on health equity and outcomes and to inform service delivery.
> 12. Conduct regular assessments of community health assets and needs, and use the results to plan and implement services that respond to the cultural and linguistic diversity of populations in the service area.
> 13. Partner with the community to design, implement, and evaluate policies, practices, and services to ensure cultural and linguistic appropriateness.
> 14. Create conflict- and grievance-resolution processes that are culturally and linguistically appropriate to identify, prevent, and resolve conflicts or complaints.
> 15. Communicate the organization's progress in implementing and sustaining CLAS to all stakeholders, constituents, and the general public.
>
> (U.S. Department of Health & Human Services Office of Minority Health, n.d.).

> **COMPETENCY CHECK-IN 9.5**
>
> **Interpersonal Skills**
>
> **Competency Assessment**
> 1. Which type of leader is receptive to employee feedback?
>    a. Laissez-faire
>    b. Democratic
>    c. Autocratic
>    d. Paternalistic
> 2. List the reasons a leader should delegate responsibilities to others.
> 3. Explain diversity and give examples of it.
> 4. What kinds of topics would be included in diversity training?

## Training and Development

**Training** is an important part of all jobs. A well-managed HIM department spends considerable time on the training and development of its employees. Training involves orientation, education, and practical application for a specific HIM job position. Development is the ongoing improvement of staff professionally. The HIM director is responsible for the hiring, training, development, and retention of employees who perform all department functions. Training is essential to the HIM department; well-trained employees provide high-quality service. Training is necessary at many times: at the beginning of employment, as procedures and policies change and processes are improved, and as technology and equipment are improved. Development is equally important because it improves the quality of service. A department that develops its employees is making an investment in the quality of its future service.

Employees obviously need training when they begin a job, but they need it just as much when processes, procedures, and equipment are changed. Training is the education of employees in techniques and processes within the organization. It is provided to employees in the health care facility through **in-service** training sessions: seminars, workshops, and CE.

**Development** is a term that can be used to describe training, but more specifically, it indicates an investment by the organization—in an employee—with the expectation that the development will indeed pay off in the future performance of the employee. For instance, an employee is hired to perform ROI. Over time and with experience, the managers recognize that this employee could be developed for a supervisor position. Development is an investment in the employee, enhancing skills and increasing his or her ability to perform necessary job duties. The organization will see their *return on investment* when the employee is able to perform a new job duty or take on additional responsibilities. Consequently, the employee is likely to feel valued and empowered.

## Planning a Training Session

### Assessment of Education Needs

Training sessions should be planned with specific goals in mind, because they are essential to successful staff development. The first step in planning a training session involves an assessment of current staff training needs. The assessment helps the HIM director identify which areas need focus. Training topics can be identified through the following means:

- **Performance standard reviews**: There may be a trend in the analysis of employee performance in an area that warrants attention through training.
- **Job analysis**: In observing staff, variations from written procedures may be observed. A job analysis will reveal whether this is a training opportunity or the procedure needs to be changed.
- **Employee surveys**: Employees may be asked to identify areas they would like to learn more about.
- **Updated or new equipment**: Any time there is a change in equipment, training must take place to ensure safe, efficient, and effective use of the equipment.
- **Legal, regulatory, policy, or procedure changes**: Role-specific training is required for changes that affect employees or the performance of their jobs.

Changes in procedure and employee desire to learn new things may be ideal opportunities for **cross-training**, which teaches employees how to perform tasks that are part of someone else's job description. Cross-training is a way to prepare a department to handle increased workloads and vacant positions when employees are on a break or lunch hour, are out sick, are on vacation, or have left their positions. It can also provide job enrichment for some employees. Care must be taken to cross-train at the same or lower pay grade to avoid employee dissatisfaction. Cross-training to a higher pay grade is generally reserved for employees who are being groomed for promotion or who have specifically asked to be cross-trained to obtain the additional skill in the target area.

### Learning Objectives

Based on the assessment of education needs, each training should have specific learning objectives. These objectives will drive the content of the training and make clear to the learner what is expected of them at the end of the training.

Examples:

The department has just installed a new photocopier. Staff are permitted to make copies, load paper, and scan documents to internal email accounts. All other tasks may only be performed by personnel with additional training. The two objectives of the general staff training might be:

At the end of the training session, each employee will be able to:

1. Demonstrate the following copier functions with 100% accuracy:
   a. Copy a single sheet
   b. Copy two-sided
   c. Copy two-sided to two-sided
   d. Scan a document to an internal email account
   e. Load a ream of letter size paper into Tray 1
2. Explain the procedure to follow to obtain assistance with any other functions with 100% accuracy.
3. Explain the procedure to follow if service is needed on the copier with 100% accuracy.

This example illustrates both the desired outcome of the hands-on training and the reinforcement of the department policy limiting the individuals who are permitted to perform other than basic tasks.

Objectives are not limited to hands-on tasks or recall/ recognition of policy and procedure. Interpersonal communication, cultural literacy, and customer service demeanor are all trainings that would require a different type of objective. For example, customer service training may require the attendee to *demonstrate a friendly, calm demeanor when confronted with an irate individual*. Remember that objectives are a communication tool. The instructor, the attendee, and the attendee's manager will all know the desired outcome of the training.

### Audience

An important part of planning a training session is learning about the audience. The presenters do not have to know each person individually, but they should know the participants' backgrounds. These backgrounds, with regard to education and work-related experience, tell the presenters how to begin the training. When the topic is new to the audience, the presenters begin with an elementary overview of the topic. If participants are knowledgeable about the topic and have practical experience, the training session can be more advanced. Additionally, knowing the backgrounds of participants affects the organization of the presentation, that is, the vocabulary and knowledge pertinent to the audience. For example, significantly different vocabulary words and examples are used to train experienced physicians (myocardial infarction) compared with those used to train the general public (heart attack).

### Format

There are many different learning styles, and it follows that training should provide information in a variety of formats. Training formats can be passive, active, or collaborative. Traditional lectures are passive; the trainer does all the talking, and the trainees just listen to learn. Active training requires that the employees/trainees participate in some activity to achieve the learning outcome, and collaborative learning puts trainees in groups to work together to learn. The best training incorporates all of these formats to ensure that employees learn what is intended by the training.

The format of a training session explains how the information or topic will be presented. For example, will the training take place as a lecture, or will it be hands-on? Will the presentation include a video or demonstration? Will there be an instructor or a self-guided manual? The format is determined by the topic of the presentation and the audience. It is very important to explain the purpose of the training to the attendees. The explanation will allow them to examine how this new skill or information will be required in the performance of their jobs. If the topic involves procedures and use of equipment, a demonstration that includes hands-on participation by each attendee will enhance their understanding. Another common training session involves explaining annual coding updates. This type of training should involve explanation, examples, and case studies so that the coders can practice applying the new coding guidelines.

The format of the presentation also determines whether the presenter needs audiovisual equipment. If the training session involves a video, access to that video must be available in the training room. Other audiovisual equipment includes overhead projectors, slide projectors, computer equipment with speakers and video capability, and microphones.

## Environment

The location of the training session is another element that can be determined by the topic of the presentation and the audience. Training sessions can be held in classrooms or auditoriums, via video conference or the Internet, or in the HIM department. If the training requires demonstration of equipment, the training should happen near the equipment, or a demonstration model should be available in the classroom. The location of the training session is also affected by the number of participants. The larger the audience, the more space is required. Sometimes multiple sessions can be held to accommodate a large number of participants. However, if the number of participants is small, the training session may be held in the HIM department. If audience members are expected to take notes, chairs at tables or desks should be considered. If a computer terminal is used for the training, make sure there is adequate seating for one person per computer.

Because of the increased performance expectations in health care organizations, many employers are looking for efficient and effective methods to train their employees. One method being used is online training. Training that can occur *asynchronously*—whenever any employee is available or able to fit it into the work schedule—is one advantage of online methods. *Synchronous* learning happens when the learner and the instructor are together, whether in person or online. Asynchronous learning can occur as a result of recorded materials or presentations (e.g., Microsoft PowerPoint).

### Technology Training

With all of the technological advances that occur in today's health care environment, equipment and computer software are continuously being updated and replaced. These changes certainly require training. Imagine the scenario in which a new time clock system for payroll is implemented. Leaders in the organization must create a presentation to explain the new time clock system and provide a method for employees to practice using the new system to clock in and out of work.

Now imagine the case of a more involved training scenario—implementation of a new computerized physician order entry (CPOE) system. Leaders in the organization need to prepare training for many different users: nurses, physicians, pharmacists, and HIM employees. For a training scenario like this, the vendor (product seller) is often very helpful in providing a test environment for practice, tutorials for online training, and onsite workshops to "train the trainers" in the organization. This training requires coordination of efforts between the health care organization and the vendor. Communication from the leadership to the employees and medical staff is needed to explain the purpose and usefulness of the CPOE. Sometimes, a webpage on the health care organization's Intranet can be created to provide additional video tutorials, information about the product, a training calendar, and contact information for technical support. At each step of the implementation process, the project leader should communicate with the organization to keep everyone informed about the progress.

## Calendar of Education

How often should employees be trained? At a minimum, all employees in the facility should receive annual role-based training in customer service, quality, safety, infection control, confidentiality and security, and body mechanics. Additional training sessions may be required for risk management, accreditation, or related to an employee's job function or as the need arises.

In addition to credential CE requirements, several HIM positions (regardless of employee credentials) require routine training, particularly in the areas of coding and ROI (Table 9.9). Coding employees should participate in quarterly training sessions. Inpatient coding changes occur twice a year, in April and October; these changes affect all of the employees responsible for inpatient coding. A training session should be organized to inform these employees of any upcoming coding changes that will affect their jobs. Outpatient coding changes occur in January. A training session should be organized accordingly to cover these changes. Additionally, other regulations, such as the implementation of prospective payment systems, occur at various times during the year and require further training sessions. Employees who handle ROI requests should receive annual training, and additional sessions should be organized when there

| TABLE 9.9 | Areas of Routine Training | | |
|-----------|--------------------------|---|---|
| Employee | Changes | | Time Frame |
| Inpatient coder | Annual coding changes | | April and October |
| Outpatient coder | Annual coding changes | | January |
| Release of information clerk | Regulatory (federal and state law) changes | | As needed; review sources daily |
| Revenue cycle manager | Regulatory (federal and state law) changes | | As needed; review sources daily |
| All employees | The Joint Commission, Health Insurance Portability and Accountability Act, and U.S. Occupational Safety and Health Administration requirements | | Annually |

are changes in federal or state laws that affect the release of health information.

It is very important that a record be kept of employee attendance at training sessions. The record of an employee's attendance supports the communication of a new policy, procedure, or method required as a part of his or her job.

A sign-in sheet should be used to document employee attendance. The heading at the top of the sign-in sheet should include the date the topic is covered and the objectives that apply. This sign-in sheet can be kept in a binder to record employee education, or the information can be transferred to each employee's file. In addition, the information can be transferred to a computer system to track employee education.

Training is an ongoing process. Often it is important to involve other departments so that employees learn the necessary information from the appropriate source. Some topics can be coordinated with members of other departments, such as quality management, nursing, infection control, and business. All of the employees who are affected by the new information, including employees who work at home, should participate in the training (Fig. 9.19).

## Evaluating the Training Program

There are several levels of evaluation that should take place with respect to training. First, the individual in-service or other training should have two levels of evaluation:

- Did the attendees achieve the objectives? If not, what should be done about that? What triggers retraining?
- What is the attendees' feedback regarding the training? A participant satisfaction survey is appropriate.

Attendee feedback is particularly important if the organization is conducting CE for the purpose of credential maintenance. The expectations of professional CE are different from an employee learning a necessary skill or compliance with a regulatory requirement.

Typically, employees attend training once; then they are expected to take role-based action on the training they received. So, one result of training on infection control would be employees paying closer attention to performing appropriate handwashing behaviors. Supervisory observation of handwashing by employees may detect a lack of compliance on the part of one or more staff. While disciplinary action may occur at that point, it is also possible that retraining would also be required. A widespread lack of compliance may indicate a deficiency in the training itself.

Some training sessions, such as HIPAA-related privacy and security, infection control, and safety, may take place every year. While it may seem as though annual trainings are "always the same," it is likely that new data will be discussed or regulatory updates be presented. The currency of these programs is at issue and the organization must ensure that it is conveying the appropriate, timely material. These trainings are typically mandatory and failure to attend needs follow-up by HR to ensure completion.

All training should be evaluated periodically for unnecessary components, appropriate audience, and outdated material. New training should be considered, for example, when there is a change in regulation, organizational or departmental policy, and compliance issues.

There is a cost involved in developing and delivering training. Some of the cost is associated with the physical preparation of materials, such as handouts. Other costs are the "opportunity cost" of the trainer or the employee–trainer lost time doing something else. For example, a coding supervisor who needs to provide quarterly coding updates to staff will have to devote a significant amount of time to that activity rather than auditing employee work or analyzing DNFB reports. That use of the employee–trainer's time can be balanced against the cost of hiring an outside trainer. Either way, the return on investment of training is not always a financial calculation. Depending on the perspective of the organization, some benefits of training can be:

**TJC Mandatory Annual Inservices**

| Topic | Date of attendance MM/DD/YYYY | Employee Initials | Witness Initials |
|---|---|---|---|
| HIPAA | | | |
| Fire and electrical safety in a health care facility (could be 2 separate) | | | |
| Cultural diversity and sensitivity | | | |
| Universal precautions | | | |
| Hazardous materials | | | |
| Infection control | | | |
| Blood-borne pathogens, hepatitis, AIDS | | | |
| Age-appropriate care | | | |
| Patient lifting, moving, restraints | | | |
| Yearly national safety goals | | | |
| N95 Respirator fitting and training | | | |

_____          _____
Signature of employee                        Signature of witness

Original to Human Resource employee file
Copy for employee and HIM Department file

• **Fig. 9.19** Form showing employee attendance at The Joint Commission's mandatory annual in-service training sessions.

- improvement in a key performance indicator, such as coding accuracy;
- compliance with regulatory requirements;
- compliance with corporate policies and procedures;
- improvement in employee retention;
- improvement in employee satisfaction; and
- improvement in employee evaluation scores.

Determining the return on investment, then, goes back to the purpose of the training in the first place.

## Educating the Public

Health care professionals are often called on to educate the public about changes in laws relating to health care or health information, as well as health-related topics, such as cancer awareness, diabetes, and infectious diseases. New technology like a personal health record, mobile apps, health information exchanges, and patient portals will also need to be explained to the community. When preparing workshops or presentations, the topics associated with planning a training session for employees can be modified for use in planning a training session for the public.

HIM professionals interact with so many people, including patients. We can no longer think of ourselves as the ones who "do not have patient contact." Our expertise and guidance are needed to help transition our patients to access their health information electronically. HIM managers can serve as leaders, providing training to patients so that meaningful uses of health information can be achieved with EHRs. We can use the same skills and talents required to manage employees or create training when we are working with patients or external customers.

## Continuing Education

Education does not stop simply because a person has completed a degree or program or obtained employment. Professionals understand that education will continue over the course of their careers. All HIM professionals should recognize that their credentials are accompanied by a commitment to lifelong learning. In all health care fields, regulations change, technology advances, and processes improve. Because of such changes, you must continue your education as it relates to your job, your career, and your special interests—whether the employer provides that education or not.

Keeping a record of professional **continuing education (CE)** hours is very important. Because CE periods vary with each association, it is difficult to remember all of the hours earned unless you maintain personal attendance records. The easiest method for keeping track of CE hours is to designate a file folder for material from the meetings you attended, journal article questionnaires you submitted, and website tutorials you completed. Using a summary form in the file folder provides a quick reference for how many hours have been completed (Fig. 9.20). This file folder and tracking form are also helpful in the

event of an audit of CE hours. Using this file folder and tracking form makes it easier to fill out the CE form when a report of your CE hours is due. Additionally, some organizations, such as the AHIMA, allow their members to track and maintain a record of their CE hours online (Fig. 9.21). HIM department managers should also maintain records of CE of credentialed employees when the job requires maintenance of credentials. It is the responsibility of the credential holder to ensure that all appropriate CE is obtained on a timely basis. Credentialing bodies publish their requirements for recertification on their websites. For example, AHIMA's recertification requirements are here: http://www.ahima.org/certification/Recertification.

Continuing education for: _____

No. of hours needed: _____

Cycle ends: _____

| Date | Topic/Title | Location | Core Content Area | No. of Hours |
|------|-------------|----------|-------------------|--------------|
|      |             |          |                   |              |
|      |             |          |                   |              |
|      |             |          |                   |              |
|      |             |          |                   |              |
|      |             |          |                   |              |
|      |             |          |                   |              |
|      |             |          |                   |              |
|      |             |          |                   |              |
|      |             |          |                   |              |
|      |             |          |                   |              |
|      |             |          |                   |              |
|      |             |          |                   |              |
|      |             |          |                   |              |
|      |             |          |                   |              |
|      |             |          |                   |              |
|      |             |          |                   |              |

• **Fig. 9.20** Continuing education tracking form.

**Personal CEU Log**

| Nature | Activity | Sponsor | Completed | CEUs Claimed | Category | Documentation |
|--------|----------|---------|-----------|--------------|----------|---------------|
| Webinar | Health Care Reform | HFMA | 11/15/20XX | 1 | External Forces | CEU form |
| In person | 2019 National Convention —General Session | AHIMA | 06/07/20XX | 2 | Management Development | CEU form |
| Author | Foundations of HIM List by chapters | Elsevier | 12/15/20XX | 30 | Management Development Performance Improvement External Forces Clinical Data Management | Copyright page Title page Table of Contents |
| Speaker | CSA meeting—Coding update | DHIMA | 09/15/20XX | 4 | Clinical Data Management | CEU form |
| In person | CSA meeting—Revenue Cycle | NJHIMA | 10/20/20XX | 3 | Performance Improvement | CEU form |

• **Fig. 9.21** Using your professional association's online CEU tracker helps to keep track of progress throughout the cycle. Here is a log that represents the information you typically need to record your CEUs into an online tracker. Review your professional association's current recertification guide for the exact number of CEUs pertaining to a particular activity.

❖ **COMPETENCY CHECK-IN 9.6**

**Training and Development**

**Competency Assessment**

1. A general term for education, instruction, or demonstration of how to perform a job is _____.
2. A name for the training provided to employees of an organization is _____.
3. _____ may be required after attaining a position, credential, or degree intended to keep those persons knowledgeable in core content areas.
4. Continuing education is critical for coding employees. Which of the following dates is critical in the education of inpatient coders?
   a. January 1
   b. October 1 and April 1
   c. December 1
   d. July 1
5. Explain the important items to consider in the preparation of a training presentation.
6. Identify two HIM functions that require annual (at a minimum) training of employees.

# Chapter Summary

The management of health information includes the management of the people performing HIM functions. Appropriate organization and management of the department's HR significantly affects the quality of health information. A great place to begin effective management is in the clear communication of the employee's responsibilities in the job description and the performance standards for the position.

HIM supervisors and managers are responsible for the daily operations of the HIM department, as well as future planning in keeping with the facility's mission and vision. Establishing mechanisms to monitor the quality and productivity of HIM functions keeps the daily operations on track. To guide the department into the future, HIM managers must plan, set goals and objectives,

and navigate the transition to the EHR. The system development life cycle—selection, design, implementation, evaluation, and support—of the EHR, transition to ICD-10, or any major changes in software products will certainly capitalize the time and attention of HIM managers. Therefore knowledge of health information, combined with management skills, sets the stage for continuous efficient and effective management of HIM departments.

Training and development are critical to the ongoing success of the HIM department. These efforts and activities make it possible for HIM employees to remain competent and knowledgeable about changing technology, policy, legislative, regulatory, and accreditation requirements. New employees in the organization, whether they are HIM, medical staff, nursing, or other professionals, must be oriented to the organization and trained in HIM-related issues, including the confidentiality and security of patient information mandated by HIPAA. Training continues beyond the orientation stage; for example, employees must participate in ongoing training efforts to maintain CE hours, remain knowledgeable about current requirements (i.e., coding and ROI), and become skilled users of new technology that is part of their job responsibilities. Annually, the entire staff must be reminded of the requirements related to their jobs and the entire health care organization as mandated by accrediting agencies. Changes that occur as a result of quality-improvement efforts are another reason for continuous training of staff. Development of the employees in the health care organization, through training, continuous education, and communication, creates an environment in which both the employees and the organization are positioned for continued success.

## Competency Milestones

### CAHIIM Competency

*I.6. **DM** Evaluate data dictionaries and data sets for compliance with governance standards. (5)*

### Rationale

Understanding of data elements and data requirements supports HIM professionals in their work. Database management skills apply that understanding to stronger support for data quality and quality compliance initiatives.

### Competency Assessment

1. Explain the difference between information governance and data governance.
2. With respect to the creation of data dictionaries, which standards would apply?
3. With respect to the reporting of data sets, which standards would apply?
4. Your HIM committee has reviewed a request from a clinical department to change the "amend data" permissions for patient demographic data to allow physician office personnel—who already have limited "view only" access—to change patient address and insurance data in the hospital system. What is your response?

### CAHIIM Competency

*VI. 1. Demonstrate fundamental leadership skills. (3)*

### Rationale

HIM professionals can lead from wherever they are. Awareness of leadership skills helps to understand weaknesses that can be overcome with CE.

### Competency Assessment

1. Explain the purpose of an organization chart.
2. Explain the difference between unity of command and span of control.
3. Explain three aspects of leadership and provide an example of how they can be accomplished.
4. Differentiate between data governance and information governance.
5. Write a policy that addresses hospital compliance with TJC incomplete chart rules.
6. Explain the importance of the meeting agenda and minutes.
7. In the United States, a handshake is a common form of greeting between business associates. Practice your handshake with classmates. What makes a good handshake?
8. You are cross-trained in ROI and analysis. Today you are working in analysis, but you know they are shorthanded in ROI today. You estimate that you can finish your work queue by 3 p.m. if you put in a little extra effort and nothing distracting happens. That would leave you a couple of hours to help out in ROI. What are you obligated to do? What would a leader do?
9. Identify some of the considerations that will affect the priority for workflow in the HIM department.

### CAHIIM Competency

*VI.3. Identify human resource strategies for organizational best practices. (3)*

## Rationale

HR are the backbone of the organization, touching every part of the employer–employee relationship. Through HR initiatives, employees are hired, trained, evaluated, disciplined, and evaluated. The HR department also ensures that the organization is in compliance with all laws and regulations governing employment.

## Competency Assessment

1. How can the HR department assist the HIM department managers/supervisors?
2. A(n) _____ works an average of 30 hours each week including overtime, earning health care benefits as offered by the health care facility.
3. The HIM department has 30 employees who work an average of 995 hours per week. If the standard hours for a full-time employee are 37.5, how many FTEs does the department have? (Round your answer to the nearest tenth.) Why are not there not 30 FTEs?
4. The patient access department has told you that they have 25 employees but 30 FTEs. What might you say in response?
5. Explain the best method of delivering an employee evaluation.
6. How is the content of the job description related to compliance with the Americans with Disabilities Act (ADA)?
7. The HIM department is allowed 450 hours per week. This equals how many FTEs, based on a 40-hour work week?
   a. 4.5
   b. 22.5
   c. 11.25
   d. 45
8. The amount of work in the HIM department is determined by:
   a. the CEO
   b. the department director
   c. admissions
   d. the number of discharges, patient type, and LOS
9. What is the purpose of performance standards?
10. Explain one method of determining performance standards for HIM functions.
11. You recently lost a coder at your facility. The department director has asked that you, the coding supervisor, create an advertisement for the local newspaper and participate in the interview for this vacant position. Using your knowledge of hiring practices, create an advertisement for this new position. Before the interview, document at least three questions that you would like to ask the applicant.

### CAHIIM Competency
*VI.6. Examine behaviors that embrace cultural diversity. (4)*

## Rationale

Cultural competence is a necessary skill in today's workforce. Eliminating discrimination and bias is not just a matter of law; it is an ethical mandate in accordance with professionalism. Moreover, working with a diverse group of people results in better patient relationships and helps eliminate health disparities.

## Competency Assessment

1. Explain cultural competence.
2. One of your registrars is registering a patient who is deaf and is accompanied by a sign language interpreter. You notice that she speaks directly to the interpreter and looks only at the interpreter when the interpreter is answering for the patient. What additional training does this registrar need? Find a resource to share with the registrar. If you are not sure, look up "communicating with the deaf and hard of hearing."
3. You are working in a multi-physician gynecologist's office and are completing the end-of-visit process with the patient. The patient seems upset and you ask her if she is OK. The patient unloads on you that she is a lesbian in a long-term, committed relationship and was offended by the intake questionnaire and the doctor's persistence in discussing "safe sex" and birth control options. What problem does this encounter highlight and how could you begin to have an appropriate conversation within your organization?
4. Create an agenda for a workshop on diversity.

### CAHIIM Competency
*VI.9. Identify processes of workforce training for health care organizations. (3)*

### Rationale

Training represents a commitment to your own success as a professional, as well as the organization's commitment to you as an investment. HIM professionals should be prepared to learn, develop, and teach others throughout their careers.

### Competency Assessment

1. The new employee attends a(n) _____to become familiar with a job and the facility.
   a. training
   b. orientation
   c. in-service
   d. department meeting
2. List and briefly explain the issues discussed in the organization-wide orientation.
3. What topics are important to cover in an HIM department physician orientation?
4. Which is the first step in planning a training, in-service, or CE program?
   a. Assessment of education needs
   b. Audience
   c. Area
   d. Inventory of skills
5. What happens if an employee is not properly trained? What are the risks associated with having an employee perform a job duty or task for which he or she has not been trained?
6. Why is it important for an effective leader to spend time developing staff members?
7. A hospital was recently purchased by a large health care organization and will implement a new enterprise-wide master patient index. Plan training for the HIM and patient access staff.
8. Plan training for coders or ROI employees. What will be covered? How will it be presented? Where will it be presented? Will it require any handouts? How will you record employee attendance? What will happen if one of the employees is not present?

## CAHIM Competency

*VI.7. Assess ethical standards of practice. (5)*

### Rationale

Although ethics permeate every aspect of HIM practice, individuals in leadership roles have a particular responsibility to demonstrate and guide ethical behavior.

### Competency Assessment

1. There are 12 students in your class, all women. You are discussing problems with physician chart completion and the difficulties some facilities have in keeping their delinquency rates down. One of the female students chimes in, "It does not matter what you do—if it is a man, he will not listen to anything you say." Most of the class finds this amusing. Do you? What would you do or say if this happened in your classroom? What should the instructor do? Would your answer be different if there were men in the class?

## Critical Thinking Questions

1. What qualities of a leader do you already possess? How have you demonstrated those qualities?
2. Poll your classmates who are employed to find out what the working hours are at their employment. Consider expanding your inquiry to include parents, friends, and relatives. Can you see a pattern or differences between industries?
3. If you were to apply for a new job next week, who would you list as references? What would those individuals say about your work? Consider having that discussion now.
4. Research the current issues associated with health information. Choose a topic that requires education of the local community (the public). Using the training session information in this chapter, perform an assessment of community education needs. In your preparation, consider the audience, the format, and the environment in which the education will be provided. Prepare a paper presentation of this information for your instructor.

# The Role of Health Information Management Professionals in the Workplace

**Professional Profile:**

### Health Information Management Director

My name is Beth Catherine, and I am the director of the health information management (HIM) department at Diamonte.

My responsibilities include overseeing the operations of the department and planning and organizing the direction of health information operations. I attend several meetings each week. I am a member of the quality management committee and the risk management committee. I am also the coordinator for the HIM committee. As coordinator, I work closely with the chairman of the committee, a member of the medical staff, to organize the meetings, coordinate record reviews, and compile minutes of the meetings.

I also attend a monthly meeting with all the department directors, at which we share important information about our department operations, perform facility-wide strategic planning, and receive communication from administration.

Once a month, I hold a department meeting for all HIM employees. During the meeting, we discuss department business and quality, and employees receive updates about various things that are occurring throughout the facility.

My education began at a community college where I earned an associate's degree in Health Information Technology. The program was accredited by CAHIIM, so I was able to sit for the RHIT exam, which I passed successfully on my first attempt. My current employer quickly realized I was a likely candidate to replace our long-time director, who was ready for retirement. I returned to school online to receive my bachelor's degree in Health Information Management. After I obtained my degree, things moved faster than I expected; our HIM director retired and I was promoted to director while working with a consultant for an interim period to make sure I was comfortable handling the department.

I really enjoy my job. Every day is a new challenge—sometimes from administration, physicians, or employees; at other times, accreditation or federal government requirements present a challenge. Working as a team, we always manage to reach our goals.

**Professional Profile:**

### Health Information Management Assistant Director

My name is Thomas, and I am the health information management (HIM) assistant director in a 220-bed facility, Oakcrest Hospital, in the same system as Diamonte Hospital. This facility provides acute care emergency services, skilled nursing services, and ambulatory services. We have an HIM department with eight clerical and release of information (ROI) employees within my responsibility, three coding employees with one coding supervisor, and eight transcription employees with one transcription supervisor.

In our department, things are very organized, to the credit of our department director. New employees participate in the organization orientation before reporting to our department for work. During the first few days of employment, each new employee is oriented to the department. We begin by explaining the employee's job description and expectations (performance standards). Then the new employee goes through the department, sitting with each current employee to learn about other HIM functions and how their jobs are related. Finally, the new employee is oriented to his or her new position. During this process, the employee also obtains a password for our computer systems and reviews the security rules associated with access to health information.

I am responsible for organizing our monthly department meetings and choosing the in-service topic. I set up the agenda, copy and distribute any necessary handouts, and record the minutes. In addition, I coordinate any training required by changes in department policy, procedure, equipment, or federal and state mandates. The employees who report to me are cross-trained in several different functions so that we can cover one another for lunch, breaks, vacations, and sick leave.

I really enjoy the training and development aspect of this position. It is rewarding to see a new employee succeed in his or her position or to have an employee move up into a new position because of appropriate training and development.

As a manager, I am also required to attend training and development workshops. I recently attended an all-day workshop on managing diversity. Before the training, I felt confident that I was culturally aware and respectful of others regardless of any differences. However, attending the workshop helped me learn things I had not considered about how others might perceive my actions or comments. I also participated in activities that allowed me to exchange ideas on how to successfully manage diverse groups so that I could improve their productivity and teamwork.

### Career Tip

Depending on state licensure regulations and the regional marketplace, the requirements for an HIM department director vary. In general, a minimum of a bachelor's degree is necessary and a master's degree is preferred. HIM professionals with an associate's degree may want to expand their skill set to obtain a bachelor's degree in business administration or computer science. HIM professionals with a bachelor's degree may choose a master's degree in business administration, public administration, health administration, information systems, or health informatics, for example. It is important to obtain experience in an HIM department. Networking with HIM professionals at professional association meetings is helpful in obtaining an understanding of the marketplace and identifying opportunities early.

**Patient Care Perspective**

### Dr. Lewis's Other Partner, Dr. Simowitz

I am a consultant with privileges at four different hospitals. Between office hours and visiting inpatients for consultations, I have very little time left in the day to make my way to the health information management (HIM) department to complete my records. It seemed to me that I was constantly in imminent danger of being suspended and was receiving warning notices almost daily. I complained to Beth that I signed my dictations electronically on a regular basis, so why was I having problems? She explained that I was not always signing my progress notes and I gave too many telephone orders, which also had to be signed. I agreed to be more careful in the future with the progress notes but the telephone orders are problematic. Since I often do not see

those patients a second time, I do not notice that the orders are not signed. Beth worked with me to identify a day and time when I would regularly be in the hospital and her staff would bring outstanding records to me on the nursing unit so that I could finish them in a timely manner. I'm not the only physician with this problem, so Beth is meeting with nursing leadership to develop and implement a process for helping physicians complete their charts while their patients are still in the hospital.

**Patient Care Perspective**

### Maria

My primary care provider referred me to a specialist, a cardiologist, for the left bundle block that was diagnosed when I had my hysterectomy. I wanted to bring my medical records with me to the visit so I contacted the HIM department, as I have in the past, to get copies. The very nice, but insistent, receptionist said they no longer make copies of records and that I would have to access my records via the patient portal. She said something about my PHR—personal health record. Since I was not happy with the receptionist's explanation, I asked to be transferred to her boss; she transferred me to Thomas, the HIM department assistant director.

## Works Cited

Beach M, Price E, Gary, et al: Cultural competence: a systematic review of health care provider educational interventions, *Med Care* 43(4): 356–373, 2005. https://doi.org/10.1097/01.mlr.0000156861.58905.96

Equity of Care Committee, American Hospital Association: *Equity of care: a toolkit for eliminating health care disparities*, 2015. https://ifdhe.aha.org/health-equity-and-value. Accessed June 22, 2022.

Guanci G: *Shared governance: what it is and is not.* Association for Nursing Professional Development website, December 12, 2018. http://www.anpd.org/blog/shared-governance-what-it-is-and-is-not. Accessed June 22, 2022.

Guerin L: *Essential job functions under the ADA*, NOLO.com website, 2019. https://www.nolo.com/legal-encyclopedia/essential-job-functions-under-the-ada.html. Accessed June 22, 2022.

2009 Internal Revenue Service: *Employers: Affordable Care Act Tax Provisions for Employers,* July 8, 2022. https://www.irs.gov/affordable-care-act/employers. Accessed February 6, 2023.

U.S. Department of Health & Human Services Office of Minority Health: *National Standards for Culturally and Linguistically Appropriate Services (CLAS) in health and health care.* National CLAS Standards website, n.d. https://www.thinkculturalhealth.hhs.gov/clas. Accessed June 22, 2022.

U.S. Department of Labor, Wages and Hours Division page: *Fair Labor Standards Act.* https://www.dol.gov/agencies/whd/flsa. Accessed June 29, 2022.

U.S. Equal Opportunity Commission (EEOC): *About EEOC.* http://www.eeoc.gov/Overview. Accessed June 22, 2022.

Wilson-Stronks A, Lee KK, Cordero CL, Kopp AL, Galvez E: *One size does not fit all: meeting the health care needs of diverse populations*, 2008. Oakbrook Terrace, IL, The Joint Commission. https://www.issuelab.org/resources/10463/10463.pdf. Accessed June 29, 2022.

## Further Reading

Davis N, Shiland B: *Practical statistics for health data management*, 2016. St. Louis, MO , Elsevier/WB Saunders, pp 172–173.

U.S. Equal Opportunity Commission: *The ADA: Your Responsibility as an Employer.* https://www.eeoc.gov/laws/guidance/ada-your-responsibilities-employer. Accessed June 22, 2022.

# 10

# Performance Improvement and Project Management

TINA CARTWRIGHT

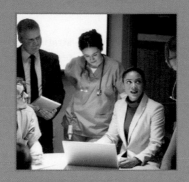

## CHAPTER OUTLINE

**Quality in Health Care**
  Patients First
  History and Evolution
  Accreditation Agencies
  International Organization for Standardization and
    American National Standards Institute
  Patient Safety Goals
  Quality Check

**Federal Health Care Quality Initiatives**
  Medicare and Medicaid's Hospital Quality Initiative
  Value-Based Purchasing
  Hospital-Acquired Condition Reduction Program
  Quality Improvement Organizations
  Hospital Compare
  Programs to Combat Fraud

**Quality Management**
  Quality Management Theories
  Components of Quality Management

**Performance Improvement**
  Methods
  Meetings, Teams, Committees, and Consensus-Building

Performance Improvement Tools
  Data-Gathering Tools
  Data Organization and Presentation Tools
  Project Management
  PERT chart

**Change Management**

**Chapter Summary**

**Competency Milestones**

**Ethics Challenge**

**Critical Thinking Questions**

**The Role of Health Information Management Professionals
  in the Workplace**
  Professional Profile: Assistant Director, Health Information
    Management
  Patient Care Perspective

**Works cited**

**Further Reading**

## CHAPTER OBJECTIVES

*By the end of this chapter, the student should be able to:*

1. Discuss the evolution of quality initiatives in health care;
2. Explain quality management efforts within the health information management (HIM) department and the facility;
3. Apply performance improvement techniques in HIM; and
4. Promote change management in the organization.

## VOCABULARY

accreditation
affinity diagram
Audit Medicaid Integrity Contractors (Audit MICs)
benchmarking
brainstorming

decision matrix
evidence-based medicine
GANTT chart
ice breaker
Lean

Medicare Administrative Contractor (MAC)
National Committee for Quality Assurance (NCQA)
National Patient Safety Goals
nominal group technique
Office of the Inspector General (OIG)
outcome
performance improvement (PI)

process control chart
quality assurance (QA)
Quality Improvement Organization (QIO)
recovery audit contractors (RACs)
sentinel event
Six Sigma
Survey

 **CAHIIM COMPETENCY DOMAINS**

VI.2.  Identify the impact of organizational change. (3)
VI.4.  Utilize data-driven performance improvement
        techniques for decision-making. (3)

## Quality in Health Care

The quality of health care data has been a running theme throughout this text. It is essential to note that high-quality data are used to monitor, verify, and improve patient care, reduce inefficiencies, and lower costs.

Some people define *quality* as "something that is excellent," based on a personal feeling, whereas others may judge quality by the outcome of the service (the result of the treatment, such as its success, or whether the patient is dead or alive). The level of quality is determined by the expectations of the customer evaluating the product or service. Thus an important concept in understanding quality is measurement.

Customers of any product or service judge its quality. In health care, there are many customers–patients, physicians, insurance companies, attorneys, accreditation agencies, and employees, to name a few. A discussion of quality management in health care can be very diverse, focusing on many different areas of service or the perspective of the person or entity assessing the quality. Patients determine quality according to their perception of the services and care they receive. Physicians perceive the quality through the eyes of their patients, their office staff, and their professional and personal interactions with employees in the facility. Insurance companies perceive the quality of a facility through the cost and outcome of the services provided to their beneficiaries. Employees may perceive the facility's quality through the competence of the staff and support from the administration. Accreditation agencies perceive quality in the facility's compliance with set standards. The facility measures quality based on its priorities, market share, and customer feedback. These are only a few examples of assessing a facility's quality, but a health care facility is certainly judged or assessed from many different perspectives.

### Patients First

Quality is perceived through the eyes of the patient according to the patient's priorities. For some patients, a prolonged life far outweighs the pain caused by a medical procedure. For example, a patient who suffers from persistent heart attacks requires bypass surgery to correct his or her heart dynamics and improve his or her chances for a longer life. The patient experiences tremendous pain from the surgery; however, if he or she no longer has heart attacks after the operation, his or her condition is improved. The patient is probably pleased with the outcome despite the intense pain that he or she experienced during recovery from the procedure. Therefore quality was not determined by the amount of pain experienced by the patient.

For another patient, the health care experience may end with a healthy new baby. However, during the patient's stay, the nurses and employees of the facility were rude, uncooperative, and of little help to the new mother. Although the experience ended well, this patient perceived the quality as poor because of her interaction with the staff.

Note that each circumstance is different, but in each case the quality of the service is determined by the customer. A powerful discussion of the patient's perception is seen in Dr. Donald Berwick's article "My Right Knee." The article describes his difficulties encountering the health care system in conjunction with a knee repair and draws attention to some fundamental premises with which patients could approach understanding health care. In the form of a request for proposal, his specifications would include the following (explanations paraphrased):

- No needless death—transparency in communicating complication rates.
- No needless pain—provides help without additional hurt and relieves unavoidable pain.
- No helplessness—by providing the patient with information and choices.
- No unwanted waiting—there are multiple models of appointments and flow that can eliminate unnecessary wait times.
- No waste—waste is an indicator of commitment to quality.

Dr. Berwick illustrates that while quality is in the eye of the patient, the delivery of quality care is the responsibility of the provider and the entire system in which that care is delivered (Berwick, 2005). Dr. Berwick's work through the Institute of Health Care Improvement led to IHI's Triple Aims for improving health care, echoed in the National Quality Strategy (Table 10.1). Thus the focus on improvement in health care, whether systematically or in the physician's office, should be on the patient.

| TABLE 10.1 | Triple Aims for improving Health Care | |
| --- | --- | --- |

| Institute for Health Care Improvement | National Quality Strategy |
| --- | --- |
| Improving the experience of care | Better Care: improve the overall quality, by making health care more patient-centered, reliable, accessible, and safe |
| Improving the health of populations | Healthy People/Healthy Communities: improve the health of the US population by supporting proven interventions to address behavioral, social, and environmental determinants of health in addition to delivering higher quality care |
| Reducing per capita costs of health care | Affordable Care: reduce the cost of quality health care for individuals, families, employers, and government |

From Agency for Healthcare Research and Quality: *About the National Quality Strategy*. Agency for Healthcare Research and Quality, 2017. https://www.ahrq.gov/workingforquality/about/index.html. Accessed January 16, 2022.

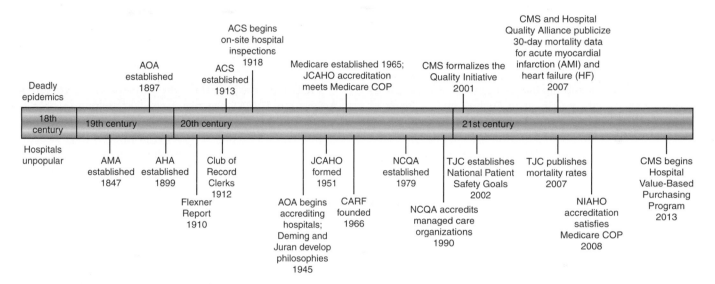

• **Fig. 10.1** Timeline of the evolution of quality in health care. *ACS*, American College of Surgeons; *AHA*, American Hospital Association; *AMA*, American Medical Association; *AOA*, American Osteopathic Association; *CARF*, Commission on Accreditation of Rehabilitation Facilities; *CMS*, Centers for Medicare and Medicaid Services; *COP*, Conditions of Participation; *JCAHO*, Joint Commission on Accreditation of Healthcare Organizations; *NCQA*, National Committee for Quality Assurance; *NIAHO*, National Integrated Accreditation for Healthcare Organizations; *TJC*, The Joint Commission.

## History and Evolution

In the 18th century, hospitals had a high incidence of deadly epidemics—due to the lack of knowledge of disease etiology and infection control—and relatively high death rates. The poor received health care in hospitals, often administered by churches or charitable organizations. The wealthy usually received care in their homes. The concept of quality in health care can be traced to the late 19th century when hospitals finally became known as places where people could go to get well because of advances in the knowledge of disease and infection control. During this time, physicians and hospital administrators began to associate for the common good. The American Medical Association (AMA) was founded in 1847. The American Hospital Association began as the Association of Hospital Superintendents in 1899. In 1906 the name was changed to the AHA. These

two associations worked diligently to promote high-quality health care through standardized medical education and hospital functions (American Hospital Association, 2021). Fig. 10.1 presents a timeline of the evolution of quality in health care.

### Medical Education

Before the existence of formal medical education, physicians trained through an apprenticeship. By the early 20th century, many medical institutions existed to educate physicians. But the education of these physicians was not standardized. Each institution could decide which courses were required to obtain a medical degree. For this reason, the health care profession increased in size and number of physicians, but the quality of patient care was not improving. Although having more physicians seemed like a good solution to an ailing population, the facts suggested that more needed to be done to improve the quality of health care. Medical institutions needed a standardized mechanism to guide the training of physicians.

Abraham Flexner studied the quality of medical education in the United States. His report in 1910 documented critical issues and discrepancies in medical education. The findings in the Flexner report prompted the closing of many training institutions, revisions of the required curriculum in those that remained, and implementation by the AMA of a mechanism for accreditation of medical education institutions. It also led to the validation of competency for medical professionals.

### Standardization and Accreditation

During this period, most patients encountered health care in hospitals for surgical intervention. Not long after the Flexner report, in 1913, the American College of Surgeons (ACS) was founded as an association of surgeons "to improve the quality of care for the surgical patient by setting high standards for surgical education and practice" (American College of Surgeons, 2021). The ACS assumed responsibility for reviewing the quality of health care provided to patients in hospitals. Its efforts to analyze quality involved a review of information from patient health records, which revealed insufficient documentation of patient care. The lack of documentation prohibited the effective study of quality to improve health care.

To standardize the contents of the patient health record so that future reviews would provide useful information, the ACS developed the Hospital Standardization Program. This program established standards, or rules, by which the ACS would survey hospitals to assess the quality of care. The first survey produced by the Hospital Standardization Program revealed that only 13% of the hospitals surveyed (with 100 beds or more) met the standards. The ACS then determined that for a facility to be considered a hospital, it must meet a set of minimum medical record documentation standards. These minimum standards required patient records to be maintained in a timely, accurate fashion and specified the minimum content, or required documentation, for a health record (Box 10.1). To this day, the saying "If it isn't documented, it didn't happen" calls to mind the importance of quality documentation in health care.

## Accreditation Agencies

By the 1950s the ACS was overwhelmed by the demand for hospital surveys. The establishment of The Joint Commission (TJC) on the Accreditation of Hospitals (JCAH) was a collaborative effort supported by the AMA, AHA, and ACS. The JCAH took over the responsibility of surveying hospitals. Over time, JCAH accreditation became popular in nonacute health care settings. In 1987 the organization was renamed the Joint Commission on Accreditation of Health Care Organizations and is now called The Joint Commission (TJC).

> ### • BOX 10.1    Medical Record Specifications— Minimum Standards
>
> A complete case record should be developed, consisting of the following information:
> - Patient identification data
> - Complaint
> - Personal and family history
> - History of current illness
> - Physical examination
> - Special examinations (consultations, radiography, and clinical laboratory)
> - Provisional or working diagnosis
> - Medical and surgical treatments
> - Progress notes
> - Gross and microscopic findings
> - Final diagnosis
> - Condition on discharge
> - Follow-up
> - Autopsy findings in the event of death

Predating the JCAH, the American Osteopathic Association (AOA) began a formal accreditation process for osteopathic hospitals in 1945. Its Hospital Facilities Accreditation Program (HFAP) continues to offer accreditation services to over 400 facilities, including acute care and critical care hospitals. The Accreditation Association for Hospitals and Health Systems (AAHHS), founded in 2012, acquired the HFAP in 2015 and administers the program in collaboration with the AOA. AAHHS was approved for deeming authority from CMS in 2019.

Accreditation is a common indicator of quality and compliance with predetermined standards in today's health care industry. TJC and the AOA are no longer the only accreditation agencies available to acute care facilities seeking deemed status from the Centers for Medicare and Medicaid Services (CMS). In 2008 the CMS approved accreditation by the National Integrated Accreditation for Health care Organizations (NIAHO) for acute care facilities. NIAHO is a subsidiary of Det Norske Veritas (DNV), a Norwegian risk management foundation. DNV focuses on the maritime, energy, food and beverage, and health care industries. NIAHO hospital accreditation is based on the International Standards Organization (ISO) 9001:2015 standards and complies with CMS's Conditions of Participation (COP). Surveys are conducted annually and focus on education and performance improvement (PI). Acute care facilities that maintain accreditation from TJC, the AOA, or the NIAHO receive deemed status from the CMS, meaning they satisfy the compliance audit portion of the COP and can receive reimbursement from Medicare and Medicaid without being subject to routine CMS audit. In Chapter 1, Table 1.6 provides a list of major accreditation agencies.

Other examples of accreditation bodies are the Commission on Accreditation of Rehabilitation Facilities, which accredits rehabilitation facilities; the AOA; HFAP;

the Accreditation Association for Ambulatory Health Care, which accredits ambulatory care facilities; and the **National Committee for Quality Assurance (NCQA)**, which accredits managed care organizations.

## International Organization for Standardization and American National Standards Institute

The International Organization for Standardization (ISO) is an independent, nongovernmental membership organization and the world's largest developer of voluntary international standards.

Established in 1947, it currently comprises the standards bodies of its 165 member countries, including the American National Standards Institute (ANSI). International standards facilitate trade by establishing products, services, and systems standards that ensure quality, safety, and efficiency (ISO).

Since its founding in 1918, ANSI has coordinated the development of voluntary consensus standards in the United States by accrediting standards developers who in turn establish consensus among qualified stakeholders. Although the resulting American National Standards are voluntary, they are increasingly cited by the US federal, state, and local bodies for regulatory or procurement purposes (ISO ANSI).

Notably, the NIAHO incorporates the ISO 9001:2015 standard into its accreditation guidelines. The ISO 9000 series of standards is supported by seven quality management principles for organizational PI, which are listed on the American Society for Quality website at: https://asq.org/quality-resources/iso-9000.

## Patient Safety Goals

TJC continued to promote quality by establishing **National Patient Safety Goals** for health care facilities in 2002. These goals were established to help TJC facilities focus on issues directly related to patient safety. TJC created an advisory group of knowledgeable patient safety experts to help them identify the goals; these experts included physicians, nurses, pharmacists, risk managers, and clinical engineers. The patient safety goals provide guidance or recommend procedures on issues such as accurate patient identification, communication among health care providers, medicine safety, health care–associated infections (HAI), reduction of patient falls, and risk assessment to ensure patient safety.

## Quality Check

In 2004 TJC also began an outcomes measurement program designed to hold health care facilities publicly accountable by publishing mortality rates for specific diseases so that consumers would have this information available when choosing a health care provider. The first published outcomes of core measures were for mortality rates of acute myocardial

infarctions (AMIs) and heart failure, followed by pneumonia in 2008. Making this information available to patients was such a success that the CMS also reports hospital data on the 30-day readmission rates for patients with these conditions and the in-hospital adverse events.

Information is made available to the public through a website called QualityCheck.org. This website provides information to consumers about the accreditation and certification of health care facilities. It offers free reports of a hospital's performance measures, National Patient Safety Goal compliance, National Quality Improvement Goal performance, patient satisfaction data, and quality awards received by the facility. It also identifies facilities that have been certified for disease-specific care and health care staffing.

## Federal Health Care Quality Initiatives

When the federal government began paying for health care through the Medicare and Medicaid programs, the quality and cost for the beneficiaries became the government's concern. The federal government began reviewing the care received by Medicare patients through audits of patient health records. Reviewers traveled to health care facilities and looked at the health record documentation to ensure Medicare patients received appropriate care. If the documentation did not comply with the Medicare regulations and reflect high-quality care, the facility was cited and its administrators had to explain why the services did not meet minimal standards; in some cases, a return of reimbursements was required.

## Medicare and Medicaid's Hospital Quality Initiative

In the 21st century, the health care industry is heavily regulated and surveyed for compliance with standards and quality. In 2001 the CMS formalized the Quality Initiative, which uses surveys and quality measures to make information about the care received at hospitals more transparent. Hospitals that can compare the quality of care they deliver with that of other hospitals and a public who can view costs and ratings of facilities create strong incentives to improve.

## Value-Based Purchasing

Always looking for ways to motivate hospitals to improve, the CMS began a plan in 2013 called the Hospital Value-Based Purchasing Program. According to the CMS (2021), the program is designed to reimburse acute care hospitals with a value-based incentive, rewarding both achievement and improvement on certain quality measures from a baseline period. As with other improvement plans, a hospital has to establish a baseline of data to measure improvement. In other words, the facility will collect data on specific performance measures, and then its improvement will be based on bettering those measures in future years. This type of plan requires that a hospital establish PI plans or programs, discussed later in this chapter. For Fiscal Year (FY) 2020, the eighth year of the program, CMS expected $1.9 billion in incentives to be available and that more hospitals would receive incentives rather than penalties (Centers for Medicare and Medicaid Services, 2019).

One aspect of value-based purchasing is the Medicare Access and CHIP Reauthorization Act of 2015 (MACRA). MACRA created the Quality Payment Program that focuses on quality over volume, initiated the Merit Based Incentive Payments System (MIPS), and established bonus payments for participation in eligible alternative payment models. For Medicare participants, MACRA also required the removal of social security numbers from Medicare cards by April 2019. To follow MACRA/MIPS development, start at their website: https://www.cms.gov/Medicare/Quality-Initiatives-Patient-Assessment-Instruments/Value-Based-Programs/MACRA-MIPS-and-APMs/MACRA-MIPS-and-APMs.html.

## Hospital-Acquired Condition Reduction Program

As discussed in Chapters 5, CMS has had in place for a decade a program in which it ignores certain conditions for payment if those conditions are acquired in the hospital (HACs). Supporting this regulation is a comprehensive program that focuses on improving hospital performance and preventing these conditions.

The HAC Reduction Program is a Medicare pay-for-performance program that supports CMS's long-standing effort to link Medicare payments to health care quality in the inpatient hospital setting. Beginning with FY 2015 discharges, CMS adjusted payments to inpatient prospective pay services (IPPS) and long-term care (LTC) hospitals which ranked in the bottom 25% of all IPPS and LTC hospitals. The ranking is based on specific HAC quality measures. The adjustment is a 1% payment reduction and occurs when CMS pays hospital claims.

For FY 2022, the Total HAC Score was based on data for six quality measures in two domains:
- Domain 1—CMS Recalibrated Patient Safety Indicator (PSI) 90 (CMS PSI 90)
- Domain 2—National Healthcare Safety Network HAI measures:
  - central line–associated bloodstream infection,
  - catheter-associated urinary tract infection,
  - surgical site infection (colon and hysterectomy),
  - methicillin-resistant *Staphylococcus aureus* bacteremia, and
  - *Clostridium difficile* infection (CDI).

These and many other quality measures are available on Medicare's Hospital Compare website: medicare.gov/hospitalcompare.

## Quality Improvement Organizations

CMS reviews are performed by a Quality Improvement Organization (QIO), a private team of health care professionals contracting with the CMS to inspect the quality of health care delivery and to address beneficiaries' concerns about the care they have received from providers. QIOs use that information to improve overall quality. QIOs are largely not-for-profit, task-specific contractors, whose 5-year contracts with the CMS are called the statement (or scope) of work (SOW) (Department of Health and Human Services, 2021).

As stated in the 2018 Report to Congress, the mission of the QIO Program is "to improve the effectiveness, efficiency, and quality of services delivered to Medicare beneficiaries" (Department of Health and Human Services, 2021). Its core functions are to improve the quality of care for Medicare beneficiaries, to ensure that CMS only pays for those services that are reasonable and necessary, and to review complaints from patients and appeals from providers.

QIOs review the aggregate and secondary data reported by facilities and perform onsite reviews of hospitals and other providers, examining health records and outcomes and conducting specific case reviews, during which they look for anomalies that may result in poor patient care. For example, a Medicare beneficiary (or an individual on his or her behalf) may file a claim if the beneficiary felt that he or she was discharged from a hospital too early. In that instance, a QIO review of the case is mandatory: The state's QIO will examine the health record, including admission date, admitting diagnosis, and treatments provided, to determine whether the patient's discharge was appropriate and whether he or she was "medically stable" at the time of discharge. Reviewers in the QIO are trained to identify certain criteria and to refer the matter to a physician within the QIO to decide whether the discharge was appropriate. These sorts of cases may also be flagged if an individual is readmitted to a facility within a certain time, usually within 30 days.

In other cases, QIOs analyze secondary data to look for trends that might indicate inefficiencies, or even fraud, both of which consume resources unnecessarily. A QIO review is prompted if a hospital requests an adjustment to a higher weighted Medicare Severity diagnosis-related group, for example, which may indicate an abuse of CMS reimbursement. But a QIO may also initiate a review based on larger patterns displayed by a particular provider over time; these patterns include the following (Centers for Medicare and Medicaid Services (CMS), 2014):

| Patterns | Example |
|---|---|
| Inappropriate, unreasonable, or medically unnecessary care (including setting of care issues) | Routine CT scans of patients when a simple radiograph is the standard of care |
| Incorrect DRG assignment | Routinely adding a code for a comorbidity/complication that was not documented |
| Inappropriate transfers | Transfer to SNF without required length of stay or appropriate evaluation |
| Premature discharges | Discharging unstable patients, who then are at high risk for readmission |
| Insufficient or poor documentation or patterns of failing to provide medical records | Patterns of failing to provide medical records upon request |

*CT,* Computed tomography; *DRG,* diagnosis-related group; *SNF,* skilled nursing facility.

The goal of all these reviews is to improve the quality of health care while reducing costs. QIOs look for ways to improve the delivery of care by interacting directly with providers, reviewing health records, examining patient outcomes, and finding trends that might provide opportunities for improvement.

The eighth and ninth SOWs (2005–08 and 2008–11) looked for specific treatments that have shown efficacy based on public health data in a variety of provider settings. Over time, AMIs, pneumonia, breast cancer, diabetes, heart failure, and end-stage renal disease have all been clinical topics of focus. The aims of the 10th SOW (2011–14) included reducing readmissions, hospital-acquired conditions, and promoting immunizations and screenings. In the 11th SOW, CMS changed the way the QIOs function. CMS separated medical case review from quality improvement work, creating two separate structures:

- Beneficiary Family Centered Care Quality Improvement Organizations (BFCC-QIOs), which perform medical case review and monitoring activities.
- Quality Innovation Network Quality Improvement Organizations (QIN-QIOs), each of which works on strategic quality initiatives. These initiatives are as varied as patient medications management, diabetes management for underserved beneficiaries, improving care for nursing home residents, and eliminating disparities in cardiovascular care—just to name a few (Centers for Medicare and Medicaid Services, 2023).

The 11th SOW ended in 2019. Under the 12th SOW, 5-year contracts were awarded to 2 BFCC-QIOs in June 2019 and to 12 regional QIN-QIOs in November 2019.

## Hospital Compare

The CMS also monitors quality from the standpoint of the patient by administering the Hospital Consumer Assessment of Health Care Providers and Systems survey. Feedback from a random selection of discharged patients is compiled based on questions about their experiences at the facility. Patients are asked to rate their communication with clinicians and other hospital staff and the cleanliness and quietness of the hospital and to give overall ratings.

With the implementation of a standardized survey on a national level, hospitals have a means to compare their performance with that of other facilities and to set goals to improve the quality of their delivery. The results of surveys are made public, at https://www.medicare.gov/care-compare/, so potential patients as consumers of health care can view ratings for each hospital and use that information to choose their providers. This availability provides strong incentives for hospitals to improve the quality of their services.

## Programs to Combat Fraud

As discussed in Chapters 5 and 6, errors in coding and billing can lead to denial of reimbursement. Third-party payers conduct numerous audits for a variety of quality attributes, particularly billing and the quality of the documentation that supports billing. The CMS conducts audits of Medicare through several contractors (Table 10.2).

Program for Evaluating Payment Patterns Electronic Report provides hospitals with a Microsoft Excel report that can be used by the health care facility to perform internal audits on medical claims. The report trends data for the facility and offers a comparison with other hospitals, helping the health care facility identify the types of bills that are susceptible to errors, overcoding (adding codes not reflected in the documentation), undercoding (failing to add codes that are appropriate based on the documentation), and questionable medical necessity admissions. With this information, hospitals can initiate internal reviews of health records in association with coding and billing to ensure accuracy. These internal reviews often give the hospital information that promotes quality improvement in areas such as physician documentation, medical coding, and patient care.

The Comprehensive Error Rate Testing program uses a random sampling of Medicare claims to measure errors associated with payments in the Medicare Fee-For-Service program (Chapter 6). The process includes reviews of health records with the associated claims to determine whether they follow the CMS coverage, coding, and billing rules. Noncompliance results in the sending of letters to the health care provider that notes the errors and overpayment or underpayment as appropriate. The health care facility can use notices from this program to identify internal areas of focus for PI.

Other audits are specifically designed to target potential bill errors, fraud, and abuse. **Audit Medicaid Integrity Contractors (Audit MICs)** and Medicaid **recovery audit contractors (RACs)** are examples of contractors whose audits are focused on identifying and correcting billing errors. Until recently, audits were entirely retrospective,

<table>
<tr><td colspan="2">TABLE 10.2    Medicare Contractor Efforts to Combat Fraud</td></tr>
<tr><th>Contractor</th><th>Role</th></tr>
<tr><td>Comprehensive Error Rate Testing (CERT) Contractors</td><td>Help calculate the Medicare Fee-For-Service (FFS) improper payment rate by reviewing claims to determine if they were paid properly.</td></tr>
<tr><td>Medicare Administrative Contractors (MACs)</td><td>Process claims and enrolls providers and suppliers.</td></tr>
<tr><td>Medicare Drug Integrity Contractors (MEDICs)</td><td>Monitor fraud, waste, and abuse in the Medicare Parts C and D Programs. Beginning January 2, 2019, the Centers for Medicare & Medicaid Services (CMS) will have two Medicare Drug Integrity Contractors (MEDICs), the National Benefit Integrity (NBI MEDIC) and the Investigations (I-MEDIC).</td></tr>
<tr><td>Recovery Audit Contractors (RACs)</td><td>Reduce improper payments by detecting and collecting overpayments and identifying underpayments.</td></tr>
<tr><td>Zone Program Integrity Contractors (ZPICs)</td><td>Formerly called Program Safeguard Contractors (PSCs). Investigate potential fraud, waste, and abuse for Medicare Parts A and B; Durable Medical Equipment Prosthetics, Orthotics, and Supplies; and Home Health and Hospice.</td></tr>
<tr><td>Unified Program Integrity Contractor (UPIC)</td><td>Combine and integrate functions of Medicare and Medicaid Program Integrity audit and investigation work into a single contract.</td></tr>
</table>

Some of these audits are conducted for benchmarking and provider performance evaluation and improvement. The Program for Evaluating Payment Patterns Electronic Report (PEPPER) and Comprehensive Error Rate Testing (CERT) are examples of such audits.
From Centers for Medicare and Medicaid Services, Medicare Learning Network, 2021.

conducted sometimes years after the dates of service and completion of the revenue cycle. In 2011 the CMS raised awareness among providers that prepayment audits were in development. Unlike a retrospective audit (review), which can recoup payment from the provider, a prepayment audit prevents the erroneous payment from taking place. Prepayment audits are driven by data-mining algorithms: software programs that compare data elements and produce exception reports of potential errors. So instead of relying on detective and corrective controls to recoup payments, CMS is developing and implementing more sophisticated preventive controls over billing errors. Effectively, the **Medicare Administrative Contractor (MAC)** runs all claims through the prepayment audit software looking for unusual patterns of billing, such as a high percentage of ED claims coded to a Level 5 with no related admission. This process is similar to what banks do to monitor a credit card account for unusual or potentially fraudulent activity. Instead of calling the customer to verify the charge, the MAC denies the claim for a stated reason, such as incorrect coding, or denies the claim and asks for documentation. In either case, the facility will have to reply and appeal the decision, send the documentation, or refile the claim (if possible) with corrected coding. Changes to the prepayment audit programs occur frequently; therefore the details are best obtained from the CMS website (www.cms.gov).

Facilities with a high number of unusual claims may be referred to the Department of Health and Human Services (DHHS) **Office of the Inspector General** (the OIG) for a fraud/abuse audit. Annually, the OIG publishes its work plan, which is derived from the analysis of common or problematic errors or issues that they have observed. The OIG updates the work plan throughout the year. In June 2017 the OIG began updating the work plan monthly.

The OIG's work spans multiple agencies under DHHS and not all of its work is focused on waste, fraud, and abuse. It also performs compliance reviews aimed at ensuring industry compliance with a variety of regulations and congressional requests. Examples of work plan topics include:
- States' Compliance with New Requirements to Prevent Medicaid Payments to Terminated Providers
- Duplicate Payments for Home Health Services Covered Under Medicare and Medicaid
- Adverse Events in Hospitals: National Incidence Among Medicare Beneficiaries-10-Year Update

Finally, the OIG also maintains a database of individuals and organizations that have been excluded from participation in Medicare and Medicaid programs as a result of their actions. The List of Excluded Individuals/Entities (or the Excludes List) is publicly available at https://oig.hhs.gov/exclusions/index.asp. Hospitals must ensure that new hires and existing employees are not on this list. Although it is a cumbersome task, there are civil monetary penalties for executing Medicare or Medicaid orders from an excluded physician, for example. In addition, the associated claim will be rejected.

Note that this section is specifically addressing the OIG that operates under the auspices of the DHHS. As of January 2022, there were 76 Inspectors General (IG) across the federal government, including the Department of Labor and the Central Intelligence Agency as well as Amtrak and the Architect of the Capital. In 2008 the Council of the Inspectors General on Integrity and Efficiency was created to support collaboration among the IG offices and provide a central point of reference on their work. A directory of the current IG incumbents is interesting reading at: https://ignet.gov/content/inspectors-general-directory

## COMPETENCY CHECK-IN 10.1

### Quality in Health Care

1. What is quality? Take a moment to define quality and then discuss your thoughts with another person. Is that person's perception of quality the same as yours?
2. Which association was the first to recognize a need for quality in health care and was organized for the purpose of promoting it?
3. Voluntary accreditation attained by a successfully undergoing survey against the standards set forth in the comprehensive accreditation manual for hospitals is given by which of the following organizations?
   a. MCOP
   b. CMS
   c. Medicare
   d. TJC
4. Which of the following groups was the predecessor of TJC?
   a. Hospital Standardization
   b. AHIMA
   c. NCQA
   d. ACS
5. The _____ preceded TJC in the survey of hospitals against set standards.
6. Which of the following is NOT a National Patient Safety Goal?
   a. Patient identification
   b. Acute myocardial infarction
   c. Communicate among health care providers
   d. Reduce falls
7. List the first two core measures established by CMS.
8. List three National Patient Safety Goals and explain why they are targeted.
9. List two outcome measures publicly reported by the CMS.
10. Which measure contributes to a facility's HAC Score?
    a. Average length of stay (ALOS)
    b. Catheter-associated urinary tract infections (CAUTIs)
    c. Mortality rates for acute myocardial infarctions (AMIs)
    d. Vaginal births after Cesarean section (VBAC)
11. Which QIO reviews medical cases for inefficiencies and fraud?
    a. Beneficiary Family Centered Care Quality Improvement Organizations (BFCC-QIOs)
    b. Quality Innovation Network Quality Improvement Organizations (QIN-QIOs)
12. Which Medicare contractor identifies excessive payments made on behalf of beneficiaries and attempts to correct the error so it does not happen again?
    a. Contractor Role Comprehensive Error Rate Testing (CERT) Contractors
    b. Medicare Administrative Contractors (MACs)
    c. Zone Program Integrity Contractors (ZPICs)
    d. Recovery Audit Contractors (RACs)

## Quality Management

In Chapter 7, we discussed the use of data to answer questions, provide decision support, and communicate information. In quality management, we use data to quantify performance for the purpose of setting standards, monitoring compliance, and measuring improvement. We will start with background from some founding theorists and follow that with a discussion of how data is used in quality management and PI.

## Quality Management Theories

Accreditation standards, regulatory requirements, and customer expectations prompted the development of methods to prevent, detect, or correct flaws in a product or service to reduce error rates. We discussed preventive, detective, and corrective controls in Chapter 4. But reducing errors is only part of the picture. Quality, from the perspective of manufacturing, is achieved through a myriad of factors. Quality management theories arose from manufacturing's drive to produce a product at the lowest possible cost that will also appeal to customers.

To understand why these quality management methods are important, you will find it helpful to know something about those who are credited with the founding theories: Deming, Juran, Shewhart, Crosby, and Donabedian. Their theories contain very similar and yet sometimes contradictory rules for managing quality. Although most of these founders did not become famous working with the health care industry, each has influenced the way the health care industry monitors quality. Therefore it would be correct to say they have inadvertently influenced the necessity to use health information to monitor quality and, in doing so, have promoted the improvement of the quality of health information.

W. Edwards Deming established his reputation when Japan used his philosophy to rebuild its industry after World War II. As consumers increasingly chose products that were made in Japan, American industry realized the value of adopting a quality management philosophy.

Deming's philosophy is process oriented, with an emphasis on how a task is performed or a product is produced. A product that does not meet company standards must be identified before it is completed. If the problem is noted after the production is completed, the company may not be able to correct it. However, if a company inspects the process as the product is being developed, problems are more likely to be addressed and corrected before it is too late. Deming developed 14 principles to implement a successful quality management program, focusing on developing and educating staff to collaborate and work together with each other and management to improve quality. While Deming's principles are focused on manufacturing production, we can glean a clear message for our purposes of facilitating collaboration, supporting workforce training and development, and focusing on accuracy (quality) over volume.

Another well-known pioneer in quality management is Joseph M. Juran. According to Juran, every quality management program should have a strong yet balanced infrastructure of quality planning, control, and improvement—the "quality trilogy." Juran applied the Pareto Principle to quality, stating that 80% of the defects are caused by 20% of the activities. He also defined a successful program as one that is acceptable to the entire organization; the program should be as important to the employees as it is to the administrators. Juran believed that many problems with quality programs arise from failure to address the human factors, including fear of change.

Walter A. Shewhart influenced both Deming and Juran. Together, these three are frequently cited as the founders of the quality movement, particularly in industry. Shewhart is credited with the widely used Plan-Do-Study-Act (PDSA) method and with process control charts, both of which are discussed later. Note that Shewhart developed and refined his work in the early to mid-1900s. His statistical process control tools gained traction toward the end of the century, evolving into Six Sigma.

Philip Crosby is best known for the term *zero defects*. Importantly, the second part of the term is sometimes left out, which is "from the standard." Like Deming, the Crosby quality management philosophy requires education of the entire organization, which requires that everyone—staff employees, supervisors, managers, and administrators—learn about the program and be motivated to participate.

Avedis Donabedian was a physician and researcher at the University of Michigan. He developed the framework for his structure–process–outcome model of evaluating quality in 1966. Specifically designed to address quality in health care, the Donabedian model is a framework for assessing the environment of care (structure), the way health care is delivered (process), and the results of the care (outcome). An illustration can be found in Fig. 10.2. In the figure, "unmeasured factors" are anything that is not a defined part of the evaluation, such as the patient dying from an unrelated accident. Donabedian's model is very useful in analyzing the components of a function. PI is seen exemplified in nursing activities across the board, from bedside care to medication administration and charting. In Chapter 9, we mentioned shared governance. An example of shared governance in health care is seen in nursing practice. Shared governance is a Magnet hospital goal for its contribution to PI. In Donabedian PI terms, the structure is shared governance, the process is professional nursing practice, and the outcomes are positive productivity data (Church, Baker, & Berry, 2008).

Unlike manufacturing, in which the steps are clearly defined from raw materials to finished product, and the outcome is subject to a clearly defined standard, health care is a fuzzier business at the patient care level. By professional

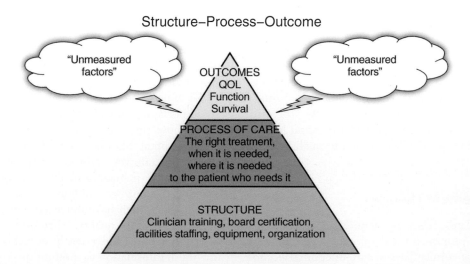

• **Fig. 10.2** Donabedian's structure–process–outcome model. *QOL*, Quality of life. (From Taneja SS: *Complications of urologic surgery*, ed 4, 2010. St. Louis, MO, Elsevier.)

practice standards and accreditation guidelines, care of the patient is supposed to be customized to the individual. We can see this in care plans, which resemble flowcharts more than lists. Nevertheless, the environment is subject to quality standards: the facilities, equipment, and supplies, and the competence of staff. The process is controlled by professional practice standards, policies, and procedures. Finally, the outcomes are measurable by several factors, including the alleviation of pain, management of disease, and (a more recent focus) patient satisfaction.

## Components of Quality Management

There are three components of quality management that represent the development, monitoring, and improvement of processes at various points in the delivery of care. They are quality control, quality assurance, and quality improvement, also known as PI.

### Quality Control

Quality control is the initial development of standards that define quality in a process. For coding, target accuracy in codes, selection of the principal diagnosis, and DRG assignment are examples of quality control standards. For nursing, one standard of quality control could be the evidence of timely administration of medications. In clinical care, quality control standards are supported by **evidence-based medicine**, or health care delivery that uses clinical research to make patient care decisions.

Quality control standards focus on the achievement of a desired outcome. For example, in scanning records, quality control standards would emphasize that 100% of appropriate records be scanned so that they are fully captured and legible.

### Quality Assurance

Once the standards have been set that identify the desired level of quality, achievement of that standard must be monitored to ensure that they are met. The monitoring of these functions is called quality assessment or **quality assurance (QA)**.

In the HIM department, all functions have some quality control standards, most of which focus on timeliness assembly, analysis, coding, abstracting, completion of records, filing/archiving, release of information (ROI), and transcription or document creation, and all must happen within specified time frames to enhance the timeliness, completion, accuracy, and validity of the record. QA is a retrospective analysis, performed at the end of a patient's visit or after discharge.

Taking into consideration all regulations governing health records, HIM department managers set the standards for performance of HIM functions. For example, let us assume that the HIM professional at a particular facility determined that assembly and analysis should occur within 24 hours of the patient's discharge and that the records should be assembled correctly 100% of the time (Table 10.3). This standard required that patient records be checked to ensure that the function was happening according to the standard. Plainly stated: Were records being assembled within 24 hours of discharge (every day) and were they assembled correctly 100% of the time? A supervisor would monitor assembly daily to monitor compliance with this standard. The results of the review would be documented for review by the HIM director. If the review revealed that the records were not being assembled correctly 100% of the time or not being assembled within the 24-hour time frame, then action was taken to correct the problem. The same process was applied to the other standards set for HIM functions; reviews were performed, compliance was noted, and any problems were actively addressed to prevent recurrence. QA reviews of coding ensured that the coding staff was accurately coding all records in a timely fashion. In a QA review of the ROI function, the HIM supervisor reviewed several requests to ensure that the release occurred in a timely fashion and that the facility's procedure for ROI was followed.

**TABLE 10.3 Quality Monitors for Health Information Management (HIM) Functions**

| HIM Function | Standard (Example) | How the Function is Audited |
|---|---|---|
| Assembly/ Scan/Index | Health records are assembled within 24 hours of discharge with 100% accuracy. | Scanned charts audited daily for legibility, completeness, and accuracy. Work queues reviewed daily for volume and timeliness. |
| Analysis | Health records are analyzed (quantitative) within 24 hours of discharge with 100% accuracy. | Work queues reviewed daily for volume and timeliness; supervisor conducts periodic reviews for accuracy. |
| Coding | All records are coded within 48 hours of discharge with 100% accuracy. | Supervisor reviews a sample of records monthly to check accuracy. DNFB is reviewed daily for uncoded records. |
| ROI | Requests for information are processed according to law and hospital policy within 48 hours of the request, 100% of the time. | Supervisor reviews a sample of requests periodically to check accuracy. Work queues are reviewed daily to monitor timeliness. |

## Outcome Measures and Monitoring

Every function in the HIM department should have its own measure of success: one or more key performance indicators (KPIs) that the process is functioning smoothly. While process monitors like Discharged, No Final Bill (DNFB) measure whether tasks are being done in a timely fashion, outcome monitors such as coding error rates measure whether the task is being done well. Routine audits of all functions help to ensure that data quality is maintained, from attribution of a physician to a case by an analyst to assignment of a code by a coder. It is through the monitoring of KPIs, as well as audits of critical functions, that the HIM department can generate department-level PI projects.

Today, the evaluation and monitoring of HIM functions remain important. TJC continues to require that facilities monitor the quality of their functions. The focus, however, is on quality improvement.

## Quality Improvement

Quality improvement, also called **performance improvement (PI)**, is a systematic approach to identifying the need for improvement, managing the development of an improvement strategy, and implementing the improvement. All of the quality management theories that we discussed previously have that one thing in common: taking a perceived problem that impairs quality and solving it to improve the process. It is not acceptable to simply meet an imposed standard; the facility should always seek to improve its performance.

Factors that would prompt a PI effort include changes in regulations, failure of a process to meet established standards, and sentinel events. A **sentinel event** is an occurrence that should never happen, such as amputating the wrong limb. This makes PI a hospital-wide function that occurs interdepartmentally and intradepartmentally. It can be multidisciplinary, involving employees to represent each area of the health care facility. Employees participate in teams to reach a solution to improve a process. All employees are encouraged to improve their work, surroundings, efforts, processes, and products. The philosophy of PI is that by improving the process, the outcome—patient care—will ultimately be improved. Through the remainder of this chapter, a Case Study feature will illustrate a real-world PI project (Case Study 10.1).

### Facility-Wide Committee

The PI process begins with a formal policy on or statement of how the facility will conduct and document improvement efforts. The organization-wide PI process is directed by a committee; typically, a committee established strictly for this purpose. This facility-wide PI Steering Committee reviews PI activities throughout the organization.

Some PI activities are driven by administrative KPIs, such as nosocomial infections. The PI Steering Committee observes an undesirable trend and initiates the process of examining the issue. The PI Steering Committee may also

## CASE STUDY 10.1

### Advance Directives PI Project

A facility is required by state law to inform its patients about advance directives. State laws regarding advance directives vary dramatically. Your state has assigned the responsibility of advance directives, patients' rights, and health care options to the hospital. This new regulation does not require the patient to have an advance directive or to make any decisions immediately; it simply states that the patient must be made aware of his or her rights. To prove compliance with the regulation, the facility requires the patient to sign an advance directive acknowledgment form at the time of admission. This acknowledgment form, signed by the patient and the admitting clerk, serves as proof that the patient was given the advance directive information. Although this process was implemented months ago, a review of compliance with the process shows that only 60% of inpatients have a signed acknowledgment form. Because this is a compliance issue, the PI Steering Committee has directed Patient Access to initiate a PI project to solve the problem.

### *NOTE*

The prefix *-inter* means "between" or "among," therefore *interdepartmental* means "between departments." The prefix *- intra* means "within," therefore *intradepartmental* means "within a department."

review customer satisfaction survey results and direct an area with an unfavorable rating to conduct a review and possibly initiate a project.

Not all unfavorable variances result in PI projects. For example, the observation of an anomaly may be the result of a known and self-correcting cause.

### Departmental Committees

While the facility designs and implements organization-wide PI efforts, all departments are required to improve processes both internally and in their relationships with other departments. At both levels, the improvement of a process is guided by a team. The teams may be made up of departmental employees or may be interdepartmental, depending on the needs of the project. Teams should have a sponsor—usually a management or administrative individual who can support the allocation of resources to the project, including political support. The team will have a leader, who organizes and runs the meetings, and a timekeeper, note-taker, or other administrative support person who facilitates the meetings. The members of the team must be chosen for their expertise in the area being reviewed, making the team multidisciplinary. They represent the active participants in the process and the users of the process output. A team working on improving patient registration data collection accuracy would likely include registrars, supervisors, HIM department personnel, patient financial service personnel, and clinical personnel.

Health care facilities have a quality management department, usually staffed by HIM and nursing professionals, to monitor and assess quality. It is the primary responsibility of this department to educate those in the health care facility about the quality management and PI process and to monitor the assessment of quality for the facility. This department monitors the facility's compliance with accreditation standards by performing a significant number of record reviews, participating in and often coordinating medical staff and facility committees, and overseeing performance (quality) improvement. This department also works closely with the HIM, risk management, and case management functions to coordinate efforts to improve quality. The department may also ultimately be responsible for coordinating the duties associated with onsite accreditation surveys, such as those conducted by TJC.

## Performance Improvement

PI projects can arise from problems identified at the facility, department, or function level. Regardless of how the project originates, the process is similar: identify the problem or issue, obtain support at the appropriate administrative level, identify the team (Case Study 10.2), develop a plan to approach the problem, then move forward as needed with the project. PI projects have a beginning and an end. While the problem addressed will likely continue to be monitored, the work of the team ends when the solution is successfully operationalized. As we will see, project management skills such as planning, coordination, and time management are useful in the PI process. This section explores PI and PI methodologies in detail.

## Methods

The theories of quality management are implemented using a variety of methods to identify, evaluate, and resolve quality issues. All quality theories and methods have in common a cyclical perspective. In other words, there is a beginning, middle, and end to a specific project; however, the monitoring and continuous search for the need to improve is never-ending.

### Plan, Do, Study, Act Method

A popular method for monitoring and improving performance is the PDSA method, also called the Plan, Do, Check, Act or PDCA method, which was developed by Shewhart and supported by Deming.

---

### COMPETENCY CHECK-IN 10.2

#### Quality Management

1. The three elements of Juran's "quality trilogy" are:
   a. planning, doing, and acting
   b. planning, control, and improvement
   c. structure, process, and outcome
   d. change, innovation, and stability
2. Your health care facility is embarking on a new quality effort. For weeks now, administrators, managers, and supervisors have been involved in meetings and training to ensure that everyone in the organization has a clear understanding of the new quality initiative message. The board has announced that this new effort will involve everyone in the organization. At the very core of this initiative is the motto "zero defects." This organization is being guided by the philosophy of which of the following thinkers?
   a. Deming
   b. Juran
   c. Crosby
   d. Donabedian
3. Which of the following philosophers emphasizes detecting problems before a product or process is completed?
   a. Deming
   b. Juran
   c. Crosby
   d. Donabedian
4. Diamonte Hospital is committed to their continuous quality improvement (CQI) philosophy. They currently have several PI teams organized to address the processes associated with the delivery of patient care. This facility is most likely being guided by the theories of:
   a. Deming
   b. Juran
   c. Crosby
   d. Donabedian
5. Explain how health information is monitored in the HIM department to ensure quality.
6. How does the supervisor know that department-level outcomes are not meeting standards?
7. For what reason(s) would a department of organization decide to begin a PI process?
8. Retrospective review of a product or service is _____.
9. _____ is an ongoing effort to improve processes within the health care facility.

**CASE STUDY 10.2**

### Advance Directives PI Project

The Patient Access Manager assembled a team consisting of an HIM coder, a patient financial services representative, two employees of physicians on staff, a clinic employee, a social services employee, and two registrars.

The health care facility may need to improve the method and accuracy by which it provides this information to its patients. To improve the collection of the acknowledgment form for advance directives, several patients will be invited to participate periodically on the committee. The customer's perspective must be considered to truly evaluate the quality of a process or product. Fig. 10.3 describes additional members of a hypothetical advance directive PI team. The employees in the social services department provide information if the patient has any questions regarding the advance directive. Therefore the social service representative must be knowledgeable of both the content of the advance directive and the patient's concerns and other related issues. An advance directive is often an end-of-life determination. Pastoral care services assist the patient and family members with spiritual and emotional concerns. Their representation on the team may provide additional insight regarding other concerns affecting the patient or family during consideration of the advance directive statements. The nurse, being very involved in the patient care process and communicating often with the patient, is also an important member of the PI team. From the HIM department, a quantitative analysis employee should be represented because of his or her knowledge of the record review process. To be effective, all staff who are a part of this process must be included on the PI team-patient access, social services, pastoral care, nursing, and HIM.

The PDSA method is easy to understand and follow, making it one of the most widely used models (Fig. 10.4). The *Plan* phase consists of data collection and analysis to propose a solution for the identified problem. The *Do*, or implementation, phase tests the proposed solution. The *Study* phase monitors the effectiveness of the solution over time. The *Act* phase formalizes or operationalizes the changes that have proved effective in the Do and Study stages, amending or developing policies and procedures around the change, for example.

The key point to remember is that a process is being improved. The area of concentration is the process itself and not any one individual's job performance. For a process to be improved, all persons who are involved in the process must be part of the team. For example, an improvement in the coding process could involve physicians, nurses, analysts, coders, patient access staff, and patient financial services staff. To illustrate, consider a hospital with delays in coding due to postdischarge physician queries and increasing denials by the payer for documentation issues (Box 10.2). The HIM staff alone can plan a work process solution to address how efficiently they deal with queries and follow up with physicians. However, the broader issue of denials requires more diverse participation. It is probably not hard to imagine how this group could settle on the development and implementation of a Clinical Documentation Improvement program as a solution to the delay and denial issues

### Statistical Process Control

One of Shewhart's major contributions to quality management was the emphasis on statistical analysis to identify variance in a process. Specifically, he is addressing the ongoing measurement of a process to establish tolerable variances and monitor for unacceptable variances. Underlying this analysis is the concept of variance from standards. Shewhart proposes that there are tolerable variances in the process (assignable or special-cause variation) that can be controlled through PI and unexpected variances (chance or common-cause variations) that might need to be addressed, but probably not by changing the process. The process is monitored using a statistical **process control chart**, a data-gathering tool that graphs the measurement of a KPI or another variable over time. For example, consider Discharged, No Final Bill (DNFB), which is a KPI for revenue cycle management. DNFB dollars tend to be high on Monday and drop during the week when the HIM Department is staffed 5 days a week. In Fig. 10.5A, the first 2 weeks illustrate that pattern. If the DNFB is creeping up—starting higher each Monday and not dropping as low on Friday—a process control chart will highlight this variance, which may indicate a problem with the process that can be corrected. The last 2 weeks in Fig. 10.5A show the pattern. An unexpected staff absence could cause this, for example, which requires filling production requirements with overtime or other staffing solutions. It could also be caused by a breakdown in the workflow delaying coding or a system upgrade that did not go well, such as the annual ICD-10-CM/PCS update in the encoder/grouper. On the other hand, if DNFB dollars are high on Monday and continue climbing rather than falling during the week due to system downtimes, as illustrated in Fig. 10.5B, then this is an unusual variation that has nothing to do with the process. Yes, it must be corrected; however, it does not require a change in process in the coding area. The process control chart does not tell us the why of the situation; it only tells us what is happening.

### Lean

With roots in efforts started by Henry Ford in 1913 on the Model T automotive assembly line, and advanced by Kiichiro Toyoda, Taiichi Ohno, and others at Toyota in the 1930s, **lean** is also a PI process that began in manufacturing but has found application in health care settings (Liker, 2004). A somewhat less formal model than PDSA, lean or "lean thinking" seeks to create value—which may be defined in this context as anything the customer would pay for—by reducing waste and wasteful activities. Lean thinking looks for ways to accomplish a task with less work, reducing inefficiencies and thereby improving the process. Because lean accepts that there are always ways to improve, it is a philosophy of continuous improvement. That is, lean philosophy embraces a culture in which individuals in the organization are constantly looking for ways to improve the

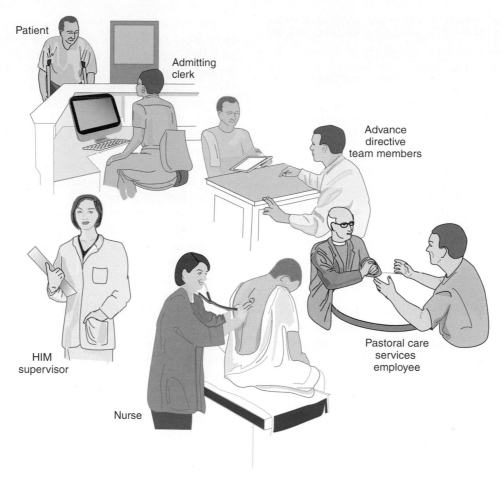

• **Fig. 10.3** Advance directive team members. *HIM*, Health information management.

**PDSA Method**

| | | |
|---|---|---|
| **P** | Plan | **In this stage you:**<br>• Coordinate a team<br>• Investigate the problem; gather data<br>• Discuss potential solutions<br>• Decide on a plan of action |
| **D** | Do | **Here's where you test the plan of action:**<br>• Educate employees on the new process<br>• Pilot the new process |
| **S** | Study | **During the Pilot be sure to:**<br>• Monitor the new process during the pilot<br>• Did the plan of action work the way the team intended?<br>• Make necessary adjustments and continue the pilot |
| **A** | Act | **Once you are certain that the process is an improvement:**<br>• Change the policy<br>• Educate and train all affected employees<br>• Implement the new process |

• **Fig. 10.4** PDSA method. *PDSA*, Plan-Do-Study-Act.

*Problem:* Queries of physician for accurate information are required for coding/billing; billing can be delayed.

*HIM Team:* Coders, analysts, and clinical documentation improvement (CDI) specialist.

**P**LAN: First review delayed bills, identify physician culprits, and examine specific diagnoses and procedures that are problematic. Review process for communicating with physicians. Brainstorm how to get physicians to answer queries.

**D**O: Implement changes necessary to resolve problems identified in planning phase.

**S**TUDY: Review coding and billing delay data to determine impact of the changes; if positive impact, proceed to ACT; if not, go back to PLAN part of the process.

**A**CT: Institutionalize the new procedures into policy and practice.

way that things are done. This continuous improvement is expected of everyone in the organization, not just managers or policymakers. Fig. 10.6 illustrates the implementation of lean, although you should note its circular pattern: improvement is not a one-time instance but is continuous.

The lean PI philosophy can be adopted by health care facilities to improve many processes, including admission and discharge processes, patient scheduling and movement between departments for treatment, clinical processes, coding and billing, and ED wait time. Let us use the ED wait time as an example. This is a common problem in many health care facilities, and improvements made here are popular among patients. A typical ED wait time project starts with monitoring the times of key activities for a period of time, say, over a week or month(s). The team would set up a method to capture information related to the time each patient presents to the ER, time of triage, time of first encounter with physician, time of any key diagnostic or treatment activities, time of departure or admission, and time to bed if admitted. Using these data, trended over time and based on peak volume as well as reason for visit, can help the PI team identify opportunities to alleviate wait times or improve timeliness of care to patients. For example, the team observes that triage places chest pain, respiratory distress, abdominal pain, and hemorrhage cases ahead of all others. While this seems logical, the wait time for a cut finger or other urgent but not critical issues can be hours. The ED staff may suggest that a separate treatment area be

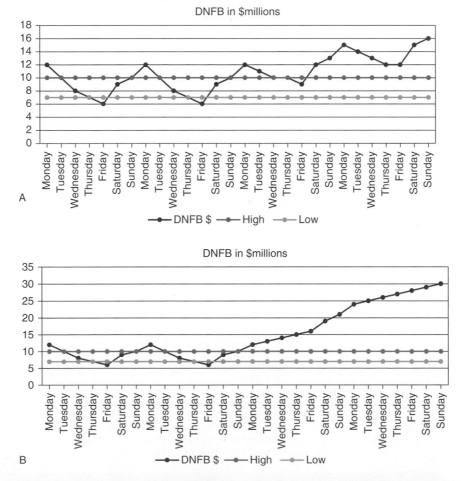

• **Fig. 10.5** Process control chart. (A) Discharged no final bill *(DNFB)* shows dollars begin high on Monday and drop by Friday, as shown in the first 2 weeks. The remaining 2 weeks shown indicate there may be a problem with the process. (B) When DNFB dollars continue to climb, there may be an unusual variation unrelated to the department's processes.

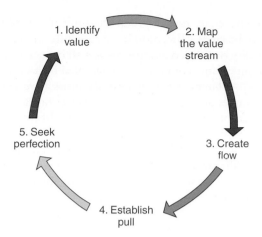

1. Identify the value in the process or product being improved.
2. Identify every step in the process or product creation and eliminate unnecessary steps that do not add value.
3. Align all of the necessary or required steps into a tightly aligned process or smooth flow.
4. Let customers "pull" the process (i.e., watch the customer's demand and respond to it).
5. Repeat these steps until perfection, a process with no waste.

• **Fig. 10.6** Steps for implementing lean techniques. (Modified from Lean Enterprise Institute: *Principles of lean.* https://www.lean.org/lexicon-terms/lean-thinking-and-practice/. Accessed January 16, 2022. Illustration Copyright 2012, Lean Enterprise Institute [www.lean.org].)

dedicated to such issues so that they can be handled apart from the critical cases. Thus is born ED Express for urgent care (George, 2003).

### Six Sigma

Originally developed by Motorola in 1986 but made famous by General Electric in 1995, **Six Sigma** is a "disciplined, data-driven approach and methodology for eliminating defects (driving toward six standard deviations between the mean and the nearest specification limit) in any process-from manufacturing to transactional and from product to service" (iSixSigma, 2022). Whereas lean thinking philosophy can be thought of as a less structured approach used

by an entire organization, Six Sigma is a highly regimented approach to PI, driven by specially trained individuals ("Black Belts" and "Green Belts") who guide others through a strict problem-solving method. Health care facilities that adopt this method of PI establish an organizational philosophy to systematically strive for PI using an approach based on statistical analysis of performance. Six Sigma uses different approaches to quality according to whether the facility is improving a current process or product—Define, Measure, Analyze, Improve, and Control (DMAIC), or creating a new process or product—Define, Measure, Analyze, Design, and Verify (DMADV). The basic steps for each approach are listed in Fig. 10.7. Six Sigma is highly data driven and does not necessarily lend itself as well to health care delivery as it does to manufacturing. However, it has gained some traction in recent years. Six Sigma is best applied to repetitive processes with little variance, such as laboratory specimen collection and analysis, pharmaceutical dispensing, food delivery, and materials management.

### Meetings, Teams, Committees, and Consensus-Building

Meetings are a very important part of the PI process. When meetings are organized and managed effectively, they are an important method for bringing people together to improve performance. Meetings can be used to gather information or share information. Meetings are used to inform the attendees of the purpose of a presentation. Everyone gets the same message at the same time. Meetings can be used to gather information about the process from the people who are involved, educate other members of the team, and keep the team focused on the goal of improving the process. Because the activity of PI teams closely mirrors that of permanent committees, the roles and functions of the members are similar. In this discussion, we will compare and contrast teams and committees as appropriate.

The meetings discussed in Chapter 9 focus on committees that are generally structured to communicate information

| DMAIC (pronounced "duh-may-ick") | DMADV (pronounced "duh-mad-vee") Also called DFSS—Design for Six Sigma |
|---|---|
| Used to improve existing process | Used to create a new process or product |
| **Define** the problem specifically | **Define** design goals |
| **Measure** the current process (collect data) | **Measure** and identify characteristics that are Critical To Quality (CTQ) |
| **Analyze** and investigate cause-and-effect relationships | **Analyze** for development and design |
| **Improve** the current process, pilot potential solutions | **Design** details |
| **Control** establish systems to monitor and maintain control of the new process | **Verify** the design, set up pilots |

• **Fig. 10.7** Two approaches for Six Sigma.

about organizational activities. PI teams are different in the sense that everyone on the team is expected to contribute and participate to the best of their ability. In administrative meetings or committees, the department chair or another organizational leader is often the clear "winner" when there are differences of opinion. On a PI team, a leader who is in a direct position of authority concerning the problem may be counter-productive. PI teams are expected to come to a consensus among group members. During PI team meetings, it is important that all members feel comfortable expressing their views. If you think the problem rests with your supervisor, who is also the PI team leader, it is unlikely that you will express that view.

On a PI team, the secretary may have other responsibilities, such as preparing the agenda, distributing communications, and collecting team feedback. Therefore it may not be appropriate to rotate the role on a PI team as it is on operational teams.

The role of a PI team that is not often seen on operational committees or teams is the facilitator. A *facilitator* plays an important role in a PI team meeting. The facilitator is the person who keeps the team focused on the goal (e.g., improvement in the collection of patient advance directives). During improvement efforts, it is common for a team to get sidetracked by equally pressing issues that need to be corrected. A facilitator makes sure that the team does not deviate too far off course. Too much deviation in a meeting could impair the team's ability to accomplish its goal (Case Study 10.3).

The members of a PI team or committee all have the responsibility to participate. That means attending meetings, speaking on the topics as appropriate, and taking action between meetings as assigned. In the organizational document of the PI team or committee, the expectations of members should be clearly stated along with the remedies for noncompliance, which should be enforced.

The work of a PI team should be collaborative. The goal is to improve a process. Therefore all members are valuable and all should be encouraged and supported to participate. The optimum result is that the team reaches consensus on the outcome of the work. To that end, both the Leader and the Facilitator have the added responsibility of ensuring that strongly opinionated individuals do not dominate the conversation or the course of the project. Group consensus-building strategies, such as brainstorming, affinity charts, and ratings, assist with consensus-building (see Brainstorming later).

**CASE STUDY 10.3**

**Advance Directives PI Project**

The team decided to meet twice a week for the first month. The Patient Access Director took responsibility for leading the group and requested volunteers to take minutes, facilitate, and act as timekeeper. In the organizational meeting, the team discussed PI models briefly and decided to employ the PDSA method.

*Committees* are formal groups that organizations use to conduct business. The committee structure of the health care facility is outlined in the medical staff bylaws, rules, and regulations. Some committees are required by accreditation agencies. Although all health care facilities have committees, the roles and functions of committees in the facilities vary. Examples of committees within a health care facility are medical staff committees, infection control, safety, surgical case review, pharmacy and therapeutics, and HIM. The following discussion briefly explains how these committees use health information and support quality initiatives in the organization.

### Medical Staff Committees

The medical staff of a health care facility is a self-governed group of physicians divided into departments based on their practices, such as the department of medicine, department of surgery, department of obstetrics, and department of pediatrics. Remember that, in hospitals, governance is shared between the administrative side and the medical side of the organization chart. This dual governance ensures that the organization has the benefit of both the process and the clinical perspective in setting strategy and caring for its patients. The medical staff structure is directed by an elected group of physicians; such positions include chief or president of the medical staff, the president-elect (incoming chief of staff), and a chairperson for each department. Each medical staff department has a committee meeting in which business directly related to that field of medicine is discussed. The committee reviews patient cases, determines appropriate documentation, and discusses standards of care, as necessary. The medical staff departments also use statistics acquired from health information to make decisions regarding physician membership, privileges, and compliance with accreditation standards.

Accreditation by TJC requires that a facility review specific cases of patient care in the areas of surgery, medication usage, and blood and tissue usage. For example, the department of surgery performs surgical case review as an accreditation requirement. The facility reviews statistics related to operations and the health records of surgical cases with unexpected outcomes (e.g., a patient who goes into cardiac arrest during an appendectomy or a case in which the wrong operation was performed). Medication usage is typically reviewed by the pharmacy and therapeutics (P&T) committee. The P&T committee is composed of members of the medical staff, with representatives from nursing, administration, and pharmacy also represented. The committee reviews medications administered to patients, specifically targeting any adverse reactions that a patient has had as a result of medication. The P&T committee also oversees the hospital formulary, which is a listing of the drugs used and approved within the facility. Blood usage is also a review that requires participation from the medical staff. This review analyzes the appropriate protocol, method, and effects for patients receiving blood transfusions (or blood products).

The business and decisions of the departments of the medical staff are reported to the medical executive committee for action, recommendation, or correspondence to the governing board. The "med exec committee," as it is commonly called, acts as a liaison to the governing board of the facility. This committee is composed of the chief of staff and elected positions, with a representative from each of the medical staff departments.

### Infection Control Committee

The infection control committee is organized to analyze the rate of infection of the patients within a facility. The committee is supported by the Infection Control Department staff. This committee meets regularly to determine whether patients are entering the facility with infections that can harm the staff or other patients or whether patients are acquiring infections within the facility, nosocomial infections that affect their care, treatment, and length of stay. The committee also reviews the regulatory reporting that is conducted by the Infection Control Department staff.

The infection control committee is also involved in preventing and investigating infections. As such, it is an important quality-related committee. Members of the infection control committee include physicians, nurses, quality management personnel, and HIM personnel. To evaluate infection control rates within a facility, the committee must analyze information from patient health records. The committee may initiate a PI project on its own or direct a department to do so. For example, the committee may track postoperative infection rates by nursing unit using a statistical control chart. In observing the postoperative infection rates, the committee may observe a spike in infections above the tolerance level in a particular unit. The committee might charge one of its nursing members to coordinate with nursing to collect data and potentially initiate a PI project.

### Safety Committee

The safety committee is organized to assist the safety officer, who is responsible for providing a program to create a safe environment for patients, visitors, the community, and staff. Health care facilities must adhere to numerous requirements from the US Occupational Safety and Health Administration, TJC, state licensing boards, and federal agencies. The safety committee evaluates the information presented by the safety officer, ensures the safety of the environment, and performs disaster planning. Occasionally, the safety committee also reviews the incident reports of cases related to the facility's environment. Members of the safety committee are appointed by administration and may include clinical and nonclinical employees.

The safety committee would naturally support quality by taking positive steps to correct issues as they arise. The Safety Officer, along with other appointed personnel, tours the facility frequently in a process called *safety rounds*. During safety rounds, the team observes the condition of the facility and looks for safety hazards such as unlit Exit signs, irregularities in carpeting, and gurneys parked on both sides of a hallway. The team will test fire doors to ensure that they stay open properly and close properly. They will also look for compliance with safety procedures such as keeping office doors closed and not propped open. The safety committee might initiate a PI project related to compliance issues or perhaps customer complaints, for example.

### Health Information Management Committee

The HIM committee, commonly referred to as the medical record committee, serves as a consultant to the director of the HIM department. The HIM committee is typically responsible for reviewing the documentation in patient health records, reviewing and advising form development, and assisting in compliance with accreditation standards. Some facilities have expanded the HIM committee into a more global quality committee, with the HIM committee reporting specific metrics at least quarterly. Many important health information issues can be addressed by this committee. Box 10.3 is a sample agenda for an HIM committee; the committee can review the findings of the record review teams, the percentage of delinquent medical records, and QA and PI activities. Members of the HIM committee include the director of HIM, physicians from each department of the medical staff, nursing staff, and quality management personnel.

The HIM committee's role inherently supports quality in its record review and forms development activities. PI projects that might be initiated include clinical documentation improvement issues and delinquent chart rates. One example of PI could be in quantitative and qualitative analysis in the EHR.

The EHR is only as good as the information that is entered. The electronic system allows an organization to evaluate key health data elements across the continuity of care in a report rather than having to retrieve individual charts; this automation helps ensure that required data elements are completed appropriately, often initiating PI activities. Another quality aspect of the EHR is the clinical decision-making system.

---

**• BOX 10.3  Agenda for Health Information Management Committee**

HIM Committee Meeting
October 17, 20XX
Agenda:
I.   Call to order
II.  Review of minutes
III. Old business
IV.  Record review
V.   New business
VI.  Reports
VII. Delinquent record count
VIII. Quality audit of HIM functions
IX.  Adjourn
*Next meeting:* November 14, 20XX

## Communication and Interpersonal Skills

As Juran surmised, many problems arise in human interactions: not just fear of change but also difficulties between individuals. Therefore, for effective team meetings, a spirit of camaraderie and collegiality is essential. Ice breakers are activities that help new team members get to know one another and can be a good social leveler in the first meeting. Ice breakers are not just introductions of the team but can also be a learning tool for team members to find ways to interact with each other that are comfortable. An ice breaker for this professional team should have a point and move the team forward. For example: group the team in pairs and have them share something relevant about themselves, including why they are on the team. Then have the pairs introduce each other with the information obtained. It is very important with ice breakers to invite the sharing of only things that are not controversial or insensitive. So, religion, marital status, and political affiliation are off the table, but giving the members a choice of sharing a hobby, favorite movie, or favorite book is likely safe.

Unless there is an organizational policy that dictates the methodology by which the team conducts its project, the team will select a model in which to conduct the project. The model not only helps the team document the PI process to support accreditation and certification standards but also provides a measure for the facility to monitor its efforts internally. The following are some models that are common in health care.

## Performance Improvement Tools

Many tools facilitate the use of data in the PI process. There are tools to organize the project, gather information, and organize or present the information in a useful manner. Project management tools, such as GANTT charts, help organize the work and are particularly helpful in controlling large implementation projects. A GANTT chart lists all of the steps in a project, the beginning and ending dates of the step, who is responsible, and the relationship among the steps (what steps must precede another). Adjacent to the list is a series of columns that represent the dates, with bars at each step showing the dates of the step. Project management software aids in the creation of this visual tool, but a simple GANTT chart can be drawn in Excel.

Data-gathering tools help the team to explore or at least acknowledge issues surrounding the process of concern. Organization and presentation tools make a statement about the information that is gathered. Two data-gathering tools, that is, brainstorming and surveys, are discussed here, as well as several organization and presentation tools: bar graphs, line graphs, pie charts, decision matrices, and flowcharts. Table 10.4 contains a comprehensive list of presentation tools and techniques.

## Data-Gathering Tools

To identify the source of the problem, the team will solicit input from a variety of sources. These sources include the team members themselves, who are stakeholders in solving the problem. There are also external sources of data that may be available for comparison to the current situation, as well as research techniques that can be applied to gather additional data.

### Brainstorming

Brainstorming is a method in which a group of people discusses ideas, solutions, or related issues on a topic or situation. It is a data-gathering tool used to identify as many aspects, events, or issues surrounding a topic as possible. This process encourages the involvement of everyone in the group. All ideas are accepted, no matter how insignificant they may appear. When brainstorming, the group should have a topic and a place to write down the ideas mentioned by the group. To begin the process, the team's facilitator explains that this tool is used to gather all ideas related to the issue regardless of how unusual they may seem.

For example, a PI team is organized to reduce the length of time that a patient waits to receive treatment in the ED. At the team's first meeting, the members brainstorm all possible factors that could have an impact on the patient's wait in the ED. The team members are encouraged to mention anything that could affect the patient's wait time. Note that at this stage, the members do not need to prove that the factors they mention actually affect the patient's wait time. Brainstorming is simply a data-gathering tool; many organization tools can be used to narrow improvement efforts, such as a fishbone chart (Fig. 10.8). Successful brainstorming sessions can result using the following guidelines:

- Establish a set time for the brainstorming session (e.g., 30 minutes).
- Collect ideas from all participants, ensuring that all ideas are welcome.
- Record all ideas. Using a whiteboard or other means of display allows all members of the group to see them.
- Do not criticize, judge, or even discuss ideas during the brainstorming session while ideas are being generated.
- The more ideas, the better. Build on the ideas of others.
- Discuss the ideas after the brainstorming session is complete.

Once ideas have been generated, they can be grouped into categories. So, if one idea for the cause of wait time is the confusion over which patient is next and another idea has to do with the lack of a "bed board" to identify waiting patients, those ideas could be grouped under the heading "Patient Identification in Workflow." Another idea about slow triage might be grouped under "Staffing" along with incomplete registration of patients. This process of grouping ideas is called an affinity diagram (Fig. 10.9).

## TABLE 10.4  Tools and Techniques for the Presentation of Data

| Tools and Techniques | Primary Function | Benefits |
|---|---|---|
| Flowchart | Displays the process | Facilitates understanding of the process |
| | | Identifies stakeholders |
| | | Clarifies potential gaps and system breakdowns |
| Run chart | Displays performance over time | Increases understanding of the problem |
| | | Identifies changes over time |
| Control chart | Displays how predictable the process is over time | Identifies change in the process as a result of intentional or unintentional changes in the process |
| | | Identifies opportunities for improvement |
| Pie chart | Displays the percentage each variable contributes to the whole | Identifies variables affecting process |
| | | Increases understanding of the problem |
| Bar chart | Compares categories of data during a single point in time | Increases understanding of the problem |
| | | Identifies differences in variables |
| | | Compares performance with known standards |
| Pareto chart | Identifies the most frequent trend within a data set | Identifies principal variables affecting the process |
| | | Identifies opportunities for improvement |
| Cause-and-effect (fishbone) chart | Displays multiple causes of a problem | Identifies root causes |
| | | Identifies variables affecting the process |
| | | Identifies opportunities for improvement |
| | | Plans for change |
| Scatter diagram | Displays relationship between two variables | Increases understanding of the relationship among multiple variables |
| Brainstorming | Rapidly generates multiple ideas | Promotes stakeholder buy-in |
| | | Increases understanding of the problem |
| | | Identifies variables affecting the process |
| Checklist | Controls data collection | Reduces errors of omission in data collection |
| Multivoting | Consolidates ideas | Achieves consensus among stakeholders |
| | | Prioritizes improvement strategies |
| Nominal group technique | Rapidly generates multiple ideas and prioritizes them | Identifies the problem |
| | | Achieves consensus among stakeholders |
| | | Prioritizes improvement strategies |
| | | Plans for change |
| Root cause analysis | Identifies the cause of the problem | Increases understanding of the problem |
| | | Identifies multicause variables affecting the process |
| | | Identifies opportunities to improve |
| | | Plans for change |
| Force field analysis | Identifies driving and restraining forces that impact proposed change | Identifies and lists variables affecting process |
| | | Plans for change |
| Consensus | Generates agreement among stakeholders | Increases understanding of the problem |
| | | Reduces resistance to change |
| | | Plans for change |

Adapted from Ogrinc GS, Headrick LA, Barton AJ, Dolansky MA, Miltner RA: *Fundamentals of health care improvement: a guide to improving your patients' care*, ed 3, 2018. Oak Brook Illinois, Joint Commission Resources. In Tracy MF, O'Grady ET, Phillips SJ: *Hamric & Hanson's advanced practice nursing: and integrative approach*, ed 7, 2023. St. Louis, Elsevier.

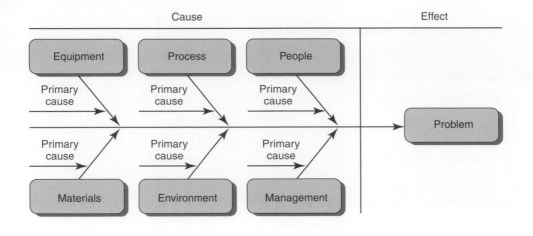

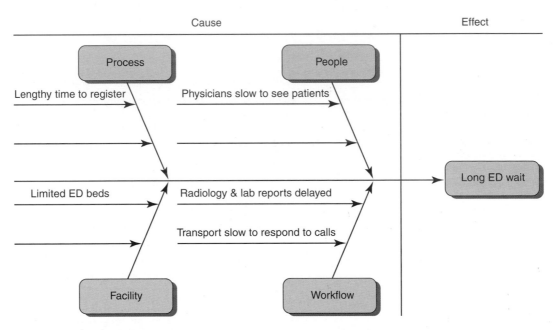

• **Fig. 10.8** This fishbone chart (top) was used during a brainstorming session to organize the possible causes of longer ED wait times (bottom). *ED*, Emergency department.

Once the groups are created, then everyone on the team will vote on their "favorite" idea. When voting on the ideas, the team is not discarding any ideas, just prioritizing them. Each team member might be given three votes, which they can place against any of the ideas. They can put all of their votes on one idea or spread them among three different ideas. The idea group with the most votes is the priority. The team may choose one or more ideas to pursue. This **nominal group technique** dampens the ability of one member to overpower the ideas of other members.

### Benchmarking

**Benchmarking** is a PI technique used by one facility to compare the performance of its processes with the same process at another facility with noted superior performance; sometimes this method is used internally to compare current performance with a previous exemplary performance. By reviewing a process that is effective in another facility,

the HIM department may discover methods or processes that would improve its own facility. Some processes are better served by throwing out the old model (the way things have always been done) and starting with a clean slate. The benchmarking technique can provide the facility with new and better methods for accomplishing the same tasks. Benchmarking internally, against previous performance, allows the facility to compare previous practices to current ones. Box 10.4 lists examples of common processes facilities use for benchmarking.

The Agency for Health Care Research and Quality (AHRQ) is an agency of the federal government charged with improving the quality of health care. The agency focuses on research into quality measures, preparing educational materials for the industry, and generating measures and data that help to inform clinicians and health care organizations. Searchable data are available on the AHRQ website at https://www.ahrq.gov/data/index.html

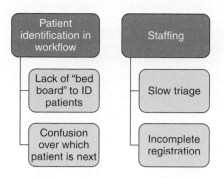

• **Fig. 10.9** The affinity diagram groups ideas from a brainstorming session. *ID*, Identify.

| TABLE 10.5 | Survey Questions | |
|---|---|---|
| **Open Question** | **Limited Answer Question** | |
| How would you describe your visit to our emergency department? | Choose one of the following to describe the emergency department during your recent visit:<br>a. Very clean<br>b. Adequately clean<br>c. Unclean<br>d. Very dirty | |
| How long did you wait in the emergency department before being seen by a physician? | How long did you wait in the emergency department before being seen by a physician?<br>a. Less than 1 hour<br>b. 1–2 hours<br>c. 2–3 hours<br>d. Longer than 3 hours | |

---

• **BOX 10.4   Examples of Benchmarks in an Acute Care Setting**

**Internal benchmarks**

- Days in accounts receivable (A/R) versus previous periods
- Discharged, not final billed (DNFB)
- Release of information (ROI) compliance

**External benchmarks**

- Average length of stay (ALOS)
- Case mix index (CMI)
- Operating margins
- Program for Evaluating Payment Patterns Electronic Report (PEPPER) reports

---

❖ **CASE STUDY 10.4**

**Advance Directives PI Project**

**Review of the Flowchart**

The team reviewed the process by creating a flowchart and discussing it. During the admission process, the patient is presented with the question: "Do you have an advance directive?" If the answer is yes, the patient is asked to provide a copy of the living will or medical power of attorney for the hospital to keep on file. If the answer is no, the patient is given additional information about making an advance directive and is asked to sign the Acknowledgment.

---

## Survey

A **survey** is a set of questions designed to gather information about a specific topic or issue. A survey can be used routinely to gather information from a group, or it can be designed as part of a PI team's efforts. For example, many facilities conduct a survey of patients after a visit to the facility. The data collectors want to find out how the patient perceived the service. This type of survey can be used to measure patient satisfaction. When significant dissatisfaction is observed, the facility may organize a PI team to address the issue. In the previously mentioned emergency department example, the PI team could develop a survey to ask patients why they think it took so long to receive treatment. The questions on a survey can be open-ended, which means that the response areas are blank. With open-ended questions, patients are free to answer the question in their own words. However, this method of questioning may not provide enough information to determine how much improvement is necessary. Table 10.5 provides an example of the same survey question asked in two different ways.

## Diagrams

A *flowchart* is a tool used to organize the steps involved in a process (Case Study 10.4). Because the PI team is interdisciplinary, some of the team members may not understand the process they are intended to improve. The flowchart

illustrates how the process works within the facility. For an example, refer to the advance directive process shown in Fig. 10.3. Fig. 10.10 is a flowchart of the advance directive process showing how the facility informs the patient about the advance directive and how the health care professional obtains the patient's signature on the acknowledgment form. Flowcharts help the team streamline a process and eliminate unnecessary steps. Flowcharts are also useful in illustrating the change in a process for reporting and training purposes. Flowcharts utilize standard symbols that are defined by ANSI so that flowcharts created adhere to standardized symbols for universal understanding.

Kaoru Ishikawa was a Japanese organizational theorist and educator who is best known in the United States as the developer of the *Ishikawa* or *fishbone* diagram for analyzing the cause of problems (Case Study 10.5). The structure of the diagram resembles a fish skeleton, hence the name. At the head of the fish is the problem, defect, or undesired outcome. Along the spine of the fish are various bones representing categories of input that affect the issue at the head. In manufacturing, there are many different bones; however, in service industries, such as health care, there are typically only four: materials (supplies), methods (process), people, and machines (equipment). The literature varies as to what

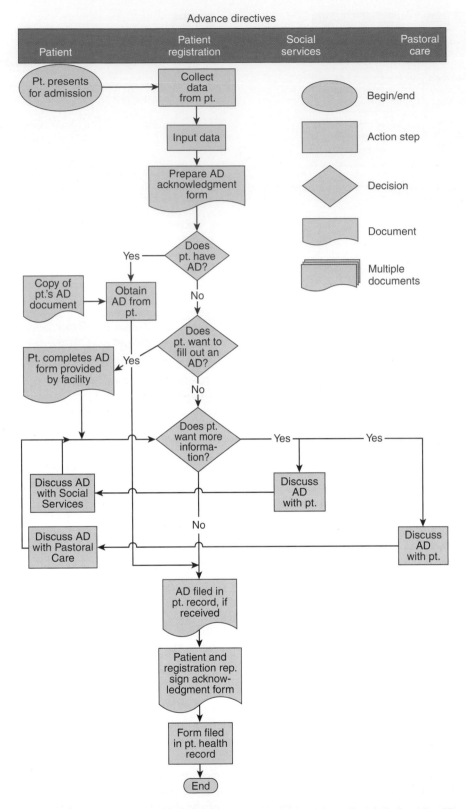

• **Fig. 10.10** Flowchart of the advance directive process showing how the facility informs the patient (pt.) about the AD and how the health care professional obtains the patient's signature on the acknowledgment form. *AD*, Advance directive; *Rep.*, representative.

## CASE STUDY 10.5

### Advance Directives PI Project

**Plan**

Through discussion with the patient access staff, review of the flowchart, and observation of a sample of patient registrations, the team learned that there are several reasons why the Acknowledgment form was not being collected.
- Patients who stated that they had advance directives, but did not provide them, were not being asked to sign the Acknowledgment.
- Some patients refused to sign the form.
- During peak registration times, sometimes the registrar forgot to ask the patient to sign.
- Some patients are not conscious on admission and there was no follow-up process.
  The team created a fishbone diagram to illustrate these issues.

the bones are called, but the concepts are the same. On each bone are the potential causes from that source that could contribute to the issue.

### Process Control Chart

A **process control chart** is a data-gathering tool that graphs the measurement of a key performance indicator or other variables over time. The indicator or variable is shown on the chart in the context of the upper and lower thresholds of tolerance of variation in the behavior of the measure. Fig. 10.5 shows an example of a process control chart depicting the DNFB. The thresholds are determined by observing the indicator over time and improving the process. The thresholds can change as the process improves or otherwise changes. This tool is most advantageous at depicting a repetitive process that is measurable and controllable. Some activities in health care do not lend themselves as well to this type of analysis, such as medication errors, for which the only truly acceptable measure is zero.

The thresholds are, effectively, tolerances for error or ranges that the organization considers appropriate. The DNFB target may be 6% of accounts receivable, but the revenue cycle committee will tolerate between 5.5% and 6.5% as variances. Typically, these percentages are expressed as a dollar amount, as depicted in Fig. 10.5.

## Data Organization and Presentation Tools

Data organization and presentation tools are used to communicate information quickly to another person or group. We discussed the construction of graphs, tables, and charts in Chapter 7. These visual tools can be quite persuasive, and the selection of title and specific data points can be used to emphasize what the preparer of the graph chooses, as illustrated in Fig. 10.11. In this example, the number of

cigarette-smoking freshmen on a college campus declined 40% between 2016 and 2020. However, overall smoking prevalence on the campus was virtually unchanged during that time. The same statement could be graphed in two different ways: The positive graph shows that the number of freshmen who smoke has decreased, and the negative graph shows that the total percentage of people who smoke remains unchanged. Thus the focus (some might say the bias) of the preparer influences the message. In a PI project, these findings might generate additional review to examine where the apparent increase in smoking is occurring and why.

### Bar and Line Graphs

Bar and line graphs are used to display discrete data elements, one axis for the group or indicator and the other axis used to plot the data for the group. For example, Fig. 10.11 is a bar graph showing the categories (2019, 2020, 2021, 2022, 2023) along the x-axis that represents the years in which freshmen smoking was measured. The data plotted along the y-axis indicate the percentage of freshmen who smoke for each year. Bar graphs depict frequency at a point in time. Therefore measurement in 5 years requires five bars. Changing the bar graph to a line graph provides an illustration of the data points across a continuum and may display a percentage of people smoking throughout the 5 years. In Fig. 10.12, the bars have been replaced with points that are connected by lines. Line graphs are used to plot data over time. This line graph is an easy way to depict the trend of the same data as they are measured continuously, month to month or year to year.

### Pie Chart

A pie chart is a graphical illustration of information as it relates to a whole. For example, a pie chart can be used to illustrate the percentages of different populations on campus who smoke. When considering this type of chart, imagine a pie, the pieces of which represent percentages. If the pie is cut into even slices, all of the pieces are equal. However, when the size of each piece represents the various smoking populations on campus, we can easily determine which group smokes the most because the sizes vary (see Fig. 10.13).

Note the labels and headings used in Figs. 10.11–10.13. The headings describe the graph or chart, giving the reader an idea of what information is included. On bar and line graphs, the labels on the axes identify what is being measured and how it is being measured. On the pie chart, a key might be used to indicate which color is associated with each group. The following is a list of reminders for creating graphs:
- Include information about the time frame of the data or the date on which the data were collected.
- Make sure the graph is legible, especially when presenting the information on an overhead projector to a large group.

| Year | 2019 | 2020 | 2021 | 2022 | 2023 | |
|---|---|---|---|---|---|---|
| # of freshmen who smoke | 1299 | 1157 | 885 | 588 | 462 | |
| *Total # of freshmen* | 2095 | 2103 | 2099 | 2100 | 2098 | |
| % of freshmen who smoke | 62% | 55% | 42% | 28% | 22% | |
| Total # of smokers on campus | 3247 | 3264 | 3254 | 3272 | 3269 | |

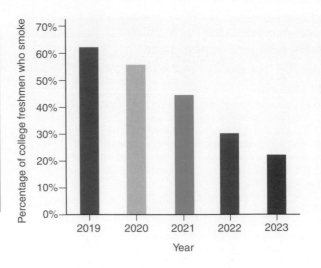

• **Fig. 10.11** Bar graph showing percentages of college freshmen who smoked cigarettes, 2019–2023.

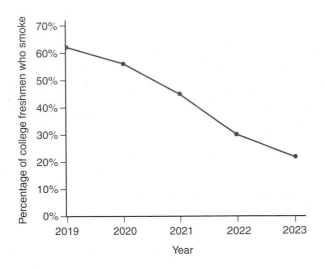

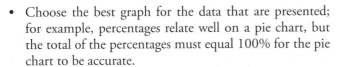

• **Fig. 10.12** Line graph of same data in Fig. 10.11.

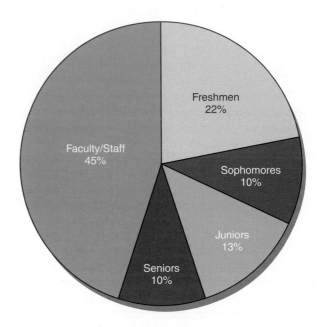

• **Fig. 10.13** Pie chart of the percentages of different populations on campus who smoke.

- Choose the best graph for the data that are presented; for example, percentages relate well on a pie chart, but the total of the percentages must equal 100% for the pie chart to be accurate.
- Be prepared to explain the graph if questioned by the audience.

Software programs such as Microsoft Excel can simplify the creation of these graphs, tables, and charts. These programs make it very easy to turn data into an easy-to-read presentation tool.

### Decision Matrix

A **decision matrix** can help a group organize information. This tool is used when the PI team must narrow its focus or choose among several categories or issues. For example, if a PI team is organized to decrease smoking on the college campus, the members may begin by brainstorming to determine all the issues that influence a person's decision to smoke. Once the team has identified the factors on campus that influence this decision, the team must decide which

influential factors they can change. A decision matrix can be used to analyze which of the factors would cause a decrease in the number of smokers if removed. Table 10.6 shows a decision matrix in which each group of smokers is analyzed to determine which issue has the greatest influence on that group's decision to smoke.

Note that the first row of the table identifies the groups of smokers and the first column identifies the issues that may influence a person's decision to smoke. To complete the decision matrix, the PI team analyzes each group according to the influences that the team identified. Team members can write their comments in the squares, or they can assign a value—in this case, 1 for least likely to influence the person to smoke, 2 for moderate influence, and 3 for most likely to influence the person to smoke. The final column on the right is a total, or decision, column.

| TABLE 10.6 | Decision Matrix | | | | | |
|---|---|---|---|---|---|---|
| | Freshmen | Sophomores | Juniors | Seniors | Faculty-Staff | Total |
| Commercials | 2 | 2 | 2 | 2 | 1 | 9 |
| Smoking areas | 3 | 3 | 3 | 3 | 3 | 15 |
| Peer pressure | 3 | 3 | 2 | 2 | 1 | 11 |

The influence with the highest rating or the influence that occurred in each of the categories would be the team's target. In this case, the first, and by far easiest, way to decrease smoking on campus would be to eliminate some of the smoking areas.

## Project Management

Project Management is a unique discipline in which practitioners develop, coordinate, and bring to completion special activities from beginning to end. The Project Management Institute supports a variety of certifications that demonstrate competence in the profession, notably the Project Management Professional. While we may not find SCRUM, XP, and Kanban useful regularly, there are tools and skills in the project management arena that are useful for administrative, PI, and planning purposes. Case Study 10.6 continues our PI project.

### Project Management Tools

A basic tool of project management is the GANTT chart. This chart is a detailed list of every step in a project and shows both the planned and actual timelines. Think about how you would describe your morning routine. You do not jump out of bed and head out the door to school or work without a few steps in between. So, a project has many steps in between the concept and the completion. There is software available to support this aspect of project management; however, for our purposes, we can illustrate a GANTT chart in an Excel worksheet. We shall talk about the columns first.

Column A is the reference number of the task. In a huge project, there may be hundreds of interrelated tasks, so we number them to enable us to easily refer back and forth.

Column B is the name of the task.

Column C is the reference of any immediate predecessor tasks—tasks that must be completed before the listed task.

Column D is the duration of the task—how long is it expected to take?

Column E is the date on which the project begins.

Column F is the date on which the project ends.

Columns to the right of the date represent a horizontal calendar in which the beginning and ending dates of the task are marked. In Excel, two rows for each task would enable the depiction of both the original estimated dates and the actual dates, for comparison.

The point of a GANTT chart is to enable the project manager to see exactly what progress has been made and where problems may be occurring. While this is in many ways a time management tool, it is also an organizational tool, because many details are required to prepare a GANTT chart in a meaningful way. Fig. 10.14 shows a simple GANTT chart of the advance directive solution.

## PERT chart

A Program Evaluation Review Technique (PERT) chart is another visual tool that helps the project manager identify the critical sequence of events in a project. As we see in the GANTT chart, some tasks can be performed at any time in the project. Other tasks are dependent on tasks that come before them to begin or end. The PERT chart takes these sequences and places them in the order in which they occur, taking into consideration all of the timelines of every task. There emerges from that analysis the shortest possible time in which the project can be completed.

### CASE STUDY 10.6

#### Advance Directives PI Project

**Do**

The team decided to rapidly test one critical adjustment to the existing process. The new requirement and the Acknowledgment form had been presented to registrars at a staff meeting; however, a revised procedure for evidencing the absence of an Advance Directive Acknowledgment form had not been developed. The team decided to move forward with this change immediately while they considered other aspects of the issue. Registrars would be required to ask whether the patient has an advance directive. If yes, and they have it, scan it in. If no, or if yes and they do not have it with them, sign the form with the appropriate response and receive a copy of the advance directive information materials. If the patient refuses to sign and/or refuses the materials, the registrar completes a section at the bottom of the form and refers the patient to social services for follow-up.

| ID | Task_Name | Predecessor | Duration | Start Date | End Date |
|---|---|---|---|---|---|
| DPP | Develop Policy & Procedure | | 5 days | 1/11 | 1/16 |
| DPP-1 | PI Committee Recommendation | DPP | 1 day | 1/16 | 1/17 |
| DPP-2 | Department Approval | DPP-1 | 1 day | 1/17 | 1/18 |
| DPP-3 | VP Approval | DPP-2 | 2 days | 1/18 | 1/20 |
| DPP-4 | CEO Approval | DPP-3 | 3 days | 1/20 | 1/23 |
| | Policy & Procedure Complete | | | | 1/23 |
| TS | Train Staff - Plan | DPP-1 | 2 days | 1/18 | 1/20 |
| TS-1 | Patient Access Days | DPP-3 | 3 days | 1/24 | 1/27 |
| TS-2 | Patient Access Nights | TS-1, TS-3 | 2 days | 1/28 | 1/30 |
| TS-3 | Other Staff | DPP-3 | 2 days | 1/25 | 1/27 |
| | Training Complete | | | | 1/30 |
| IMP | Write Implementation Memos | DPP -1 | 2 days | 1/19 | 1/21 |
| IMP-1 | Go Live | TS-2 | 3 days | 1/31 | 2/3 |
| IMP-2 | Data Collection | IMP-1 | 30 days | 2/4 | 3/6 |
| IMP-3 | PI Team Analyze Data | IMP-1 | 30 days | 2/4 | 3/6 |
| | **Implementation Complete** | | | | **3/6** |

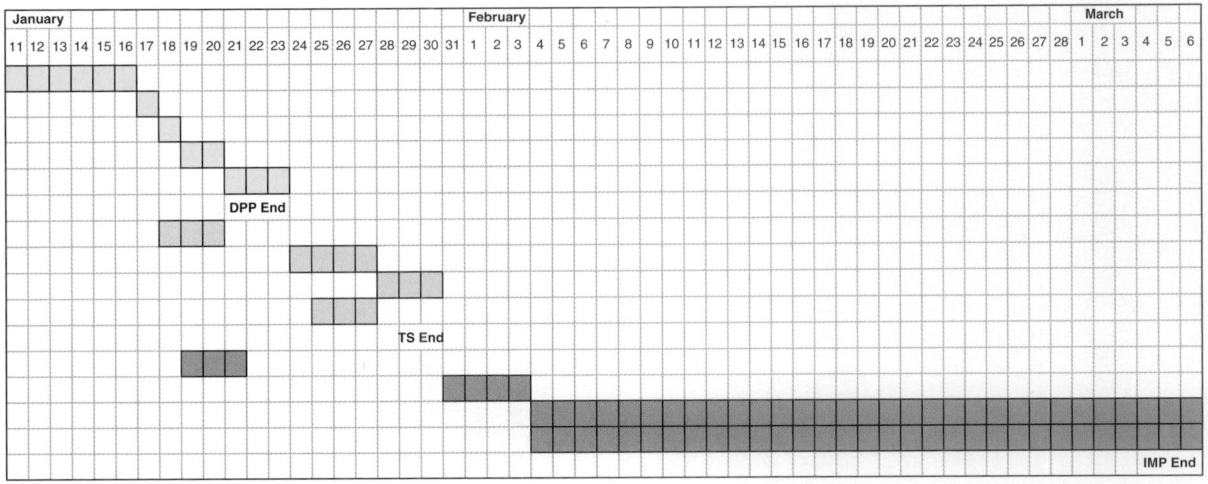

• **Fig. 10.14** Advance directive policy and procedure GANTT chart.

For our advance directive solution (Case Study 10.7), the PERT chart shows that the solution project will take a minimum of 49 days from initiation to sign-off.

## Skills

SCRUM is a methodology for delivering software projects using an iterative process. XP is Extreme Programming, an agile framework for software development. Kanban is a lean method of improving performance and is named for a schedule that facilitates process improvement and just-in-time manufacturing. These are some of the tools in the Agile Project Management toolbox, which we mention to demonstrate that Project Management is not just about time management.

As we have discussed, PI activities involve aspects of these competencies: identifying the problem, initiating the project, analyzing the problem, planning the solution, implementing the solution, and operationalizing the solution. Throughout the PI project, the leader must monitor and control the activities so that the team is focused on the problem at hand (Case Study 10.8).

There are myriad points in which project management skills are useful generally. For example, any time there is a change of any kind, there is an opportunity for project management skills: initiating communication about the change, planning, executing, and monitoring the change. Consider the implementation of ICD-10-CM/PCS a few years ago and the potential future implementation of ICD-11-CM/PCS. This was a vast project that required extensive communication, multidepartment education, software changes, and a federal amendment of the HIPAA code sets. Thus there were many opportunities to demonstrate interpersonal communication, leadership, and planning skills.

---

### ❖ CASE STUDY 10.7

**Advance Directives PI Project**

**Act**

To roll out the implementation, a GANTT chart was developed. The Patient Access Director would own the implementation of the new process. The updated procedure needed approval by the VP and the CEO. The Director would train the day staff and supervisors in two batches over 3 days and social services at the same time over 2 days. To ensure consistent training, the Director would train the night staff on subsequent days. Once all staff were trained, the procedure would go live and the supervisory staff would begin 100% review and data collection for feedback to the PI team. A PERT chart demonstrated that from procedure to feedback would take a minimum of 49 days (Fig. 10.15).

### ❖ CASE STUDY 10.8

**Advance Directives PI Project**

**Wrap-up**

The team ultimately decided to implement two additional processes. During the supervisory review of all inpatient registrations, a qualitative review of the advance directive documentation is now required. Follow-up with patients who were unconscious on arrival is required and the advance directive discussion documented within 24 hours of admission by social services. After 3 months of data collection, the process was working well and qualitative review was cut back to random checks of current registrars and 100% review for 3 months of new registrars. The team reported its project to its VP champion and the PI Committee at its quarterly meeting.

---

| Develop P&P | DPP |  DPP-1 | DPP-2 | DPP-3 | DPP-4 | | | |
|---|---|---|---|---|---|---|---|---|
| | 5 days | 1 day | 1 day | 2 days | 3 days | | | |
| | 1/11 – 1/16 | 1/16 – 1/17 | 1/17 – 1/18 | 1/18 – 1/20 | 1/20 – 1/23 | | | |
| | | | | | | | | |
| Train Staff | | | | TS | TS | | | |
| | | | | 2 days | 3 days | | | |
| | | | | 1/18 – 1/20 | 1/24 – 1/27 | TS | | |
| | | | | | | 2 days | | |
| | | | | TS | TS | 1/28 – 1/30 | | |
| | | | | 2 days | | | | |
| | | | | 1/25 – 1/27 | | | | |
| | | | | | | | | |
| Implement | | | | IMP | | IMP-1 | IMP-2 | |
| | | | | 2 days | | 3 days | 30 days | |
| | | | | 1/19 – 1/21 | | 1/31 – 2/03 | 2/04 – 3/06 | |
| | | | | | | | | 49 |
| | | | | | | | | DAYS |
| | | | | | | IMP 3 | | |
| | | | | | | 30 days | | |
| | | | | | | 2/04 – 3/06 | | |

• **Fig. 10.15** Advance directive Policy & Procedure implementation PERT chart.

## COMPETENCY CHECK-IN 10.3

### Performance Improvement

1. In the popular PDSA quality improvement method, which step of the process involves monitoring effectiveness of the solution over a period of time?
   a. Plan
   b. Do
   c. Study
   d. Act

2. Which of the following abbreviations is used to describe the continuous improvement of processes within a facility?
   a. QA
   b. QM
   c. PI/QI
   d. UM

3. In addition to PDCA methods, list two other PI methods that are popular among health care facilities.

4. To improve quality according to a standard, a health care facility may use _____ comparing its performance to that of a similar facility.

5. Which graph would you use to show that the overall percentage of people smoking on campus has remained unchanged?

6. _____ is a PI technique used to solicit participation and information from an entire group.

7. A supervisor and team of employees are confronted with two solutions to a problem. Each solution involves time, money, and space; which quality management tool might the supervisor use to choose a solution?

8. Which committee is often responsible for reviewing health care records according to accreditation standards, checking physician record completion statistics, and acting as the consultant to the director of HIM?
   a. HIM committee
   b. Safety committee
   c. Infection control committee
   d. P&T committee

9. Infections acquired by patients while they are in the hospital are known as:
   a. Nosocomial infections
   b. Comorbidities
   c. Secondary infections
   d. Opportunistic infections

10. Which of the following committees acts as liaison to the governing board of the facility?
    a. Surgical case review
    b. P&T committee
    c. Medical executive committee
    d. Credentials committee

11. Which of the following medical staff committees reviews medication usage?
    a. Surgical case review
    b. P&T committee
    c. Medical executive committee
    d. Credentials committee

12. What does the PERT chart show?
    a. The shortest possible time in which the project can be completed
    b. The longest possible time in which the project will take
    c. The number of people required to work on a project
    d. The unity of command within the project

13. A supervisor and team of employees are confronted with two solutions to a problem. Each solution involves time, money, and space. Which quality management tool might the supervisor use to help the team choose a solution?

14. Which is a characteristic of a process control chart?
    a. Upper and lower thresholds
    b. Standardized symbols showing an action
    c. The display of factors that can change a variable
    d. The sequence of events of a project

## Change Management

To summarize some of what we have learned in the last nine chapters, consider change. Change is inevitable in the health care industry: organizations merge, technology advances, coding systems are updated, laws are promulgated, and regulations ensue. Throughout all of this, the health information management professional must learn, absorb, and adapt.

Not everyone embraces change. For example, consider the coder who has used a code book for 20 years and is now required to adapt to computer-assisted coding. Resistance, denial, and, ultimately, the failure to adapt can be career-limiting. So, it is important as HIM professionals to understand how change affects us and to learn how to manage change for ourselves and those around us.

Change management, like project management, is a distinct discipline with its own skillset—some of which we already know. While the discipline is evolving, there are certificate programs available, and the Change Management Institute, with chapters in seven countries, offers multiple levels of "accreditation" based on its Change Management Body of Knowledge (Change Management Institute, n.d.).

Change management refers to the broad range of processes and skills needed to effect change. Change can be on a personal level, such as a job or position change. Change can be thrust upon us, like a new manager. We can be the drivers of change in PI, for example. Wherever we are in the process, the first thing to understand is that there are at least two sides to every change: the changer(s), who is the initiator of the change, and those upon whom the change is imposed. Thus it becomes obvious from the start that communication is a key change management skill.

There are numerous "principles" of change management, varying from a handful to over a dozen cited in the literature. They all have some key elements, which are highlighted in Table 10.7. When change is known, some steps can be taken to ameliorate the impact of change on staff and the organization. Two key elements of change management are communication and transparency. Keep management abreast of issues that are impacting the organization so that change is not a surprise. For example, the coding system change from ICD-9 to ICD-10 was not just an HIM issue. It impacted departments across the hospital and required staffing and resources to manage far in advance of the actual go-live. This works both ways. If the organization is losing money and looking for ways to streamline and cut costs, it is beneficial for administration to be candid with managers regarding how the issue is being addressed and to engage their participation in seeking solutions where appropriate.

So, in our discussion of change, you may be thinking that it sounds like a project. Well, it is. So, the tools and skills we learn for PI and project management can be employed in managing change. Our advance directive project, for example, did not necessarily have to be a PI project. The Patient Access Director could have had another staff meeting and imposed discipline on staff who were not completing the forms correctly. There would still be missing forms and staff would be disgruntled. Further, social services would not have been engaged and participated to support the effort. So, creating a project engages the critical thinking skills of new observers, who can bring new ideas to the table.

Failure to effectively manage change can lead to widespread lack of productivity and staff dissatisfaction. Consider that the most likely staff to leave, in the face of general dissatisfaction, are the staff who are the most desirable employees—the ones who will have the easiest time finding a new position elsewhere. Therefore employing positive leadership in a changing environment will help mitigate that problem. Communicate the need for the change and engage staff in understanding the impact of the change.

Just as change is inevitable in an organization, so are industry changes ongoing. The best strategy for anticipating change and preparing for it is to actively participate in career planning and continuing education. Maintaining currency in the profession through continuing education provides value to your employer, enhances job satisfaction, and facilitates career planning.

| TABLE 10.7 | Principles of Change Management |
|---|---|
| *Communication* | Communicate clearly and often. |
| *Top down* | Start at the top and ensure that everyone is on board and clear with the plan. |
| *Engagement at all levels* | Ensure that employees are reasonably aware of issues administration is facing before a change is necessary and keep all levels of staff apprised of steps to be taken, soliciting their feedback as appropriate. |
| *Support the process* | Provide policy, procedure, budget, training, and recognition. |
| *Adapt* | Provide leadership through unexpected issues that arise. |

## COMPETENCY CHECK-IN 10.4

### Change Management

1. Revenue Cycle Committee has observed an increase in Medicare denials for lack of medical necessity. The hospital cannot always bill the patient, because the patient did not always sign an ABN. Who should be on the PI project to investigate and solve the problem?
2. Prepare a fishbone diagram identifying potential sources of problems with Medicare denials for lack of medical necessity.
3. Consider that one outcome of the PI Project is the installation of a preregistration software module that checks for Medicare's medical necessity requirements before the service is rendered. List the main tasks, in order, that would have to be completed in order to implement this solution.

# Chapter Summary

Health information is widely accepted as an important part of the health care industry, and people take for granted that it will be timely, complete, accurate, and valid. As specifically noted in this chapter, the uses of health information are not limited to the internal needs of a health care facility. Patient health information is valuable to many outside the facility. Notably, this chapter reflects the importance of continued efforts to ensure high-quality health information so that it may be used effectively to make decisions about patient care, to establish compliance with standards, and to improve patient care. Having standardized information for all patients, as first required by ACS minimum standards, is important. With standardized information, health care professionals can compare one patient's care with another's and determine the quality of each. Standardized information allows for similar information to be shared as well as compared.

With ongoing PI initiatives like National Patient Safety Goals and outcomes measures, the health care record and health information provide the data needed for reporting and compliance. Likewise, PI efforts often rely on documentation in patient records to investigate, monitor, and ensure quality.

Ensuring that health information is of high quality allows others to use this vital information for the benefit of patients, communities, payers, and providers.

# Competency Milestones

### CAHIIM Competency

*VI.2. Identify the impact of organizational change. (3)*

### Rationale
Change is frequent in health care. HIM professionals need to build their skill set to include weathering and managing change.

### Competency Assessment
1. List and describe key strategies for managing change.
2. List and describe three events that could involve organizational change.
3. In response to recent abuses of break time, staff and management are now required to swipe their badges in the time clock if they leave the building for lunch or a break. What can you do, as a supervisor, to support your staff through this change?
4. One of your employees has just asked you whether it is true that your hospital is about to be merged with another organization. This is the first you have heard of a merger. You call your manager right away to confirm, but he does not know anything. Later in the day, he gets back to you, explaining that administration is keeping it quiet for now and not to say anything. The next morning, there is an article in the local paper announcing the merger. What is wrong with this scenario? What should have happened? What is likely to happen now?
5. Your hospital is merging with another hospital in the area. Management of the HIM department will be consolidated into one Director. No staff layoffs are anticipated, but some functions will be shifted to be "housed" in only one facility to eliminate redundancy and some staff will be cross-trained. As the new corporate Director of HIM, what skills and tools could you use to efficiently reorganize the department to achieve this goal?

### CAHIIM Competency

*VI.4. Utilize data-driven performance improvement techniques for decision-making. (3)*

### Rationale
Health care facilities have a quality management department, usually staffed by health information management (HIM) and nursing professionals, to monitor and assess quality. It is the primary responsibility of this department to educate those in the health care facility about the quality management and PI process and to monitor the assessment of quality for the facility.

### Competency Assessment
1. Briefly explain the philosophies of Deming, Juran, and Crosby.
2. Explain the PDSA method for quality improvement.
3. Describe the lean performance improvement process.
4. Identify the Six Sigma steps for improvement of an established process.
5. List and explain the tools used for data gathering.
6. List and explain the tools used for data organization and presentation.

7. Identify three committees and how they use health information.
8. Explain the structure of the medical staff committee in a health care facility.
9. Explain the purpose and composition of the HIM committee in a health care facility.

## Ethics Challenge

*VI.7. Assess ethical standards of practice. (5)*

1. You are a member of a PI team working on a materials management project. One aspect of the project is to observe the delivery and storage of supplies to nursing units. Several internal TJC compliance audits have revealed outdated materials on the units, which is one of the indicators that prompted your project. You are paired with a team member from nursing: a unit clerk who is very opinionated on the subject and thinks that materials management is being unfairly targeted. Instead of just collecting the data, she has already "supervised" the process several times and ensured that the delivery person rotated the stock every time. What do you do?

## Critical Thinking Questions

1. You are a revenue cycle specialist in the HIM Department of a Community Hospital. One of your daily tasks is to compile and review the Uniform Hospital Discharge Data Set (UHDDS) data that is transmitted daily to the data collection agency. You work about a week post discharge in order to ensure that processing is complete. You are noticing an increase in the number of errors that need to be corrected: missing data that is necessary for the Uniform Bill (UB). This data is collected in Patient Access and the UB will not "drop" (complete processing and transmit to the payor) without this data. In reviewing the patient account, you can see that the data is missing; however, a review of the UB shows that the data is present but is not always correct.
   a. What is your first step in determining what to do about this data quality issue?
   b. What departments should be involved in analyzing and evaluating solutions to this issue?
   c. What quality tools would be most effective in analyzing the cause?

## The Role of Health Information Management Professionals in the Workplace

### Professional Profile: Assistant Director, Health Information Management

My name is Kim, and I am the assistant director of the HIM department. My role involves coordinating the operations of the HIM department with the supervisors of the three key areas: coding, chart completion, and release of information. I meet daily with the supervisors to ensure that processes are on track and to assist with any outstanding problems. I coordinate with other departments, as needed, to evaluate the need for training in overlapping areas, to resolve problems, and to participate in hospital-wide initiatives. For example, I meet with Patient Access to discuss coding training for registrars and work with them to resolve revenue cycle problems that can arise from registrar errors. I also sit on the Clinical Documentation Improvement Committee—an interdisciplinary committee that reviews and evaluates CDI monthly reports and oversees provider education.

I am responsible for coordinating review of health records (ongoing record review) to ensure compliance with TJC standards. Record review is performed on a monthly basis at Diamonte. According to standards, my staff and I review 50 records each month. I make sure that all of the records are pulled before the meeting and prepare enough forms for review of the 50 records. During the multidisciplinary review meeting, I help the team members when they have a problem interpreting a standard or locating information in the health record. After all 50 records have been reviewed, I collect the forms and tabulate the scores to determine the compliance with each standard. I then present the results of this review to the HIM committee for recommendation and action, as necessary. If the committee suggests a corrective action to improve compliance with a standard, I coordinate that effort. After the implementation of the corrective action, I report back to the HIM committee to show whether compliance has been achieved.

### Career Tip

Ongoing record review is a TJC requirement, and HIM-credentialed professionals are logical leaders for record review and quality auditing. Preparation for this challenge includes a thorough understanding of TJC standards, including the interrelationship among the standards: Provision of Care and Record of Care, for example. Monthly review of TJC's newsletter, *Perspectives*, and annual, thorough review of the standards that affect HIM practice are essential.

**Patient Care Perspective**

**Dr. Lewis's Partner, Dr. Milque**

I sit on the ongoing record review committee. It is a very interesting process. At first, I thought it was a waste of time to look at these records and that the regulators were making us jump through hoops. However, now that I have

seen for myself the problems that users of the records have when documentation is missing or inaccurate, I have become an advocate of record review. I recently addressed the medical staff on the importance of completing records as soon as possible after discharge. In this electronic environment, 30 days is much too long to wait for a completed record.

## Works Cited

American College of Surgeons: *About ACS*, 2021. https://www.facs.org/about-acs. Accessed January 9, 2022.

American Hospital Association: *History AHA*, 2021. https://www.aha.org/about/history. Accessed January 9, 2022.

Berwick D: Improving patient care. My right knee, *Ann Intern Med* 142(2):121–125, 2005.

Centers for Medicare and Medicaid Services (CMS): *Quality improvement organization manual, revision 18, Chapter 4: Case review*, 2014. https://www.cms.gov/Regulations-and-Guidance/Guidance/Manuals/Downloads/qio110c04.pdf. Accessed January 22, 2022.

Centers for Medicare and Medicaid Services: CMS hospital value-based purchasing program results for fiscal year 2020. *CMS.gov Newsroom.*, 2019. https://www.cms.gov/newsroom/fact-sheets/cms-hospital-value-based-purchasing-program-results-fiscal-year-2020. Accessed February 10, 2023.

Centers for Medicare and Medicaid Services: *The Hospital Value-Based Purchasing (VBP) Program*, 2021. https://www.cms.gov/Medicare/Quality-Initiatives-Patient-Assessment-Instruments/Value-Based-Programs/HVBP/Hospital-Value-Based-Purchasing. Accessed February 10, 2021.

Centers for Medicare and Medicaid Services: *Current work: QIO Program 11th SOW (2014–2019)*, 2023. https://www.cms.gov/medicare/quality-initiatives-patient-assessment-instruments/qualityimprovementorgs/current. Accessed February 10, 2023.

Change Management Institute: *Change manager competency models: preview document*, n.d. https://www.change-management-institute.com/sites/default/files/uploaded-content/field_f_content_file/cmi_change_manager_competency_models_preview_sept17.pdf. Accessed January 9, 2022.

Church J, Baker P, Berry D: Shared governance: a journey with continual mile markers, *Nurs Manage* 39(4 ):34, 2008. 36, 38 passim doi:10.1097/01.NUMA.0000316058.20070.8c

Department of Health and Human Services: *Report to Congress: the administration, cost, and impact of the quality improvement organization program for Medicare beneficiaries for fiscal year 2018, 2021*. Washington, DC, Department of Health and Human Services. https://www.cms.gov/Medicare/Quality-Initiatives-Patient-Assessment-Instruments/QualityImprovementOrgs/Downloads/Annual-Report-to-Congress-QIO-Program-Fiscal-Year-2018.pdf.

George ML: *Lean Six Sigma for service*, 2003. New York, McGraw-Hill. Accessed February 15, 2019.

iSixSigma: *What is Six Sigma?*, June 14, 2022 http://www.isixsigma.com/new-to-six-sigma/getting-started/what-six-sigma/. Accessed January 9, 2022.

Liker JK: *The Toyota Way: 14 management principles from the world's greatest manufacturer*, 2004. New York, McGraw-Hill.

## Further Reading

Agency for Healthcare Research and Quality: *About the National Quality Strategy*. Agency for Healthcare Research and Quality, 2021. https://www.ahrq.gov/workingforquality/about/index.html. Accessed January 9, 2022.

Centers for Medicare and Medicaid Services: CMS hospital value-based purchasing program results for fiscal year 2020. *CMS.gov Newsroom*, October 29, 2019. https://www.cms.gov/newsroom/fact-sheets/cms-hospital-value-based-purchasing-program-results-fiscal-year-2020. Accessed January 22, 2022.

Centers for Medicare and Medicaid Services, Medicare Learning Network: Medicare fraud & abuse: prevent, detect, report. *MLN booklet*, January 2021. https://www.cms.gov/Outreach-and-Education/Medicare-Learning-Network-MLN/MLNProducts/Downloads/Fraud-Abuse-MLN4649244-Print-Friendly.pdf. Accessed January 9, 2022.

Centers for Medicare and Medicaid Services, QualityNet: Hospital value-based purchasing (HVBP) program. Overview. *About the Hospital VBP Program*, 2021. https://qualitynet.cms.gov/inpatient/hvbp. Accessed January 9, 2022.

Davoudi S, et al: Data Quality management model (2015 update), *J AHIMA*. 86(10), 2015. http://library.ahima.org/doc?oid=107773. Accessed January 9, 2022.

Department of Health and Human Services, National Institutes of Health: *National Institute for Research on Safety and Quality (NIRSQ)*, 2021. https://www.ahrq.gov/sites/default/files/wysiwyg/cpi/about/mission/budget/2021/FY_2021_CJ_NIRSQ.pdf.

Institute for Healthcare Improvement: *About Us | History*, 2021. http://www.ihi.org/about/Pages/History.aspx. Accessed January 9, 2022.

ISO: International Organization for Standardization: *About ISO*, 2022. https://www.iso.org/about-us.html. Accessed January 9, 2022.

ISO. Member: *ANSI United States; Membership: Member body*. n.d. https://www.iso.org/member/2188.html. Accessed February 6, 2023.

Lean Enterprise Institute: *A brief history of lean*. n.d. https://www.lean.org/explore-lean/a-brief-history-of-lean/. Accessed April 16, 2022.

# Appendix A

# Paper Health Records

## CHAPTER OUTLINE

**From Paper to Electronic Health Records**
The Push for EHRs
Meaningful Use

**Organization of a Paper-Based Health Record**
Integrated Record
Source-Oriented Record
Problem-Oriented Record
Problem List
Advantages and Disadvantages

**Postdischarge Paper-Based Processing**
Chart Assembly
Quantitative Analysis
Retrieval

**Record Storage: Legacy Systems**
Identification of Physical Files
Filing Methods

**Work Cited**

**Sample Paper Records**
Inpatient Admission Form/Face Sheet
Conditions of Admission

Advance Directive Acknowledgment
Emergency Department Record
History
Physical
Provider's Order Form
Provider's Progress Notes
Informed Consent
Consultation Record
Medication Administration Record
Insulin Administration Record
Analgesic Pain Management Assessment
Intake/Output Record
Nursing Progress Notes
Operative Report Progress Notes
Discharge Orders
Nursing Discharge Summary
Certificate of Live Birth
Certificate of Death
Report of Fetal Death

## VOCABULARY

chart assembly
countersignature
Health Information Technology for Economic and Clinical
    Health Act (HITECH)
integrated record
legacy system
loose sheets
meaningful use

outguide
problem list
problem-oriented record
quantitative analysis
source-oriented record
terminal-digit filing system
universal chart order

## From Paper to Electronic Health Records

Historically, patient records have been maintained in a paper format. Each clinical department within a facility may develop one or more forms to document treatment, tests, and other results pertinent to that department's functions. The paper record is initiated at the time of the patient's admission or encounter and may move with the patient as he or she receives treatment throughout the health care facility. The paper record is assembled after discharge, analyzed, coded, completed, and then filed in the health information management (HIM) department. Due to limited storage space, older records are typically stored elsewhere or scanned to an alternative storage medium, such as microfiche. One advantage of a paper record is that it is reasonably secure within a locked file room; however, there is always some delay in obtaining data from prior visits, because it takes a bit of time to retrieve a record. Further, a paper record format prohibits more than one person at a time from working with the entire record. A need for increased accessibility for a variety of purposes has led to a trend away from paper records and toward the electronic health record (EHR).

## The Push for EHRs

One specific natural disaster event highlighting the need for EHRs was Hurricane Katrina in 2005, when millions of health records were displaced and destroyed, leaving patients without access to their medical records. This made it difficult to impossible for the physicians and other providers to deliver continued care based on established patient care plans. Responding in part to this disaster, more public and private efforts were initiated, and attention was focused on the development of an EHR system.

The US federal government, through the Centers for Medicare and Medicaid Systems (CMS), has provided financial incentives to the health care providers who use certified EHRs in a "meaningful" way, called meaningful use, to hasten the widespread use of the EHRs. These incentives provide a driving force for the adoption of EHRs to achieve the vision of a transformed health care that uses technology in the right way to save time and money, improve patient care, and ensure that each American can have a secure EHR.

Through the Health Information Technology for Economic and Clinical Health Act (HITECH), which focused on various aspects of health information technology, the federal government allotted a total of $27 billion over 10 years through the CMS to clinicians and hospitals when they used EHRs that met meaningful use guidelines (Gold and McLaughlin, 2016). Providers who utilized qualified technologies would receive an incentive or payment from the CMS. Hospital reimbursement for meeting meaningful use criteria was significant and provided substantial financial incentives in the millions of dollars. Meaningful use benchmarks and guidelines were rolled out in stages and are now part of the Merit-Based Incentive Payment System (MIPS). The current state of this and other federal quality

initiatives can be examined at the HealthIT Web site: http://www.healthit.gov/providers-professionals/meaningful-use-definition-objectives.

## Meaningful Use

The American Recovery and Reinvestment Act (ARRA) and its HITECH legislation provided a financial incentive for the meaningful use of certified EHR technology to achieve quality health care and efficiency goals. By applying meaningful use, the health care providers not only reaped financial benefits but also improved the quality of care by reducing medical errors and gaining clinical decision-making system (CDS) support and electronic prescribing-even though they might not be able to otherwise afford the technology. The ARRA laid out three main components of meaningful use in the EHR incentive program, as follows (Centers for Medicare and Medicaid Services, 2012):

1. The use of a certified EHR in a meaningful manner, such as e-prescribing.
2. The use of certified EHR technology for electronic exchange of health information to improve quality of health care.
3. The use of certified EHR technology to submit clinical quality and other measures.

Because the widespread use of a fully functional and interoperable electronic health care documentation and delivery system represents tremendous investments of time and energy, meaningful use requirements were set up in three stages over a period of 5 years. Although physicians, hospitals, and other providers who meet meaningful use guidelines received cash incentives from the CMS, those who did not embrace these technologies were slated to suffer a penalty in the payments they receive from Medicare, beginning with a 1% reduction in 2015.

There were 25 meaningful-use objectives in Stage 1, 20 of which had to be met for a health care provider to qualify for increased reimbursement. The provider had to choose 15 core objectives, and the remaining 5 objectives could be chosen from the set of 10 menu-set objectives. The objectives have been summarized in Boxes A1 and A2, which show the set of 15 core objectives and 10 menu objectives, respectively.

Each of the three stages of meaningful use is essentially built upon the EHR. Stage 1, which started in 2011, required the major functionality of a certified EHR, such as documenting visits, diagnosis, prescriptions, and other relevant health information, including reminders and alerts, and sharing patient information, reporting quality measures, and other public health information. Stage 2, which began in 2013, included all the functionality from Stage 1, in addition to sending and receiving laboratory orders and results. Implementation deadlines for Stage 2 were set at 2016. With the implementation of the Medicare Access and CHIP Reauthorization Act (MACRA), the Meaningful Use Program has been transitioned into the Merit-Based Incentive Payment System (MIPS), which includes the Physician

Quality Reporting System (PQRS) and Value-Based Payment Modifier (VBM). The goals of meaningful use remain in MIPS, including: quality, safety, efficiency, patient engagement, improved care coordination, and maintaining privacy and security of protected health information.

As we have moved into a more EHR-oriented environment, the need for paper-based processing has diminished considerably. However, it has not disappeared. The use of paper for data collection during down-times and in non-EHR settings makes it necessary for HIM professionals to be familiar with the issues surrounding paper-based processing. We discussed the use and development of paper forms in Chapter 2; however, our later discussion of processing focused on scanning those pages into a document management system associated with an EHR. What follows, largely unedited from previous editions, is our discussion of paper-based processing and record storage.

## Organization of a Paper-Based Health Record

Although we are in a transition period from mostly paper records to mostly electronic records, there is still a significant amount of paper that needs to be dealt with, as well as vast amounts of stored records in paper format. This section discusses the way paper-based records are organized, but it also helps you to understand why paper documentation needs to be carefully organized when storing pages in a computer for future retrieval.

Data are collected in an organized fashion. In a paper-based environment, the data collection device is a form. Forms are specific to their purpose, as discussed previously. As the forms are collected into the record, they must be put into some kind of order so that users will be able to locate and retrieve the data. Paper records are sorted in one or a combination of three ways: by date, source, or diagnosis.

### Integrated Record

Pages in the record can be organized by order of date. In a completely integrated record, the data themselves are also collected by date order (i.e., chronologically), regardless of the source of the data. The first piece of data is recorded with its date, and each subsequent piece of data is organized sequentially after the preceding piece of data. This method of maintaining data is particularly useful when we need to know when events happen in relation to one another. For practical purposes, different types of data are recorded on separate forms, but those forms are also placed in date order. Fig. A1 illustrates the chronological organization of data.

This method of recording data in date order can also be called *date-oriented*. The organization of the data in date order is a fairly useful and efficient way to collect data sequentially during each episode of care and from one episode to the next. In a paper record, it is easier to place the most recent pages on top; an integrated paper record organized in reverse chronological order is still considered an integrated record.

Because of the ease of filing and the chronological picture such records provide, many physicians and other ambulatory care providers use an integrated record.

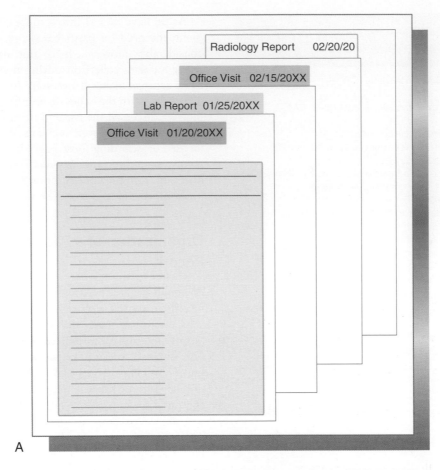

A

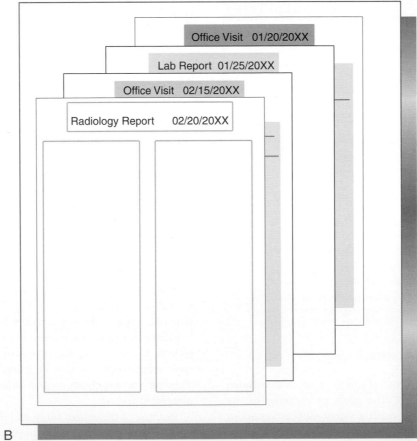

B

• **Fig. A1** (A) Integrated record. (B) Integrated record in reverse chronological order.

## Source-Oriented Record

In addition to being organized by date, data may be organized by source. In other words, all of the data obtained from the physician can be grouped together, all of the data obtained from the nurse can be grouped together, and all of the laboratory data can be grouped together. This method of organizing data produces a source-oriented record.

Organizing data by source is useful when there are many items of data coming from different sources. For example, a patient who is in the hospital for several days may require numerous laboratory and blood tests, and many pages of physician and nursing notes are compiled. If all of these pieces of data are organized in date order, as an integrated record, one would have to know the exact date on which something occurred to find the desired data. Furthermore, it would be very difficult to compare laboratory results from one date to the next. Consequently, in records that have numerous items from each type of source, the records tend to be organized in a source-oriented manner. Fig. A2 illustrates a source-oriented record. Notice that within each source, the data are organized in chronological order so that specific items are more easily located and the record shows the patient's progress chronologically.

## Problem-Oriented Record

The data can also be organized by the patient's diagnosis or problem. For instance, all of the data on a patient's appendicitis and appendectomy can be organized together. Similarly, all of the data that pertain to the patient's congestive heart failure can be organized together. Such a method greatly facilitates the monitoring of individual patient conditions. This method of organizing data produces a problem-oriented record and is useful when the patient has several major chronic conditions that may be addressed at different times. For example, if a patient has congestive heart failure, diabetes, and hypertension, the patient might not be treated for all three simultaneously. Therefore the records for each of the conditions may be kept separately. Problems that have been resolved are easily flagged, and current problems are more easily referenced. Fig. A3 illustrates a simple problem-oriented record. The problem-oriented record format is most often used by physician offices or clinics.

## Problem List

After several visits to an ambulatory care facility, a list of the patient's problems (diagnoses or complaints) is compiled. This problem list facilitates management of the patient's care and improves communication among caregivers. In a problem-oriented record, this list becomes an index to the record, as well as a historical summary of patient care management. Therefore, the problem list is an integral part of a problem-oriented record. However, a problem list is required regardless of the organization of the record. A simple problem list is shown in Fig. A4. Maintaining a problem list is a requirement for the Joint Commission (TJC) accreditation. Note that, in an EHR, a problem list is also accumulated for inpatients.

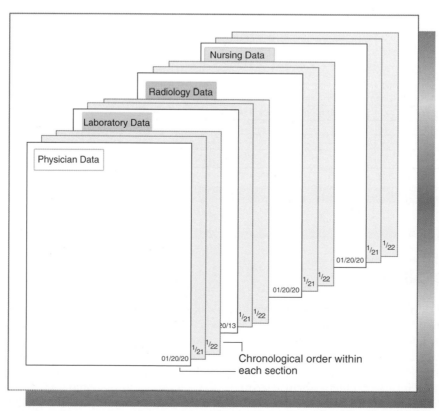

• **Fig. A2** Source-oriented record.

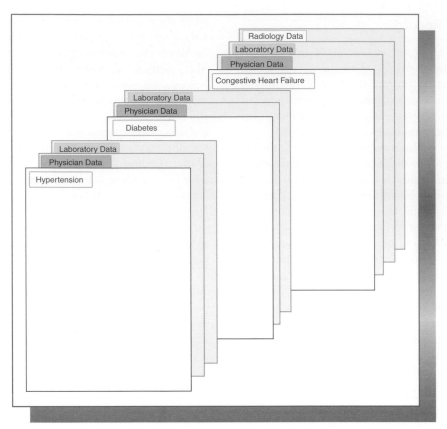

• **Fig. A3** Problem-oriented record.

| Problem List | | | | | |
|---|---|---|---|---|---|
| **Date** | **Problem #** | **Description** | **Date of Initial Diagnosis** | **Current Treatment** | **Comments** |
| 01/20/20XX | 1 | Hypertension | 11/27/20XX | Diet | Follow-up 01/20XX |
| 02/15/20XX | 2 | Sprain/right ankle | 02/15/20XX | Wrap and rest Tylenol 1000 mg as needed | |
| 03/15/20XX | 2 | Sprain/right ankle | 02/15/20XX | None | Resolved |
| | | | | | |
| | | | | | |
| | | | | | |

• **Fig. A4** Problem list.

## Advantages and Disadvantages

Each of these methods of organizing patient records has its own advantages and disadvantages. The integrated record is simple to file, but subsequent retrieval and comparison of data are more difficult. The source-oriented record is more complicated to file, but this method facilitates the retrieval and comparison of source data. The problem-oriented record lends itself best to the long-term management of chronic illnesses; however, filing is complicated, and duplication of data may be necessary so that laboratory reports related to different problems are included in all relevant sections. All of these methods are essentially paper-based record organization systems. A well-designed computer-based system can solve filing and retrieval inefficiencies.

It should be noted that the method of organizing a record is not patient specific. In other words, all patients' records are recorded in the same way. The method of organization is determined by its overall suitability to the particular environment and the needs that it satisfies.

## Postdischarge Paper-Based Processing

### Chart Assembly

**Chart assembly** is the set of procedures by which a paper record is reorganized after discharge and prepared for further processing. The extent to which a record is reorganized varies among facilities. The need to reorganize the record arises from the differences between the order of the sections and documents of the record as filed on the patient unit and the order of the sections and documents of the record used in postdischarge processing. The patient care unit staff may place all sections pertaining to physician documentation in the beginning of the record so that the physicians do not have to search through other sections in order to find their section. In addition, the documentation is generally organized within sections in reverse chronological order, with the most recent date on top. Reverse chronological order makes sense while the record is on the patient unit, but after the patient is discharged, this method may actually hamper record review and understanding of the hospitalization because most people are used to reading events in chronological order from front to back, like a book. Similarly, sections that were considered sufficiently important to be placed up front for ease of documentation, such as physician's orders, may be shifted after the patient is discharged so that the overall record may be more easily read.

Reorganization of a paper record is done manually by HIM staff members, who are often called *assemblers*. Some administrators question the cost-effectiveness of this function. Why take an organized record and reorganize it? The answer is that the needs of the users on the patient unit, while the patient is being treated, are different from the needs of the users after the patient has been discharged. Nevertheless, the cost of reorganizing the paper record may be prohibitive, so the paper record can be stored in the same order as it is kept on the patient unit. This approach is called **universal chart order**. In theory, universal chart order is a practical solution. However, it does require cooperation and coordination among the staff of the patient units and the HIM department. Further, the principal users of the record must agree on the universal order. Without such collaboration and agreement, universal chart order cannot be successfully implemented.

Once the paper record has been organized, it is bound. Binding consists of affixing the pages of the record within a permanent cover, usually a manila folder. The front of the folder usually contains the name of the facility. It may also contain warnings about the confidentiality of the record and other pertinent facility record policies. The front and tabs of the folder contain the patient's name, medical record number (MRN), and the discharge date. Because health records are generally stored on open shelves, the tab is on the short side of the folder. This position enables the user to identify the contents of the folder when the folder is placed on a shelf.

## Quantitative Analysis

Another important detective control that takes place in the HIM department is quantitative analysis. **Quantitative analysis** is the process of reviewing a health record to ensure that the record is complete according to organization policies and procedures for a complete medical record. As previously discussed, *completeness* refers to the entirety of data: are all of the data elements present? Sample job titles for this HIM professional are *medical record analyst, medical record analysis specialist, health information specialist,* or *health information analyst.*

This professional's responsibility is to review the patient's record and determine whether any reports, notes, or necessary signatures are missing. In many facilities, assembly and analysis are both performed by the same individual. In general, this analysis occurs after discharge. Review of the chart after the patient has gone home is called a retrospective, or postdischarge, analysis.

The extent of quantitative analysis performed in a facility depends on the type of facility and the rules of its licensure and accreditation. However, there are three guiding principles:

*Existence*: The record must contain all of the elements required by the licensure and accrediting bodies for the particular type of facility and all of the elements required by the clinical services pertaining to that patient's treatment, as well as the elements common to all patients.

*Completeness*: The existing documents must be complete and must not be missing data elements.

*Authentication*: Each element of the record must be properly dated, timed, and authenticated in accordance with the rules and regulations of state or accrediting agencies that apply to the facility, with the authors clearly identified.

### Elements of the Health Record

Different clinical services typically have special forms that pertain to those services. Physical therapy may have special assessment and progress forms that differ from those used by nursing. The analyst must know which forms are used in each service and must be able to identify any forms that are missing. Again, the complete absence of the data element is easier to identify than the partial absence. For example, a history and physical (H&P) must be documented on every inpatient record. Failure to perform an H&P is a serious error. If either the history portion or the physical portion of the transcribed report is missing, it may not have been performed. More often, however, the H&P was performed, noted in the record, and dictated, but the dictated report has not yet been matched with the chart. The same is true of operative reports and consultation reports. No rule or regulation states that reports must be dictated, so on some records, depending on hospital policy, a handwritten H&P is acceptable. The analyst must know the rules and must be able to identify noncompliance. The analyst must also be able to identify forms that are incomplete.

The absence of the author's authentication or of identification of authorship is easily recognized if the analyst is aware of when and where the authentication must appear. However, the analyst must also know who should have authenticated the document. This knowledge becomes critical if a document has been signed but not by the correct individual. Perhaps a countersignature is required. A countersignature is authentication by an individual in addition to the author. For example, an unlicensed resident may write (author) a progress note, which the attending physician must then countersign to provide evidence that the resident was supervised.

Finally, the analyst ensures that the record is complete according to licensure, accreditation rules, and hospital policy. For example, the H&P, discharge summary, and progress notes are required elements. Sometimes, this requirement overlaps with the requirement for authentication. Table A1 summarizes the major record elements for which quantitative analysis acts as a detective control.

There is more to record completeness than compliance with external standards. Because the health record is part of the hospital's business records, the hospital must determine what constitutes its legal record for the purpose of communication or distribution.

As the analyst identifies missing elements, the pages are flagged and the missing elements are noted, along with the party responsible for correction. *Flagging* consists of affixing stickers to the pages of the record. The stickers come in multiple colors so that various clinicians can be identified, each with a different color, in a single record. In many facilities, the policy is to analyze only the physician portions of the record, such as orders, progress notes, and all dictated reports. In other facilities, the policy is to analyze many sections or all of the clinical documentation, which would include nursing progress notes.

## Loose Sheets

In a paper-based record, some reports, test results, and other data have not been compiled with the record before the patient's discharge. Suppose, for example, that the results of a radiology examination were communicated verbally to the physician but the transcribed report did not arrive at the nursing unit before the patient's discharge. Because the record is used primarily for communication and is a legal document, the lack of a report must be resolved. These noncompiled pages are frequently called loose sheets or loose reports. If an excessive amount of documentation is still being received by the HIM department after discharge, organizational issues may have to be resolved with the other departments involved. Filing this trailing documentation, or loose sheets, is not an effective use of HIM staff members' time if the reports should have been filed by patient unit personnel while the patient was still in-house. While the patient is in the facility, it is the responsibility of the clinical staff, usually nursing or patient unit clerks, to compile these pages into the record. Because many reports and other data are delivered to the area that requested them, typically the nursing unit, a delay may occur in rerouting the data to the HIM department.

Loose sheets may arrive in the HIM department hours, days, or weeks after the patient has been discharged. By that time, the paper record has been processed and must be located in order to file the paperwork. If the record is stored electronically, the loose sheets will be scanned into the record. Filing of loose sheets should not be a huge issue in a completely electronic record, although we have discussed that there may be a small volume of documents that it will be necessary to scan. Handling the volume of loose sheets arriving daily may be a full-time job in a large facility. Regular, systematic sorting and filing or scanning of loose sheets is necessary to ensure a complete record.

## Deficiency Tracking

Incomplete charts are routinely maintained in a special area of the department to allow clinicians easy access to complete the charts and correct deficiencies. The organization of this area depends on the extent to which the record has been computerized and on the level of staffing available. If physicians are expected to retrieve their own charts, the area is typically organized alphabetically, by physician's last name. As each physician associated with an incomplete chart completes his or her deficiencies, the paper record is shifted from physician to physician until the chart is complete. If the HIM department is sufficiently well staffed that the charts can be gathered (pulled) for the physician on request, then all the charts are filed together by MRN.

When a record appears to be complete, it is analyzed again to ensure that nothing was missed. When the record is complete, it is transferred to permanent storage. Incomplete records remain in the incomplete chart area until completed.

## Retrieval

It is appropriate to mention here that in a paper environment, storage is a very critical function in the facility. The

| TABLE A1 | Elements of Quantitative Analysis | |
|---|---|---|
| Element | Analysis to Determine | Common Deficiencies |
| Existence | Do the data exist? | Missing operative report<br>Missing discharge summary |
| Completeness | Are the data entirely present, or are there missing components? | Missing reason for consultation |
| Authentication | Is the author's or other appropriate signature/ password present? | Unsigned H&P<br>Unsigned discharge summary<br>Unsigned order |

storage and retention of health records, and the ability to retrieve those records efficiently, are traditionally the responsibility of HIM professionals.

Once the records are complete and filed, the need for retrieval is based on a number of factors. If no one would ever need to look at the record again after the patient has gone home, it would not need to be organized, analyzed, or stored. As previously mentioned, however, the health record is the business record that supports treatment and payment and is a critical communication tool; it will be reviewed many times after the patient leaves the facility. For example, the function of retrieving the health record and providing it, or parts of it, to individuals who need it is commonly called release of information (ROI) and requires access to the stored records.

## Record Storage: Legacy Systems

A legacy system is a method or computerized system formerly used by health care facilities (or any organization). As changes occur in health care, this term is used by HIM professionals to refer to the "old" way or system used. For many organizations, the manual/paper filing methods discussed in this appendix are legacy systems. It is important to recognize the value of these systems and to understand them so that the information they contain can be retrieved and used as needed for patient care.

## Identification of Physical Files

Prior to the EHR, paper health record documents were stored in physical file folders. Some health care environments may retain patient health records in manila folders, binders, envelopes, or expandable pocket files. For easy identification and filing, the file folder containing the patient's health information was labeled with alphanumeric characters. In a small health care facility or a physician's office, the file folder might have been identified alphabetically with the patient's name. In a large health care facility, the MRN may have been used to identify the patient's health record file. MRNs vary in length: some are only six digits, others are eight or nine digits, and some may even be longer. Currently, the number of digits or type of number used by a facility is not mandated. However, accreditation agencies such as TJC require facilities to use a system that ensures timely access to patient information when requested for patient care or other authorized use. Additionally, the facility chooses the system that best suits its purpose for identification and storage of patient files. Five types of health record identification are discussed here: alphabetical filing, unit numbering, serial numbering, serial-unit numbering, and family unit numbering. While you are learning these identification methods, keep in mind that a numbering system is not the same as a filing method.

Before computerized technology, health care forms were manually stamped with the patient's name, MRN, account number, patient account number, and room number by means of an addressograph. The addressograph is a machine that uses a plastic card imprinted with the patient's identification information. The imprint on the card resembles the name imprinted on a credit card. The plastic card is put into the addressograph machine, the patient's forms are placed one at a time on top of the card, and an ink roller is passed over the paper and card to mark the patient's information on each piece of the record. The addressograph card contains enough information to identify the patient so that the forms can be placed in the correct patient record. Although this system is still used, technology has replaced it in many facilities with printed labels, computer-generated forms, and bar codes.

### Alphabetical Filing

In a small physician's office, clinic, home health care facility, or nursing home, the patient health record file folders are often labeled using the patients' names. Thus, the "numbering" and "alphabetical" filing systems are the same. The health record file for the patient John Adams is identified thus: Adams, John. File folders are arranged on the shelf in alphabetical order, beginning with the patient's last name (Fig. A5). For those records stored on a shelf, the patient's name is color coded on the side tab, often using the first three letters of the patient's last name. The records are still filed alphabetically, but the labeling is different. In the alphabetical system in which records are filed in a cabinet, the folder is labeled with the patient's name, preferably on the top tab (Fig. A6A-B). Alphabetical filing works well in health care environments where the number of patient visits or records is relatively low. The file folders are easy to label, and pulling a patient's file can be accomplished if the patient's name is known. Health care professionals in facilities using this system must take special care to protect the privacy of patient records because the patient health information is easily identified. Alphabetical filing does not require an additional system, such as the master patient index (MPI), to correlate patient names and numbers to identify a particular file folder.

Problems can arise when two patients have the same name. Common names require careful attention to be certain that the correct patient record is found. Think about the names Michael, Joe, and Ann. How many other ways may these names be identified? Mike, Michael, Jo, Joe, Joseph, José, Josef, Ann, Anne, Annie, and Annette are common versions of Michael, Joe, and Ann, respectively. When duplicate names occur in an alphabetical filing system, procedures must be specified to further organize the records by the patient's middle name, by titles (Jr., Sr., III), or by the patient's date of birth (DOB). Common rules for alphabetical filing are as follows:

- Personal names are filed last name first; for example, the name John Adams is filed by Adams first, followed by John: Adams, John. The first name is followed by the middle initial (e.g., E) or name if necessary: Adams, John E.
- All punctuation and possessives are ignored. Disregard commas, hyphens, and apostrophes. In the last name, prefixes, foreign articles, and particles are combined with

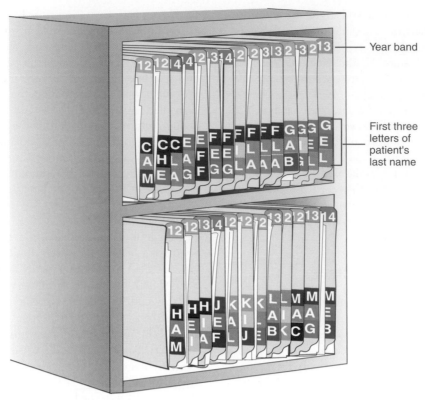

• **Fig. A5** File folders in a cabinet in alphabetical order.

the name following it, omitting spaces (e.g., De Witt is filed as dewitt).

• Abbreviations, nicknames, and shortened names are filed as written (e.g., Wm., Bud, Rob).

• Suffixes are considered after the middle name or initial. Titles are considered after suffixes. Royal or religious titles follow the given name and surname; the title is indexed last.

• When identical names occur, consider the DOB for filing order and proceed chronologically.

Patients' files must be clearly labeled. It is important to print clearly when labeling the patient's file folder. This is not an occasion for fancy script or calligraphy. Illegible or fancy handwriting may cause a file folder to be misfiled. Table A2 lists the advantages and disadvantages of alphabetical filing.

Space is a common problem in the alphabetical filing system. The shelves or cabinets holding the files of patients' names beginning with common letters become full very quickly, so HIM departments must allow adequate file space for these letters of the alphabet. Filing in a section that is full of records is difficult and requires shifting of the records for further filing. Alphabetical filing systems can become inefficient in a facility that serves a large population with a high volume of patient records.

Another consideration with this system is the spelling of patient names. In an alphabetical file system, a folder labeled incorrectly because of misspelling will not be filed correctly. When the HIM employee attempts to locate the patient's folder, efforts will involve searching for a misspelled, misfiled record. When unsure of the spelling of the patient's

name, the person taking the information from the patient should ask for identification to clarify the spelling.

### Unit Numbering

In a unit numbering system, a patient receives the same medical record number for each admission to the facility. Therefore the numeric identification of each individual patient is always patient specific. For example, if a person is born in a facility that uses unit numbering, at birth (which is considered an admission) the patient is assigned a number (e.g., MRN 001234). Any subsequent admissions of this patient to the facility would use the same MRN. In a unit numbering identification system, the patient's MRN remains the same, within the facility, throughout the lifetime of the patient. MRNs are not shared and are not reused after a patient dies.

Consider the following scenario: Molly Brabant is born at Diamonte Hospital on January 1, 2001. At birth, Molly is assigned MRN 001234. Her birth record is filed in a folder identified with MRN 001234. At age 7, Molly returns to the same facility to have a tonsillectomy. Molly's new records are stored in the same folder identified as MRN 001234. Any subsequent admissions (e.g., for a hip replacement later in life) are filed under the same number (Fig. A7).

In a unit numbering system, extra care must be taken to identify whether the patient already has an MRN from a previous admission. Name change due to marriage/divorce, misspelling of name, or failure to search the system, even when the patient asserts that they have not been to the facility before, are common reasons that the MRN from a

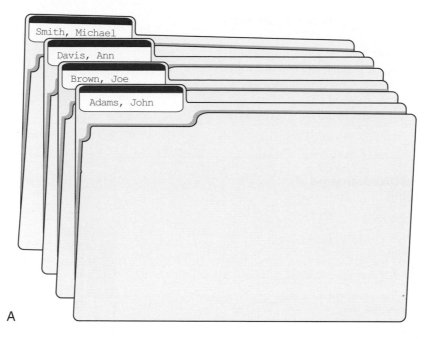

A

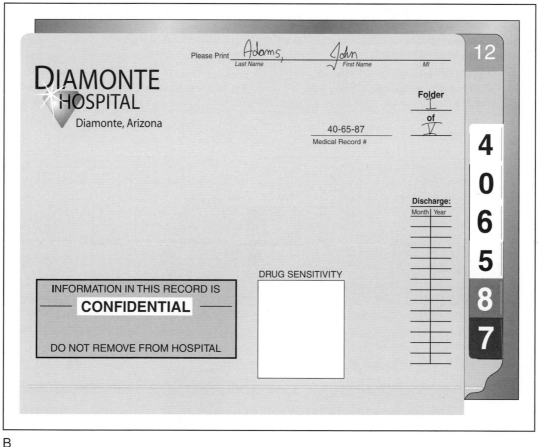

B

• **Fig. A6** File folder labeling showing top (A) and side (B) tabs.

previous admission might not be located. Failure to identify a previously assigned number results in duplicate entries into the MPI for the same patient (i.e., more than one MRN for the same patient). This redundancy will create problems for anyone trying to locate the patient's medical record.

## Serial Numbering

In a serial numbering system, a new MRN is assigned each time a patient has an encounter at the facility. In this type of system, the patient's file folders containing the health record for each encounter are not filed in the same folder.

Therefore the records are not typically located together on the file shelf.

In the previous scenario but with a serial numbering system, Molly Brabant is assigned MRN 001234 at birth. However, when she returns at age 7 for a tonsillectomy, a new number, MRN 112233, is assigned (Fig. A8). In this system, Molly's records are not stored in the same folder, and

| TABLE A2 | Advantages and Disadvantages of Alphabetical Filing |
|---|---|
| Advantages | Easy to learn |
| | Does not require additional cross-reference |
| | Works well in smaller facilities |
| Disadvantages | Illegible handwriting may cause problems with filing |
| | Space within the popular letters of the alphabet to locate a patient chart can fill quickly |
| | Can be inefficient for a large facility with a large patient population |
| | Many alternative spellings of names exist, which can cause problems with retrieval |

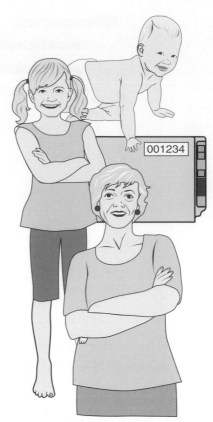

• **Fig. A7** Example of unit medical record numbering for one patient.

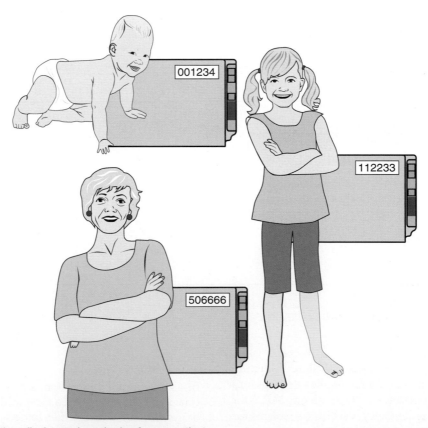

• **Fig. A8** Example of serial medical record numbering for one patient.

they are not located near one another on the file shelf. Molly now has two separate folders containing her health record, and she receives a third MRN and a new folder when she visits the facility for a hip replacement in later years. The number assigned during each one of Molly's encounters is recorded in the MPI under her name.

### Serial-Unit Numbering

A serial-unit numbering system is a combination of the previous two numbering systems. In this system, the patient receives a new MRN each time he or she comes into a facility. The difference is that each time the patient receives health care, the old records are brought forward and filed with the most recent visit, under a new MRN. This system requires a cross-reference system from the old MRN to the new number so that records can be located. For cross-referencing, the MPI must be updated so each encounter reflects the corresponding MRN, and a file guide is placed in the old file location alerting HIM employees to look for the current MRN to locate the patient's health record.

In the previous scenario using a serial-unit numbering system, Molly is assigned MRN 001234 at birth, and on return 7 years later for a tonsillectomy, she is assigned a new number, MRN 112233. When Molly returns for the tonsillectomy, the birth record (MRN 001234) is retrieved from its place in the files and combined with the file folder MRN 112233. A cross-reference should be set up by insertion of an **outguide** (Fig. A9) in place of the old MRN 001234 to indicate that the record is now filed at MRN 112233 (Fig. A10). Molly's records are transferred and cross-referenced a third time when Molly has a hip replacement later in life.

### Family Unit Numbering

In rare cases in health care settings where it is common for an entire family to visit a physician or clinic and to have the same insurance carrier, an entire family's records may be identified using one MRN. Each family member's file is then identified by the one MRN of the entire family (parents and children). This system is called a family unit numbering system. A modifier-a number attached to the MRN using a hyphen-unique to each member of the family is placed at the end of the family unit number. Each member of the family can be identified by a modifier associated with his or her position in the family: head of household, 01; spouse, 02; first born, 03; second born, 04; and so on. With this system, all of the family members' records may be contained in one file folder.

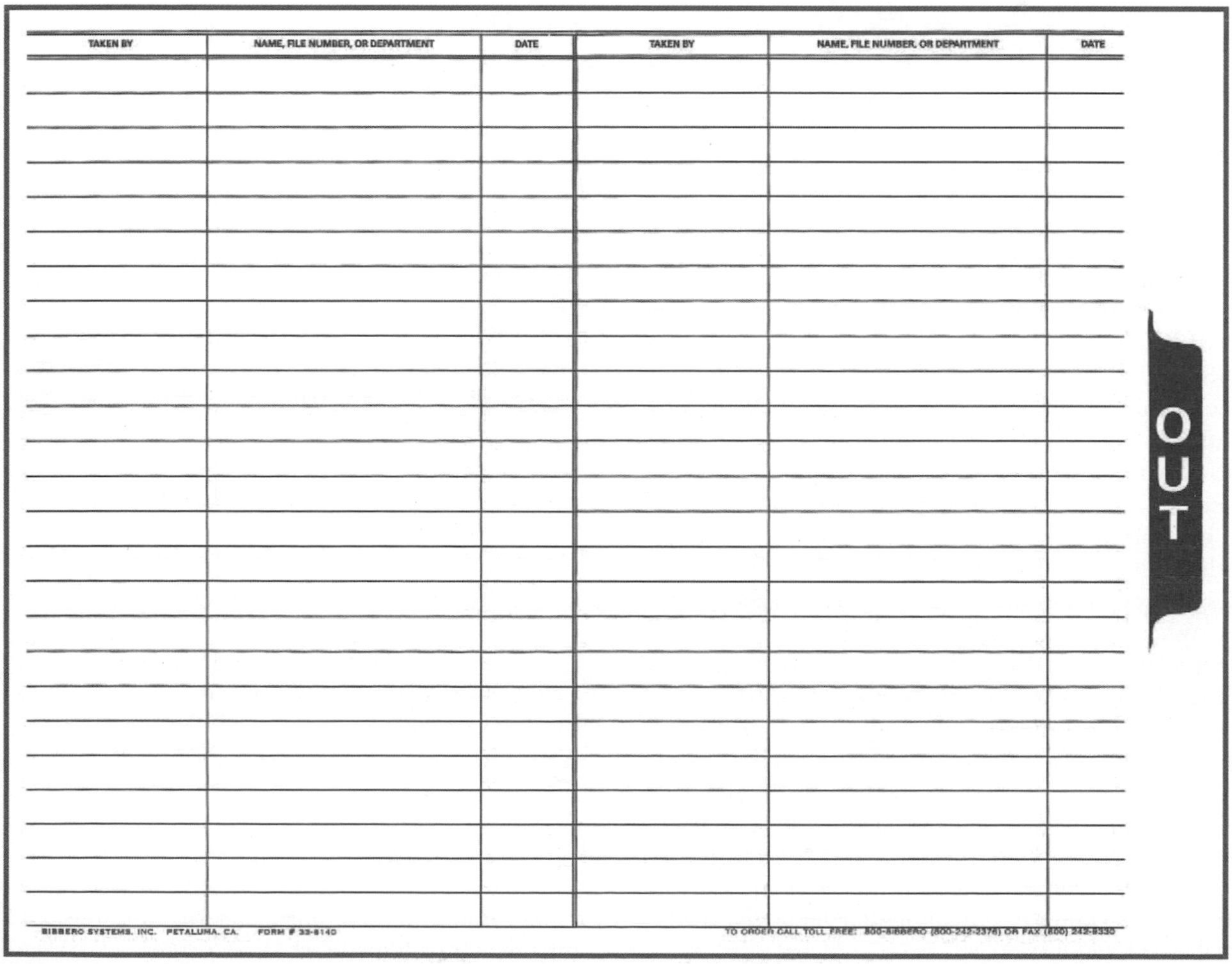

| TAKEN BY | NAME, FILE NUMBER, OR DEPARTMENT | DATE | TAKEN BY | NAME, FILE NUMBER, OR DEPARTMENT | DATE |
|---|---|---|---|---|---|

OUT

BIBBERO SYSTEMS, INC. PETALUMA, CA. FORM # 33-8140

TO ORDER CALL TOLL FREE: 800-BIBBERO (800-242-2376) OR FAX (800) 242-9330

• **Fig. A9** The outguide identifies a record removed from its usual location. (Courtesy Bibbero Systems, Inc., Atlanta, Georgia.)

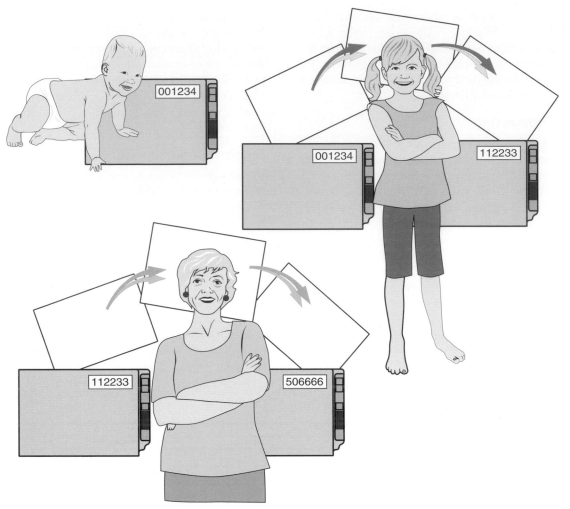

• **Fig. A10** Example of serial-unit medical record numbering for one patient.

In our example, Molly's family unit number is MRN 123456. At birth, Molly, being the first-born child, is assigned MRN 123456-03. Molly's mother has MRN 123456-02. The last two numbers after the hyphen indicate to which family member the record belongs. Table A3 provides an example of family unit numbering.

This system is also beneficial in a small clinic or physician's office setting where clinical and financial records are combined for claim processing. There are potential problems with this numbering system, however. Families change, couples divorce, and grown children marry and adopt other names. When members of the family divorce, die, marry, or remarry, the medical records for those patients must be renumbered. This process can be quite tedious. Even in a family unit numbering system, the facility is responsible for maintaining the confidentiality of each patient's health information. Safeguards must be taken to ensure that family members are allowed access to each other's information only with appropriate authorization (see Chapter 8). Furthermore, procedures should exist to safeguard the confidentiality of a child's information after he or she reaches the legal age of majority.

Each facility should examine the positive and negative aspects of each numbering identification system to choose

**TABLE A3   Family Unit Numbering.**

| Family Member | Family Number | Modifier | Patient Number |
|---|---|---|---|
| John Smith | 123456 | 01 | 123456-01 |
| Mary Smith | 123456 | 02 | 123456-02 |
| Molly Smith | 123456 | 03 | 123456-03 |
| Tommy Smith | 123456 | 04 | 123456-04 |

the system that allows the most efficient delivery of health care for its patients. The system should have a positive impact on both employee and facility productivity. Table A4 summarizes the advantages and disadvantages of each numbering system.

## Filing Methods

*Filing* is the process of organizing the health record folders on a shelf, in a file cabinet, or in a computer system. There are some common methods for organizing paper-based health records in a file area: alphabetical, middle-digit,

**TABLE A4   Advantages and Disadvantages of Numbering Systems**

| System | Advantages | Disadvantages |
|---|---|---|
| Unit | All patient records can be located under one number. | Filing of all encounters in one folder can cause problems with incomplete records. |
| Serial | Each admission is filed in a single folder. | Retrieving all the records for one patient involves going to multiple places in the files. |
| Serial-unit | Each admission has a unique number, but they are all filed with the most recent. | This method is time consuming. |
| Family unit | Records are filed together for clinical and financial processing of claims. | Confidentiality can be compromised; divorce, remarriage, and other factors can create complications. |

straight numeric, and terminal-digit. Alphabetical filing was described previously in the discussion on identification of files. In an electronic system, patient health information is indexed; this issue is discussed at the end of this section.

## Straight Numeric Filing

Straight numeric filing involves placing the folders on the shelf in numeric order (e.g., MRN 001234, MRN 001235, MRN 001522). This filing system is easy for HIM staff to understand. Straight numeric filing is best used in a system in which there is minimal activity in the records once they are filed in the permanent file area.

Straight numeric methods usually work well in long-term care facilities. In this filing method, the activity is concentrated at the end of the file shelf. The filing shelves are filled as records are added. Increased filing in the older records (lower numbers) will cause growth in shelves that may already be full, engendering a need to shift records. Shifting records involves the systematic physical relocation of files so that they are more evenly distributed on the shelves. In large file rooms, this is a time-consuming task.

## Terminal-Digit Filing

A **terminal-digit filing system** is a system in which the patient's MRN is divided into sets of digits for filing purposes. Each set of digits is used to file the health record numerically within sections of the files, beginning with the last set. Terminal-digit filing and other variations of digit filing are very common in health care facilities. The easiest example of terminal-digit filing uses a six-digit MRN. The six-digit number is separated into three sets of two numbers before filing. For example, for MRN 012345, the sets would look like this: 01-23-45. The sets of digits have names: The first two numbers are called the *tertiary* digits, the second two numbers are called the *secondary* digits, and the last two numbers are called the *primary* digits (Table A5). To file in terminal-digit (TD) order, one must locate the section of files that corresponds with the sets, beginning with the primary digits, then within the primary section locate the secondary digits, and finally file the record in numeric order by the tertiary digits. Filing in TD order is easy once

**TABLE A5   Terminal-Digit Sorting of Medical Record Number 01-23-45.**

| Medical Record Number | Number in Section | Filing |
|---|---|---|
| 0 | Tertiary | Finally, file in numerical order by this number |
| 1 | | |
| 2 | Secondary | Then find number 23 in section 45 |
| 3 | | |
| 4 | Primary | First, find section 45 in the files |
| 5 | | |

one understands how to separate the digits in the MRN and then which digit set to use first (Fig. A11).

In this example, one begins to file by using the last two numbers of the medical record number, the primary digits, as follows:

*Step 1*: Separate the MRN into the necessary sections. This example uses a six-digit number separated into three sections with two numbers each: MRN 012345 converts to 01-23-45. To file this health record (#01-23-45), begin with the primary digits 45, the last two digits of MRN 01-23-45. In the file area, locate the primary section 45. All files in primary section 45 will end with the number 45.

*Step 2*: In primary section 45, next search for the middle digits, 23. Remain in section 45, where the bottom two numbers are all the same, and be sure not to venture into another primary section on the shelf. Find middle digits 22 to 24 because 23 is going to be filed between middle digits 22-45 and 24-45.

*Step 3*: Once the appropriate middle-digit section is located, file the record in this TD section numerically by the first two digits.

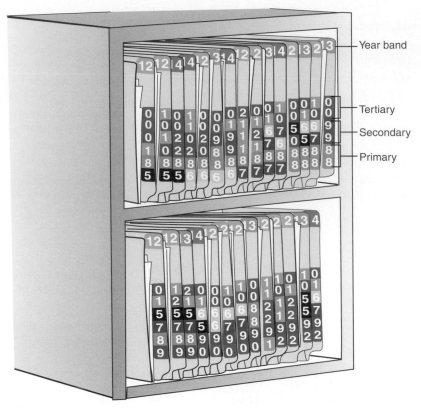

• **Fig. A11** Filing by terminal digit.

TD filing can be modified in several different ways. Some facilities use a larger nine-digit MRN. There are several ways to separate a nine-digit MRN for filing. One method is to have three sections with three numbers each-for example, MRN 111222333 converts to 111-222-333 for filing.

In a six-digit filing scenario, there are 100 primary sections of records, 00 through 99. In a nine-digit filing system, there are 1000 primary sections, 000 through 999. Primary sections reaching 1000 require a tremendous file area.

### Middle-Digit Filing

TD filing can be modified into another filing method, middle-digit filing. As in TD filing, the six-digit number is separated into three sets of two numbers before filing; MRN 012345 sets would look like this: 01-23-45. The sets of digits, however, have been renamed; the first two numbers are the secondary digits, the second two numbers are the primary digits, and the last two numbers are the tertiary digits (Table A6).

The following shows the process of filing MRN 012345 in a middle-digit filing system:

*Step 1*: Separate the MRN into three sections with two numbers each. MRN 012345 converts to 01-23-45. In middle-digit filing, begin with the middle set of digits and use that set as the primary digits; in our example, it is number 23. Locate the primary section (middle digits) 23 in the file area. All files in primary section 23 will have middle sets with the number 23.

*Step 2*: Remain in section 23. Be sure not to move into another primary section on the shelf. Find the secondary set of digits, 01.

| TABLE A6 | Middle-Digit Sorting of Medical Record Number 01-23-45. | |
|---|---|---|
| Medical Record Number | Number in Section | Filing |
| 0 | Secondary | Then find number 01 in section 23 |
| 1 | | |
| 2 | Primary | First, find section 23 in the files |
| 3 | | |
| 4 | Tertiary | Finally, file in numeric order by this number |
| 5 | | |

*Step 3*: Remain in section 01-23, and then file the record numerically by the tertiary digits 45.

Fig. A12 shows an example of middle-digit filing.

Each facility should examine both the positive and the negative aspects of each filing method. An organized filing system allows efficient retrieval of patient health records. Quick retrieval of health records can improve the quality of patient care. A good system should have a positive impact on both employee and facility productivity. Table A7 lists the advantages and disadvantages of each filing method.

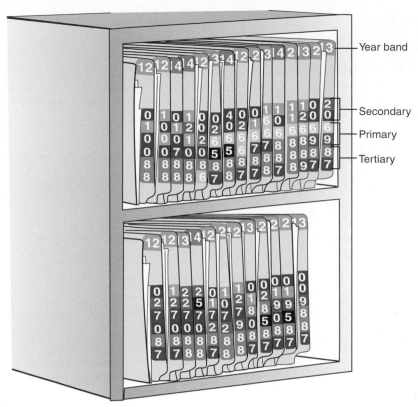

• **Fig. A12** Filing by middle digit.

| TABLE A7 | Advantages and Disadvantages of Filing Methods | |
|---|---|---|

| Filing Method | Advantages | Disadvantages |
|---|---|---|
| Alphabetical | Easy to learn; does not require additional cross-reference to identify a file number | Illegible handwriting can cause problems; space requirements for popular letters also problematic |
| Straight numerical | Easy to learn | File activity is concentrated |
| Terminal-digit | Equalizes filing activity throughout the filing sections. Can be a security feature because those who are unfamiliar with terminal-digit filing will be unable to identify a patient's record | Challenging for some file clerks to learn. Misfiles are often difficult to locate |
| Middle-digit | Equalizes filing activity throughout the filing sections | Even more challenging for some file clerks to learn; misfiles are often difficult to locate |

## Works Cited

Centers for Medicare and Medicaid Services. CMS Finalizes Definition of Meaningful Use of Certified Electronic Health Records (EHR) Technology. From CMS.gov: https://www.cms.gov/newsroom/fact-sheets/cms-finalizes-definition-meaningful-use-certified-electronic-health-records-ehr-technology. Retrieved April 17, 2023. Published July 16, 2010.

Gold M, McLaughlin C: Assessing HITECH Implementation and Lessons: 5 Years Later, *Milbank Q* 94(3):654–687, 2016. https://doi.org/10.1111/1468-0009.12214.

Office of the National Coordinator for Health Information Technology (ONC): Meaningful use and the shift to the merit-based incentive payment system. From HealthIT.gov: https://www.healthit.gov/topic/meaningful-use-and-macra/meaningful-use. Retrieved October 6, 2022. Published January 9, 2019.

## Sample Paper Records

Following are paper forms to serve as examples of the paper documentation found in a variety of settings. These may be photocopied from the book and used for practice. They may also be printed from the Evolve website. Included here are:

Inpatient Admission Form/Face Sheet, 431
Conditions of Admission, 433
Advance Directive Acknowledgment, 434
Emergency Department Record, 435
History, 436
Physical, 437
Provider's Order Form, 438
Provider's Progress Notes, 439
Informed Consent, 440
Consultation Record, 443
Medication Administration Records, 444
Intake/Output Record, 449
Nursing Progress Notes, 450
Operative Report Progress Notes, 451
Discharge Orders, 453
Nursing Discharge Summary, 454
Certificate of Live Birth, 455
Certificate of Death, 457
Report of Fetal Death, 458

# INPATIENT ADMISSION

| | |
|---|---|
| MED REC #: | ENCOUNTER #: |

**INSURANCE**

| PATIENT NAME: | SSN: | FC: | TYPE: | PHONE-HOME: | PHONE-WORK: |
|---|---|---|---|---|---|
| ADDRESS: | | | | DATE OF BIRTH: | AGE: / SEX: / RACE: / MS: |
| | | | | MAIDEN NAME: | ETHNICITY: |

**GUARANTEE NAME EMP**

| | MAIDEN NAME: | PRIMARY LANGUAGE: |
|---|---|---|
| | PHONE-HOME: | PHONE-WORK: |

**NOTIFY**

| EMERGENCY NOTIFICATION: | RELATION: | PHONE-HOME: | PHONE-WORK: |
|---|---|---|---|

**INSURANCE**

| INSURANCE COMPANY: | POLICY #: | GROUP #: | CONTRACT HOLDER: | REL: |
|---|---|---|---|---|

**ADMISSION**

| ICD9 CODE: | ADMITTING DIAGNOSIS: | | | | |
|---|---|---|---|---|---|
| ACCOM. ROOM | BED | SERVICE: | VIA | SRC | INFORMANT: | ADMIT BY: | ADMIT DATE: | ADMIT TIME: |
| ADMITTING PHYSICIAN: | ATTENDING PHYSICIAN / AHP: | PRINCIPAL PHYSICIAN: | DISCHARGE DATE: |

## NARRATIVE

**PRINCIPAL DIAGNOSIS:** THE CONDITION ESTABLISHED AFTER STUDY TO BE CHIEFLY RESPONSIBLE FOR OCCASIONING THE ADMISSION OF THE PATIENT TO THE HOSPITAL.

**OTHER DIAGNOSIS:**
SEQ #:
SEQUENCE IN ORDER OF SIGNIFICANCE TO THE CASE; INCLUDE ALL RELEVANT COMPLICATIONS AND COMORBIDITIES.

TNM STAGING CLASSIFICATION: (APPLIES ONLY TO NEWLY DIAGNOSED CANCER CASES WITH SOLID TUMORS)

T _____

N _____

M _____

**PRINCIPAL PROCEDURE:** PERFORMED FOR DEFINITIVE TREATMENT, RATHER THAN FOR DIAGNOSTIC OR EXPLORATORY PURPOSES; USUALLY MOST RELATED TO PRINCIPAL DIAGNOSIS.

DATE

**OTHER DIAGNOSIS:**
SEQ #:
SEQUENCE IN ORDER OF SIGNIFICANCE TO THE CASE; INCLUDE ALL RELEVANT COMPLICATIONS AND COMORBIDITIES.

DATE

CONSULTANTS:

DISPOSITION: ☐ Home   ☐ SNF   ☐ ICF   ☐ HOME CARE   ☐ OTHER HOSPITAL   ☐ AMA   ☐ OTHER INSTITUTION

☐ UNDER 48 HRS   ☐ OVER 48 HRS   AUTOPSY: ☐ YES   ☐ NO

| RESIDENT / AHP | ATTENDING PHYSICIAN | I certify that the narrative description of the principal and secondary diagnoses and the major procedures performed are accurate and complete to the best of my knowledge. |
|---|---|---|
| SIGNATURE | SIGNATURE | |
| PRINTED NAME | PRINTED NAME | DATE    CHART COPY |

## PART OF THE MEDICAL RECORD

8850534 Rev. 05/05              Inpatient Admission Record_CASE MANAGEMENT              PAGE 1 of 1

Inpatient Admission Form/Face Sheet

PERMISSION FOR AUTOPSY

Permission is hereby given to perform an autopsy upon _____
and to remove and retain whole or parts of organs for study as necessary.

Witness _____    Signed _____    Relationship _____

_____    _____

Date _____    _____

DEPARTURE AGAINST MEDICAL ADVICE

This is to certify that I, _____ , a Patient in
YOUR HOSPITAL, am leaving against the advice of the attending Physician and faculty authorities. I also acknowledge
that I have been informed of the risk involved and hereby release the attending Physician and hospital from all responsibility
for any of its effects which may result.

Witness _____    Signed _____

_____

Date _____

APPLICATION FOR ADMISSION & RELEASE OF HOSPITAL RECORDS

1. I, _____ , hereby apply for admission to YOUR HOSPITAL as a patient and request
that I be furnished appropriate hospital care and services for the condition(s) for which I am being admitted. My Physician,
Dr. _____ , is authorized to utilize the facilities of YOUR HOSPITAL on my behalf, and
I hereby authorize YOUR HOSPITAL to furnish and administer to me such diagnostic procedures, treatments, medications,
and other services as my said physician may direct.

2. I am aware that the practice of medicine and surgery is not an exact science and I acknowledge that no guarantees have
been made to me as to the result of the examination or treatment in the hospital.

3. If a health care worker is exposed significantly to my blood or body fluids, I consent to a test of my blood for hepatitis and
antibodies to the virus that causes AIDS.

4. The Hospital records concerning the patient are the property of YOUR HOSPITAL and are maintained for the benefit of
the patient, the medical staff and the Hospital. I hereby authorize YOUR HOSPITAL to release these records to the patient's
personal physician and to any other individual and private or governmental agency responsible for payment of the patient's
care and treatment.

Witness _____    Signed _____

On behalf of _____ , who is a minor and/or unable to grant permission or sign the document

and/or in need of emergency treatment, I, _____ , hereby make the aforementioned

requests and give the aforementioned authority to YOUR HOSPITAL on his/her behalf.

Signature _____    Age _____
          PERSON ACTING FOR THE PATIENT

Relationship _____

Address _____

Witness _____    Date _____    Was Hospital policy on placing patient's name on
                                                their door explained to patient?    ☐ Yes    ☐ No

FOR CHAPLAIN'S USE

Sacraments received?  ☐ Yes  ☐ No    Date _____ Signature _____

## PART OF THE MEDICAL RECORD

Inpatient Admission Form/Face Sheet (cont'd)

DIAMONTE HOSPITAL
Diamonte, Arizona

**CONDITIONS of
ADMISSION**

**I.   LEGAL RELATIONSHIP BETWEEN DIAMONTE HOSPITAL AND PHYSICIAN**

I understand that many of the physicians on the staff of this hospital, including the attending physician(s), are not employees or agents of Diamonte Hospital but, rather, are independent contractors who have been granted privileges of using its facility for the care and treatment of their patients. I also realize that among those who attend patients at this facility are medical, nursing, and other health care professionals in training who, unless otherwise requested, may be present during patient care as part of their education.

**II.   CONSENT TO TREATMENT**

The patient, identified above, hereby consents and authorizes Diamonte Hospital and its staff and the patient's physician(s) to perform or administer the diagnostic and treatment procedures (including, but not limited to, radiology examinations, blood tests and other laboratory examinations and medication) as may be required by the Hospital or as may be ordered by the patient's physician(s). The patient acknowledges that Diamonte Hospital is a teaching institution. The patient agrees that he/she may participate as a teaching subject unless the patient otherwise notes in writing to the contrary.

**III.   RELEASE OF RECORDS**

The undersigned authorizes Diamonte Hospital to release any part or all patient medical records to such insurance company (companies), health care plan administrator, workmen's compensation carrier, welfare agency, or their respective authorized auditor or agents, or to any other person or party that is under contract or liable to Diamonte Hospital for all or any part of the hospital charges for this admission. The undersigned further authorizes Diamonte Hospital to release all or part of the patient's medical record or financial record to such physicians involved in the care of the patient, hospital committees, consultants, subsidiaries or physician hospital organizations, including but not limited to any committee, subsidiary, or physician hospital organization in which the patient's physician is a member or their respective agents.

**IV.   ASSIGNMENT OF BENEFITS**

In consideration of the care and services to be provided to the patient by Diamonte Hospital, the undersigned assigns and authorizes, whether as agent or patient, direct payment to Diamonte Hospital or hospital-based physicians of all insurance and health plan benefits otherwise payable to or on behalf of the patient for this hospitalization and services. It is understood by the undersigned that he/she is financially responsible for charges not covered by this assignment.

**V.   VALUABLES**

The undersigned understands fully that Diamonte Hospital is not responsible for the safety or security of and personal property or valuables.

**VI.   PHOTOGRAPHS**

The undersigned hereby authorizes and consents to Diamonte Hospital for the taking of photographs, images, or videotapes of such diagnostic, surgical, or treatment procedures of the patient as may be required by Diamonte Hospital or ordered by the patient's physician(s). With the exception of radiological images, Diamonte is not required to keep videotapes or photographs for any period of time if the medical record contains a record of the surgical, diagnostic, or treatment procedure. The patient hereby consents to the taking of pictures of newborns for possible purchase or for security purposes.

Conditions of Admission

DIAMONTE HOSPITAL
Diamonte, Arizona

**Advance Directive
Acknowledgment**

Instructions:    This form should be initiated upon admission to the facility and completed by the
admitting RN. All patients receive an Advance Directive Booklet upon admission

| | YES | NO |
|---|---|---|
| 1. Is the patient registering him/herself?<br><br>   If NO, please give reason: | | |
| 2. Does the patient have an advance directive?<br><br>   If NO, skip to question 5. | | |
| 3. Does the patient have a living will?<br><br>   Has the patient supplied a copy of the living will?<br>      Placed on chart by _____ Date/Time: _____ | | |
| 4. Does the patient have a durable power of attorney for health care?<br><br>   Has the patient supplied a copy of the durable power of attorney for health care?<br>      Placed on chart by _____ Date/Time: _____ | | |
| 5. Does the patient request additional information or wish to execute an advance directive at this time?<br><br>   If YES, please consult Social Services, x 4435. | | |

_____

Form completed by                                                    Date   Time

Advance Directive Acknowledgment

Your Hospital's Logo Here

### Hospital Dr  |  Princeton, ZZ 12345  |  T 202/555-1212  |  F 202/555-1212

# EMERGENCY DEPT RECORD

HOSPITAL #:

EMERGENCY ROOM #:

| PATIENT NAME: | Last | First | Middle | SEX: ☐ F ☐ M | AGE: | ADMIN DATE: | TIME IN: |
|---|---|---|---|---|---|---|---|

| HEIGHT: | WEIGHT: | IMMUNIZATIONS CURRENT: ☐ Y ☐ N | ALLERGIES: |
|---|---|---|---|

CONDITION ON ADMISSION: ☐ Critical ☐ Good ☐ Fair ☐ Stable ☐ Guarded

BROUGHT IN BY: ☐ Other_____ ☐ Self ☐ Police ☐ EMS ☐ Family

BROUGHT IN BY: ☐ Other_____ ☐ Amb ☐ Stretcher ☐ W/C ☐ Parent's Arms

ER MD:                FAMILY MD:                LAST TETNUS:

| TIME: | | | | | CURRENT PRESCRIPTION MEDICATION | SIGNIFICANT MEDICAL HISTORY |
|---|---|---|---|---|---|---|
| TEMP | | | | | | |
| PULSE | | | | | | |
| RESP | | | | | | |
| B / P | | | | | | |
| PULSE OX | | | | | | PREGNANT? ☐ Y ☐ N |
| GCS | | | | | | ____ EDC |
| | | | | | | ____ FHT |
| TS | | | | | | LACTATING? ☐ Y ☐ N |

USED ANY OF THE FOLLOWING IN THE PAST 72 HRS?

| | Yes | No |
|---|---|---|
| OTC Meds | ☐ | ☐ |
| Herbs / Vitamins | ☐ | ☐ |
| Street Drugs | ☐ | ☐ |
| Alcohol | ☐ | ☐ |
| Tobacco | ☐ | ☐ |

If "Yes", name & amount:

NURSING ASSESSMENT AND HISTORY

**PHYSICAL FINDINGS**

PROBLEM ORIENTED PHYSICAL EXAM:

**LAB & X-RAY**

☐ CBC   ☐ CXR
☐ CHEM_____   ☐ URINALYSIS (Voided, CCMS, Cath)
☐ EKG   ☐ OTHER:

**DIAG**

**PHYSICIANS ORDERS and TX**

I _____

O _____

☐ Attending MD of Transfer / Admit
☐ Instruction Sheet Given

DISPOSITION OF CASE:
☐ Critical ☐ Admitted: **RM#**_____
☐ Guarded ☐ Transferred _____ *FACILITY*

CONDITION ON DISCHARGE:
☐ Improved ☐ Stable ☐ Guarded
☐ Good ☐ Critical ☐ Deceased

MODE OF DISCHARGE:
☐ Ambulatory ☐ W/C ☐ Ambulance ☐ Stretcher
☐ Parents Arms ☐ Other_____

| TIME OF DISCHARGE: | PHYSICIAN'S SIGNATURE | DATE: | NURSE'S SIGNATURE: | DATE: |
|---|---|---|---|---|

*WHITE - Medical Records*          *GREEN - Family Physician*          *CANARY - Emergency Dept*

Emergency Department Record

**DIAMONTE HOSPITAL**
**Diamonte, Arizona**

**History**

(Page 1 of 2)

| | |
|---|---|
| Chief Complaint | |
| History of Present Illness | |
| History of Past Illness | |
| Family History | |
| Social History | |
| Review of Systems | |
| General | |
| Skin | |
| HEENT | |
| Neck | |
| Respiratory | |
| Cardiovascular | |
| GI | |
| GU | |
| GYN | |
| Neuropsychiatric | |
| Musculoskeletal | |

History

**DIAMONTE HOSPITAL**
**Diamonte, Arizona**

**Physical Exam**

(Page 2 of 2)

| Blood Pressure | Pulse | Resp. | | Temp. | Weight |
|---|---|---|---|---|---|
| General | | | | | |
| Skin | | | | | |
| Eyes | | | | | |
| Ears | | | | | |
| Nose | | | | | |
| Mouth | | | | | |
| Throat | | | | | |
| Neck | | | | | |
| Chest | | | | | |
| Heart | | | | | |
| Abdomen | | | | | |
| Genitalia | | | | | |
| Lymphatic | | | | | |
| Blood Vessels | | | | | |
| Musculoskeletal | | | | | |
| Extremities | | | | | |
| Neurological | | | | | |
| Rectal | | | | | |
| Vaginal | | | | | |
| **Diagnosis Plan of Care** | | | | | |
| Signature | | | Date | | |

Physical

○ *PLEASE PUNCH HERE* ○

| Diamonte Hospital<br>Phoenix, Arizona 12345-6789<br>Phone: (999) 123-XXXX Fax: (999) 123-XXXX | Patient Name Label |
|---|---|

## *Provider's Order Form*

| Date/<br>Time | Order | Physician's<br>Signature | Date/<br>Time | Nurse<br>Initials |
|---|---|---|---|---|
| | | | | |
| | | | | |
| | | | | |
| | | | | |
| | | | | |

Provider's Order Form

O *PLEASE PUNCH HERE* O

| Diamonte Hospital<br>Phoenix, Arizona 12345-6789<br>Phone: (999) 123-XXXX Fax: (999) 123-XXXX | Patient Name Label |
|---|---|

## Provider's Progress Notes

| Date | Time | Progress note | Physician signature | Discipline |
|---|---|---|---|---|
| | | | | |
| | | | | |
| | | | | |
| | | | | |
| | | | | |
| | | | | |
| | | | | |
| | | | | |
| | | | | |
| | | | | |
| | | | | |
| | | | | |
| | | | | |
| | | | | |
| | | | | |
| | | | | |
| | | | | |
| | | | | |
| | | | | |
| | | | | |

Provider's Progress Notes

**DIAMONTE HOSPITAL**
**Diamonte, Arizona**

**Informed Consent**

(example only)

**PATIENT CONSENT TO MEDICAL TREATMENT/SURGICAL PROCEDURE
AND ACKNOWLEDGMENT OF RECEIPT OF MEDICAL INFORMATION**

**READ CAREFULLY BEFORE SIGNING**

**TO THE PATIENT:** You have been told that you should consider medical treatment/surgery. State law requires this facility to tell you (1) the nature of your condition, (2) the general nature of the procedure/treatment/surgery, (3) the risks of the proposed treatment/surgery, as defined by the state or as determined by your doctor, and (4) reasonable therapeutic alternatives and risks associated with such alternatives.

You have the right, as a patient, to be informed about your condition and the recommended surgical, medical, or diagnostic procedure to be used so that you may make the decision whether or not to undergo the procedure after knowing the risks and hazards involved.

In keeping with the State law of informed consent, you are being asked to sign a confirmation that we have discussed all these matters. We have already discussed with you the common problems and risks. We wish to inform you as completely as possible. Please read this form carefully. Ask about anything you do not understand, and we will be pleased to explain it.

1. Patient name: _____

2. Treatment/procedure:
    (a)  Description, nature of the treatment/procedure: _____
    _____

    Purpose: _____
    _____

3. Patient condition: Patient's diagnosis, description of the nature of the condition or ailment for which the medical treatment, surgical procedure, or other therapy described in Item 2 is indicated and recommended:
    _____
    _____

4. Material risks of treatment procedure:
    (a)  All medical or surgical treatment involves risks. Listed below are those risks associated with this procedure that members of this facility believe a reasonable person in your (patient's) position would likely consider significant when deciding whether to have or forego the proposed therapy. Please ask your provider if you would like additional information regarding the nature or consequences of these risks, their likelihood of occurrence, or other associated risks that you might consider significant but may not be listed below.

        - See attachment for risks identified by the State
        - See attachment for risks determined by your provider

Informed Consent

Page 2 of 3

    (b)  Additional risks (if any) particular to the patient because of a complicating medical
        condition:

        _____

        _____

    (c)  Risks generally associated with any surgical treatment/procedure, including
        anesthesia are death, brain damage, disfiguring scars, quadriplegia (paralysis from
        neck down), paraplegia (paralysis from waist down), the loss or loss of function of
        any organ or limb, infection, bleeding, and pain.

5.  Therapeutic alternatives, risks associated therewith, and risks of no treatment:
    Reasonable therapeutic alternatives and the risks associated with such alternatives:

    _____

    _____

## ACKNOWLEDGMENT
## AUTHORIZATION AND CONSENT

6.  (a)  No guarantees: All information given me and, in particular, all estimates made as to the
        likelihood of occurrence of risks of this or alternate procedures or as to the prospects of
        success are made in the best professional judgment of my physician. The possibility and
        nature of complications cannot always be accurately anticipated, and therefore there is and can
        be no guarantee, either express or implied, as to the success or other results of the medical
        treatment or surgical procedure.

    (b)  Additional information: Nothing has been said to me, no information has been given to me, and I
        have not relied upon any information that is inconsistent with the information set forth in this
        document.

    (c)  Particular concerns: I have had an opportunity to disclose to and discuss with the provider
        communicating such information those risks or other potential consequences of the medical treatment or
        surgical procedure that are of particular concern to me.

    (d)  Questions: I have had an opportunity to ask, and I have asked, any questions I may have about the
        information in this document and any other questions I have about the proposed treatment or
        procedure, and all such questions were answered in a satisfactory manner.

    (e)  Authorized provider: The provider (or physician group) authorized to administer or perform the
        medical treatment, surgical procedures or other therapy described in Item 2 is

    _____

        (Name of authorized provider or group)

    (f)  Physician certification: I hereby certify that I have provided and explained the information set forth
        herein, including any attachment, and answered all questions of the patient or the patient's
        representative concerning the medical treatment or surgical procedure, to the best of my knowledge
        and ability.

_____

    (Signature of Provider)               Date            Time

Informed Consent (cont'd)

Page 3 of 3

## Consent

I hereby authorize and direct the designated authorized provider/group, together with associates and assistants of his/her choice, to administer or perform the medical treatment or surgical procedure described in Item 2 of this consent form, including any additional procedures or services as they may deem necessary or reasonable, including the administration of any general or regional anesthetic agent, x-ray or other radiological services, laboratory services, and the disposal of any tissue removed during a diagnostic or surgical procedure, and I hereby consent thereto.

I have read and understand all information set forth in this document, and all blanks were filled in prior to my signing. This authorization for and consent to medical treatment or surgical procedure is and shall remain valid until revoked.

I acknowledge that I have had the opportunity to ask any questions about the contemplated medical procedure or surgical procedure described in Item 2 of this consent form, including risks and alternatives, and acknowledge that my questions have been answered to my satisfaction.

_____     _____
Witness                              Date/time        Patient or person          Date/time
                                                      authorized to consent


If consent is signed by someone other than patient, indicate relationship: _____

Informed Consent (cont'd)

**Your
Hospital's
Logo
Here**

**CONSULTATION
RECORD**

**Consult Notified:**   Date:_____

TIME _____   Initials:_____
(Military Time)

☐  Done by: _____ **MD**

☐  Fax: _____

☐  Telephone:_____

☐  Answering Svc:_____

PATIENT IDENTIFICATION

TO CONSULTING SERVICE
AND / OR PROVIDER:

REASON FOR REQUEST

_____   _____
SIGNATURE OF REQUESTING PROVIDER        DATE

PLEASE CHECK:   ☐ **A**                ☐ **B**
WRITE ORDERS NOW          **DO NOT** WRITE ORDERS

REPORT

**DICTATED**

☐ YES        ☐ NO

**TESTS, PROCEDURES, INTERVENTIONS, ETC. WHICH ARE FOR GENERAL DIAGNOSTIC USE AND WILL NOT ALTER THE
ACUTE INPATIENT MANAGEMENT, SHOULD BE PERFORMED AS AN OUTPATIENT WITH APPROPRIATE FOLLOW-UP.**

**RECOMMENDATIONS**

| INPATIENT | OUTPATIENT |
|---|---|
| | |

DATE        TIME                          SIGNATURE OF CONSULTANT

WHITE - Medical Records        YELLOW - Attending Physician        PINK - Consultant

**PART OF THE MEDICAL RECORD**

8850101 Rev. 05/05                Consultation Record NCR_MEDICAL AFFAIRS                PAGE 1 of 1

Consultation Record

**RECOPIED BY:**

DATE: _____

MILITARY TIME: _____

RN SIGNATURE/TITLE: _____

Page ___ of ___

ALL ENTRIES MUST BE PRINTED IN INK

Your Hospital's Logo Here

Your Hospital
Washington, DC

**MEDICATION ADMINISTRATION RECORD**

**ALLERGIES**

PATIENT IDENTIFICATION

**DATES**

| MEDICATION, DOSE, FREQUENCY, ROUTE | MILITARY TIME | DATE | INITIAL | MILITARY TIME | DATE | INITIAL | MILITARY TIME | DATE | INITIAL |
|---|---|---|---|---|---|---|---|---|---|
| | | | | | | | | | |

INITIAL ORDER DATE | RENEWAL DATE

**SIGNATURE RECORD**

| SIGNATURE | TITLE | INIT'L | SIGNATURE | TITLE | INIT'L |
|---|---|---|---|---|---|
| | | | | | |

Medication Administration Record

# INSULIN ADMINISTRATION RECORD

| BLOOD GLUCOSE MONITORING | | | | INITIAL ORDER | RENEWAL DATE | MEDICATION, DOSE, FREQUENCY ROUTE | DATE | TIME | SITE | INITIAL | DATE | TIME | SITE | INITIAL | DATE | TIME | SITE | INITIAL | DATE | TIME | SITE | INITIAL | DATE | TIME | SITE | INITIAL | DATE | TIME | SITE | INITIAL | DATE | TIME | SITE | INITIAL | DATE | TIME | SITE | INITIAL | DATE | TIME | SITE | INITIAL | DATE | TIME | SITE | INITIAL | DATE | TIME | SITE | INITIAL |
|---|---|---|---|---|---|---|---|---|---|---|---|---|---|---|---|---|---|---|---|---|---|---|---|---|---|---|---|---|---|---|---|---|---|---|---|---|---|---|---|---|---|---|---|---|---|---|---|---|---|---|
| DATE | TIME | LEVEL | INIT'L | | | | | | | | | | | | | | | | | | | | | | | | | | | | | | | | | | | | | | | | | | | | | | | | |

Insulin Administration Record

## ANALGESIC PAIN MANAGEMENT ASSESSMENT

| DATE | TIME | PAIN LOCATION | SEDATION RATING | PAIN SCALE | PAIN RATING | INTERVENTION | COMFORT GOAL | INIT'LS | REASSESSMENT PAIN RATING | TIME | INIT'LS |
|------|------|---------------|-----------------|------------|-------------|--------------|--------------|---------|--------------------------|------|---------|
|      |      |               |                 |            |             |              |              |         |                          |      |         |
|      |      |               |                 |            |             |              |              |         |                          |      |         |
|      |      |               |                 |            |             |              |              |         |                          |      |         |
|      |      |               |                 |            |             |              |              |         |                          |      |         |
|      |      |               |                 |            |             |              |              |         |                          |      |         |
|      |      |               |                 |            |             |              |              |         |                          |      |         |
|      |      |               |                 |            |             |              |              |         |                          |      |         |
|      |      |               |                 |            |             |              |              |         |                          |      |         |
|      |      |               |                 |            |             |              |              |         |                          |      |         |
|      |      |               |                 |            |             |              |              |         |                          |      |         |
|      |      |               |                 |            |             |              |              |         |                          |      |         |
|      |      |               |                 |            |             |              |              |         |                          |      |         |

ROOM #: ___   PATIENT Last Name: ___   PATIENT First Name: ___   Middle ___   DIAGNOSIS: ___   PHYSICIAN: ___

Analgesic Pain Management Assessment

**PAIN SCALES:**

**WONG-BAKER:** *(Faces)*

0  1  2  3  4  5

**0-10 VISUAL:** *(Numeric)*

0  1  2  3  4  5  6  7  8  9  10

**VERBAL:** No Hurt    Hurts Little Bit    Hurts Little More    Hurts Even More    Hurts Whole Lot    Worst Pain

WONG-BAKER FACES PAIN SCALE from Wong DL, Hockenberry-Eaton M, Wilson D, Winkelstein ML, Ahmann E, DiVito-Thomas PA, Whaley & Wong: Care of Infants & Children, 6th ed, St. Louis, MO; Mosby-Year Book Inc., 1996; 1153. Copyrighted by Mosby-Year Book, Inc. Reprinted with permission.

**NON-COGNITIVE:**

**SEDATION SCALE:**

S = NORMAL SLEEP, EASY TO AROUSE, ORIENTED WHEN AWAKENED, APPROPRIATE COGNITIVE BEHAVIOR

1 = WIDE AWAKE - ALERT (OR AT BASELINE), ORIENTED, INITIATES CONVERSATION

2 = DROWSY, EASY TO AROUSE, BUT ORIENTED AND DEMONSTRATES APPROPRIATE COGNITIVE BEHAVIOR WHEN AWAKE

3 = DROWSY, SOMEWHAT DIFFICULT TO AROUSE, BUT ORIENTED WHEN AWAKE

4 = DIFFICULT TO AROUSE, CONFUSED, NOT ORIENTED

5 = UNAROUSABLE

**FLACC SCALE:** *(Non-Cognitive)*

1. Sum of FACE, LEGS, ACTIVITY, CRY AND CONSOLABILITY Scores = FLACC
2. Record FLACC Score using the 0-10 VISUAL (NUMERIC) Scale above

**= FACE Score**
0 = No particular expression or smile
1 = Occasional grimace or frown, withdrawn, disinterested
2 = Frequent to constant frown, clenched jaw, quivering chin

**= LEGS Score**
0 = Normal position, or relaxed
1 = Uneasy, restless, tense
2 = Kicking, or legs drawn up

**= ACTIVITY Score**
0 = Lying quietly, normal position, moves easily
1 = Squirming, shifting back and forth, tense
2 = Arched, rigid, or jerking

**= CRY Score**
0 = No crying (asleep or awake)
1 = Moans or whimpers, occasional complaint
2 = Crying steadily, screams or sobs, frequent complaints

**= CONSOLABILITY Score**
0 = Content, relaxed
1 = Reassured by touching/hugging/talking to, distractable
2 = Difficult to console or comfort

**INTERVENTION:**

1 = Discuss Pain Management Plan with MD
2 = Pharmacological (See MED KARDEX)
3 = Non-Pharmacological
   A. Position Changed
   B. Relaxation Technique
   C. Splinting
   D. Imagery
   E. Music
   F. Education
   G. Other: _____

| DATE | TIME | MEDICATION | REASON FOR OMISSION | INIT'L | INIT'L |
|------|------|------------|---------------------|--------|--------|
|      |      |            |                     |        |        |
|      |      |            |                     |        |        |
|      |      |            |                     |        |        |
|      |      |            |                     |        |        |
|      |      |            |                     |        |        |
|      |      |            |                     |        |        |
|      |      |            |                     |        |        |
|      |      |            |                     |        |        |

**SIGNATURE RECORD**

| SIGNATURE | TITLE |
|-----------|-------|
|           |       |
|           |       |
|           |       |
|           |       |

Analgesic Pain Management Assessment (cont'd)

## PRN / ANALGESIC PAIN MEDICATION ADMINISTRATION RECORD

| INITIAL | MEDICATION | DOSAGE | FREQUENCY ROUTE OF ADMINISTRATION |

DATE
TIME
SITE
EFF
INIT'L

Date Ord.    Exp. Date

## SINGLE ORDER / PRE-OPS

| INITIAL | MEDICATIONS | | GIVEN | | |
| | DOSE AND ROUTE OF ADMINISTRATION | SITE | Date | Milit. Time | INIT'L |
| ORDER DATE | | | | | |

**EFFECTIVENESS:**

Y = YES          N = NO

* If "NO", document interventions on Nurse's Notes

A B C D E F G H I J K L M N

8850417 Rev. 08/06

Medication Administration Kardex_NURSING

Analgesic Pain Management Assessment (cont'd)

**DIAMONTE HOSPITAL**
Diamonte, Arizona

**Intake/Output
Record**

Date: _____

| Time a.m./p.m. | IV Fluid/Rate | Absorbed 7 a.m.-3 p.m.  3 p.m.-11 p.m.  11 p.m.-7 a.m. | | | Comments: |
|---|---|---|---|---|---|
| | | | | | |
| | | | | | |
| | | | | | |
| | | | | | |
| | | | | | |
| | | | | | |
| | | | | | |
| | | | | | |
| | | | | | |
| | | | | | |
| | | | | | |
| | | | | | |

**INTAKE** — **OUTPUT**

| Time | Oral | Tube | IV | Blood | Total | Urine Voided | Catheter | Suction | Drains | Emesis | Total |
|---|---|---|---|---|---|---|---|---|---|---|---|
| 7 a.m.-3 p.m. | | | | | | | | | | | |
| 3 p.m.-11 p.m. | | | | | | | | | | | |
| 11 p.m.-7 a.m. | | | | | | | | | | | |
| Total | | | | | | | | | | | |

IV START/RESTART      Time: _____      IV START/RESTART      Time: _____

CATHETER SIZE# USED: _____ / _____      CATHETER SIZE# USED: _____ / _____

| TIME | APPEARANCE | SITE |
|---|---|---|
| 7 a.m.-3 p.m. | | |
| 3 p.m.-11 p.m. | | |
| 11 p.m.-7 a.m. | | |

| 7 a.m.-3 p.m. Shift | | 3 p.m.-11 p.m. Shift | |
|---|---|---|---|
| Initials | Signature/Title | Initials | Signature/Title |
| | | | |
| | | | |

| 11 p.m.-7 a.m. Shift | | | |
|---|---|---|---|
| Initials | Signature/Title | | |
| | | | |
| | | | |

Intake/Output Record

Your Hospital's Logo Here

**NURSING PROGRESS NOTES**

**Print NAME and SIGN all entries**

Patient identification

| Abbreviations | | Date | NOTES |
|---|---|---|---|
| **DO NOT USE** | **USE** | Military Time | |
| QD | Daily | | |
| QOD | Every other day | | |
| QID | 4 times a day | | |
| U | Units | | |
| UG | Microgram | | |
| CC | mL | | |
| .2mg | 0.2 mg | | |
| 10.0mg | 10 mg | | |
| MS or MSO₄ | Morphine sulfate | | |
| MG or MgSO₄ | Magnesium sulfate | | |
| OS | Left eye | | |
| OU | Both eyes | | |
| OD | Right eye | | |
| AS | Left ear | | |
| AU | Both ears | | |
| AD | Right ear | | |

## PART OF THE MEDICAL RECORD

Nursing Progress Notes

| Operative Report |
| :---: |
| **PROGRESS** |
| **NOTES** |

**Your Hospital's Logo Here**

**Print NAME and SIGN all entries**

Patient identification

| Abbreviations | | Date | Military Time | NOTES |
| :---: | :---: | :---: | :---: | :--- |
| DO NOT USE | USE | | | |
| QD | Dally | | | |
| QOD | Every other day | | | **OPERATIVE REPORT** |
| QID | 4 times a day | | | Pre operative Dx: |
| | | | | Post operative Dx: |
| U | Units | | | Procedure: |
| UG | Microgram | | | Attending Surgeon: |
| | | | | Assistant: |
| CC | mL | | | Anesthesia: |
| | | | | Cord gas:  ☐ Yes  ☐ No |
| .2mg | 0.2 mg | | | Estimated blood loss: _____ mL |
| 10.0mg | 10 mg | | | Urine Output: _____ mL |
| | | | | IV Fluids: _____ mL |
| MS or MSO₄ | Morphine Sulfate | | | Drains: |
| MG or MgSO₄ | Magnesium Sulfate | | | Complications: |
| | | | | Disposition: |
| OS | Left eye | | | |
| OU | Both eyes | | | |
| OD | Right eye | | | Operative findings: |
| AS | Left ear | | | |
| AU | Both ears | | | |
| AD | Right ear | | | |

**PART OF THE MEDICAL RECORD**

8850499 Rev. 05/05    Operative Report Progress Notes_MIH_MEDICAL AFFAIRS    PAGE 1 of 2

Operative Report Progress Notes

Your Hospital's Logo Here

**Operative Report
PROGRESS
NOTES**

**Print NAME and SIGN all entries**

Patient identification

| Abbreviations | | Date / Military Time | **NOTES** |
|---|---|---|---|
| DO NOT USE | USE | | |
| QD | Daily | | |
| QOD | Every other day | | |
| QID | 4 times a day | | |
| U | Units | | |
| UG | Microgram | | |
| CC | mL | | |
| .2mg | 0.2 mg | | |
| 10.0mg | 10 mg | | |
| MS or MSO$_4$ | Morphine sulfate | | |
| MG or MgSO$_4$ | Magnesium sulfate | | |
| OS | Left eye | | |
| OU | Both eyes | | |
| OD | Right eye | | |
| AS | Left ear | | |
| AU | Both ears | | |
| AD | Right ear | | |

**PART OF THE MEDICAL RECORD**

Operative Report Progress Notes (cont'd)

**Your Hospital's Logo Here**

**DISCHARGE ORDERS**

PATIENT IDENTIFICATION

DISCHARGE ORDERS FOR: _____

DISCHARGE PHYSICIAN: _____

**ACTIVITY:** ☐ NO RESTRICTIONS        ☐ RESTRICTIONS

_____        _____

**MEDICATIONS**      Ejection Fraction: _____%      (CHF Patients only)

Ace Inhibitor: _____        _____

Beta Blocker: _____        _____

_____        _____

_____        _____

**TREATMENT/PAIN MANAGEMENT:**

_____        _____

_____        _____

_____        _____

**CALL YOUR DOCTOR IF YOU HAVE:**

_____        _____

_____        _____

**DIET:**

REGULAR _____ ** _____ CALORIE ADA _____ ** _____ Copy of diet given, as ordered by Physician

SOFT _____ ** _____ LOW SODIUM ** OTHER _____

**FOLLOW UP REFERRALS:**

Patient Education Booklet: _____

Home Care: _____

Return to MD: _____

Other: _____

**EQUIPMENT:** Supplies can be bought at: _____

**I HAVE RECEIVED THE ABOVE INSTRUCTIONS AND WAS GIVEN THE OPPORTUNITY TO ASK QUESTIONS**

_____        _____        _____

Discharging Physician's Signature        Date        Patient/Responsible Person's Signature

_____        _____

Physician's Phone        Discharging Nurse's Signature/Title

**WHITE** = Chart        **YELLOW** = Patient        **PINK** = Physician

**PART OF THE MEDICAL RECORD**

Discharge Orders

**DIAMONTE HOSPITAL**
Diamonte, Arizona

Patient Name:

Medical Record No.

**Nursing
Discharge Summary**

(addressograph)

Date of discharge:_____    Time of discharge:_____    Accompanied by:_____
Disposition: ____ Home    ____ Death    ____Other (Please specify) _____
Discharged:____ Ambulatory    ____Wheelchair    ____Stretcher    ____Ambulance
Vital signs: Blood pressure:_____    Pulse:_____    Resp:_____    Temp:_____
Mental status:____ Alert    ____ Confused    ____Other (specify)_____
Social worker:_____    Phone number:_____

**Services Needed**
**Equipment/Supplies:** Company:_____    Phone:_____
Type of service:_____    Date service is to start:_____

**Home Health:** Company:_____    Phone:_____
Type of service:_____    Date service is to start:_____

**Other:** Company:_____    Phone:_____
Type of service:_____    Date service is to start:_____

| **Medication** | **Dose** | **Time of Day** | **Special Instruction** |
|---|---|---|---|
| | | | |
| | | | |
| | | | |

____ Medication/diet Counseling for above drugs, signature of dietitian_____Date:_____
____ Prescription given to patient                ____ Medication from pharmacy returned____Yes    ____No

**Diet**        ____Regular
  ____ Other:_____ Diet Instructions:_____
  _____ Signature of dietitian:_____Date:_____

**Treatment/Wound Care**                ____ No treatments prescribed
  Treatment/wound care
  Site 1 _____
  Site 2 _____
  ____ Patient instructed        ____Significant other        Date:_____

**Activity**
  ____ Special precautions:_____
  ____ Gradually resume daily activities
  ____ Do not lift object heavier than _____
  ____ Use the following devices to move safely:_____
  ____ Remain on bed rest except for:  ___bathroom    ___meals

**Follow-up**
  ____ No appointment needed                ____Patient teaching form discussed with patient/family
  See doctor _____ on _____Phone _____ Appointment made: Yes/No
  See doctor _____ on _____Phone _____ Appointment made: Yes/No
  Call doctor if:_____
  _____
  I have received and understand the above instructions:
  Patient signature:_____ Date:_____ Nurse signature:_____ Date:_____

Nursing Discharge Summary

TYPE/PRINT IN PERMANENT BLACK INK FOR INSTRUCTIONS SEE HANDBOOK

**CHILD**

DEATH UNDER ONE YEAR OF AGE Enter State File Number of death certificate for this child

**MOTHER**

**FATHER**

**INFORMANT**

**U.S. STANDARD**
## CERTIFICATE OF LIVE BIRTH

LOCAL FILE NUMBER                          BIRTH NUMBER

1. CHILD'S NAME *(First, Middle, Last)*

2. DATE OF BIRTH *(Month, Day, Year)*

3. TIME OF BIRTH

4. SEX

5. CITY, TOWN, OR LOCATION OF BIRTH

6. COUNTY OF BIRTH

7. PLACE OF BIRTH: ☐ Hospital   ☐ Freestanding Birthing Center   ☐ Clinic/Doctor's Office   ☐ Residence   ☐ Other *(Specify)* _____

8. FACILITY NAME *(If not institution, give street and number)*

**CERTIFIER/ATTENDANT**

9. I certify that this child was born alive at the place and time and on the date stated.

Signature ▶

10. DATE SIGNED *(Month, Day, Year)*

11. ATTENDANT'S NAME AND TITLE *(If other than certifier) (Type/Print)*
Name _____
☐ M.D.   ☐ D.O.   ☐ C.N.M.   ☐ Other Midwife
☐ Other *(Specify)* _____

12. CERTIFIER'S NAME AND TITLE *(Type/Print)*
Name _____
☐ M.D.   ☐ D.O.   ☐ Hospital Admin.   ☐ C.N.M.   ☐ Other Midwife
☐ Other *(Specify)* _____

13. ATTENDANT'S MAILING ADDRESS *(Street and Number or Rural Route Number, City or Town, State, Zip Code)*

14. REGISTRAR'S SIGNATURE ▶

15. DATE FILED BY REGISTRAR *(Month, Day, Year)*

16a. MOTHER'S NAME *(First, Middle, Last)*

16b. MAIDEN SURNAME

17. DATE OF BIRTH *(Month, Day, Year)*

18. BIRTHPLACE *(State or Foreign Country)*

19a. RESIDENCE–STATE

19B. COUNTY

19c. CITY, TOWN, OR LOCATION

19d. STREET AND NUMBER

19e. INSIDE CITY LIMITS? *(Yes or no)*

20. MOTHER'S MAILING ADDRESS *(If same as residence, enter Zip Code only)*

21. FATHER'S NAME *(First, Middle, Last)*

22. DATE OF BIRTH *(Month, Day, Year)*

23. BIRTHPLACE *(State or Foreign Country)*

24. I certify that the personal information provided on this certificate is correct to the best of my knowledge and belief.
Signature of Parent of Other Informant ▶

INFORMATION FOR MEDICAL AND HEALTH USE ONLY

MULTIPLE BIRTHS Enter State File Number for Mates(s) LIVE BIRTH (S)

FETAL DEATH (S)

25. OF HISPANIC ORIGIN? *(Specify No or Yes—if yes, specify Cuban, Mexican, Puerto Rican, etc.)*

26. RACE–American Indian, Black, White, etc. *(Specify below)*

27. EDUCATION *(Specify only highest grade completed)*
Elementary/Secondary (0-12) | College (1-4 or 5 +)

**MOTHER**
25a.   ☐ No   ☐ Yes   Specify:

26a.

27a.

**FATHER**
25b.   ☐ No   ☐ Yes   Specify:

26b.

27b.

| 28. PREGNANCY HISTORY *(Complete each section)* | | | 29. MOTHER MARRIED? (At birth, conception, or any time between) *(Yes or no)* | 30. DATE LAST NORMAL MENSES BEGAN *(Month, Day, Year)* |
|---|---|---|---|---|
| LIVE BIRTHS *(Do not include this child)* | | OTHER TERMINATIONS *(Spontaneous and induced at Any time after conception)* | | |

| 28a. Now Living | 28b. Now Dead | 28d. | 31. MONTH OF PREGNANCY PRENATAL CARE BEGAN  First, Second, Third, etc. *(Specify)* | 32. PRENATAL VISITS–Total Number *(If none, so state)* |
|---|---|---|---|---|
| Number  ☐ None | Number  ☐ None | Number  ☐ None | | |
| 28c. DATE OF LAST LIVE BIRTH *(Month, Year)* | | 28e. DATE OF LAST OTHER TERMINATION *(Month, Year)* | 33. BIRTH WEIGHT *(Specify unit)* | 34. CLINICAL ESTIMATE OF GESTATION *(Weeks)* |
| | | | 35a. PLURALITY- Single, Twin, Triplet, etc. *(Specify)* | 35b. IF NOT SINGLE BIRTH–Born First, Second, Third, etc. *(Specify)* |

| 36. APGAR SCORE | | 37a. MOTHER TRANSFERRED PRIOR TO DELIVERY?  ☐ NO   ☐ YES   If Yes, enter name of facility transferred from: |
|---|---|---|
| 36a. 1 Minute | 36b. 5 Minutes | 37b. INFANT TRANSFERRED?  ☐ No   ☐ Yes   If Yes, enter name of facility transferred to: |

Certificate of Live Birth

**38a. MEDICAL RISK FACTORS FOR THIS PREGNANCY**
*(Check all that apply)*

Anemia (Hct. < 30/Hgb. <101 . . . . . . . . . . . . . . . . . . . .01 ☐
Cardiac disease . . . . . . . . . . . . . . . . . . . . . . . . . . .02 ☐
Acute or chronic lung disease . . . . . . . . . . . . . . .03 ☐
Diabetes . . . . . . . . . . . . . . . . . . . . . . . . . . . . . . . 04 ☐
Genital herpes . . . . . . . . . . . . . . . . . . . . . . . . . . .05 ☐
Hydramnios/Oligohydramnios . . . . . . . . . . . . . . . . .06 ☐
Hemoglobinopathy . . . . . . . . . . . . . . . . . . . . . . . .07 ☐
Hypertension, chronic . . . . . . . . . . . . . . . . . . . . . .08 ☐
Hypertension, pregnancy-associated . . . . . . . . . . . . .09 ☐
Eclampsia . . . . . . . . . . . . . . . . . . . . . . . . . . . . . . 10 ☐
Incompetent cervix . . . . . . . . . . . . . . . . . . . . . . . .11 ☐
Previous infant 4000 + grams . . . . . . . . . . . . . . . . 12 ☐
Previous preterm or small for-gestational-age
   infant . . . . . . . . . . . . . . . . . . . . . . . . . . . . . . . . .13 ☐
Renal disease . . . . . . . . . . . . . . . . . . . . . . . . . . . .14 ☐
Rh sensitization . . . . . . . . . . . . . . . . . . . . . . . . . . .15 ☐
Uterine bleeding . . . . . . . . . . . . . . . . . . . . . . . . . .16 ☐
None . . . . . . . . . . . . . . . . . . . . . . . . . . . . . . . . . .00 ☐
Other _____ 17 ☐
         *(Specify)*

**38b. OTHER RISK FACTORS FOR THIS PREGNANCY**
*(Complete all items)*

Tobacco use during pregnancy . . . . . . . . . . Yes ☐ No ☐
   Average number cigarettes per day _____
Alcohol use during pregnancy . . . . . . . . . . Yes ☐ No ☐
   Average number drinks per week _____
Weight gained during pregnancy _____ lbs.

**39. OBSTETRIC PROCEDURES**
*(Check all that apply)*

Amniocentesis . . . . . . . . . . . . . . . . . . . . . . . . . .01 ☐
Electronic fetal monitoring . . . . . . . . . . . . . . . . . . . .02 ☐
Induction of labor . . . . . . . . . . . . . . . . . . . . . . . ...03 ☐
Stimulation of labor . . . . . . . . . . . . . . . . . . . . . ...04 ☐
Tocolysis . . . . . . . . . . . . . . . . . . . . . . . . . . . . . ...05 ☐
Ultrasound . . . . . . . . . . . . . . . . . . . . . . . . . . . . . 06 ☐
None . . . . . . . . . . . . . . . . . . . . . . . . . . . . . . . . 00 ☐
Other _____ 07 ☐
         *(Specify)*

**40. COMPLICATIONS OF LABOR AND/OR DELIVERY**
*(Check all that apply)*

Febrile (> 100°F. or 38°C.) . . . . . . . . . . . . . . . . . . . .01 ☐
Meconium, moderate/heavy . . . . . . . . . . . . . . . . . .02 ☐
Premature rupture of membrane (> 12 hours) . . . . . ..03 ☐
Abruptio placenta . . . . . . . . . . . . . . . . . . . . . . . . .04 ☐
Placenta previa . . . . . . . . . . . . . . . . . . . . . . . . . . .05 ☐
Other excessive bleeding . . . . . . . . . . . . . . . . . . . .06 ☐
Seizures during labor . . . . . . . . . . . . . . . . . . . . . . .07 ☐
Precipitous labor (< 3 hours) . . . . . . . . . . . . . . . 08 ☐
Prolonged labor (> 20 hours) . . . . . . . . . . . . . . . .09 ☐
Dysfunctional labor . . . . . . . . . . . . . . . . . . . . . . . .10 ☐
Breech/Malpresentation . . . . . . . . . . . . . . . . . . . . .11 ☐
Cephalopelvic disproportion . . . . . . . . . . . . . . . . . .12 ☐
Cord prolapse . . . . . . . . . . . . . . . . . . . . . . . . . . .13 ☐
Anesthetic complications . . . . . . . . . . . . . . . . . . . .14 ☐
Fetal distress . . . . . . . . . . . . . . . . . . . . . . . . . . . .15 ☐
None . . . . . . . . . . . . . . . . . . . . . . . . . . . . . . . . . .00 ☐
Other _____ 16 ☐
         *(Specify)*

**41. METHOD OF DELIVERY** *(Check all that apply)*

Vaginal . . . . . . . . . . . . . . . . . . . . . . . . . . . . . . . .01 ☐
Vaginal birth after previous C-section . . . . . . . . . . .02 ☐
Primary C-section . . . . . . . . . . . . . . . . . . . . . . . . .03 ☐
Repeat C-section . . . . . . . . . . . . . . . . . . . . . . . . .04 ☐
Forceps . . . . . . . . . . . . . . . . . . . . . . . . . . . . . . . .05 ☐
Vacuum . . . . . . . . . . . . . . . . . . . . . . . . . . . . . . . .06 ☐

**42. ABNORMAL CONDITIONS OF THE NEWBORN**
*(Check all that apply)*

Anemia (Hct. < 39/Hgb. < 13) . . . . . . . . . . . . . . . . .01 ☐
Birth injury . . . . . . . . . . . . . . . . . . . . . . . . . . . . . .02 ☐
Fetal alcohol syndrome . . . . . . . . . . . . . . . . . . . . .03 ☐
Hyaline membrane disease/RDS . . . . . . . . . . . . . . .04 ☐
Meconium aspiration syndrome . . . . . . . . . . . . . . . .05 ☐
Assisted ventilation < 30 min . . . . . . . . . . . . . . . . .06 ☐
Assisted ventilation ≥ 30 min . . . . . . . . . . . . . . . . .07 ☐
Seizures . . . . . . . . . . . . . . . . . . . . . . . . . . . . . . . .08 ☐
None . . . . . . . . . . . . . . . . . . . . . . . . . . . . . . . . . .00 ☐
Other _____ 09 ☐
         *(Specify)*

**43. CONGENITAL ANOMALIES OF CHILD**
*(Check all that apply)*

Anencephalus . . . . . . . . . . . . . . . . . . . . . . . . . . .01 ☐
Spina bifida/Meningocele . . . . . . . . . . . . . . . . . . . . 02 ☐
Hydrocephalus . . . . . . . . . . . . . . . . . . . . . . . . . . 03 ☐
Microcephalus . . . . . . . . . . . . . . . . . . . . . . . . . . 04 ☐
Other central nervous system anomalies
   *(Specify)* _____ 05 ☐

Heart malformations . . . . . . . . . . . . . . . . . . . . . . . 06 ☐
Other circulatory/respiratory anomalies
   *(Specify)* _____ 07 ☐

Rectal atresia/stenosis . . . . . . . . . . . . . . . . . . . . . 08 ☐
Tracheo-esophageal fistula/Esophageal atresia . . 09 ☐
Omphalocele/Gastroschisis . . . . . . . . . . . . . . . . . . 10 ☐
Other gastrointestinal anomalies
   *(Specify)* _____ 11 ☐

Malformed genitalia . . . . . . . . . . . . . . . . . . . . . . . 12 ☐
Renal agenesis . . . . . . . . . . . . . . . . . . . . . . . ... 13 ☐
Other urogenital anomalies
   *(Specify)* _____ 14 ☐

Cleft lip/palate . . . . . . . . . . . . . . . . . . . . . . . . . . 15 ☐
Polydactyly/Syndactyly/Adactyly . . . . . . . . . . . . . .16 ☐
Club foot . . . . . . . . . . . . . . . . . . . . . . . . . . . . . 17 ☐
Diaphragmatic hernia . . . . . . . . . . . . . . . . . . . . . .18 ☐
Other musculoskeletal/integumental anomalies
   *(Specify)* _____ 19 ☐

Down's syndrome . . . . . . . . . . . . . . . . . . . . . . . . 20 ☐
Other chromosomal anomalies
   *(Specify)* 21 ☐

None . . . . . . . . . . . . . . . . . . . . . . . . . . . . . . . . .00 ☐
Other _____ 22 ☐
         *(Specify)*

Certificate of Live Birth (cont'd)

TYPE/PRINT IN PERMANENT BLACK INK FOR INSTRUCTIONS SEE HANDBOOK

LOCAL FILE NUMBER

**U.S. STANDARD**
**CERTIFICATE OF DEATH**

STATE FILE NUMBER

**DECEDENT**

1. DECEDENT'S NAME (First, Middle, Last)

2. SEX

3. DATE OF DEATH (Month, Day, Year)

4. SOCIAL SECURITY NUMBER | 5a. AGE–Last Birthday (Years) | 5b. UNDER 1 YEAR — Months / Days | 5C. UNDER 1 DAY — Hours / Minutes | 6. DATE OF BIRTH (Month, Day, Year) | 7. BIRTHPLACE (City and State or Foreign Country)

8. WAS DECEDENT EVER IN U.S. ARMED FORCES? (Yes or no)

9a. PLACE OF DEATH (Check only one: see instructions on other side)
HOSPITAL: ☐ Inpatient  ☐ ER/Outpatient  ☐ DOA    OTHER: ☐ Nursing Home  ☐ Residence  ☐ Other (Specify)

9b. FACILITY NAME (If not institution, give street and number)

9c. CITY, TOWN, OR LOCATION OF DEATH

9d. COUNTY OF DEATH

10. MARITAL STATUS–Married, Never Married, Widowed, Divorced (Specify)

11. SURVIVING SPOUSE (If wife, give maiden name)

12a. DECEDENT'S USUAL OCCUPATION (Give kind of work done during most of working life. Do not use retired.)

12b. KIND OF BUSINESS/INDUSTRY

13a. RESIDENCE–STATE

13b. COUNTY

13c. CITY, TOWN, OR LOCATION

13d. STREET AND NUMBER

13e. INSIDE CITY LIMITS? (Yes or no)

13f. ZIP CODE

14. WAS DECEDENT OF HISPANIC ORIGIN? (Specify No or Yes–If yes, specify Cuban Mexican, Puerto Rican, etc.) ☐ No  ☐ Yes  Specify:

15. RACE–American Indian, Black, White, etc. (Specify)

16. DECEDENT'S EDUCATION (Specify only highest grade completed)
Elementary/Secondary (0-12) | College (1-4 or 5 +)

**PARENTS**

17. FATHER'S NAME (First, Middle, Last)

18. MOTHER'S NAME (First, Middle, Last)

**INFORMANT**

19a. INFORMANT'S NAME (Type/Print)

19b. MAILING ADDRESS (Street and Number or Rural Route Number, City or Town, State, Zip Code)

**DISPOSITION**

20a. METHOD OF DISPOSITION
☐ Burial  ☐ Cremation  ☐ Removal from State  ☐ Donation  ☐ Other (Specify) _____

20b. PLACE OF DISPOSITION (Name of cemetery, crematory, or other place)

20c. LOCATION–City or Town, State

21a. SIGNATURE OF FUNERAL SERVICE LICENSEE OR PERSON ACTING AS SUCH ▶

21b. LICENSE NUMBER (Of Licensee)

22. NAME AND ADDRESS OF FACILITY

**PRONOUNCING PHYSICIAN ONLY**

Complete items 23a-c only when certifying physician is not available at time of death to certify cause of death.

23a. To the best of my knowledge, death occurred at the time, date, and place stated.
Signature and Title ▶

23b. LICENSE NUMBER

23c. DATE SIGNED (Month, Day, Year)

**ITEMS 24-26 MUST BE COMPLETED BY PERSON WHO PRONOUNCES DEATH**

24. TIME OF DEATH

25. DATE PRONOUNCED DEAD (Month, Day, Year)

26. WAS CASE REFERRED TO MEDICAL EXAMINER/CORONER? (Yes or no)

**CAUSE OF DEATH**

27. PART I. Enter the diseases, injuries, or complications that caused the death. Do not enter the mode of dying, such as cardiac or respiratory arrest, shock, or heart failure. List only one cause on each line.

Approximate Interval Between Onset and Death

IMMEDIATE CAUSE (Final deceased or condition resulting in death)

a. _____
   DUE TO (OR AS A CONSEQUENCE OF):

Sequentially list conditions, if any, leading to immediate cause. Enter UNDERLYING CAUSE (Disease or injury that initiated events resulting in death LAST

b. _____
   DUE TO (OR AS A CONSEQUENCE OF):

c. _____
   DUE TO (OR AS A CONSEQUENCE OF):

d. _____

PART II. Other significant conditions contributing to death but not resulting in the underlying cause given in Part I.

28a. WAS AN AUTOPSY PERFORMED? (Yes or no)

28b. WERE AUTOPSY FINDINGS AVAILABLE PRIOR TO COMPLETION OF CAUSE OF DEATH? (Yes or no)

29. MANNER OF DEATH
☐ Natural  ☐ Pending Investigation
☐ Accident  ☐ Could not be Determined
☐ Suicide
☐ Homicide

30a. DATE OF INJURY (Month, Day, Year)

30b. TIME OF INJURY   M

30c. INJURY AT WORK? (Yes or no)

30d. DESCRIBE HOW INJURY OCCURRED

30e. PLACE OF INJURY–At home, farm, street, factory, office building, etc. (Specify)

30f. LOCATION (Street and Number or Rural Route Number, City or Town, State)

**CERTIFIER**

31a. CERTIFIER (Check only one)
☐ CERTIFYING PHYSICIAN (Physician certifying cause of death when another physician has pronounced death and completed item 23)
To the best of my knowledge, death occurred due to the cause(s) and manner as stated.

☐ PRONOUNCING AND CERTIFYING PHYSICIAN (Physician both pronouncing death and certifying to cause of death)
To the best of my knowledge, death occurred at the time, date, and place, and due to the cause(s) and manner as stated.

☐ MEDICAL EXAMINER/CORONER
On the basis of examination and/or investigation, in my opinion, death occurred at the time, date, and place, and due to the cause(s) and manner as stated.

31b. SIGNATURE AND TITLE OF CERTIFIER ▶

31c. LICENSE NUMBER

31d. DATE SIGNED (Month, Day, Year)

32. NAME AND ADDRESS OF PERSON WHO COMPLETED CAUSE OF DEATH (ITEM 27) (Type/Print)

**REGISTRAR**

33. REGISTRAR'S SIGNATURE ▶

34. DATE FILED (Month, Day, Year)

PHS-T-003
REV. 1/89

NAME OF DECEDENT For use by physician or institution

SEE INSTRUCTIONS ON OTHER SIDE

SEE DEFINITION ON OTHER SIDE

SEE INSTRUCTIONS ON OTHER SIDE

SEE DEFINITION ON OTHER SIDE

DEPARTMENT OF HEALTH AND HUMAN SERVICES • PUBLIC HEALTH SERVICE • NATIONAL CENTER FOR HEALTH STATISTICS • 1989 REVISION

Certificate of Death

TYPE/PRINT IN PERMANENT BLACK INK FOR INSTRUCTIONS SEE HANDBOOK

**U.S. STANDARD**
## REPORT OF FETAL DEATH

STATE FILE NUMBER

| 1. FACILITY NAME (If not institution, give street and number) |
|---|

| 2. CITY, TOWN, OR LOCATION OF DELIVERY | 3. COUNTY OF DELIVERY | 4. DATE OF DELIVERY (Month, Day, Year) | 5. SEX OF FETUS |
|---|---|---|---|

**PARENTS**

| 5a. MOTHER'S NAME (First, Middle, Last) | 5b. MAIDEN SURNAME | 7. DATE OF BIRTH (Month, Day, Year) |
|---|---|---|

| 8a. RESIDENCE-STATE | 8b. COUNTY | 8c. CITY, TOWN, OR LOCATION | 8d. STREET AND NUMBER |
|---|---|---|---|

| 8e. INSIDE CITY LIMITS? (Yes or no) | 8f. ZIP CODE | 9. FATHER'S NAME (First, Middle, Last) | 10. DATE OF BIRTH (Month, Day, Year) |
|---|---|---|---|

| 11. OF HISPANIC ORIGIN? (Specify No or Yes—if yes, specify Cuban, Mexican, Puerto Rican, etc.) | 12. RACE–American Indian, Black, White, etc. (Specify) | 13. EDUCATION (Specify only highest grade completed) | | 14. OCCUPATION AND BUSINESS/INDUSTRY (Worked during last year) | |
|---|---|---|---|---|---|
| | | Elementary/Secondary (0-12) | College (1-4 or 5 +) | Occupation | Business/Industry |

**MOTHER**

| 11a. ☐ No  ☐ Yes  Specify: | 12a. | 13a. | | 14a. | 14b. |
|---|---|---|---|---|---|

**FATHER**

| 11b. ☐ No  ☐ Yes  Specify: | 12b. | 13b. | | 14c. | 14d. |
|---|---|---|---|---|---|

MULTIPLE BIRTHS
Enter State File Number for Mate(s)
LIVE BIRTHS

FETAL DEATH(S)

| 15. PREGNANCY HISTORY (Complete each section) | | | 16. MOTHER MARRIED? (At delivery, conception, or any time between) (Yes or no) | 17. DATE LAST NORMAL MENSES BEGAN (Month, Day, Year) |
|---|---|---|---|---|
| LIVE BIRTHS | | OTHER TERMINATIONS (Spontaneous and induced at Any time after conception) | | |
| 15a. Now Living  Number ____  ☐ None | 15b. Now Dead  Number ____  ☐ None | 15d. (Do not include this fetus)  Number ____  ☐ None | 18. MONTH OF PREGNANCY PRENATAL CARE BEGAN  First, Second, Third, etc. (Specify) | 19. PRENATAL VISITS–Total Number (If none, so state) |
| | | | 20. WEIGHT OF FETUS (Specify unit) | 21. CLINICAL ESTIMATE OF GESTATION (Weeks) |
| 15c. DATE OF LAST LIVE BIRTH (Month, Year) | | 15e. DATE OF LAST OTHER TERMINATION (Month, Year) | 22a. PLURALITY- Single, Twin, Triplet, etc. (Specify) | 22b. IF NOT SINGLE BIRTH–Born First, Second, Third, etc. (Specify) |

**MEDICAL AND HEALTH INFORMATION**

**23a. MEDICAL RISK FACTORS FOR THIS PREGNANCY** (Check all that apply)

Anemia (Hct. < 30/Hgb. < 10)................ 01 ☐
Cardiac disease ......................... 02 ☐
Acute or chronic lung disease .............. 03 ☐
Diabetes ............................... 04 ☐
Genital herpes .......................... 05 ☐
Hydramnios/Oligohydramnios ............. 06 ☐
Hemoglobinopathy ...................... 07 ☐
Hypertension, chronic .................... 08 ☐
Hypertension, pregnancy-associated .......... 09 ☐
Eclampsia ............................. 10 ☐
Incompetent cervix .......................11 ☐
Previous infant 4000 + grams ............ 12 ☐
Previous preterm or small for-gestational-age
 infant ............................... 13 ☐
Renal disease .......................... 14 ☐
Rh sensitization ........................ 15 ☐
Uterine bleeding ........................ 16 ☐
None .................................. 00 ☐
Other _____ 17 ☐
 (Specify)

**23b. OTHER RISK FACTORS FOR THIS PREGNANCY** (Complete all items)

Tobacco use during pregnancy ......... Yes ☐ No ☐
 Average number cigarettes per day ____
Alcohol use during pregnancy .......... Yes ☐ No ☐
 Average number drinks per week ____
Weight gained during pregnancy ____ lbs.

**24. OBSTETRIC PROCEDURES** (Check all that apply)

Amniocentesis ......................... 01 ☐
Electronic fetal monitoring .................. 02 ☐
Induction of labor ....................... 03 ☐
Stimulation of labor ..................... 04 ☐
Tocolysis .............................. 05 ☐
Ultrasound ............................. 06 ☐
None .................................. 00 ☐
Other _____ 07 ☐
 (Specify)

**25. COMPLICATIONS OF LABOR AND/OR DELIVERY** (Check all that apply)

Febrile (> 100°F. or 38°C.) .................. 01 ☐
Meconium, moderate/heavy ............... 02 ☐
Premature rupture of membrane (> 12 hours) .... 03 ☐
Abruptio placenta ....................... 04 ☐
Placenta privia ......................... 05 ☐
Other excessive bleeding .................. 06 ☐
Seizures during labor .................... 07 ☐
Precipitous labor (< 3 hours) .............. 08 ☐
Prolonged labor (> 20 hours) ............. 09 ☐
Dysfunctional labor ..................... 10 ☐
Breech/Malpresentation .................. 11 ☐
Cephalopelvic disproportion .............. 12 ☐
Cord prolapse ......................... 13 ☐
Anesthetic complications ................. 14 ☐
Fetal distress .......................... 15 ☐
None .................................. 00 ☐
Other _____ 16 ☐
 (Specify)

**26. METHOD OF DELIVERY** (Check all that apply)

Vaginal ............................... 01 ☐
Vaginal birth after previous C-section ..........02 ☐
Primary C-section ....................... 03 ☐
Repeat C-section ....................... 04 ☐
Forceps ............................... 05 ☐
Vacuum ............................... 06 ☐
Hysterotomy/Hysterectomy ............... 07 ☐

**27. CONGENITAL ANOMALIES OF FETUS** (Check all that apply)

Anencephalus .......................... 01 ☐
Spina bifida/Meningocele ................. 02 ☐
Hydrocephalus ......................... 03 ☐
Microcephalus ......................... 04 ☐
Other central nervous system anomalies
 (Specify) _____ 05 ☐

Heart malformations ..................... 06 ☐
Other circulatory/respiratory anomalies
 (Specify) _____ 07 ☐

Rectal atresia/stenosis ................... 08 ☐
Tracheo-esophageal fistula/Esophageal atresia .. 09 ☐
Omphalocele/Gastroschisis ............... 10 ☐
Other gastrointestinal anomalies
 (Specify) _____ 11 ☐

Malformed genitalia ..................... 12 ☐
Renal agenesis ......................... 13 ☐
Other urogenital anomalies
 (Specify) _____ 14 ☐

Cleft lip/palate ......................... 15 ☐
Polydactyly/Syndactyly/Adactyly .............. 16 ☐
Club foot .............................. 17 ☐
Diaphragmatic hernia .................... 18 ☐
Other musculoskeletal/integumental anomalies
 (Specify) _____ 19 ☐

Down's syndrome ....................... 20 ☐
Other chromosomal anomalies
 (Specify) _____ 21 ☐

None .................................. 00 ☐
Other _____ 22 ☐
 (Specify)

**CAUSE OF FETAL DEATH**

28.

**PART I.** Fetal or maternal condition directly causing fetal death.

Enter only one cause per line for a, b, and c.

IMMEDIATE CAUSE
a. _____ Specify Fetal or Maternal

Fetal and/or maternal conditions, if any, giving rise to the immediate cause(s), stating the underlying cause lost.

DUE TO (OR AS A CONSEQUENCE OF):
b. _____ Specify Fetal or Maternal

DUE TO (OR AS A CONSEQUENCE OF):
c. _____ Specify Fetal or Maternal

**PART II.** Other significant conditions of fetus or mother contributing to fetal death but not resulting in the underlying cause given in Part I.

_____

_____

29. FETUS DIED BEFORE LABOR DURING LABOR OR DELIVERY, UNKNOWN (Specify)

| 30. ATTENDANT'S NAME AND TITLE (Type/Print) | 31. NAME AND TITLE OF PERSON COMPLETING REPORT (Type/Print) |
|---|---|
| Name _____ | |
| | Name _____ |
| ☐ M.D.  ☐ D.O.  ☐ C.N.M.  ☐ Other Midwife | |
| ☐ Other (Specify) _____ | Title _____ |

PHS-T-007

DEPARTMENT OF HEALTH AND HUMAN SERVICES • PUBLIC HEALTH SERVICE • NATIONAL CENTER FOR HEALTH STATISTICS • 1989 REVISION

# Appendix B

# Electronic Documentation

## Sample Electronic Health Record

The following screenshots are examples of data collection within the electronic health record using the web-based program SimChart for the Medical Office.

- Patient demographic data, p. 459
- Patient financial data, p. 460
- Patient socioeconomic data, p. 461
- Allergy list, p. 461
- Health history, Medical, p. 462
- Health history, Social, p. 463

- Immunization record, p. 464
- Medication list, p. 465
- Vital signs, p. 465
- Progress notes in SOAP format, p. 466
- Computerized physician order entry (CPOE), p. 467
- Office visit summary, p. 468

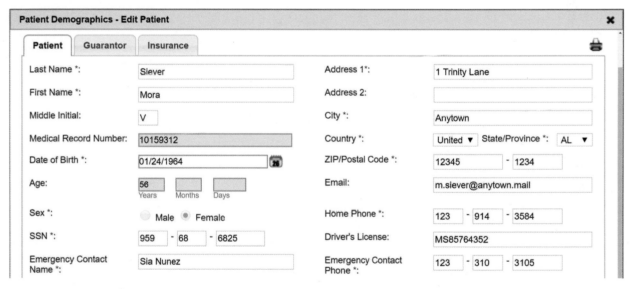

Patient demographic data. (Courtesy SimChart for the Medical Office, Elsevier, Inc., 2022.)

Fields with * are required to complete the patient registration

| Patient | Guarantor | Insurance |

**PRIMARY INSURANCE**

<u>Primary Insurance Card</u>

Primary Insurance *: Aetna

Claims Address 1 *: 1234 Insurance Way

Name of Policy Holder *: Mora Siever

Claims Address 2:

SSN of Policy Holder *: 959 - 68 - 6825

City *: Anytown

Policy/ID Number *: MS3379480

Country *: United ▾   State/Province *: AL ▾

Group Number: 38870S

ZIP/Postal Code *: 12345 - 1234

Claims Phone *: 180 - 012 - 3222

**SECONDARY INSURANCE**

<u>Upload Insurance Card</u>

Insurance: Select or Type New

Claims Address 1:

Name of Policy Holder:

Claims Address 2:

SSN of Policy Holder:   -   -

City:

Policy/ID Number:

Country: -Selec ▾   State/Province: -Sel ▾

Group Number:

ZIP/Postal Code:   -

Claims Phone:   -   -

**DENTAL INSURANCE**

<u>Upload Insurance Card</u>

Insurance: Aetna PPO (Dental)

Claims Address 1: 1234 Insurance Way

Name of Policy Holder: Mora Siever

Claims Address 2:

SSN of Policy Holder: 959 - 68 - 6825

City: Anytown

Policy/ID Number: 0000000151517

Country: United ▾   State/Province: AL ▾

Group Number: 65467

ZIP/Postal Code: 12345 - 1234

Claims Phone: 800 - 123 - 3434

**WORKERS' COMPENSATION**

Insurance: Peerless Insurance Company

Claims Address 1: 175 Berkeley Street

Employer: Quality Masonry Products

Claims Address 2:

Contact: Steven Rhodes

City: Boston

Policy / ID Number: 54448564

Country: United ▾   State/Province: MA ▾

Claims Phone: 800 - 262 - 8238

ZIP/Postal Code: 02116 - 1111

Patient financial data. (Courtesy SimChart for the Medical Office, Elsevier, Inc., 2022.)

Patient Status:       ☑ Single  ☐ Married  ☐ Other
                      ☐ Employed  ☐ Full-Time Student
                      ☑ Part-Time Student

Employer Name:   Quality Masonry Products

School Name:     Alabama Polytechnic

Language:    Spanish

Race:        African American

Ethnicity:   Hispanic

Image Upload:   Upload

View Large

Patient socioeconomic data. (Courtesy SimChart for the Medical Office, Elsevier, Inc., 2022.)

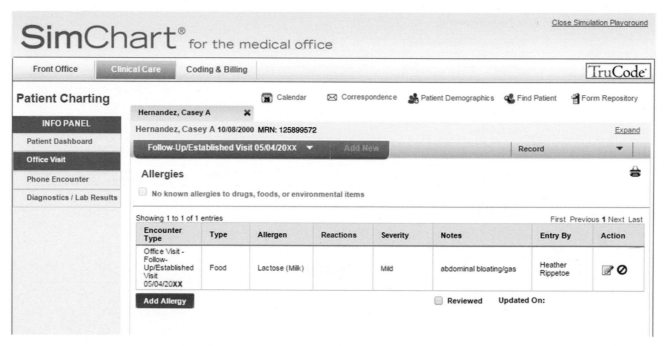

Allergy list. (Courtesy SimChart for the Medical Office, Elsevier, Inc., 2022.)

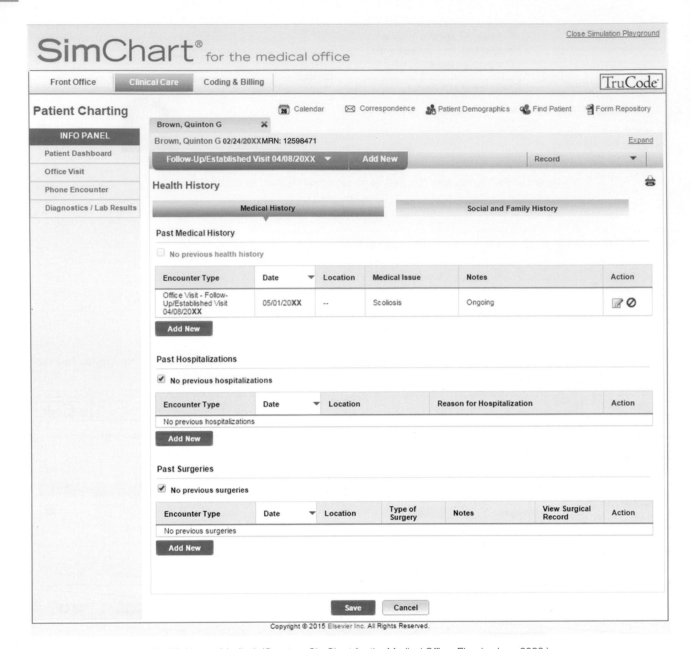

Health history, Medical. (Courtesy SimChart for the Medical Office, Elsevier, Inc., 2022.)

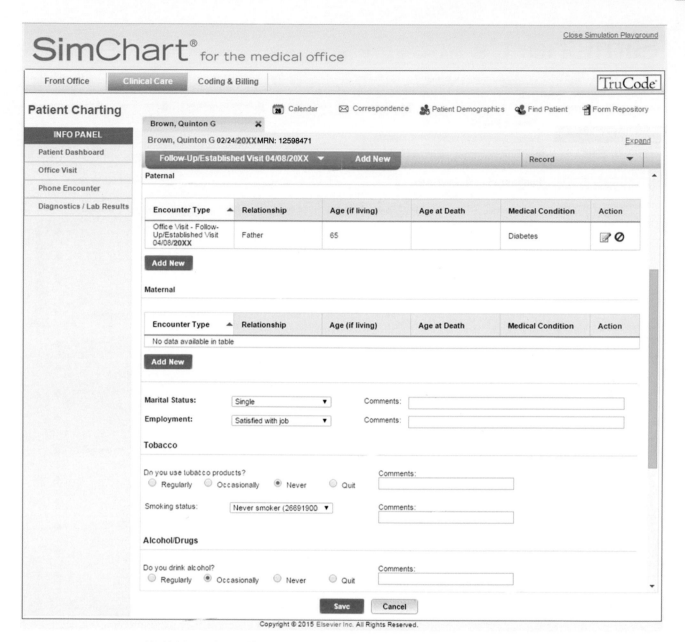

Health history, Social. (Courtesy SimChart for the Medical Office, Elsevier, Inc., 2022.)

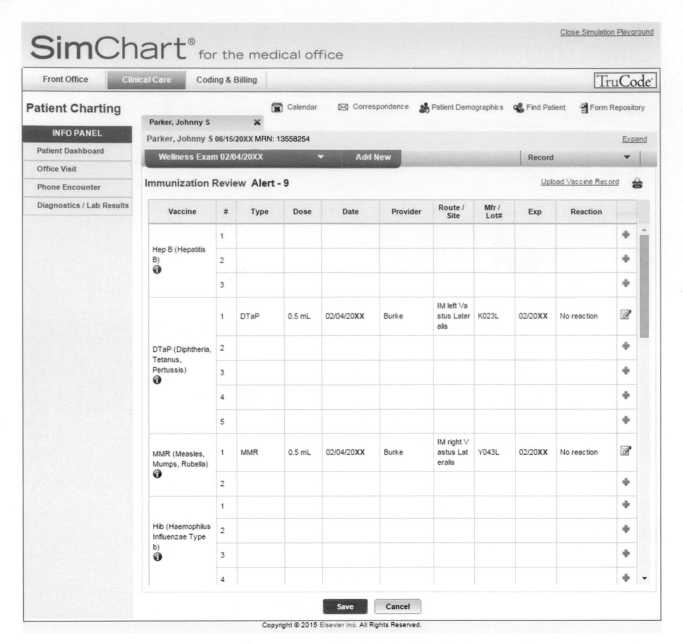

Immunization record. (Courtesy SimChart for the Medical Office, Elsevier, Inc., 2022.)

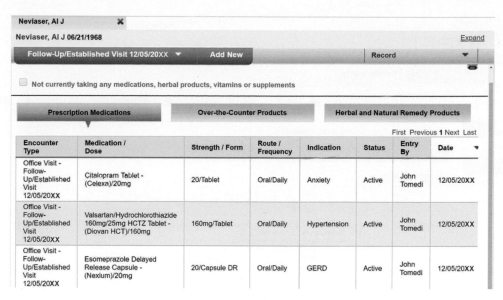

Medication list. (Courtesy SimChart for the Medical Office, Elsevier, Inc., 2022.)

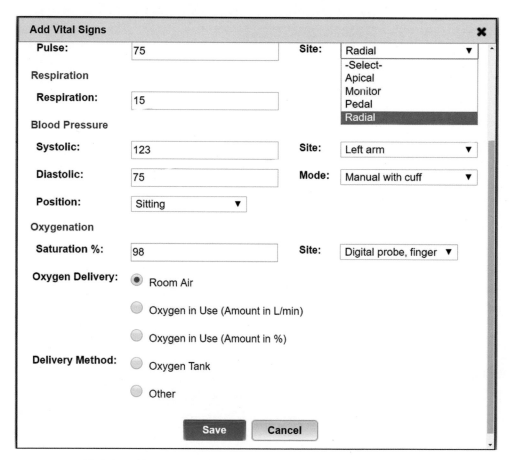

Vital signs. (Courtesy SimChart for the Medical Office, Elsevier, Inc., 2022.)

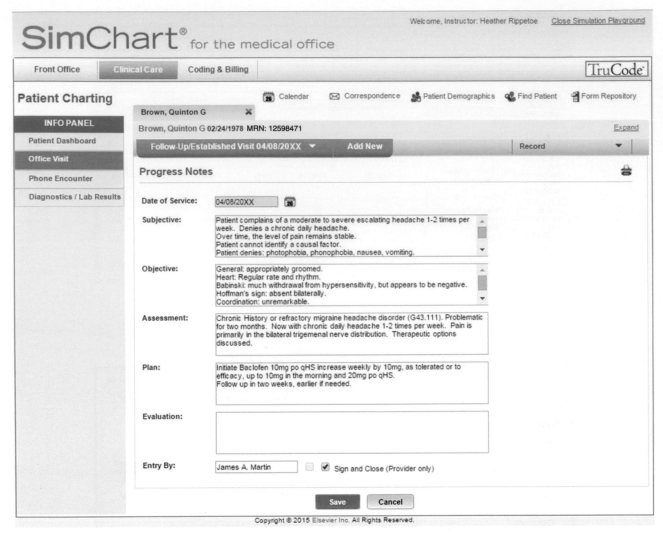

Progress notes in SOAP (subjective, objective, assessment, and plan) format. (Courtesy SimChart for the Medical Office, Elsevier, Inc., 2022.)

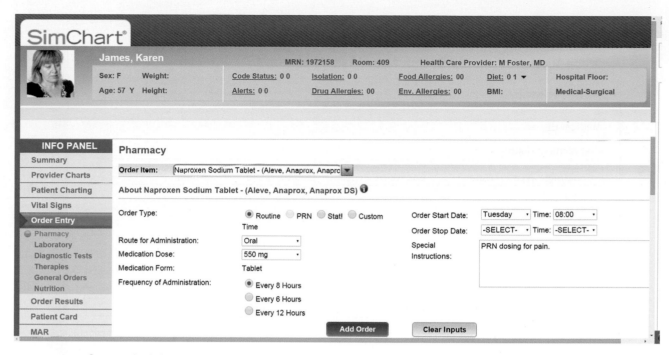

Computerized physician order entry (CPOE). (Courtesy SimChart for the Medical Office, Elsevier, Inc., 2022.)

**Brown, Quinton G**
**MRN: 12598471**
**Office Visit - Follow-Up/Established Visit 04/08/20XX**

## Health History

### Medical History

**Past Medical History**

| Encounter Type | Date | Location | Medical Issue | Notes |
|---|---|---|---|---|
| Office Visit - Follow-Up/Established Visit 04/08/20XX | 05/01/20XX | -- | Scoliosis | Ongoing |

**Past Hospitalizations**

**No previous hospitalizations**

| Encounter Type | Date | Location | Reason for Hospitalization |
|---|---|---|---|
| No previous hospitalizations | | | |

**Past Surgeries**

**No previous surgeries**

| Encounter Type | Date | Location | Type of Surgery | Notes | View Surgical Record |
|---|---|---|---|---|---|
| No previous surgeries | | | | | |

### Social and Family History

**Paternal**

| Encounter Type | Relationship | Age (if living) | Age at Death | Medical Condition |
|---|---|---|---|---|
| Office Visit - Follow-Up/Established Visit 04/08/20XX | Father | 65 | | Diabetes |

**Maternal**

| Encounter Type | Relationship | Age (if living) | Age at Death | Medical Condition |
|---|---|---|---|---|
| No Data Saved | | | | |

| | | | |
|---|---|---|---|
| **Marital Status:** | Single | **Comments:** | -- |
| **Employment:** | Satisfied with job | **Comments:** | -- |

**Tobacco**

| | | | |
|---|---|---|---|
| **Do you use tobacco products?** | Never | **Comments:** | -- |
| **Smoking status:** | Never smoker (266919005) | **Comments:** | -- |

Office visit summary. (Courtesy SimChart for the Medical Office, Elsevier, Inc., 2022.)

# Appendix C

# Using Microsoft Excel to Perform Calculations

When we are working with a small number of items or a simple, two-figure calculation, using a calculator is probably the easiest way to complete the computations. However, when we have a large number of figures or if we are going to be performing the same computation multiple times, it is very useful to know how to use Microsoft Excel to help with the computations.

In this appendix, we will explain some common calculations, the purpose of the computations, and how to complete those calculations in Microsoft Excel.

- First Quarter Discharges, p. 470
- Health Information Department Staffing, p. 471
- Full-time Equivalent Staff, p. 471
- Patient Census 12/15/20XX, p. 472
- Cafeteria Survey, p. 472
- Length of Stay, p. 473–475

| | A | B | C | D | E | F |
|---|---|---|---|---|---|---|
| 1 | Community Hospital | | | | | |
| 2 | First Quarter Discharges | | | | | |
| 3 | | | | | | |
| 4 | | 19,021 | *January* | | | |
| 5 | | 18,945 | *February* | | | |
| 6 | | 21,439 | *March* | | | |
| 7 | | 59,405 | *Total First Quarter Discharges* | | | |
| 8 | | | | | | |
| 9 | The formula to obtain the total of 59,405 is: =SUM(B4:B6) | | | | | |
| 10 | This yields the same result as: =B4+B5+B6 | | | | | |
| 11 | | | | | | |
| 12 | A quarter is 1/4 of a year (3 months) | | | | | |
| 13 | A fiscal year is the organization's tax year (a business cycle) | | | | | |
| 14 | | | | | | |
| 15 | In this example, we might want to calculate the discharges, | | | | | |
| 16 | by quarter, for the entire year: | | | | | |
| 17 | | | | | | |
| 18 | On the right are the data entry and the formulas. On the left are the results. | | | | | |
| 19 | | | | | | |
| 20 | As you are preparing your worksheet, you can reveal the formulas by | | | | | |
| 21 | pressing Ctrl` (The Control key and the accent grave, located to the left of | | | | | |
| 22 | the number 1 on your keyboard.) | | | | | |
| 23 | | | | | | |
| 24 | Community Hospital | | | | | |
| 25 | 20XX Discharges | | | | | |
| 26 | | | | | | |
| 27 | | 19,021 | *January* | | | 19,021 |
| 28 | | 18,945 | *February* | | | 18,945 |
| 29 | | 21,439 | *March* | | | 21,439 |
| 30 | | 59,405 | *Total First Quarter Discharges* | | | =SUM(A27:A29) |
| 31 | | | | | | |
| 32 | | 18,435 | *April* | | | 18,435 |
| 33 | | 18,854 | *May* | | | 18,854 |
| 34 | | 19,146 | *June* | | | 19,146 |
| 35 | | 56,435 | *Total Second Quarter Discharges* | | | =SUM(A32:A34) |
| 36 | | | | | | |
| 37 | | 20,564 | *July* | | | 20,564 |
| 38 | | 20,437 | *August* | | | 20,437 |
| 39 | | 19,111 | *September* | | | 19,111 |
| 40 | | 60,112 | *Total Third Quarter Discharges* | | | =SUM(A37:A39) |
| 41 | | | | | | |
| 42 | | 19,021 | *October* | | | 19,021 |
| 43 | | 18,945 | *November* | | | 18,945 |
| 44 | | 21,439 | *December* | | | 21,439 |
| 45 | | 59,405 | *Total Fourth Quarter Discharges* | | | =SUM(A42:A44) |
| 46 | | | | | | |
| 47 | | 235,357 | *Total Discharges for the Year* | | | =A30+A35+A40+A45 |

| ⊿ | A | B | C | D | E | F | G | H |
|---|---|---|---|---|---|---|---|---|
| 1 | **Community Hospital** | | | | | | | |
| 2 | **Health Information Department Staffing** | | | | | | | |
| 3 | | | | | | | | |
| 4 | | 75 | Total Staff | | In this calculation, we enter the total staff into | | | |
| 5 | | 6 | Part-time Staff | | cell B4 and the number of part-time staff in | | | |
| 6 | | 69 | Full-time Staff | | cell B5. To determine the number of full-time | | | |
| 7 | Formula is: | =B4−B5 | | | staff, we enter the subtraction calculation into | | | |
| 8 | | | | | cell B6. The actual formula is noted below. | | | |
| 9 | | | | | | | | |
| 10 | | | | | | | | |
| 11 | If you are having problems understanding this calculation, you may not be using the | | | | | | | |
| 12 | correct sequence of instructions, because your calculator may require a different | | | | | | | |
| 13 | sequence of entries. Some calculators want you to enter the operation BEFORE | | | | | | | |
| 14 | the number. Other calculators want you to enter the operation AFTER the number. | | | | | | | |

| ⊿ | A | B | C | D | E | F | G | H | I |
|---|---|---|---|---|---|---|---|---|---|
| 1 | **Community Hospital** | | | | | | | | |
| 2 | **Full-time Equivalent Staff** | | | | | | | | |
| 3 | | | | | | | | | |
| 4 | | | | | | | | | |
| 5 | | Number | Hours | Total | | | | | |
| 6 | Part-time | 6 | 20 | 120 | =B6*C6 | | | | |
| 7 | Full-time | 69 | 40 | 2760 | =B7*C7 | | | | |
| 8 | | | | | | | | | |
| 9 | Total Hours Worked | | | 2880 | =SUM(D6:D7) | | | | |
| 10 | Normal Work Hours | | | 40 | | | | | |
| 11 | Full-time Equivalents | | | 72 | =D9/D10 | | | | |
| 12 | | | | | | | | | |
| 13 | FTE = Full-time Equivalents | | | | | | | | |
| 14 | FTEs = Total number of hours worked per week, divided by number of normal work hours | | | | | | | | |
| 15 | | | | | | | | | |
| 16 | In this example, we calculated the total hours worked by the part-time employees and | | | | | | | | |
| 17 | the total hours worked by the full-time employees. We then divided the total number | | | | | | | | |
| 18 | of hours worked by all employees by the number of hours in the normal work week. This | | | | | | | | |
| 19 | calculation of Full-time Equivalents provides management with a number of employees | | | | | | | | |
| 20 | that can be compared to other departments and evaluated based on other volume | | | | | | | | |
| 21 | measurements, such as the number of discharges. | | | | | | | | |

| ◢ | A | B | C | D | E | F | G |
|---|---|---|---|---|---|---|---|
| 1 | | | **Community Hospital** | | | | |
| 2 | | | **Patient Census 12/15/20XX** | | | | |
| 3 | | | | | | | |
| 4 | | 175 | *Patients 12/14/20XX* | | In this example, we have a series of | | |
| 5 | + | 3 | *Births* | | calculations in which the values in | | |
| 6 | − | 8 | *Deaths* | | some rows are added and others are | | |
| 7 | + | 11 | *Admitted* | | subtracted. The formula used in cell | | |
| 8 | − | 9 | *Discharged* | | B9 is illustrated below. | | |
| 9 | | 172 | *Patients 12/15/20XX* | | =B4+B5−B6+B7−B8 | | |
| 10 | | | | | | | |
| 11 | Be careful with the sequence of instructions in the formula. In this sequence, the instruction to add or subtract goes BEFORE the number to be operated on. | | | | | | |
| 12 | | | | | | | |

| ◢ | A | B | C | D | E | F | G |
|---|---|---|---|---|---|---|---|
| 1 | | **Community Hospital Cafeteria Survey** | | | | | |
| 2 | | | | | | | |
| 3 | | Total Patients Responding | Liked Food | Percent Who Liked Food | | | |
| 4 | | | | | | | |
| 5 | *2022* | 500 | 394 | 79% | =C5/B5 | | |
| 6 | *2023* | 2,000 | 1,645 | 82% | =C6/B6 | | |
| 7 | *Hospital B* | 20,011 | 15,492 | 77% | =C7/B7 | | |
| 8 | | | | | | | |
| 9 | | | | | | | |
| 10 | Percentages are useful in comparing results between different years or groups. In this example, Community Hospital is comparing its cafeteria satisfaction between 2022 and 2023. It is also comparing its cafeteria satisfaction with a survey taken at another hospital (Hospital B). Because the satisfaction is expressed as a percentage, we can easily see that Community Hospital's satisfaction results are improving and that they are superior to Hospital B. | | | | | | |
| 11 | | | | | | | |
| 12 | | | | | | | |
| 13 | | | | | | | |
| 14 | | | | | | | |
| 15 | | | | | | | |
| 16 | | | | | | | |
| 17 | Notice that the formula yields a decimal, not a percentage. In order to display the results as a percentage, the cell must be formatted to recognize the number as a percentage. To format the cell, click on the following series of options from the main menu at the top of the screen (Or click on the % icon on the home page, if available.) | | | | | | |
| 18 | | | | | | | |
| 19 | | | | | | | |
| 20 | | | | | | | |
| 21 | | **Format** | | | | | |
| 22 | | **Cell** | | | | | |
| 23 | | **Number** | | | | | |
| 24 | | **Percentage** | | | | | |
| 25 | Another way to obtain the percentage (without the % sign) is to multiply the decimal times 100; e.g. =C5/B5*100. | | | | | | |
| 26 | | | | | | | |

| | A | B | C | D | E | F | G | H | I | J | K | L | M | N | O | P | Q |
|---|---|---|---|---|---|---|---|---|---|---|---|---|---|---|---|---|---|
| 1 | | | | | **Community Hospital** | | | | | | | | | | | | |
| 2 | | | | | **Length of Stay** | | | | | | | | | | | | |
| 3 | | | | | | | | | | | | | | | | | |
| 4 | 1 | 2 | 3 | 3 | 3 | 4 | 4 | 5 | 5 | 6 | | | | | | | |
| 5 | 1 | 2 | 3 | 3 | 3 | 4 | 4 | 5 | 5 | 6 | | | | | | | |
| 6 | 1 | 2 | 3 | 3 | 4 | 4 | 4 | 5 | 5 | 6 | | | | | | | |
| 7 | 1 | 2 | 3 | 3 | 4 | 4 | 4 | 5 | 5 | 6 | | In this example, there is a large amount of data, but we can still | | | | | |
| 8 | 1 | 2 | 3 | 3 | 4 | 4 | 4 | 5 | 5 | 6 | | use our formulas to compute the answers to the following | | | | | |
| 9 | 1 | 2 | 3 | 3 | 4 | 4 | 4 | 5 | 5 | 6 | | questions. Under each question is the formula that yields the | | | | | |
| 10 | 1 | 2 | 3 | 3 | 4 | 4 | 4 | 5 | 5 | 6 | | numerical answer shown next to the question. | | | | | |
| 11 | 1 | 2 | 3 | 3 | 4 | 4 | 4 | 5 | 5 | 6 | | *How many patients?* | | 250 | | | |
| 12 | 1 | 2 | 3 | 3 | 4 | 4 | 4 | 5 | 5 | 6 | | =COUNT(A4:J28) | | | | | |
| 13 | 1 | 2 | 3 | 3 | 4 | 4 | 4 | 5 | 5 | 7 | | *What is the average length of stay?* | | | | 3.864 days | |
| 14 | 1 | 2 | 3 | 3 | 4 | 4 | 4 | 5 | 5 | 7 | | =AVERAGE(A4:J28) | | | | | |
| 15 | 1 | 2 | 3 | 3 | 4 | 4 | 4 | 5 | 5 | 7 | | This is the mean, which could | | | | | |
| 16 | 1 | 2 | 3 | 3 | 4 | 4 | 4 | 5 | 5 | 7 | | also be calculated as | | | | | |
| 17 | 1 | 2 | 3 | 3 | 4 | 4 | 4 | 5 | 5 | 7 | | =SUM(A4:J28)/250 | | | | | |
| 18 | 1 | 2 | 3 | 3 | 4 | 4 | 4 | 5 | 5 | 7 | | | | | | | |
| 19 | 1 | 2 | 3 | 3 | 4 | 4 | 4 | 5 | 5 | 7 | | *What is the median length of stay?* | | | | 4 days | |
| 20 | 1 | 2 | 3 | 3 | 4 | 4 | 4 | 5 | 5 | 7 | | =MEDIAN(A4:J28) | | | | | |
| 21 | 1 | 2 | 3 | 3 | 4 | 4 | 5 | 5 | 5 | 7 | | | | | | | |
| 22 | 1 | 2 | 3 | 3 | 4 | 4 | 5 | 5 | 5 | 7 | | *What is the mode?* | | | | 4 days | |
| 23 | 1 | 2 | 3 | 3 | 4 | 4 | 5 | 5 | 6 | 8 | | =MODE(A4:J28) | | | | | |
| 24 | 1 | 3 | 3 | 3 | 4 | 4 | 5 | 5 | 6 | 8 | | | | | | | |
| 25 | 1 | 3 | 3 | 3 | 4 | 4 | 5 | 5 | 6 | 8 | | | | | | | |
| 26 | 1 | 3 | 3 | 3 | 4 | 4 | 5 | 5 | 6 | 8 | | | | | | | |
| 27 | 1 | 3 | 3 | 3 | 4 | 4 | 5 | 5 | 6 | 9 | | | | | | | |
| 28 | 1 | 3 | 3 | 3 | 4 | 4 | 5 | 5 | 6 | 9 | | | | | | | |

**Community Hospital**
**Length of Stay**

| | A | B | C | D | E | F | G | H | I | J |
|---|---|---|---|---|---|---|---|---|---|---|
| 5 | 1 | 2 | 3 | 3 | 3 | 4 | 4 | 5 | 5 | 6 |
| 6 | 1 | 2 | 3 | 3 | 3 | 4 | 4 | 5 | 5 | 6 |
| 7 | 1 | 2 | 3 | 3 | 4 | 4 | 4 | 5 | 5 | 6 |
| 8 | 1 | 2 | 3 | 3 | 4 | 4 | 4 | 5 | 5 | 6 |
| 9 | 1 | 2 | 3 | 3 | 4 | 4 | 4 | 5 | 5 | 6 |
| 10 | 1 | 2 | 3 | 3 | 4 | 4 | 4 | 5 | 5 | 6 |
| 11 | 1 | 2 | 3 | 3 | 4 | 4 | 4 | 5 | 5 | 6 |
| 12 | 1 | 2 | 3 | 3 | 4 | 4 | 4 | 5 | 5 | 6 |
| 13 | 1 | 2 | 3 | 3 | 4 | 4 | 4 | 5 | 5 | 6 |
| 14 | 1 | 2 | 3 | 3 | 4 | 4 | 4 | 5 | 5 | 7 |
| 15 | 1 | 2 | 3 | 3 | 4 | 4 | 4 | 5 | 5 | 7 |
| 16 | 1 | 2 | 3 | 3 | 4 | 4 | 4 | 5 | 5 | 7 |
| 17 | 1 | 2 | 3 | 3 | 4 | 4 | 4 | 5 | 5 | 7 |
| 18 | 1 | 2 | 3 | 3 | 4 | 4 | 4 | 5 | 5 | 7 |
| 19 | 1 | 2 | 3 | 3 | 4 | 4 | 4 | 5 | 5 | 7 |
| 20 | 1 | 2 | 3 | 3 | 4 | 4 | 4 | 5 | 5 | 7 |
| 21 | 1 | 2 | 3 | 3 | 4 | 4 | 4 | 5 | 5 | 7 |
| 22 | 1 | 2 | 3 | 3 | 4 | 4 | 5 | 5 | 5 | 7 |
| 23 | 1 | 2 | 3 | 3 | 4 | 4 | 5 | 5 | 5 | 7 |
| 24 | 1 | 2 | 3 | 3 | 4 | 4 | 5 | 5 | 6 | 8 |
| 25 | 1 | 3 | 3 | 3 | 4 | 4 | 5 | 5 | 6 | 8 |
| 26 | 1 | 3 | 3 | 3 | 4 | 4 | 5 | 5 | 6 | 8 |
| 27 | 1 | 3 | 3 | 3 | 4 | 4 | 5 | 5 | 6 | 8 |
| 28 | 1 | 3 | 3 | 3 | 4 | 4 | 5 | 5 | 6 | 9 |
| 29 | 1 | 3 | 3 | 3 | 4 | 4 | 5 | 5 | 6 | 9 |

Frequency distribution

EXCEL will calculate the frequency distribution of a data set. It sorts the data into class intervals that we describe. In this example, we will use the individual lengths of stay as our target, which EXCEL calls "BINS."

**BINS (L9–L18)**

| BINS |
|------|
| 1 |
| 2 |
| 3 |
| 4 |
| 5 |
| 6 |
| 7 |
| 8 |
| 9 |

*Step 1: List the BINS in order.
(THIS BINS ARRAY IS LOCATED IN CELLS L10 THROUGH L18.)*

**BINS (L21 area)**

| BINS | |
|------|---|
| 1 | =FREQUENCY(A5:J29,L10:L18) |
| 2 | |
| 3 | |
| 4 | |
| 5 | |
| 6 | |
| 7 | |
| 8 | |
| 9 | |

*Step 2: Enter the formula.
Specify the range for the data; press Enter.
Specify the range for the BINS.*

**BINS**

| BINS | |
|------|---|
| 1 | =FREQUENCY(A5:J29,L10:L18) |
| 2 | |
| 3 | |
| 4 | |
| 5 | |
| 6 | |
| 7 | |
| 8 | |
| 9 | |

*Step 3: Click and drag to highlight the entire area in which you wish to display the results, including your formula cell and one extra cell at the bottom to catch any values that don't match the bin values.*

**BINS**

| BINS | |
|------|-----|
| 1 | 25 |
| 2 | 20 |
| 3 | 57 |
| 4 | 65 |
| 5 | 52 |
| 6 | 15 |
| 7 | 10 |
| 8 | 4 |
| 9 | 2 |

*Step 4: Press F2. Then, press and hold:
Ctrl   Shift   Enter*

*The frequencies of each BIN will appear next to the BIN they represent. These frequencies can then be used to prepare informative tables and graphs.*

|   | A | B | C | D | E | F |
|---|---|---|---|---|---|---|
| 1 | | | | | | |
| 2 | | Community Hospital | | | | |
| 3 | | Length of Stay | | | | |
| 4 | | | | | | |
| 5 | | *Frequencies:* | | *Percentage:* | | |
| 6 | | 1 | 25 | 10% | =C6/$C$15 | |
| 7 | | 2 | 20 | 8% | =C7/$C$15 | |
| 8 | | 3 | 57 | 23% | =C8/$C$15 | |
| 9 | | 4 | 65 | 26% | =C9/$C$15 | |
| 10 | | 5 | 52 | 21% | =C10/$C$15 | |
| 11 | | 6 | 15 | 6% | =C11/$C$15 | |
| 12 | | 7 | 10 | 4% | =C12/$C$15 | |
| 13 | | 8 | 4 | 2% | =C13/$C$15 | |
| 14 | | 9 | 2 | 1% | =C14/$C$15 | |
| 15 | | *Total* | 250 | | | |
| 16 | | | =SUM(C6:C14) | | | |

In this example, we calculate the percentage of patients with each length of stay. The percentage is the frequency of patients for each length of stay, divided by the total number of patients to get the decimal. To complete the operation and get the percentage, we formatted the percentage column to show the percentage rather than the decimal. If you don't want to format, then you need to multiply the decimal times 100, for example: =(C6/$C$15)*100. Notice that we anchored the total in the percentage formula by placing a dollar sign in front of each element of the cell.

The graph below is a "Scatter" graph with a line connecting the dots. It represents the data fields **B6:B14, C6:C14.**

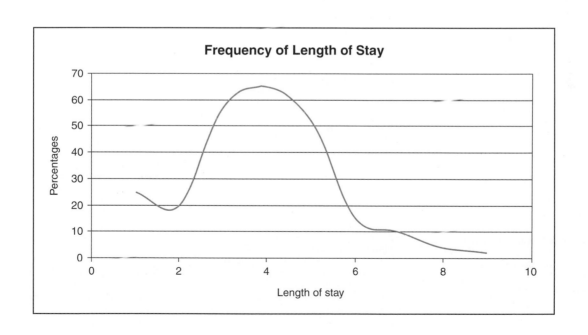

Frequency of Length of Stay

# Glossary

**abstract**   A summary of the patient health record.

**abstracting**   The recap of selected fields from a health record to create an informative summary. Also refers to the activity of identifying such fields and entering them into a computer system.

**access**   The ability to learn the contents of a record by obtaining it or having the contents revealed.

**accessibility**   In data quality, the characteristic that data can be obtained when needed by authorized individuals.

**accounting of disclosures**   The listing of the identity of those to which certain protected health information has been disclosed.

**accreditation**   Voluntary compliance with a set of standards developed by an independent agent, who periodically performs audits to ensure compliance.

**accrual basis**   An accounting method in which income and expenses are recorded when they are incurred, regardless of when the money is actually exchanged.

**accuracy**   The characteristic that data are correct.

**activities of daily living (ADLs)**   Refer to self-care, such as bathing, as well as cooking, shopping, and other routines requiring thought, planning, and physical motion.

**acute care facility**   A health care facility in which patients have an average length of stay of less than 30 days and that has an ED, operating suite, and clinical departments to handle a broad range of diagnoses and treatments.

**Administrative data**   Data assigned by a provider to facilitate the capture, storage, retention, and reporting of a patient's visit.

**admission**   The act of accepting a patient into care in a health care facility, including any nonambulatory care facility. Admission requires a physician's order.

**admission consent form**   A form signed by the patient in an inpatient facility granting permission to the hospital to provide general diagnostic and therapeutic care as well as to release patient information to a third-party payer, if applicable. Also known as a *general consent form*.

**admission denial**   Occurs when the payer or its designee (such as UR staff) will not reimburse the facility for treatment of the patient because the admission was deemed unnecessary.

**admission record**   The demographic, financial, socioeconomic, and clinical data collected about a patient at registration. Also refers to the document in a paper record that contains these data.

**admitting diagnosis**   The reason given by the physician for initiating the order for the patient to be placed into care in a hospital.

**admitting physician**   The physician who gives the order to observe or admit a patient.

**advance directive**   A written document, like a living will, that specifies a patient's wishes for his or her care and dictates power of attorney, for the purpose of providing clear instructions in the event the patient is unable to do so.

**affinity diagram**   A method of organizing ideas (e.g. from brainstorming) based on their relationships.

**against medical advice (AMA)**   The discharge disposition of a patient who chooses to leave the facility prior to clearance from the physician.

**agenda**   A tool used to organize the topics to be discussed during a meeting.

**aggregate data**   A group of like data elements compiled to provide information about the group.

**algorithm**   A procedure (set of instructions) for accomplishing a task.

**allied health professionals**   Health care professionals who support patient care in a variety of disciplines, including occupational therapy and physical therapy.

**ambulatory care**   Care provided on an outpatient basis, in which the patient is not admitted: arriving at a facility, receiving treatment, and leaving within 1 day.

**ambulatory care facility**   An outpatient facility, such as an ED or physician's office, in which treatment is intended to occur within 1 calendar day.

**ambulatory surgery**   Surgery performed on an outpatient basis; the patient returns home after the surgery is performed. Also called *same-day surgery*.

**amendment**   A change to the original document.

**American Health Information Management Association (AHIMA)**   The professional organization supporting the health care industry by promoting high-quality information standards through a variety of activities, including, but not limited to, continuing education, professional development and educational publications, and legislative and regulatory advocacy.

**American Medical Association (AMA)**   National professional organization involved in supporting all medical decision makers; the AMA also owns and maintains the Current Procedural Terminology (CPT) code set.

**American Psychiatric Association (APA)**   National professional organization involved in supporting licensed psychiatrists; maintains the DSM-5.

**American Recovery and Reinvestment Act (ARRA)**   Also called the "stimulus bill." 2009 federal legislation providing many stimulus opportunities in different areas. The portion of the law that finds and sets mandates for health information technology is called the HITECH Act.

**amortization**   The periodic writing off of the cost of an asset or paying off of a loan, often represented by a fixed schedule.

**anesthesia report**   An anesthesiologist's documentation of patient evaluations before, during, and after surgery, including the specifics of the administration of anesthesia.

**applied research**   Study done to solve an existing or anticipated problem.

**arithmetic mean**   The measure of central tendency that represents the arithmetic average of the observations.

**assault**   An intentional attempt to cause bodily harm to another.

**assessment**   An evaluation. In medical decision-making, the physician's evaluation of the subjective and objective evidence. Also refers to the evaluation of a patient by any clinical discipline.

**assisted living**   A type of LTC in which the resident is significantly independent in ADLs and does not need high levels of skilled nursing.

**attending physician**   The physician who is primarily responsible for coordinating the care of the patient in the hospital; it is usually the physician who ordered the patient's admission to the hospital.

**attribution**   The assignment to a case of a clinician and the clinician's relationship to the case.

**Audit Medicaid Integrity Contractor (Audit MIC)**   A contractor who works with CMS to identify fraud and waste through claims audits and other data collection activities.

**audit trail**   Software that tracks and stores information related to the activity of users in the system.

**authenticate**   To assume responsibility for data collection or the activities described by the data collection by signature, mark, code, password, or other means of identification.

**authentication**   To assume responsibility for data collection or the activities described by the data collection by signature, mark, code, password, or other means of identification.

**authorization**   A written direction by or on behalf of the patient to release the patient's information to a third party.

**average length of stay (ALOS)**   The arithmetic mean of the lengths of stay of a group of inpatients.

## B

**balance sheet**   A snapshot of the organization's financial status at a point in time.

**bar code**   The representation of data using parallel lines or other patterns in a way readable to a machine, such as an optical bar code scanner or a smartphone.

**bar graph** A chart that uses bars to represent the frequencies of items in the specified categories of a variable.

**basic research** Study done to answer a question just for the sake of obtaining an answer.

**batch control form** A listing of charts in process, postdischarge, that identifies which steps have been completed.

**batch scanning** The automated digitization of multiple documents.

**battery** An intentional act of contact with another that causes harm or offends the individual being touched or injured.

**BCSW** Board-certified social worker.

**bed control** The function of assigning beds in an acute care facility.

**bed count** The actual number of beds that a hospital has staffed, equipped, and otherwise made available for occupancy by patients for each specific operating day.

**behavioral health facility** An inpatient or outpatient health care facility that focuses on the treatment of psychiatric conditions.

**benchmarking** An improvement technique that compares one facility's process with that of another facility that has been noted to have superior performance.

**billing** The process of submitting health insurance claims or rendering invoices.

**blended rate** A weighted component of MS-DRG assignment that consists of the hospital-specific rate and additional factors such as regional labor costs and graduate medical education.

**brainstorming** A data-gathering performance improvement tool used to generate ideas and information on a topic, process, or problem.

**breach** An incident of unauthorized access to protected health information.

**business associates** Under HIPAA, a contracted vendor that uses confidential health information to perform a service on behalf of a covered entity.

**business record rule** An exception to the hearsay rule. Allows health records to be admitted as evidence in legal proceedings because they are kept in the normal course of business, are recorded concurrently with the events that they describe, and are recorded by individuals who are in a position to know the facts of the events that are described.

## C

**capital budget** Money set aside for larger purchases, usually over a certain dollar amount, the use of which will span multiple fiscal years.

**capitation** A uniform reimbursement to a health care provider based on the number of patients contractually in the physician's care, regardless of diagnoses or services rendered.

**case management** The coordination of the patient's care and services, including reimbursement considerations.

**case mix** Statistical distribution of patients according to their utilization of resources. Also refers to the grouping of patients by clinical department or other meaningful distribution, such as health insurance type.

**case mix index (CMI)** The arithmetic average (mean) of the relative DRG weights of all health care cases in a given period.

**cash basis accounting** A method of tracking finances in which transactions are recorded at the time currency is exchanged.

**cash flow** The balance of money in and money out of the department.

**census** The actual number of inpatients in a facility at a point in time, for comparative purposes, usually midnight.

**Centers for Medicare and Medicaid Services (CMS)** The division of the DHHS that administers Medicare and Medicaid.

**central limit theorem** The tendency of a large number of means to distribute symmetrically, approaching a normal distribution.

**certification** The custodian's authentication that the copies of medical records used in litigation are true and complete.

**chain of command** The formal authority and decision-making structure within an organization.

**character** A single letter, number, or symbol.

**charge** Fee for or cost of services rendered.

**charge capture** The systematic collection of specific charges for services rendered to a patient.

**Chargemaster** The database that contains the detailed description of charges related to all potential services rendered to a patient.

**chief complaint** The main reason a patient has sought treatment.

**claim** The application to an insurance company for reimbursement.

**class intervals** Groups, categories, or tiers of the highest and lowest values that are meaningful to the user.

**classification** Systematic organization of elements into categories. ICD-10-CM is a classification system that organizes diagnoses into categories, primarily by body system.

**clinic** A facility-based ambulatory care department that provides general or specialized services, such as those provided in a physician's office.

**clinical data** All of the medical data that have been recorded about the patient's stay or visit, including diagnoses and procedures.

**clinical decision-making system (CDS)** A computer application in the EHR that advises clinicians on the treatment of the patient.

**clinical outcome analysis** Clinical outcome analysis the study of the results of treatment or other management of a condition.

**clinical pathway** A predetermined standard of treatment for a particular disease, diagnosis, or procedure designed to facilitate the patient's progress through the health care encounter.

**code set** A standardized list of alphanumeric representations of diagnoses, procedures, data elements, and medical concepts used to communicate health care data.

**coding** The assignment of numeric or alphanumeric character values to a word, phrase, or other nonnumeric expression. In health care, coding is the assignment of numeric or alphanumeric character values to diagnosis and procedure descriptions.

**coding compliance plan** The development, implementation, and enforcement of policies and procedures to ensure that coding standards are met.

**cognitive definition** What the survey participant or other reader thinks is the meaning of a term.

**cognitive remediation** A type of therapy for judgment, reasoning, perception, or memory impairments.

**coinsurance** A cost-sharing reduction in which an individual is responsible for a percentage of the amount owed to the provider.

**Commission on Accreditation for Health Informatics and Information Management (CAHIIM)** The organization that accredits and sets quality and educational standards for HIM higher education programs.

**Commission on Accreditation of Rehabilitation Facilities (CARF)** An organization that accredits aging services, behavioral health, and rehabilitation facilities.

**Community Health Accreditation Program (CHAP)** An organization that accredits home health care agencies.

**competent** The quality of being able weigh alternatives and make reasonable decisions.

**completeness** The data quality of existence. If a required data element is missing, the record is not complete.

**compliance** Meeting standards. Also the development, implementation, and enforcement of policies and procedures, which ensure that standards are met.

**computerized physician order entry (CPOE)** A health information system in which physicians enter orders electronically. Includes decision support and alerts.

**concurrent analysis** Any type of record analysis performed during the patient's stay (i.e., after admission but before discharge).

**concurrent coding** Coding performed during the patient's stay (i.e., after admission but before discharge).

**concurrent review** Review occurring during the act or event (i.e., a chart review during the patient's stay in the facility).

**Conditions of Admission** The legal agreement between the health care facility and a patient (or the patient's legal agent) to perform routine services. May also include the statement of the patient's financial responsibility and prospective consent for release of information and examination and disposal of tissue.

**Conditions of Participation (COP)** The terms under which a facility is eligible to receive reimbursement from Medicare.

**confidential communication** The sharing of patient health information protected from disclosure in court, such as patient/physician. Also refers to transmission of information to minimize the risk of inadvertent disclosure, such as patient requesting mailing to an alternative address.

**confidentiality** Discretion regarding the disclosure of information.

**consent** An agreement or permission to receive health care services.

**consistency** In data quality, the characteristic that data are the same wherever they appear.

**consultant** A medical professional who provides clinical expertise in a specialty at the request of the attending physician.

**consultation** The formal request by a physician for the professional opinion or services of another health care professional, usually another physician, in caring for a patient. Also refers to the opinion or services themselves as well as the activity of rendering the opinion or services.

**continued stay denial** Similar to admission denial; however, it is the additional payment for the length of stay that is not approved rather than the entire admission.

**continuing education (CE)** Education required after a person has attained a position, credential, or degree, intended to keep the person knowledgeable in his or her profession.

**continuity of care** The coordination among caregivers to provide, efficiently and effectively, the broad range of health care services required by a patient during an illness or for an entire lifetime. May also refer to the coordination of care provided among caregivers/services within a health care organization.

**continuum of care**    The broad range of health care services required by a patient during an illness or for an entire lifetime. May also refer to the continuity of care provided by a health care organization.

**Cooperating Parties**    The four organizations responsible for maintaining the ICD-10-CM: CMS, NCHS, AHA, and AHIMA.

**copay**    A fixed amount paid by the patient at the time of service.

**corrective controls**    Procedures, processes, or structures that are designed to fix errors when they are detected. Because errors cannot always be fixed, corrective controls also include the initiation of an investigation into future error prevention or detection.

**correspondence**    Written communication between parties.

**countersignature**    Evidence of supervision of subordinate personnel, such as physician residents.

**countersigned**    Evidence of supervision of subordinate personnel, such as physician residents.

**court order**    The direction of a judge who has made a decision that an order to produce information (on the record) is necessary.

**covered entity**    Under HIPAA and HITECH provisions, any organization that collects and manages health information.

**credentials**    An individual's specific professional qualifications. Also refers to the letters that a professionally qualified person is entitled to list after his or her name.

**cross-training**    Training of employees for additional jobs or functions within the department so that they can help with those jobs when necessary.

**cultural competence**    The ability to work with others and deliver care to patients in a way that meets their needs: culture, language, and customs.

**Current Procedural Terminology (CPT)**    A nomenclature and coding system developed and maintained by the American Medical Association (AMA) to facilitate billing for physicians and other services.

**custodian**    The person entrusted with the responsibility for the confidentiality, privacy, and security of medical records.

## D

**data**    The smallest elements or units of facts or observations. Also refers to a collection of such elements.

**data analytics**    The process of analyzing and exploring data to create information.

**data collection device**    Paper form or computer data entry screen designed to capture data elements in a standardized format or the physical computer hardware/software that facilitates the data collection process.

**data dictionary**    A list of details that describe each field in a database.

**Data Elements for Emergency Department Systems (DEEDS)**    Minimum data set for emergency services.

**data entry**    The process of recording elements into a collection device.

**data repository**    Where data are stored from different, unrelated software programs.

**data set**    A group of data elements collected for a specific purpose.

**data warehouse**    Where information from different databases is collected and organized to be used for ad hoc reports and analytical research.

**database**    An organized collection of data in a computer.

**decision matrix**    A quality improvement tool used to narrow focus or choose between two or more related possible decisions.

**deductible**    A specified dollar amount for which the patient is personally responsible before the payer reimburses for any claims.

**deemed status**    The Medicare provision that an approved accreditation is sufficient to satisfy the compliance audit element of the COP.

**defendant**    The party or parties against whom the plaintiff has initiated litigation.

**deficiencies**    Required elements that are missing from a record.

**deficiency system (incomplete system)**    The policies and procedures that form the corrective control of collecting the missing data identified in quantitative analysis. Includes the recording and reporting of deficiencies. Also called an **incomplete system**.

**delegation**    The transfer of a responsibility, task, or project from a manager to a lower level employee.

**delinquent**    Status accorded to a record that has not been completed within a specified time frame, such as within 30 days of discharge.

**demographic data**    Provides identification, those elements that distinguish one patient from another, such as name, address, and birth date.

**Department of Health and Human Services (DHHS)**    The US federal agency with regulatory oversight of American health care, which also provides health services to certain populations through several operating divisions.

**depreciation**    The loss of value over time due to wear from use and obsolescence.

**designated record set**    A specific portion of the patient's health information, consisting of medical records, reimbursement, and payer information, and other information used to make health care decisions, all of which may be accessed by the patient under HIPAA provisions.

**detective controls**    Procedures, processes, or structures that are designed to find errors after they have been made.

**deterministic matching**    An identity matching algorithm that relies on exact matching of individual fields, such as date of birth.

**Deterministic method**    An identity matching algorithm that relies on exact matching of individual fields, such as date of birth.

**diagnosis**    The name of the patient's condition or illness.

**diagnosis-related group (DRG)**    A collection of health care descriptions organized into statistically similar categories.

***Diagnostic and Statistical Manual of Mental Disorders*, Fifth Edition (DSM-5)**    Used for classifying behavior and mental health care disorders and coding these disorders using ICD-10-CM.

**dialysis center**    An ambulatory care facility that specializes in blood-cleansing procedures to treat, for example, chronic kidney (renal) failure.

**differential diagnosis**    The list of possible conditions or diseases that are causing the patient's symptoms.

**Digital Imaging and Communications in Medicine (DICOM)**    A standard that enables the storage and use of clinical digital imaging, making their exchange among physicians and other providers possible.

**direct admission**    An expedited inpatient admission arranged in advance by a physician's office or other entity due to a patient's urgent medical condition.

**discharge**    The act of releasing the patient from the care of the facility to go home, for transfer to another health care facility, or because of death.

**discharge disposition**    The setting to which a patient went after discharge from the facility.

**discharge planning**    The multidisciplinary, coordinated effort to ensure that a patient is discharged to the appropriate level of care and with the appropriate support.

**discharge register (list)**    A list of all patients discharged on a specific date or during a specific period. Also called a **discharge list**.

**discharge summary**    The recap of an inpatient stay, usually dictated by the attending physician and transcribed into a formal report.

**disclosure**    When patient health information is given to someone.

**discounted fee for service**    The exchange of cash for professional services rendered, at a rate less than the normal fee for the service.

**discovery**    The process of investigating the circumstances surrounding a lawsuit.

**discrete data**    Named and identifiable pieces of data that can be queried and reported in a meaningful way.

**diversity**    The differences that exist among or between team members.

**document imaging**    Scanning or faxing of printed papers into a computer system.

**dual governance**    In hospitals, a shared organization structure consisting of the administration, headed by the CEO, and the medical staff, headed by the Chief of Medical Staff.

## E

**electronic data interchange (EDI)**    A standard in which data can be transmitted, communicated, and understood by the sending and receiving computer systems, allowing the exchange of information.

**electronic document management system (EDMS)**    Computer software and hardware, typically scanners, that allow health record documents to be stored, retrieved, and shared.

**electronic health record (EHR)**    A secure real-time point-of-care patient-centric information resource for clinicians that allows access to patient information when and where needed and that incorporates evidence-based decision support.

**emancipation**    Consideration of a patient as an adult even though the patient is younger than the statutory age.

**encounter**    A unit of a health professional's service to a patient.

**encounter form**    A data collection device that facilitates the accurate capture of ambulatory care diagnoses and services.

**encryption**    A security process that blocks unauthorized access to patient information.

**entitlement program**    Government financial support based on an individual's age, medical condition, employment status, or other circumstances.

**epidemiology**    The study of morbidity trends and occurrences.

**error report**    An electronically generated report that lists deficient or erroneous data. Also called an *exception report*.

**ethics**    A system of beliefs about acceptable behavior; a standard of moral excellence that all

HIM professionals must uphold while managing patient information.

**evaluation and management (E/M) code**  A subset of CPT coding that represents the amount of time and skill needed to treat the patient.

**evidence-based medicine**  A decision-making methodology for patient care that makes conscientious, explicit, and judicious use of current best research.

**exception**  In HIPAA, use and disclosure of PHI for certain public priorities without patient authorization.

**exception report**  An electronically generated report that lists deficient or erroneous data. Also called an error report.

**expenses**  The costs incurred by the organization in the process of earning income.

## F

**Federal Drug and Alcohol Abuse Regulations**  Regulations at the national level addressing requirements for disclosure of chemical and alcohol abuse patient information.

*Federal Register*  The publication of the proceedings of the US Congress.

**fee for service**  The exchange of monies, goods, or services for professional services rendered at a specific rate, typically determined by the provider and associated with specific activities (such as a physical examination).

**fee schedule**  The list of charges that a physician expects to be paid for services rendered. Also, a list of the amounts a payer will remit for certain services.

**field**  A collection or series of related characters. A field may contain a word, a group of words, a number, or a code, for example.

**file**  Numerous records of different types of related data. Files can be large or small, depending on the number of records they contain.

**financial accounting**  The process of measuring, recording, reporting, and analyzing financial data.

**financial data**  Elements that describe the payer and the services rendered to the patient. For example, the name, address, telephone number, group number, and member number of the patient's insurance company as well as the charges incurred.

**fiscal intermediaries**  Organizations that administer the claims and reimbursements for the funding agency. Medicare uses fiscal intermediaries to process its claims and reimbursements.

**fixed expense**  Expense in the operational budget that does not change with changes in volume.

**frequency distribution**  The grouping of observations into a small number of categories.

**full-time equivalent (FTE)**  A unit of staffing that equals the regular 30- to 40-hour work week as defined by the organization.

**functional organization**  An administrative structure in which each employee has only one superior for reporting and supervisory purposes.

## G

**GANTT chart**  A project management tool for planning and controlling in which a list of all the steps in a project, the beginning and ending dates of the step, who is responsible, and the order of the steps are laid out.

**gatekeeper**  A primary care provider who sees the patient first to control access to other parts of the health care delivery system.

**geometric mean**  The measure of central tendency calculated by taking the *n*th root of the product of *n* values.

**goal**  Desired achievement or outcome.

**granularity**  The level of detail with which data are collected, recorded, or calculated.

**group plan**  A pool of covered individuals that averages the risk for a third-party payer, used to leverage lower premiums for the group as a whole.

**group practice model HMO**  An HMO that contracts with a group or network of physicians and facilities to provide health care services.

**group practice**  Multiple physicians who share facilities and resources and may also cooperate in rendering patient care.

**grouper**  The software used to derive the DRG from the ICD-10-CM diagnoses and procedures.

**guarantor**  The individual or organization that promises to pay for the rendered health care services after all other sources (such as insurance) are exhausted.

## H

**health data**  Elements related to a patient's diagnosis and procedures as well as factors that may affect the patient's condition.

**health informatics**  The interdisciplinary development and application of technology-based solutions to generate and use data to improve the delivery, management, and planning of health care services.

**health information**  Organized data that have been collected about a patient or a group of patients.

**health information exchange (HIE)**  The database of a network of health care providers (physicians, hospitals, laboratories, and public health organizations) allowing access to patient records within the network from approved points of care.

**health information management (HIM)**  The profession that manages the sources and uses of health information, including the collection, storage, retrieval, and reporting of health information.

**health information technology (HIT)**  The specialty in the field of health information management that focuses on the day-to-day activities of HIM that support the collection, storage, retrieval, and reporting of health information.

**Health Information Technology for Economic and Clinical Health (HITECH) Act**  A subset of the American Recovery and Reinvestment Act (2009) legislation providing federal funding and mandates for the use of technology in health care.

**Health Insurance Portability and Accountability Act (HIPAA)**  Public Law 104-191, federal legislation passed in 1996 that outlines the guidelines of managing patient information in terms of privacy, security, and confidentiality. The legislation also outlines penalties for noncompliance.

**Health Level-Seven (HL7)**  A health information systems compliance organization, the goal of which is to standardize the collection of patient information in the EHR.

**health literacy**  The ability of a patient to obtain, process, and understand basic information about their condition or that of an individual for whom they are caring.

**health maintenance organization (HMO)**  Managed care organization characterized by the ownership or employer control over the health care providers.

**health record**  All the personal and health data collected about a patient by one or more providers.

**Healthcare Common Procedure Coding System (HCPCS)**  The CMS coding system, of which CPT-4 is Level I. Used for drugs, equipment, supplies, and other auxiliary health care services rendered.

**hearsay rule**  The court rule that prohibits most testimony regarding events by parties who were not directly involved in the event.

**histogram**  A modified bar graph representing continuous data. Each bar represents a class interval; the height of the bar represents the frequency of observations.

**history**  The physician's record of the patient's chief complaint, history of present illness, pertinent family and social history, and review of systems.

**history and physical (H&P)**  Health record documentation comprising the patient's history and physical examination; a formal, dictated copy must be included in the patient's health care record within 24 hours of admission for inpatient facilities.

**hospice**  Palliative health care services rendered to the terminally ill, their families, and their friends.

**hospital**  An organization having permanent facilities that deliver inpatient health care services through 24-hour nursing care, an organized medical staff, and appropriate ancillary departments.

**Hospital-Acquired Condition (HAC)**  A condition (e.g., infection, traumatic injury) contracted by the patient as a result of being in the facility. CMS ignores certain HACs for reimbursement purposes.

**hospitalist**  A physician employed by a hospital, whose medical practice is focused primarily on patient care situations specific to the acute care setting.

**hybrid record**  A record in which both electronic and paper media are used.

**hypothesis**  A tentative explanation for an observation or scientific problem that can be tested by further investigation.

## I

**ice breaker**  An activity that helps new team members get to know one another.

**incidence**  The number of new and existing cases of a disease or disorder in a population.

**income statement**  A summary of revenue and expenses over a period of time.

**indemnity insurance**  Assumption of the payment for all or part of certain specified services. Characterized by out-of-pocket deductibles and caps on total covered payments.

**independent practice association (IPA) model HMO**  An HMO that contracts with individual physicians, portions of whose practices are devoted to the HMO.

**index**  A list of all patients in a time period, sorted by a specific characteristic, e.g.: admission date, discharge date, principal diagnosis, attending physician.

**indexing**  The process of identifying a paper document so that, when scanned into a document management system, it is associated with the correct patient, encounter, and type of documentation.

**information**  Processed data (i.e., data that are presented in an appropriate frame of reference).

**informed consent**  A permission given by a competent individual, of legal age, with full knowledge or understanding of the risks, potential benefits, and potential consequences of the permission.

**infrastructure** The interrelated components of a system.

**inpatient** The status of a patient who is admitted to a hospital with the intention of staying overnight.

**inpatient service day (IPSD)** A measure of the use of hospital services, representing the care provided to one inpatient during a 24-hour period.

**inservice** Training provided to employees of an organization for continued or reinforced education.

**Institutional Review Board (IRB)** A committee within a facility charged with ensuring that research conducted within the facility conforms to all applicable rules and regulations.

**insurance** A contract between two parties in which one party assumes the risk of loss on behalf of the other party in return for some, usually monetary, compensation.

**insurer** The party that assumes the risk of paying some or all of the cost of providing health care services in return for the payment of a premium by or on behalf of the insured.

**integrated delivery system (IDS)** A health care organization that provides services through most or all of the continuity of care.

**integrity** The data quality characteristic displayed when alteration of a finalized document is not permitted.

**intensity of service (IS)** In UR, a type of criterion consisting primarily of monitoring and diagnostic assessments that must be met in order to qualify a patient for inpatient admission.

**Interactive Map-Assisted Generation of ICD-10-CM Codes (I-MAGIC) algorithm** An algorithm used to map EHR-generated SNOMED CT codes to the more specific ICD-10-CM code set, seeking input from a coder to supply missing information as necessary.

**interface** Computer configuration allowing information to pass from one system to another.

**International Classification of Diseases, Tenth Revision, Clinical Modification (ICD-10-CM).** A unique classification system, developed in the United States, for reporting diagnoses. It is a HIPAA-mandated code set.

**International Classification of Diseases, Tenth Revision, Procedural Coding System (ICD-10-PCS).** A unique classification system, developed in the United States, for reporting procedures performed in inpatient settings. It is a HIPAA-mandated code set.

**International Classification of Diseases—Oncology (ICD-O)** The coding system used to record and track the occurrence of neoplasms (i.e., malignant tumors, cancer).

**International Health Terminology Standards Development Organisation (IHTSDO)** A multinational organization that supports the standardized exchange of health information through the development of clinical terminologies, notably SNOMED CT.

**interoperability** The ability of different software and computer systems to communicate and share data.

**interval data** Are numeric, ordered, and have a continuous array of values; however, there is no absolute zero.

**J**

**job analysis** Review of a function to determine all of the tasks or components that make up an employee's job.

**job description** A list of the employee's responsibilities.

**jurisdiction** The authority of a court to decide certain cases. May be based on statutory authority, geography, money, or type of case.

**K**

**key performance indicator (KPI)** A pre-determined target value (e.g., average DNFB, ALOS, CMI, employee turnover rate) against which an outcome is measured to evaluate success.

**L**

**laboratory** The physical location of the specialists who analyze body fluids.

**Lean** A performance improvement process that seeks to add value through the reduction of waste and wasteful activities.

**length of stay** The duration of an inpatient visit, measured in whole days; the number of whole days between the inpatient's admission and discharge.

**liability** The legal responsibility for wrongdoing.

**licensed beds** The maximum number of beds that a facility is legally permitted to have, as approved by state licensure.

**licensure** The mandatory government approval required for performing specified activities. In health care, the state approval required for providing health care services.

**line graph** A chart that represents observations over time or between variables by locating the intersection of the horizontal and vertical values and connecting the dots signifying the intersections.

**litigation** The term used to indicate that a matter must be settled by the court and the process of engaging in legal proceedings.

**local coverage determination (LCD)** A list of diagnostic codes used by Medicare contractors to determine medical necessity.

**longitudinal record** The compilation of patient health data from all providers over a period of time, ideally birth to death.

**long-term care (LTC) facility** A hospital that provides services to patients over an extended period; an average length of stay is in excess of 30 days. Facilities are characterized by the extent to which nursing care is provided.

**M**

**major diagnostic categories (MDCs)** Segments of the DRG assignment flowchart (grouper).

**malpractice** In health care, harm to a patient caused by a failure to practice within the standards of professional competence.

**managed care** A type of insurer (payer) focused on reducing health care costs, controlling expensive care, and improving the quality of patient care provided.

**master forms file** A file containing blank copies of all current paper forms used in a facility.

**master patient index (MPI)** A system containing a list of patients who have received care at the health care facility and their encounter information, often used to correlate the patient with the file identification.

**matrix reporting** An employee reports to more than one manager.

**maximization** The process of determining the highest possible DRG payment.

**median** The measure of central tendency that represents the observation that is exactly halfway between the highest and lowest observations.

**Medicaid** A federal/state funded program of health coverage for eligible low-income individuals, administered by states, under federal regulation.

**medical record number (MRN)** A unique number assigned to each patient in a health care system; this code will be used for the rest of the patient's encounters with that specific health care system.

**Medicare** Federally funded health care insurance program for older adults and for certain categories of chronically ill patients.

**Medicare administrative contractor (MAC)** Regional, private contractor who processes reimbursement claims for CMS.

**Medicare Code Editor (MCE)** A part of grouping software that checks for valid codes in claims data.

**Medicare Severity diagnosis-related group (MS-DRG)** A collection of health care descriptions organized into statistically similar categories.

**medication administration** Clinical data including the name of the medication, dosage, date and time of administration, method of administration, and name of the nurse who administered it.

**memorandum (memo)** A written communication in a specified formate, typically used to provide intra-organizational information.

**minimum data set (MDS)** The detailed data collected about patients receiving long-term care. It is collected several times, and it forms the basis for the Resource Utilization Group.

**minimum necessary** A rule requiring health providers to disclose only the minimum amount of information necessary to accomplish a task.

**minutes** A written record of the events, topics, and discussions of a meeting.

**mission statement** The strategic purpose of the organization documented in a formal statement.

**mixed method research** A type of study in which both quantitative and qualitative methods are used.

**mode** The measure of central tendency that represents the most frequently occurring observation.

**modifier** A two-digit addition to a CPT or HCPCS code that provides additional information about the service or procedure performed.

**morbidity** In public health, information concerning disease or illness.

**mortality** In public health, information concerning death.

**multi-axial** A code structure in which the position of a character has a specific meaning.

**N**

**National Committee for Quality Assurance (NCQA)** A nonprofit entity focusing on quality in health care delivery that accredits managed care organizations.

**national coverage determination (NCD)** A process using evidence-based medicine to determine whether Medicare will cover an item or service on the basis of medical necessity.

**National Drug Code (NDC)** A transaction code set field used to identify drugs by the firm, labeler, and batch.

**National Integrated Accreditation for Healthcare Organizations (NIAHO)** A compliance and accreditation entity partnered with CMS to ensure quality and standards in acute care settings. Facilities maintaining NIAHO accreditation receive *deemed status* from CMS.

**National Library of Medicine (NLM)** The medical library operated by the US government under the National Institutes of Health. Serves as representative for the United States in the international standards organization IHTSDO.

**National Patient Safety Goals** Guidance created by TJC to recommend patient safety measures in accredited facilities.

**Nationwide Health Information Network (NHIN)** A system of nationally shared health data, composed of a network of providers, consumers, and researchers, that aims to improve health care delivery through the secure exchange of information.

**negligence** Carelessness or lack of foresight that leads to harm or damage.

**network** A group of providers serving the members of a managed care organization; the payer will generally not cover health care services from providers outside the network.

**nomenclature** A formal method of naming used by a scientific or technical profession; in medical coding, users of the nomenclature determine the definition of each code.

**nominal data** A type of categorical data with no inherent numeric or relative value.

**nominal group technique** A problem-solving and decision-making process in which group members offer solutions which are then ranked by favorability.

**nonrepudiation** A process that provides irrefutable identification of the user.

**normal curve** The symmetric distribution of observations around a mean; usually in the shape of a bell.

**nosocomial infection** An infection contracted by the patient at the health care facility.

**Notice of Privacy Practices** A notice, written in clear and simple language, summarizing a facility's privacy policies and the conditions for use or disclosure of patient health information.

**nurse** A medical professional who has satisfied the academic, professional, and legal requirements to care for patients at state-specified levels. Although usually delivering patient care at the direction of physicians, nurse practitioners may also deliver care independently.

**nursing assessment** The nurse's evaluation of the patient.

**nursing progress notes** Routine documentation of the nurse's interaction with a patient.

## O

**objective** (1) A measurable and defined statement of an action that, when completed, will help to achieve a goal; (2) in the SOAP format for medical decision-making, the physician's observations and review of diagnostic tests.

**observation** A patient not admitted to the hospital but monitored in the facility for a period of time.

**occupancy** In a hospital, the percentage of available beds that have been used over time.

**Office of the Inspector General (OIG)** Of the 57 inspectors general, the OIG associated with the DHHS is the largest, having oversight of Medicare and Medicaid programs.

***Official Guidelines for Coding and Reporting*** Instructions for the use of ICD-10-CM codes, updated at least annually.

**operational budget** Costs related to the operation of the department, such as payroll, utilities, and supplies.

**operational definition** The specific criteria by which the researcher will measure a variable.

**operative report** The surgeon's formal report of surgical procedure(s) performed.

**optimization** The process of determining the most accurate DRG payment.

**order set (protocol)** A predetermined plan of care that guides the health care professional toward best practices in diagnosing or treating the condition. Also called a *protocol*.

**ordinal data** A type of categorical data with inherent relative value but no numeric value.

**organization chart** An illustration used to describe the relationships among departments, positions, and functions within an organization.

**orientation** Training to familiarize a new employee with the job.

**outcome** The result of a patient's treatment.

**Outcome and Assessment Information Set (OASIS)** Data set most associated with home health care. This data set monitors patient care by identifying markers over the course of patient care.

**outlier** A patient whose length of stay or cost is far lower or higher than the average expected by the prospective payment system, notably the DRG.

**outlier payment** An unusually high payment within a given case mix group.

**outpatient** A patient whose health care services are intended to be delivered within 1 calendar day or, in some cases, a 24-hour period.

**outpatient PPS (OPPS)** A Medicare PPS used to determine the amount of reimbursement for outpatient services.

**outsource** Procure services from external organizations or individuals who are not employees of the facility for which the services are being provided.

## P

**palliative care** Health care services that are intended to soothe, comfort, or reduce symptoms but are not intended to cure.

**patient account number** A numerical identifier assigned to a specific encounter or health care service received by a patient; a new number will be assigned to each encounter, but the patient will retain the same medical record number.

**patient assessment instrument (PAI)** A tool used to identify patients with greater needs and for the treatment of whom the long-term care or skilled nursing facility will receive higher reimbursement.

**patient care plan** The formal directions for treatment of the patient, which involves many different individuals, including the patient. It may be as simple as instructions to "take two aspirin and drink plenty of fluids," or it may be a multiple-page document with delegation of responsibilities. Care plans may also be developed by discipline, such as nursing.

**patient portal** A website on which a patient can interact and communicate with their provider, view lab results, and track, monitor, and send information regarding their personal health.

**payback period** The amount of time it will take for the savings or revenues generated by a purchase to exceed the price of the purchase.

**payer** The individual or organization that is primarily responsible for the reimbursement for a particular health care service. Usually refers to the insurance company or third party.

**per diem** Each day, daily. Also refers to part time or casual workers.

**percentage** Standardization of data so that unlike groups can be compared. Can be calculated by dividing the observations in the category by the total observations and multiplying by 100.

**performance improvement (PI)** Also known as *quality improvement* (*QI*) or *continuous quality improvement* (*CQI*). Refers to the process by which a facility reviews its services or products to ensure quality.

**performance improvement plan (PIP)** A plan to explain the required responsibilities and competencies expected of an employee's job performance.

**performance standards** Set guidelines explaining how much work an employee must complete.

**permitted disclosure** Disclosure authorized by the patient or allowed for treatment, payment, or health care operations.

**personal health record (PHR)** A patient's record of his or her own health information.

**physiatrist** A physician who specializes in physical medicine and rehabilitation.

**physical examination** The physician's record of examination of the patient.

**physician** A medical professional who has satisfied the academic, professional, and legal requirements to diagnose and treat patients at state-specified levels and within a declared specialty. A physician directs the care of a patient.

**physician's assistant** A clinical professional who provides primary care under the supervision of a physician.

**physician–patient privilege** The legal foundation that private communication between a physician and a patient is confidential. Only the patient has the right to give up this privilege.

**physician's office** A setting for providing ambulatory care in which the primary provider is the physician.

**physician's orders** The physician's directions regarding the patient's care. Also refers to the data collection device on which these elements are captured. Physician's orders are a required part of the health care record.

**Picture archiving and communication system (PACS)** A system that allows many different kinds of diagnostic images (e.g., radiographs, magnetic resonance images, ultrasound scans, and computed tomography scans) produced by many different kinds of machines to be archived and accessed from any computer terminal in the network.

**pie chart** A circular chart in which the frequency of observations is represented as a wedge of the circle.

**plaintiff** The party who initiates litigation.

**plan of care (treatment)** In the SOAP format for documentation of medical decision-making, the diagnostic, therapeutic, or palliative measures that are taken to investigate or treat the patient's condition or disease.

**point-of-care documentation** Clinical data recorded at the time the interaction with the patient occurs.

**policy** A statement of something that is done or expected in an organization.

**population** An entire group; every actual and potential element, item, or individual under study.

**postdischarge processing** The procedures designed to prepare a health record for retention.

**potentially compensable event (PCE)** An event that could cause the facility a financial loss or lead to litigation.

**power of attorney**   The legal document that identifies someone as the legal representative to make decisions for the patient when the patient is unable to do so.

**preemption**   The legal principle that federal law invalidates conflicting state law; pertaining to HIPAA, the regulation or law that gives the patient more rights or is more restrictive prevails.

**preferred provider organization (PPO)**   A managed care organization that contracts with a network of health care providers to render services to its members.

**premium**   Periodic payment to an insurance company made by the patient for coverage (an insurance policy).

**prevalence**   Rate of incidence of an occurrence, disease, or diagnosis or the number of existing cases.

**preventive controls**   Procedures, processes, or structures that are designed to minimize errors at the point of data collection.

**primary care provider (PCP)**   In insurance, the provider who has been designated by the insured to deliver routine care to the insured and to evaluate the need for referral to a specialist, if applicable. Colloquial use is synonymous with "family doctor."

**primary caregiver**   The individual who is principally responsible for the daily care of a patient at home, usually a friend or family member.

**primary data**   Data taken directly from the patient or the original source. The patient's health record contains primary data.

**principal diagnosis**   According to the UHDDS, the condition that, after study, is determined to be chiefly responsible for occasioning the admission of the patient to the hospital for care.

**principal procedure**   According to the UHDDS, the procedure that was performed for definitive treatment rather than one performed for diagnostic or exploratory purposes or necessary to take care of a complication. If two procedures appear to meet this definition, then the one most related to the principal diagnosis should be selected as the principal procedure.

**privacy**   The right of an individual to control access to medical information.

**privacy officer**   The designated official in the health care organization who oversees privacy compliance and handles complaints.

**privileges**   The set of standards allowing a physician or other provider to perform services in a hospital.

**Probabilistic method**   An identity matching algorithm that compares multiple fields in records, such as date of birth, name, and address, to calculate the chance that the records refer to the same patient.

**procedure**   A process that describes how to comply with a policy. Also, a medical or surgical treatment. Also refers to the processing steps in an administrative function.

**process control chart**   A data-gathering tool that graphs the measurement of a key performance indicator or other variable over time.

**productivity**   The amount of work produced by an employee in a given time frame.

**profession**   A type of occupation requiring mastery of knowledge and skills, the members of which adhere to ethical principles in the service of the society.

**progress notes**   The physician's record of each interaction with the patient.

**prospective consent**   Permission given prior to having knowledge of the event to which the permission applies. For example, a permission to release information before the information is gathered (i.e., before admission).

**prospective payment system (PPS)**   Any of several reimbursement methods that pay an amount predetermined by the payer on the basis of statistical analysis of the diagnosis, procedures, and other factors (depending on setting) rather than actual, current resources expended by the provider.

**protected health information (PHI)**   Individually identifiable health information that is transmitted or maintained in any form or medium by covered entities or their business associates.

**protocol (order set)**   A predetermined plan of care that guides the health care professional toward best practices in diagnosing or treating the condition. Also called an *order set*.

**provider number**   The number assigned to a participating facility by Medicare for identification purposes.

## Q

**qualitative research**   A type of study that uses observation rather than numerical values.

**quality assurance (QA)**   A method for reviewing health care functions to determine their compliance with predetermined standards that requires action to correct noncompliance and then follow-up review to ascertain whether the correction was effective.

**Quality Improvement Organization (QIO)**   An organization that contracts with payers, specifically Medicare and Medicaid, to review care and reimbursement issues.

**quantitative analysis**   The process of reviewing a health record to ensure that the record is complete according to organization policies and procedures for a complete medical record.

**quantitative research**   A type of study in which the observations can be quantified numerically.

**query**   To question the database for specific elements, information, or a report.

**queue**   In an electronic work management system, the listing of work and its status.

## R

**radiology**   The study of internal body structures using radiographs (X-rays) and other imaging technologies. In a health care facility, the department responsible for maintaining radiographic and other types of diagnostic and therapeutic equipment as well as analyzing diagnostic images.

**random selection**   In sampling of a population, a method that ensures that all cases have an equal chance of being selected and that the cases are selected in no particular order or pattern.

**rate**   A value in relation to a different unit.

**ratio data**   Are true numeric data; continuous values and absolute zero.

**record**   A collection of related fields. Also refers to all of the data collected about a patient's visit or all of the patient's visits.

**recovery audit contractor (RAC)**   An entity that contracts with CMS to audit providers, using DRG assignment and other data to identify overpayments and underpayments.

**redact**   To remove patient-identifying information from a health record.

**registry**   A database of health information specific to disease, diagnosis, or implant used to improve the care provided to patients with that disease, diagnosis, or implant.

**reimbursement**   The amount of money that the health care facility receives from the party responsible for paying the bill.

**relational database**   Data organized into linked tables of related data that can be retrieved in different ways without changing the data's organization.

**relative weight (RW)**   A number assigned yearly by CMS that is applied to each DRG and used to calculate reimbursement. This number represents the comparative difference in the use of resources by patients in each DRG.

**release of information (ROI)**   The term used to describe the health information management department function that provides disclosure of patient health information.

**reliability**   A characteristic of quality exhibited when codes are consistently assigned by one or more coders for similar or identical cases.

**remote patient monitoring (RPM)**   A type of telemedicine in which the patient transmits physiological health data outside of a health care setting (such as at home) to a provider.

**report**   The result of a query. A list from a database.

**request for proposal (RFP)**   A document presented to a vendor that describes what services are required, such as the system and functionality requirements of an EHR product.

**required disclosure**   A disclosure to the patient and to the secretary of the Department of Health and Human Services for compliance auditing purposes.

**resident**   A person who, after attending college and medical school, performs professional duties under the supervision of a fully qualified physician.

**Resident Assessment Instrument (RAI)**   A data set collected by SNFs that includes elements of MDS 3.0, along with information on patient statuses and conditions in the facility.

**Resident Assessment Protocol (RAP)**   A detailed, individualized evaluation and plan for patients in LTC.

**resource intensity (RI)**   A weight of the resources used for the care of an inpatient in an acute care setting that result in a successful discharge.

**resource utilization group (RUG)**   These constitute a prospective payment system for long-term care. Current Medicare application is a per diem rate based on the RUG III grouper.

**resource-based relative value system (RBRVS)**   The system used to determine reimbursements to physicians for the treatment of Medicare patients.

**respite care**   Services rendered to an individual who is not independent in ADLs, for the purpose of temporarily relieving the primary caregiver.

**restriction**   Under HIPAA's Privacy Rule, the right of patients to limit the use of their protected health information.

**retail care**   Preventive health services and treatment for minor illnesses offered in large retail stores, supermarkets, and pharmacies.

**retention**   The procedures governing the storage of records, including duration, location, security, and access.

**retrospective consent**   Permission given after the event to which the permission applies. For example, permission to release information after the information is gathered (i.e., after discharge).

**return on investment (ROI)**   The percentage of the capital expenditure recovered each year.

**revenue**  Earnings from the activities or investments of the organization.

**revenue code**  A Chargemaster code required for Medicare billing.

**revenue cycle**  The groups of processes that identify, record, and report the financial transactions that result from the facility's clinical relationship with a patient.

**revenue cycle management (RCM)**  All the activities that connect the services being rendered to a patient with the provider's reimbursement for those services.

**right to complain**  The patient's right to discuss his or her concerns about privacy violations.

**right to revoke**  The right to withdraw consent or approval for a previously approved action or request.

**risk**  The potential exposure to loss, financial expenditure, or other undesirable events; used to determine potential reimbursement of health care services.

**risk management (RM)**  The coordination of efforts within a facility to prevent and control inadvertent occurrences.

**root cause analysis (RCA)**  The process of determining the cause of an error.

**rule out**  The process of systematically eliminating potential diagnoses. Also refers to the list of potential diagnoses.

## S

**same-day surgery**  Surgery performed on an outpatient basis; the patient returns home after the surgery is performed. Also called *ambulatory surgery*.

**sample**  A group within a population.

**secondary data**  Data taken from the primary source document for use elsewhere.

**security**  The administrative, physical, and technologic safeguards used to protect patient health information.

**self-pay**  A method of payment for health care services in which the patient pays the provider directly, without the involvement of a third-party payer (e.g., insurance).

**sentinel event**  An unwanted occurrence that should never happen.

**severity of illness (SI)**  In utilization review, a type of criterion, based on the patient's condition, that is used to screen patients for the appropriate care setting.

**shared governance**  The empowerment of all staff to be responsible for their particular areas.

**Six Sigma**  Performance improvement methodology that uses structured steps and measurable targets to eliminate defects from a process.

**skewed**  Frequency distributions that are not symmetric, sometimes because of a small sample.

**skilled nursing facility (SNF)**  An LTC facility providing a range of nursing and other health care services to patients who require continuous care, typically those with a chronic illness.

**socioeconomic data**  Elements that pertain to the patient's personal life and personal habits, such as marital status, religion, and culture.

**span of control**  The number of employees who report to one supervisor, manager, or administrator.

**staff model HMO**  An HMO in which the organization owns the facilities, employs the physicians, and provides essentially all health care services.

**stakeholder**  Regarding EHR implementation and selection, an individual or department with an interest in the process, either in the implementation or the outcome.

**standard deviation**  A measure of the average distance of observations from a mean.

**standards for transactions and code sets**  Standards that must be used under HIPAA for the electronic exchange of data for certain transactions—namely, encounter and payment data.

**Standards of Ethical Coding**  Guidelines from the AHIMA to guide professional coders toward ethical decisions.

**statistics**  Analysis, interpretation, and presentation of information in numeric or pictorial format derived from the numbers.

**statute**  A law that has been passed by the legislative branch of government.

**store-and-forward**  A type of telemedicine in which images or video of a patient is recorded to be viewed by a specialist at a later time.

**subjective**  In the SOAP format of medical decision-making documentation, the patient's description of the symptoms or other complaints.

**subpoena ad testificandum**  A direction from an officer of the court to provide testimony.

**subpoena duces tecum**  A direction from an officer of the court to provide documents.

**subpoena**  A direction from an officer of the court.

**Substance Abuse and Mental Health Services Administration (SAMHSA)**  An agency under the US Department of Health and Human Services (DHHS) facilitating research and care for the treatment of patients with substance abuse and mental health problems.

**superbill**  An ambulatory care encounter form on which potential diagnoses and procedures are preprinted for easy checkoff at the point of care.

**superuser**  An individual trained in all aspects of a computer system who can offer on-site support to others.

**Surveillance, Epidemiology and End Results (SEER) Program**  The National Cancer Institute's program that collects cancer statistics using the ICD-O-3 code set.

**survey**  A data-gathering tool for capturing the responses to queries. May be administered verbally or by written questionnaire. Also refers to the activity of querying, as in "taking a survey."

**symptom**  The patient's report of physical or other complaints, such as dizziness, headache, and stomach pain.

**system development life cycle (SDLC)**  The process of planning, designing, implementation, and evaluation used in updating and improving or implementing a new health information system.

**Systemized Nomenclature of Medicine—Clinical Terms (SNOMED CT)**  Systematized nomenclature of human and veterinary medicine clinical terms; a reference terminology that, among other things, links common or input medical terminology and codes with the output reporting systems in an electronic health record.

## T

**Tax Equity and Fiscal Responsibility Act of 1982 (TEFRA)**  A federal law with wide-reaching provisions, one of which was the establishment of the Medicare PPS.

**telemedicine**  The delivery of health care to individuals who are physically remote from the provider.

**The Joint Commission (TJC)**  An organization that accredits and sets standards for acute care facilities, ambulatory care networks, LTC facilities, and rehabilitation facilities, as well as certain specialty facilities, such as hospice and home care. Facilities maintaining TJC accreditation receive *deemed status* from CMS.

**third-party payer**  An entity that pays a provider for part or all of a patient's health care services; often the patient's insurance company.

**timeliness**  The quality of data's being obtained, recorded, or reported within the time frame appropriate for that data.

**tort**  Harm, damage, or wrongdoing that entitles the injured party to compensation.

**tracer methodology**  TJC method of on-site review of open records in which the surveyors follow the actual path of documentation from start to finish.

**training**  Education in, instruction in, or demonstration of how to perform a job.

**treatment**  A procedure, medication, or other measure designed to cure or alleviate the symptoms of disease.

**trend**  The way in which a variance of values behaves over time.

**triage**  In emergency services, the system of prioritizing patients by severity of illness.

**TRICARE**  A US program of health benefits for military personnel, their families, and military retirees.

## U

**Uniform Ambulatory Care Data Set (UACDS)**  The mandated data set for ambulatory care patients.

**Uniform Bill (UB-04)**  The standardized form used by hospitals for inpatient and outpatient billing to CMS and other third-party payers.

**Uniform Hospital Discharge Data Set (UHDDS)**  The mandated data set for hospital inpatients.

**unity of command**  Sole management of one employee by one manager.

**Urgent Care Association (UCA)**  A professional organization representing those working in urgent care settings, serving as an advocate for the role of urgent care facilities in health care delivery.

**urgent care center**  A facility that treats patients whose illness or injury requires immediate attention but is not life threatening.

**use**  The employment of protected health information for a purpose.

**usual customary and reasonable (UCR) fee**  The amount a payer reimburses for a medical service based on what providers usually charge in a geographic area.

**utilization review (UR)**  The process of evaluating medical interventions against established criteria, on the basis of the patient's known or tentative diagnosis. Evaluation may take place before, during, or after the episode of care for different purposes.

## V

**validity**  In data quality, the characteristic that data reflect the known or acceptable range of values.

**variable expense**  Expense in the operational budget that change based on the volume of activity.

**variance**  A deviation from the projected spending in the budget.

**verification**  Confirming accuracy.

**vision**    The goal of the organization, above and beyond the mission.

**visit**    A unit of service in an ambulatory care setting.

**vital signs**    Measurements of the patient's health status such as heart rate, body temperature, respiration rate, oxygen saturation, and blood pressure.

**vital statistics**    Public health data collected through birth certificates, death certificates, and other data-gathering tools.

## W

**workers' compensation**    An employer's coverage of an employee's medical expenses due to a work-related injury or illness.

**workflow**    The process of work flowing through a set of procedures to complete the health record.

**workflow analysis**    A careful examination of how work is performed in order to identify inefficiencies and make changes.

**working DRG**    The DRG that reflects the patient's current diagnosis and procedures while still an inpatient.

**working MS-DRG**    The concurrent DRG. The DRG that reflects the patient's current diagnosis and procedures while still an inpatient.

**wraparound policy**    Insurance policies that supplement Medicare coverage. Also called *secondary insurance*.

# Index

*Note*: The Abbreviations start on p. 498.

*Note*: Page numbers followed by "*f*" and "*t*" refer to figures and tables, respectively.

## A

Abstract, 136–137, 240, 246
Abstracting, 136–137, 240
  as component of postdischarge processing, 136, 138–139
  for data retrieval, 139–140
Access, 305–314
  confidentiality and, 303, 306
  continuing patient care and, 305–306
  health care operations and, 305–306
  litigation and, 293, 306–307
  reimbursement and, 305
Accessibility, data quality and, 120*t*, 121–122
Accountability, in organizational structure, 328
Accountable care organizations (ACOs), 17
Accounting concepts, 222–229
  financial accounting, 222–223
  management accounting, 223–229
    capital budget, 225–227
    operational budget, 227–229
    strategic budget, 225
Accounting of disclosures, 244, 304
Accreditation, 21–23, 236–237, 272, 382–383
  agencies for, 382–383
  ambulatory surgery and, 99, 102
  of behavioral health facilities, 105
  compliance and, 314–316
  history and evolution of, 381–382
  home health care and, 110
  hospice and, 109
  of long-term care facilities, 105
  patient safety goals and, 383
  quality check and, 383
  for rehabilitation facilities, 108
Accrual method, 222–223
Accuracy
  in coding quality, 179–180
  data quality and, 120–121
ACDIS. *See* Association of Clinical Documentation Improvement Specialists
ACOs. *See* Accountable care organizations
ACS. *See* American College of Surgeons
Activities of daily living (ADLs), 13, 103
Acute care facilities, 260, 314–315
  definition of, 12
ADA. *See* American Dental Association
Adjusted mean, 252
ADLs. *See* Activities of daily living
Administration, 148
Administrative data, 68–71
Admission, 259–260
  ambulatory care and, 12
  definition of, 11
  discharge, transfer (ADT) data, 66
  medical treatment consent and, 296
  statistics for, 258–259
Admission consent form, 74
Admission denial, 91, 272
Admission record, 73, 239–240
  data collection and, 41

Admitting diagnosis, 72, 246, 384
Admitting physician, 71
Advance directives, 74, 240, 296, 392
Advanced practice registered nurse (APRN), 6
Affinity diagram, 398
Affordable Care Act, 201
Against medical advice (AMA), 76
Agencies, communicating with, 358
Agency for Healthcare Research and Quality (AHRQ), 20
Aggregate data
  definition of, 244
  retrieval of, 244–247
  secondary sources and, 238–239
AHA. *See* American Hospital Association
AHIMA, 208. *See also* American Health Information Management Association
AHIP. *See* America's Health Insurance Plans
AHRQ. *See* Agency for Healthcare Research and Quality
Algorithm, in electronic health records, 48–49
Allied health professionals, 6
ALOS. *See* Average length of stay
Alpha-numeric field, in database building, 35
AMA. *See* American Medical Association
Ambulatory care, 93–94
  care providers in, 95–97
  physicians' offices and, 94
  services in, 93–95
  settings for, 94–95
Ambulatory care facility, 314–315
  definition of, 11
  emergency department and, 11
  health information management and, 11
Ambulatory payment classification, 210–211
Ambulatory surgery
  care providers in, 102
  data collection issues in, 97–98
  data sets and, 98–99
  definition of, 102–103
  length of stay and, 102
  licensure and accreditation for, 102
  services of, 101–102
  settings for, 101
Ambulatory surgery center (ASC), 99
Ambulatory surgery coding notes, 211
Amendment, to health information, 303
American Academy of Professional Coders, 208
American College of Surgeons (ACS), 382
American Dental Association (ADA), 169
American Health Information Management Association (AHIMA), 9, 183, 301–302
  Standards of Ethical Coding and, 157
American Hospital Association (AHA), 218, 381
American Medical Association (AMA), 163, 381
American National Standards Institute (ANSI), 383
American Occupational Therapy Association, 107
American Osteopathic Association (AOA), 382
American Psychiatric Association (APA), 168

American Recovery and Reinvestment Act (ARRA), 290
  health information technology and, 149
American Trauma Society (ATS), 274
America's Health Insurance Plans (AHIP), 165
Amortization, 227
Ancillary departments, in data collection, 47
Anesthesia data, 88
Anesthesia report, 88
ANSI. *See* American National Standards Institute
AOA. *See* American Osteopathic Association
APA. *See* American Psychiatric Association
Applied research, 267
APRN. *See* Advanced practice registered nurse
Arithmetic mean, 250–251
ARRA. *See* American Recovery and Reinvestment Act
ASC. *See* Ambulatory surgery center
Assault, 291
Assembly, 131
Assessment
  clinical data and, 68
  nursing, 86–87
Assisted living, 103
Association of Clinical Documentation Improvement Specialists (ACDIS), 183
ATS. *See* American Trauma Society
Attending physician, 84, 239–240
  consultations and, 84
  discharge summary and, 84–86
  orders and, 80–84
  progress notes and, 84
  registration process and, 72
  SOAP structure and, 75
Attribution, 272
Audience, in training session, 368
Audit Medicaid Integrity Contractors (Audit MICs), 385–386
Audit trail, 122, 244, 305–306
Authentication
  in data collection, 44–45
  physician, H&P creation, 80
  quantitative analysis and, 132
Authorization form, 307
Authorized disclosures, 307–308
Autocratic leader, 364–365
Autopsy, 86
  reports, 89
Average, 250
AVERAGE function in Microsoft Excel, 250*f*
Average length of stay (ALOS), 237
  statistics and, 260–262

## B

Backup file, 320
Balance sheet, 223
Bar (Excel), 275–276
Bar codes, registration process and, 73
Bar graph, 275–276, 278*f*, 403
Basic research, 267

Bassinet, 263
Batch control form, 141
Batch scanning, 130
Battery, 291
BCBSA. *See* Blue Cross and Blue Shield
    Association
Bed control, 129, 263
Bed count, 13, 264
Bed occupancy rate, 264
Beds, number of, on facility size, 13
Behavioral health facilities, 5
    care providers in, 105–106
    data collection issues in, 106
    data sets and, 106–108
    definition of, 105–106
    drug and alcohol rehabilitation in, 105
    length of stay in, 105
    licensure and accreditation for, 106
    services in, 105
    settings for, 105
Benchmarking, 400
Bertillon Classification of Causes of Death, 159
Billing, 215, 272, 385
    charge capture and, 216–218
    chargemaster and, 215–216
    claim denials and, 222
    claim rejections and, 218–222
    CMS-1500 and, 218, 221*f*
    collection and, 222
    error correction and, 222
    impact of coding on reimbursement and, 218
    for inpatients and outpatients, 71
    patient financial services and, 215
    UHDDS data elements and, 218, 220*f*
    Uniform Bill and, 218
Billing number, 37
Biomedical informatics, 237
Biometric technology, 319
Bit, database building and, 35
Blended rate, 209
Blue Cross and Blue Shield Association (BCBSA),
    163–164
Board and care homes, 104*t*
Brainstorming, 398–400, 401*f*
Breach, 145
Budgets, 223–229
Business associate, 301, 304–305
Business record rule, 293

## C

"C-suite," in organizational structure, 327
CABG. *See* Coronary artery bypass graft
CAHIIM. *See* Commission on Accreditation for
    Health Informatics and Information
    Management
CAHIIM competency domains, 193
Cahiim competency domains, 326
CAHs. *See* Critical Access Hospitals
Cameras, 319
Cancer treatment centers, 109
Capital budget, 225–227
Capital expenditure approval form, 226*f*
Capitation, 206–207
CARF. *See* Commission on Accreditation of
    Rehabilitation Facilities
Case management, 72, 89–90, 272
    personnel, 72
Case mix, 205
    analysis of, 178
Case Mix Assessment Tool (CMAT), 106
Case mix index (CMI), 209–210
Cash basis, 222–223

Cash flow, 223
CCCs. *See* Convenient care clinics
CCHIT. *See* Certification Commission for
    Health Information Technology
CCU. *See* Coronary care unit
CDC. *See* Centers for Disease Control and
    Prevention
CDI. *See* Clinical Documentation Improvement
CDM. *See* Charge Description Master
CDS. *See* Clinical decision-making system
CE. *See* Continuing education
CEHERT. *See* Certified electronic health
    technology
Census, 129, 259, 262–263, 264*t*
Centers for Disease Control and Prevention
    (CDC), 20
    health care data and, 57
    mission of, 148
    vital statistics and, 274
Centers for Medicare and Medicaid Services
    (CMS), 20, 49, 68
    data sets and, 37–40
    ICD-10-PCS and, 159
    verbal or telephone order authentication and,
    82
Central limit theorem, 256
Central tendency, measures of, 249–252,
    254
CEO. *See* Chief Executive Officer
CERT. *See* Comprehensive Error Rate Testing
Certification, 293, 314
    of information for release, 310
Certification Commission for Health Information
    Technology (CCHIT), 54
Certified Coding Specialist and Certified Coding
    Assistance Credential, 208
Certified electronic health technology
    (CEHERT), 49
Certified Inpatient Coder, 208
Certified Outpatient Coder, 208
Certified Professional Coder, 208
Certified Risk Adjustment Coder (CRC),
    208
Certified Tumor Registrars (CTRs), 273
Chain of command, 326–327
CHAMPVA. *See* Civilian Health and Medical
    Program of the Veterans Administration
Change management, 408–410
CHAP. *See* Community Health Accreditation
    Program
Characters, database building and, 35
Charge capture, 216–218
Charge Data Master, 216
Charge Description Master (CDM), 216
Charge ticket, 216
Chargemaster, 216
Charges, 206
Charity care, 204–205
Chemical systems, fire damage and, 318
Chief complaint, 78–79
Chief Executive Officer (CEO), 327
Children's Health Insurance Program (CHIP),
    204
CHIP. *See* Children's Health Insurance Program
Civilian Health and Medical Program of the
    Veterans Administration (CHAMPVA),
    205
Claims, 385
    denials, 222
    health care payment and, 194
    rejections of, 211, 218–222
Class interval, 252–254, 263

Classification, 158
Clinic, 95
Clinical data, 47, 68, 71
    coded, 178–179
        case mix analysis and, 179
        code sets and, 176*t*, 178
        comparative analysis and, 179
        exercise in, 181–182
        reimbursement and, 179
        reporting and, 179
    laboratory data and, 87
    nurses and, 86–87
    radiology data and, 87
    special records and, 88–89
Clinical data analyst, 286
Clinical decision-making system (CDS), in
    electronic health records, 48–49
Clinical documentation, 78–91, 96–97, 113
Clinical documentation improvement (CDI),
    136, 183–185
    monitoring, 184
    outcomes reporting, 184–185
    physician query process, 183–185
    purpose, 183
    staffing, 183
Clinical flow of data, exercises for, 71–78
Clinical outcome analysis, 267
Clinical oversight, 89–91
    case management and, 89–90
    patient care plan and, 89
    utilization review and, 90–91
Clinical pathway, 89
CMAT. *See* Case Mix Assessment Tool
CMI. *See* Case mix index
CMS. *See* Centers for Medicare and Medicaid
    Services
CMS-1500, 218, 221*f*
Code modifier, 211
Code of ethics, in professional standards, 23
Code sets
    coding and, 158
    dental terminology codes and, 168
    general purpose of, 159–165
    special purpose classifications of, 165–169
    uses for coded clinical data and, 178–179
Coded clinical data, 178
    case mix analysis and, 178
    code sets and, 176*t*, 178
    comparative analysis and, 179
    exercise in, 181–182
    reimbursement and, 179
    reporting and, 178
Coded data, 155–156
Coder, 189
Coder training, in coding quality, 179
Coding, 256, 389
    classification, 158
    clinical vocabulary, 158–159
    competency milestones, 185–188
    critical thinking, 188–189
    definition of, 156
    ethics challenge, 188
    exercise in, 157
    fraud and, 385–386
    inpatient, 135–136
    interim, 136
    nomenclature, 157–158
    patient care perspective, 189–190
    postdischarge processing and, 134–137
    principles and applications, 156–159
    retrospective, 136
    taxonomy, 159

Coding compliance, 181–183
Coding compliance plan, 181
Coding quality, 178–185
  achieving, 179–180
  coding compliance, 181
  computer-assisted coding, 179
Coding supervisor, 330
Cognitive definition, 268–269
Cognitive remediation, 106–107
Coinsurance, 194
Collection, and billing, 222
Column (Excel), 274
Commission on Accreditation for Health
    Informatics and Information
    Management (CAHIIM), 23
Commission on Accreditation of Rehabilitation
    Facilities (CARF), 23, 105, 382–383
Committees, 395–398
Communication, 358–364
  meetings, 359–363
  oral, 358
  with outside agencies or parties, 358
  with physicians, 358
  of work teams, 363
  written, 358–359
Communication skills, 398
Community awareness, 149
Community Health Accreditation Program
    (CHAP), 110
Comorbidity, 175
Comparative analysis, coded clinical data and,
    179
Compensation, for record preparation, 310
Competency, informed consent and, 295–296
Completeness
  data quality and, 120t, 123
  quantitative analysis and, 132
Compliance, 290
  accreditation and, 314–316
  data collection and, 44–45
  federal, corporate, and facility, 314–316
  legal and legislative landscape, 290, 295
Comprehensive Error Rate Testing (CERT),
    385
Comprehensive examination, 164
Computer-assisted coding, 179
Computer passwords, 319
Computerized physician order entry (CPOE)
  data and, 71
  data collection and, 43–44
Computerized productivity reports, 350
Concept (SNOMED CT), 166
Concierge medicine, 202
Concurrent analysis, 133–134
Concurrent coding, 136
Concurrent review, 315
Conditions of admission, 296, 306
Conditions of Participation (COP), 20, 93, 123,
    382
Confidential communication, 299
Confidentiality, 289, 299–306
  agreement, 299, 300f
  computer screen and, 299–300
  definition of, 299
  legal foundation for, 299
  scope of, 299–301
Consent, 247, 295–299
  admission and, 296
  informed consents and, 295
  medical procedures and, 297–299
  special, 309
  for surgery, 297–299

Consistency, data quality and, 120t, 122
Consultant, 84
Consultation, 84, 85t
Continued stay denial, 91
Continuing care retirement communities, 104t
Continuing education (CE), in health care
    industry, 7–8
Continuity of care, 14–16, 94–95, 305–306,
    314–315
Controls
  corrective, 126–127, 385–386
  data quality and, 87, 124–128
  detective, 125–126, 385–386
  preventive, 124–125, 385–386
Convenient care clinics (CCCs), 109
Cookbook medicine, 200
Cooperating Parties, 161
COP. *See* Conditions of Participation
Copay, 194
Copy/paste function, 125
Coronary artery bypass graft (CABG), 250
Coronary care unit (CCU), 89
Corporate Trainer-Coding Specialist Division, 190
Correction of errors, 127–128
Corrective controls
  data quality and, 126–127
  discharge register and, 129
  quality management theories and, 385–386
Correspondence, 309–310
  tracking log, 309–310
Cost, health care, insurance and, 199
Countersignature, 132
Countersigned, 44–45, 84
Court order, 294–295
Covered entity, 305
  HITECH and, 301
Covered services, 198
COVID-19 pandemic, 19, 55, 160
CPOE. *See* Computerized physician order
    entry
CPT. *See* Current Procedural Terminology
CRC. *See* Certified Risk Adjustment Coder
Credentials, in health care industry, 7–8
Criminal law, 291–292
Critical Access Hospitals (CAHs), 49
Crosby, Philip, 388
Cross-training, 368
CTRs. *See* Certified Tumor Registrars
Cultural competence, 365
Currency, data quality and, 120t, 123
Current Dental Terminology Codes, 169
Current Procedural Terminology (CPT), 157–
    158, 163–165
  procedure, in ambulatory payment
      classification, 210
Custodian, 310
Customer Service Representative, 323

**D**

*Darling v. Charleston Community Memorial
    Hospital*, 292
Dashboard, 280–281, 280f
Data
  aggregate, 34
  architecture, 34–40
  basic concepts of, 30–34
  classifying, 247–248
  clinical, 47
  clinical flow of, 71–78
  definition of, 31
  dictionary, 35, 245
  health, 32–34, 66

Data (*Continued*)
  interval, 249
  mapping, 57
  nominal, 248
  optimal source of, 246–247
  ordinal, 248–249
  presentation of, 274–281
    bar graphs as, 275–276, 278f
    dashboard as, 280–281, 280f
    histograms as, 276, 279f
    line graphs as, 275, 278f
    organization tools for, 398
    pie charts as, 276–280, 279f
    pivot tables as, 274–275, 277f
    tables as, 274
    tools for, 275t
  ratio, 249
  repository, 55–56, 56f
  retrieving, 245
  review of, 239
  types of, 247–249
  warehouse, 56–57, 56f
Data analytics, 34, 237
  in health care, 237
Data collection
  basic concepts of, 31
  database creation and, 240
  device, 34–35, 43t
  electronic, 43
  health care, 31
  health records and, 66–71
  issues with
    in ambulatory surgery, 101, 103
    in behavioral health facilities, 105
    in home health care, 108
    in hospice, 108–109
    in rehabilitation facilities, 107–108
  organized, primary and secondary data in, 238
  sources of, 64
  storage and, 40–57
    compliance of, 44–45
    content of, 40–57
    formatting of, 41–44
    forms of, 40–46
    other considerations in, 45–46
Data Elements for Emergency Department
    Systems (DEEDS), 101
Data entry, 97–98, 119
Data-gathering tools, 398
  brainstorming as, 398
  survey as, 401
Data governance, 128, 333
Data quality, 34–35, 37, 119–128
  accuracy, 120t
  characteristics, 120–124, 127
    accessibility, 120t, 121–122
    accuracy and validity, 120–121
    completeness and, 120t, 123
    consistency, 120t, 122
    currency, 120t, 123
    data definition, 120t, 123–124
    granularity, 120t, 124
    precision, 120t, 123
    relevancy, 120t, 124
    timeliness, 120t, 122–123
  controls and, 87, 124–128
  data sets in, 37–40
  entering data and, 34–35
  master patient index and, 36–39
Data reporting
  to individual departments, 270–272
  to outside agencies, 272

Data request form, 245*f*
Data retrieval
    aggregate data and, 244–247
    optimal source for, 246–247
    populations and samples for, 245–246
Data sets
    ambulatory surgery and, 103
    behavioral health facilities and, 106
    data architecture and, 37–40
    defined, 38–40
    home health care and, 110
    long-term care facilities and, 105
    rehabilitation facilities and, 108
Database
    abstracting from, 240
    building a, 35–36
    creation of, 240
    data collection and, 34–35
    data retrieval from, 244–247
    definition of, 34
    optimal source of data and, 246
    value of, 239–240
Decimal, 255–256
Decision-making process, 307–308
Decision matrix, 404–405
Deductible, 194, 199
DEEDS. *See* Data Elements for Emergency
        Department Systems
Deemed status, 23, 314–315
Defective authorization, 308–309
Defendant, 306–307
Deficiencies, 132
Deficiency system, 133–134, 135*f*
Delinquent, 133–134
Deming, W. Edwards, 388
Democratic leader, 365
Demographic data, 66, 67*f*, 246
Department of Health and Human Services
        (DHHS), 20, 145
Departmental committees, 390–391
Depreciate, 227
Designated record set, 303
Destruction, of health information, 319–320
Det Norske Veritas (DNV), 382
Detailed examination, 164
Detective controls, 125–126, 385–386
Deterministic method of patient matching,
        138
Development, 367–373
DHHS. *See* Department of Health and Human
        Services
Diagnosis
    clinical data and, 68
    in health care industry, 3
Diagnosis-related groups (DRGs), 169, 178,
        246–247, 276, 384–385
    assignment, 169–172, 176
    coder's role in, 176
    MDC 05 diseases & disorders of the
        circulatory system, 174–176
    MS-DRG grouper logic, 172–173
Diagnostic and Statistical Manual of Mental
        Disorders, Fifth Edition (DSM-5), 106,
        168
Diagnostic resource groups, 207–209
Dialysis, 150
Dialysis centers, 109
DICOM. *See* Digital imaging and
        communication in medicine
Differential diagnosis, 75
Digital imaging and communication in medicine
        (DICOM), 51

Direct admission, 71
Direct care standards, of Health level 7 (HL7),
        54
Disaster planning
    fire damage and, 318
    health data management and, 316
    water damage and, 318
Discharge, 259, 314, 384
    ambulatory care and, 12
    definition of, 11
    disposition of, 259
    on facility size, 13–14
    statistics for, 266
    summary of, 84–86
Discharge data set, 91–92
Discharge disposition, 76
Discharge list, 128–129
Discharge planning, 90–91
Discharge register, 128–129
Discharge summary, 84–86
Disciplines, 237–238
Disclosures, 302–303
    accounting of, 244, 304
Discounted fee for service, 206
Discovery, 293
Discrete data, 240
Distribution, of information, 311
Diversity, 365–366
DME. *See* Durable medical equipment
DNFB (discharged, no final bill, or discharged,
        not final billed), 216
DNV. *See* Det Norske Veritas
Document imaging system, for hybrid
        record, 47
Documentation committee, data collection and,
        41
Documentations, 382
Donabedian, Avedis, 388
Donabedian's structure-process-outcome model,
        388*f*
DRG 981, 175
DRG 987, 176
DRG 998, 175
DRG creep, MS-DRG and, 176
DRGs. *See* Diagnosis-related groups
Drop-down menus, 68
Dropped bill, 216
Drug and alcohol rehabilitation, 105
DSM-5. *See* Diagnostic and Statistical Manual of
        Mental Disorders, Fifth Edition
Dual governance, 11, 327
Durable medical equipment (DME), 107

**E**

E-PHI. *See* Electronic protected health
        information
EBM. *See* Evidence-based medicine
ED. *See* Emergency department
EDI. *See* Electronic data interchange
EDMS. *See* Electronic document management
        system
Education, health information uses and,
        147
eHealth Exchange, 53
EHR. *See* Electronic health record
Elective, 71
Electronic communication, 358–359
Electronic data collection, 40–41
Electronic data interchange (EDI), 54,
        157
Electronic document management system
        (EDMS), 47, 130

Electronic health record (EHR), 46–55, 119,
        133–134
    features of, 48–49
    health information exchange and, 51–55
    hybrid record and, 46–47
    interoperability of, 50–51
    migration of, planning for, 57, 59
        design of, 58
        evaluation in, 59
        implementation in, 58–59
        selection in, 58
        support and, 59–60
    patient access to, 55
    storing health care data in, 55
Electronic protected health information (E-PHI),
        144
Emancipation, 295
Emergency, 71
Emergency department (ED), 11, 99–101
Employee, classification, by hours worked,
        339–340
Employee patients, 306
Employment laws, 339*t*
Encounter, 12, 94, 199
Encounter form, 217
Encryption, 144–145
Enhanced Nurse Licensure Compact (eNLC), 6
eNLC. *See* Enhanced Nurse Licensure Compact
Entitlement programs, 18
    federal coverage for specific populations as,
        205
    as insurance, 203–206
    Medicaid as, 18, 204–205
    Medicare as, 18, 203–204
    Tax Equity and Fiscal Responsibility Act of
        1982 as, 205–206
Environment, in training session, 369
Epidemiology, 34
Error correction, and billing, 222
Error report, 125–126
Etiology, 381
Evaluation, employee, 351, 352*f*
Evaluation and management (E/M) codes, 164
Evidence-based medicine (EBM), 48–49, 89,
        389
Exception report, 125–126
Exceptions, 293, 302, 302*t*
Existence, 131
Expanded problem focused examination, 164
Expenses, 223
Extensible Markup Language (XML), 160
External forces, in health care industry, 19–25
    accreditation and, 21–23
    federal government as, 19–20
    local government as, 21
    state government as, 20–21

**F**

Facilitator, 396
Facility closure, 312–314
Facility-wide committee, 390
Family care physician, 105
Farr, William, 157
Faxed information, 312*f*
FDA. *See* Food and Drug Administration
Federal Drug and Alcohol Abuse Regulations,
        309
*Federal Register*, 161
Fee for service, 206
Fee schedule, 214
Fields, database building and, 35–36
Files, database building and, 36–37

Final bill, 216
Financial accounting, 222–223
Financial data, 66–68, 194
Financial loss, 196
Financial management, 192
  competency milestones, 229–232
  critical thinking, 232
  ethics challenge, 232
  patient care perspective, 233
Financial statements, 223, 224f
Fire damage, 318
Fiscal intermediary, 195t, 204
Fiscal year, 264
Fishbone chart, 398, 400f
Fixed expenses, 227
Flexible spending account (FSA), 202
Flexner, Abraham, 382
Flowchart, 401
Food and Drug Administration (FDA), 20
Form CMS-1450, 218
Format, in training session, 368–369
Forms committee, data collection and, 41, 45
Fraud, 385–387
Frequency distribution, 252–256, 276
FSA. See Flexible spending account
Full-time equivalents, 340
Functional organization, 328

**G**

GANTT chart, 398, 407
Gatekeeper model, 200
General consent form, 74
General purpose code sets, 159–165
  Healthcare Common Procedure Coding
    System/Current Procedural Terminology
    (HCPCS/CPT), 163–165
    HCPCS level I and, 163–164
    HCPCS level II and, 165
  International Classification of Diseases, Tenth
    Revision, Procedural Coding System
    (ICD-10-PCS), 156, 165–166
  International Classification of Diseases,
    Tenth Revision-Clinical Modification
    (ICD-10-CM)
    general purpose code sets and, 156,
      159–162, 166
    grouping and, 173t
    MS-DRGs and, 172
  *Official Guidelines for Coding and Reporting,*
    161
Geometric mean, 252, 254f
Geometric mean length of stay (GMLOS),
  252
GMLOS. See Geometric mean length of stay
Goals, in operational planning, 334–335
Granularity, data quality and, 120t, 124
Graph, 403
Group plans, 196–197
Group practice, 94–95
Group practice model HMO, 201
Grouper software, 169–172
Guarantor, 68, 194

**H**

HAC. See Hospital-acquired conditions
HCPCS. See Healthcare Common Procedure
  Coding System
Health, 30–31
Health care, quality in, 380–383, 387
  health care data and, 380
  history and evolution of, 381–382
  medical education and, 381–382

Health care, quality in *(Continued)*
  outcomes measurement program for, 383
  patients first and, 380
  Quality Initiative and, 383–387
  standardization and accreditation in, 382
  timeline of, 381f
Health care costs, insurance and, 199
Health care industry, 2
  continuing education in, 7–8
  credentials in, 7–8
  customer satisfaction in, 19
  employers of, 18
  external forces of, 19–25
    accreditation, 21–23
    federal government, 19–20
    local government, 21
  federal and state government in, 18
  health information management in, 6–8
  independent organizations in, 24–25
  insurance companies in, 18
  interdisciplinary collaboration and, 9–10
  manufacturing and distribution in, 19
  medical specialties and subspecialties
    of, 4t
  patients of, 18–19
  payers of, 18
  professional associations in, 8–9
  professional standards of, 23, 25
  professionals in, 2
    allied, 6
    nurses, 5–6
    physician assistants, 6
    physicians, 3–5
  providers of, 11
    continuity of care and, 14–16
    evolving organizational models and, 17
    facility size and, 13–14
    inpatient, 11
    outpatient, 12
    ownership, 16
    patient population and, 12–13
    services and, 13
    tax status of, 16–17
Health care operation, access to information and,
  306
Health Care Professionals Advisory Committee,
  163–164
Health data. *See also* Data
  basic concepts in, 32–34
  collecting, 31
    basic concepts of, 30–34
    building a database in, 35–36
    data architecture and, 34–40
    data quality and, 34–35
    data sets and, 37–40
    electronic health record and, 46
    forms for, 40–46
    master patient index in, 36–37
    planning for EHR migration and imple-
      mentation in, 57–60
    storage and, 40
Health facilities, behavioral, 13
  care providers in, 105–106
  data collection issues in, 106
  data sets and, 106
  definition of, 105
  drug and alcohol rehabilitation in, 105
  length of stay in, 105
  licensure and accreditation for, 106
  services in, 105
  settings for, 105
Health informatics, 237–238

Health information
  basic concepts in, 30–31, 34
  destruction of, 319–320
  quality of, monitoring of, 389t
  retrieval of, 139–140
  uses of, 146–150
    administration as, 148
    community awareness as, 149
    education as, 147
    improving patient care as, 147
    internal or external facilities and, 146
    litigation as, 149
    managed care as, 149–150
    marketing as, 150
    mortality and morbidity as, prevalence and
      incidence of, 148
    national policy and legislation as, 148–149
    reimbursement support and collection as,
      147–148
    research as, 149
Health information management (HIM), 6–7,
  236–237
  abstracting and, 137
  in analysis, 238
  committee for, 397
  department workflow, 330–332
  organization, 329–330
  processing of, data quality and, 119
Health information services, 329
Health information technologies (HIT), 237
Health Information Technology for Economic
    and Clinical Health (HITECH) Act, 290
Health Insurance Portability and Accountability
    Act (HIPAA), 19–20, 289, 303
  confidentiality and, 300, 303
  data sets and, 39
  notice of privacy practices and, 303
  patient rights and, 303
  privacy regulations and, 301
  protected health information and, 302
  standards for code sets and, 156–157
  uses and disclosures under, 302–303
Health level 7 (HL7), 54
Health literacy, 147
Health Maintenance Organization Act of 1973,
  200–201
Health maintenance organizations (HMOs), 198,
  200–201
Health record, 238, 299, 382
  clinical flow of data, 71–78
  completion of, 134, 136
  confidentiality and, 299
  data collection and, 40
  defined, 66–71
  elements of, 132–133
  in health care industry, 9–10
  key data categories, 66–71
  retention of, 143
  timeliness and, 122–123
Health Resources and Services Administration
    (HRSA), 20
Health savings account (HSA), 202
Healthcare Common Procedure Coding System
    (HCPCS), 157–158
Healthcare Common Procedure Coding System/
    Current Procedural Terminology
    (HCPCS/CPT), 163–165
  in ambulatory payment classification, 210
  HCPCS level I and, 163–164
  HCPCS level II and, 165
Healthcare Financial Management Association, 72
Healthy people 2020, 19

Hearsay rule, 293
Help desk, 59–60
HH PPS. *See* Home Health Prospective Payment System
HIM. *See* Health information management
HIPAA. *See* Health Insurance Portability and Accountability Act
Hiring process, for recruitment, 343–345
Histograms, 276, 279*f*
History
    clinical documentation and, 78–91
    patient, clinical data and, 78–80
History and physical (H&P), 246
    physician's data and, 80
    timeliness and, 122
HMOs. *See* Health maintenance organizations
Home health care, 13, 109–110
    care providers in, 110
    data collection issues in, 110
    data sets and, 110
    licensure and accreditation for, 110
    services in, 110, 111*t*
    settings for, 109–110
Home Health Care Coding Notes, 213
Home health organizations, data sets and, 39
Home Health Prospective Payment System (HH PPS), 213
Hospice, 13
    care providers in, 108
    data collection issues in, 108
    length of stay in, 108
    licensure and accreditation for, 110
    services in, 108
Hospice in Skilled Nursing Facility Coding Notes, 213
Hospital, 11
Hospital-acquired conditions (HAC), 178
Hospital compare, 385
Hospital Consumer Assessment of Health Care Providers and Systems (HCAHPS) survey, 385
Hospital Value-Based Purchasing Program, 383–384
Hospitalists, 3–4, 76
H&P. *See* History and physical
HRSA. *See* Health Resources and Services Administration
HSA. *See* Health savings account
Human resources, 338–358
    clinical staff orientation, 356–357
    discipline and, 357
    employee evaluations in, 351, 352*f*
    HIM department orientation, 355–356
    job analysis and description in, 340–342
    legal aspects of, 338–340
    organization-wide orientation, 351–355
    outsourcing in, 357–358
    performance standards in, 347–348
    recruitment and retention in, 342–347
    workflow and process monitor in, 349–351
    workload and, 348–349
Hypothesis, 267

**I**

ICD-10, 159
ICD-10-CA Canada, 157
ICD-10-CM codes, in ambulatory payment classification, 210
ICD-O-3, 167–168
Ice breakers, 398
IDSs. *See* Integrated delivery systems
IHS. *See* Indian Health Service
Incidence, 148, 272

Incident report, 317
Income statement, 223
Incomplete system, 133
Indemnity insurance, 198–199
Independent practice association (IPA) model HMO, 201
Index, 272
Index to Diseases and Injuries, ICD-10-CM and, 160
Indexing, 130
Indian Health Service (IHS), 20, 205
Infection control, committee for, 397
Information, 31–32, 66
Information governance, 333–334
Information infrastructure standards, of Health level 7 (HL7), 54
Informed consent, 295
Infrastructure, definition of, 58
Inpatient, 11, 296
Inpatient Behavioral Health Coding Notes, 212
Inpatient coding, 190
Inpatient Psychiatric Facility Prospective Payment System (IPF PPS), 106, 211–212
Inpatient Rehabilitation Facility Coding Notes, 212
Inpatient Rehabilitation Facility Patient Assessment Instrument (IRF-PAI), 212
Inpatient Rehabilitation Facility Prospective Payment System, 212
Inpatient service days (IPSDs), 263–264
Institutional Review Board (IRB), 244, 269
Insurance
    assumption of risk and, 194, 198–199
    competency check-in for, 202
    contract, 196
    definition of, 194
    history of, 194
    terminology for, 195*t*
    types of, 198–201
        Affordable Care Act in, 201
        health maintenance organizations as, 200–201
        indemnity as, 198–199
        managed care as, 199–201
        preferred provider organizations as, 201
        self-insurance as, 201–203
Insurer, 194
Integrated care, 16
Integrated delivery systems (IDSs), 17
Integrity, record, 144
Intensity of service (IS), 91
Intensive care unit records, 88–89
Interactive Map-Assisted Generation of ICD-10-CM Codes (I-MAGIC) algorithm, 167
Interdepartmental, 390
Interim coding, 136
International Classification of Diseases (ICD), 159
International Classification of Diseases, Tenth Revision, Procedural Coding System (ICD-10-PCS), 156, 165–166
International Classification of Diseases, Tenth Revision-Clinical Modification (ICD-10-CM), 51
    general purpose code sets and, 156, 159–160, 166
    grouping and, 173*t*
    MS-DRGs and, 172
International Health Terminology Standards Development Organisation (IHTSDO), 165
International Standards Organization (ISO), 382
    quality management principles, 383
International Statistics Institute (ISI), 159
Internist, 107

Interpersonal skills, 364–367, 398
    diversity and, 365–367
    in leadership, 364–365
Interpretation, 247–248
Interviewing, for recruitment, 345–346
Intradepartmental, 390
IPF PPS. *See* Inpatient Psychiatric Facility Prospective Payment System
IPSDs. *See* Inpatient service days
IRB. *See* Institutional Review Board
IRF-PAI. *See* Inpatient Rehabilitation Facility Patient Assessment Instrument
IS. *See* Intensity of service
ISI. *See* International Statistics Institute
ISO. *See* International Standards Organization

**J**

JCAHO. *See* Joint Commission on Accreditation of Health Care Organizations
Job analysis, 340–342
Joint Commission on Accreditation of Health Care Organizations (JCAHO), 382
Juran, Joseph M., 388
Jurisdiction, 293

**K**

Kanban, 405
Key code entry system, 319
Key data categories, 66–71
    administrative data, 68–71
    clinical data, 68
    demographic data, 66, 67*f*
    financial data, 66–68
    socioeconomic data, 66–67
Key performance indicators (KPIs), 237
KPIs. *See* Key performance indicators

**L**

Labor laws, 338
Laboratory data, 87
Laboratory tests, 87
Laissez-faire leader, 365
LCD. *See* Local coverage determination
LCSW. *See* Licensed Clinical Social Worker
Lean technique, 395*f*
Leapfrog group, 24
Legal age, 295
Legal aspects, of human resources, 338–340
Legal files, 306
Legislation, health care, 148–149
Length of stay (LOS), 244, 259–260
    average, 12–14, 15*f*, 260
    statistics for, 259–260
Liability, 292
Licensed beds, 13, 264
Licensed Clinical Social Worker (LCSW), 106
Licensed Master Social Worker (LMSW), 106
Licensed practical nurse (LPN), 5–6
Licensed vocational nurse (LVN), 104
Licensure, 314
    ambulatory surgery and, 103
    of behavioral health facilities, 106
    compliance and, 314–316
    definition of, 21
    in health care industry, 21
    home health care and, 110
    hospice and, 109
    of long-term care facilities, 105
    for rehabilitation facilities, 108
Line graphs, 275, 278*f*, 403
Litigation, 149
    access to information and, 293–295, 306–307

LMSW. *See* Licensed Master Social Worker
Local coverage determination (LCD), 211
Long-term care, 103–105
Long-term care (LTC) facilities, 12–13, 314–315
  care providers in, 102–103
  data collection issues in, 106
  data sets and, 106
  definition of, 103
  examples of, 104*t*
  length of stay in, 103
  licensure and accreditation for, 106
  services of, 103
  setting for, 102–103
Long-Term Care Facility Coding Notes, 213
Long-term Care Prospective Payment System (LTCH-PPS), 212–213
Longitudinal record, 50, 66
LOS. *See* Length of stay
LPN. *See* Licensed practical nurse
LTCH-PPS. *See* Long-term Care Prospective Payment System
LVN. *See* Licensed vocational nurse

**M**

MACs. *See* Medicare Administrative Contractors
Major diagnostic category (MDC), 173
Malpractice, medical, 292
Managed care, 199–201
  health information and, 149–150
Management accounting, 223–229
  capital budget, 225–227
  operational budget, 227–229
  strategic budget, 225
Management and leadership, 325–326
  communication, 358–364
    meetings, 359–363
    oral, 358
    with outside agencies or parties, 358
    with physicians, 358
    of work teams, 363
    written, 358–359
  human resources, 338–358
    clinical staff orientation, 356–357
    discipline and, 357
    employee evaluations in, 351, 352*f*
    HIM department orientation, 355–356
    job analysis and description in, 340–342
    legal aspects of, 338–340
    organization-wide orientation, 351–355
    outsourcing in, 357–358
    performance standards in, 347–348
    recruitment and retention in, 342–347
    workflow and process monitor in, 349–351
    workload and, 348–349
  interpersonal skills, 364–367
    diversity and, 365–367
    in leadership, 364–365
  operational planning, 334–338
    customer satisfaction in, 336–338
    goals and objectives in, 334–335
    policies and procedures for, 335–336
  organizational structure, 326–332
    accountability in, 328
    HIM department organization, 329–330
    HIM department workflow in, 330–332
    management responsibilities in, 329
    shared governance in, 328–329
  strategic planning, 332–334
    data and information governance, 333–334
    mission, vision, and values, 332–333
    rolling out the strategic plan, 334

Management and leadership *(Continued)*
  training, 367–373
    calendar of education, 369–370
    continuing education and, 371–373, 372*f*
    educating the public, 371
    evaluation of, 370–371
    program, evaluating, 370–371
    session, planning for, 368–369
    technology, 369
Management responsibilities, in organizational structure, 329
Manual productivity reports, 349–350
Marketing, health information and, 150
Markle Foundation, 53
Master forms file, 45
Master patient index (MPI), 36–37, 38*f*, 272
  data collection and, 36–38
  maintenance, postdischarge processing and, 137–138
  table, 66
Matrix organization, 328
Matrix reporting, 328
Maximizing, MS-DRG and, 176
MCE. *See* Medicare Code Editor
MDC. *See* Major diagnostic category
MDS. *See* Minimum Data Set
Mean
  median and, 240
  mode and, 252
  with outlier, 252
Measures of frequency, 252, 256
  frequency distribution as, 252–255
  percentages, decimals, rates, and ratios as, 255–256
Median, 251–252
Medicaid, 18, 193–194, 204–205, 291
Medicaid Integrity Contractors (MICs), 385–386
Medicaid's hospital quality initiative, 383
Medical assistant, 14–16
Medical decision making, 75–78, 80*f*
Medical education, 382
Medical examiner, 89
Medical home model, 17, 55
Medical malls, 109
Medical procedure consent, 297–299
Medical record, 40, 66. *See also* Health record
Medical record department, 329
Medical record number (MRN), 37, 68, 245, 299
Medical record specifications, 382
Medical Records Manager, 115
Medical staff, committees, 396–397
Medical Staff Office, 68
Medical staff organization chart, 328*f*
Medical statistician, 157
Medicare, 18, 193–194, 203–204, 240, 255, 291, 383
Medicare Administrative Contractors (MACs), 203, 385–386
Medicare Code Editor (MCE), 172
Medicare Physician Fee Schedule final rule (2019), 164–165
Medication administration, 86–87, 108
  data collection and, 41
Medication errors, 87
Meetings, 359–363
  agenda of, 360
  conducting and documenting, 359
  minutes of, 360–363
  for performance improvement, 390, 395–396
Memorandum, 359
Memos, 359

Mental health facility. *See* Behavioral health facilities
Metathesaurus, 159
Micromanagers, 364–365
MICs. *See* Medicaid Integrity Contractors
Minimum Data Set (MDS), 105, 212–213
Minimum Data Set 3.0 (MDS 3.0), 39
Minimum necessary, 299, 306
Mixed method research, 268
Mode, 252
Morbidity, 34, 272
  prevalence and incidence of, 148
Morphology axis, 168
Mortality, 272
  data, 34
  prevalence and incidence of, 148
MPI. *See* Master patient index
MRN. *See* Medical record number
MS-DRG grouper, 207–208
Multi-axial code structure, 162

**N**

NAM. *See* National Academy of Medicine
National Academy of Medicine (NAM), 24
National Association of Healthcare Access Management, 72
National Association of Social Workers, 106
National Cancer Institute's Surveillance, Epidemiology, and End Results (SEER) Program, 168
National Cancer Registry Association, 273
National Center for Health Statistics (NCHS), 274
National Committee for Quality Assurance (NCQA), 106, 150, 382–383
National Correct Coding Initiative (NCCI), 211
National coverage determination (NCD), 211
National Drug Codes (NDCs), 168–169
National Hospice and Palliative Care Organization (NHPCO), 108
National Institute of Mental Health, 106
National Institutes of Health (NIH), 20
National Integrated Accreditation for Healthcare Organizations (NIAHO), 23, 382
National Library of Medicine (NLM), 166
National Patient Safety Goals, 383
National policy, in health care, 148–149
National Trauma Data Bank, 274
National Uniform Billing Committee (NUBC), 218
National Vital Statistics System, 274
Nationwide Health Information Network (NHIN), 52–53
NCCI. *See* National Correct Coding Initiative
NCD. *See* National coverage determination
NCHS. *See* National Center for Health Statistics
NCQA. *See* National Committee for Quality Assurance
NDCs. *See* National Drug Codes
Negligence, 292
Neonatal records, 88
Network, 199
Network policies, 146
Newborns, admittance of, 71
NHIN. *See* Nationwide Health Information Network
NHPCO. *See* National Hospice and Palliative Care Organization
NIAHO. *See* National Integrated Accreditation for Healthcare Organizations
NIH. *See* National Institutes of Health
NLM. *See* National Library of Medicine

Nomenclature, 157–158
Nominal group technique, 400
Nonacute care providers, documentation in, 93–114
Nonrepudiation, 132
Normal curve, 256
Nosocomial infections, 87, 264
Notice of Privacy Practices, 303, 306
NUBC. *See* National Uniform Billing Committee
Nurse anesthetist, 6
Nurse midwife, 6
Nursery, 263
Nurses, 86–87
    clinical data and, 68
    in health care industry, 5–6
    patient plan of care and, 76
Nursing assessment, 86
Nursing home, 104*t*
Nursing Home Reform Act (1987), 105
Nursing progress notes, 86

## O

OASIS. *See* Outcome and Assessment Information Set
Objective, 75–76
    in operational planning, 334–335
Observation, 71–72
Obstetric records, 88
Occupancy, 14, 264
Occupational therapists (OTs), 107
Occupational therapy assistants (OTA), 107
OCE. *See* Outpatient code editor
Office of Inspector General (OIG), 20
Office of Population Censuses and Surveys (OPCS-4) Classification of Interventions and Procedures, 157
Office of the Inspector General, 386
Office of the National Coordinator for Health Information Technology (ONC), 20, 52–53
*Official Guidelines for Coding and Reporting*, 161
OIG. *See* Office of Inspector General
Operation, 88
Operational budget, 227–229
Operational planning, 334–338
    customer satisfaction in, 336–338
    goals and objectives in, 334–335
    policies and procedures for, 335–336
Operative definition, 268–269
Operative records, 88
    anesthesia data as, 88
    clinical data and, 88
    operative data as, 88
Operative report, 88
OPPS. *See* Outpatient Prospective Payment System
Optimizing, MS-DRG and, 176
Oral communication, 358
Order sets, 81–82
Order to admit
    clinical data flow and, 71–75
    patient registration department and, 72
    precertification and, 72, 73*f*
    registration process and, 73–75
Organization-wide orientation, 351–355
    building safety and security in, 354
    confidentiality in, 355
    customer service, 354
    infection control in, 354–355
    information systems in, 355
    personnel consideration in, 354
    quality in, 354

Organizational chart, 326
    medical staff, 328*f*
Organizational structure, 326–332
    accountability in, 328
    HIM department organization, 329–330
    HIM department workflow in, 330–332
    management responsibilities in, 329
    shared governance in, 328–329
OTA. *See* Occupational therapy assistants
OTs. *See* Occupational therapists
Out-of-pocket, 194, 199
Out-of-pocket costs, 18
Outcome, 76–78, 237, 273, 380
    measures and monitoring of, 390
Outcome and Assessment Information Set (OASIS), data sets and, 39, 110
Outlier payment, 209
Outliers, 251
    mean with, 252
Outpatient, 12
Outpatient Behavioral Health Coding Notes, 212
Outpatient code editor (OCE), 211
Outpatient Prospective Payment System (OPPS), 210
Outpatient Rehabilitation Coding Notes, 212
Outpatient status, 71–72
Outsourcing, 340

## P

PACS. *See* Picture archiving and communication system
PAI. *See* Patient assessment instrument
Pain management treatment centers, 109
Palliative care, 108
    in health care industry, 13
Paper-based record, data collection and, 40–41
Paper records, 130
    data collection and, 41
    optimum data source and, 246
Paperless environment, 113
PAs. *See* Physician assistants
Pathologists, 89
Patient account number, 37, 245
Patient assessment instrument (PAI), 212
Patient care
    continuity of, 305–306
    improvement of, 147
    plan, 9, 89
Patient education, health information uses and, 147
Patient financial services, 215–222
Patient information, statistical analysis of
    central tendency measures and, 249–252, 254
    measures of frequency and, 252, 256
    measures of variance and, 256–258
Patient-matching algorithms, 138
Patient portal, in electronic health records, 49
Patient Protection and Affordable Care Act (PPACA), 201
Patient registration, department for, 72
Patient Self-Determination Act, consent and, 296
Payback period, 225
Payers, 18, 66, 193–194, 240, 255, 255*t*, 310
Payment status indicator (SI), 211
PDF. *See* Printer-downloadable format
PDSA. *See* Plan, do, study, act method
Peer Review Organizations (PROs), 205
PEPPER. *See* Program for Evaluating Payment Patterns Electronic Report
*Per diem* (daily) rates, 206, 339–340
Percentage, 255–256, 276
    calculation of, 255–256

Performance improvement (PI), 244, 272, 391–408
    meetings, teams, committees, and consensus-building, 395–398
    plan, do, study, act method of, 391–392
    quality and, health care, 380–383
    Six Sigma and, 395, 395*f*
    tools for, 398
Performance improvement plan, 351
Performance standards, 347–348
Permitted disclosure, 302
Personal health record (PHR), 55
    confidentiality and, 303
Personal representative, 307
PERT chart, 405–408, 407*f*
Pharmacy and therapeutics (P&T) committee, 396
PHI. *See* Protected health information
Photocopying, 307
Photographs, 74
PHR. *See* Personal health record
Physiatrist, 107
Physical examination, 80
Physical therapists (PTs), 107
Physician, 78–86
    attending, 84, 239, 305–306
        consultations and, 84
        discharge summary and, 84–86
        orders and, 80–84
        progress notes and, 84
        registration process and, 72
        SOAP structure and, 75
    attribution, 272
    clinical data and, 75
    communicating with, 358
    in health care industry, 3–5
    special records and, 88–89
Physician assistants (PAs), 6
Physician-patient privilege, 299
Physician's orders, 3, 71
    form for, 41–42, 48
    nurse authentication of, 82, 86
PI. *See* Performance improvement
Picture archiving and communication system (PACS), 51
Pie charts, 276–280, 279*f*, 398
Pilot phase implementation, in EHR migration and implementation, 58
Pivot tables, 274–275, 277*f*
Plaintiff, 306–307
Plan, do, study, act method (PDSA), 391–392
Plan of care, 76
Planning
    operational, 334–338
        customer satisfaction in, 336–338
        goals and objectives in, 334–335
        policies and procedures for, 335–336
    strategic, 332, 334
        data and information governance, 333–334
        mission, vision, and values, 332–333
        rolling out the strategic plan, 334
POA. *See* Present on admission
Point-of-care documentation, 46–47
Point-of-care documentation system, 78–79
Policies
    in health care, 148–149
    in operational planning, 335–336
Population, 245–246
    retrieving data from, 245
    sampling of, 245–246

Postdischarge processing, 128–143
  abstracting and, 138–139
  identification of records and, 128–130
  master patient index and, 136
  quantitative analysis and, 131–134
  scanning, 130–131
  tracking records and, 141
  transcription and, 141
  workflow and, 141–143, 143f
Power of attorney, confidentiality and, 295–296
PPACA. See Patient Protection and Affordable
    Care Act
PPOs. See Preferred provider organizations
PPS. See Prospective payment system
Practice manager, 232–233
Precertification, 72, 73f
Precision, data quality and, 120t, 123
Preemption, 290
Preferred provider organizations (PPOs), 198,
    201
Premium, 194
  in insurance companies, 18
Present on admission (POA), 177–178, 184
Prevalence, 148, 272, 403
Preventive care, managed care as, 200
Preventive controls, 124–125, 385–386
Primary care physician (PCP), 105
  managed care and, 200
Primary care provider, 5, 94
Primary caregiver, 109
Primary data, 238
Primary payer, 67–68
Principal diagnosis, 172, 272
  definition of, 39–40
Principal procedure, 172–173, 272
Printer-downloadable format (PDF), 160
Privacy, confidentiality and, 299–305
Privacy officer, 301–302
Privacy regulations, HIPAA and, 301
Privileges, of physician, 4
Probabilistic method, 138
Problem focused examination, 164
Procedure
  clinical data and, 68
  in health care industry, 2
  in operational planning, 335–336
Process control chart, 392, 403
Productivity, 349
  calculations, 350–351
Profession, in health care industry, 2
Professional Standards Review Organizations
    (PSROs), 205
Professionals, in health care industry, 2
  allied, 6
  nurses, 5–6
  physician assistants, 6
  physicians, 3–5
Program for Evaluating Payment Patterns
    Electronic Report (PEPPER), 385
Progress notes, 108
  nursing, 86
  physicians and, 84
Project management, 379, 405, 409
  tools for, 405
Promoting Interoperability Program, 49
PROs. See Peer Review Organizations
Prospective consent, 306
Prospective payment system (PPS), 207, 213–214
Protected health information (PHI), 144
  HIPAA and, 301
Protocols, 81–82
Provider number, 210

Providers, of health care industry, 10–18
  continuity of care and, 14, 16
  evolving organizational models and, 17
  facility size and, 13–14
  inpatient, 11
  outpatient, 12
  ownership, 16
  patient population and, 12–13
  services and, 13
  tax status of, 16–17
PSROs. See Professional Standards Review
    Organizations
Psychiatric facility. See Behavioral health facilities
PTs. See Physical therapists
Public Law, 301

Q
QA. See Quality assurance
QIO. See Quality Improvement Organization
Qualitative research, 268
Quality
  coding, 178–185
    achieving, 179–180
    coding compliance, 181
    computer-assisted coding, 179
  in data collection, 34
    data sets in, 37, 39
    entering data and, 34–35
    master patient index and, 36–39
  in health care, 380–383, 387
    health care data and, 380
    history and evolution of, 381–382
    medical education and, 381–382
    outcomes measurement program for, 383
    patients first and, 380
    Quality Initiative and, 383–387
    standardization and accreditation in, 382
    timeline of, 389
Quality assurance (QA), 389
Quality control, 389
Quality improvement, 390–391
Quality Improvement Organization (QIO), 183,
    205, 384–385
Quality initiative
  CMS and, 384
  hospital-acquired condition reduction
    program, 384
  programs combating fraud, 385
  quality improvement organizations and,
    384–385
  value-based purchasing and, 383–384
Quality management, components of, 389–391
  outcome measures and monitoring, 390
  quality assurance, 389
  quality control, 389
  quality improvement, 390–391
Quality management theories, 387–389
  Crosby and, 388
  Deming and, 388
  Donabedian and, 388
  Juran and, 388
Quantitative analysis, 131–134
Quantitative research, 268
Query, 239–240, 246
Queues, 141–142

R
RACs. See Recovery Audit Contractors
Radiology and laboratory services, 101–102
Radiology data, 87
Radiology examinations, 87
RAI. See Resident Assessment Instrument

Random selection, 246, 385
RAPs. See Resident Assessment Protocols
Rate of occurrence, 264
Ratio, 255–256
RBRVS. See Resource-based relative value system
RCA. See Root cause analysis
RCM. See Revenue cycle management
Record retention schedule, 320
Record review, 315
  team, 315
  tracer methodology for, 318
  value of, 316
Records
  database building and, 36
  electronic chart completion tracking and, 134
  integrity and access, 143–146
  retrieval, 131
  security and privacy, 144–145
  sensitive, 306
    employee patient as, 307
    legal files as, 306
  storage and retention, 143–144
Recovery Audit Contractors (RACs), 183,
    385–386
Recredentialing, 272
Recruitment, 342–347
  assessment for, 346–347
  hiring process in, 343–345
  interviewing in, 345–346
Redacted, 239
Referral, 200
  of physicians, 4
Registered nurse (RN), 6, 104
Registrars, 72
Registration process, 73–75
Registry, 140
  definition of, 272
  other, 274
  trauma, 273–274
  tumor or cancer, 272–273
  vital statistics and, 274
Rehabilitation, physical medicine and, 13
Rehabilitation facilities, 13, 106–108, 314–315
  care providers in, 107
  data-collection issues, 108
  data sets and, 108
  length of stay in, 107
  licensure and accreditation for, 109
  services in, 107
  settings for, 107
Reimbursement, 18, 193–194, 214–215, 306
  access to health information and, 305–314
  calculation for MS-DRG, 209
  coded clinical data and, 178
  forms of, 194
  impact of coding on, 216
  methodologies of, 206–215
    capitation as, 206–207
    charges as, 206
    comparison of, 214–215
    discounted fee for service as, 206
    fee for service as, 206
    prospective payment systems as, 207–214
  paying for health care and, 193–206
  support and collection of, 147–148
Relational database, 36–37
Relative weight (RW), 209
Release of information (ROI), 145, 307–311
  authorized disclosures and, 307–308
  defective authorizations and, 308–309
  preparation of records for, 309–311
    certification of, 310

Release of information (ROI) (Continued)
  compensation of, 310
  distribution of, 311
  reproduction of, 310
  retrieval of, 310
  steps in, 311t
  validation and tracking of, 309–310
  special consents and, 309
Relevancy, data quality and, 120t, 124
Reliability, 179, 218
Remote patient monitoring, 112
Report, 239
  database and, 239
Reporting
  of coded clinical data, 178
  in health care industry, 21
Reproduction, of information for release, 310
Request for information, internal, 306
Request for proposal (RFP), 58
Required disclosure, 302
Research, 266–269, 271
  design, 268–269
  health information and, 149
Resident, in health care industry, 3
Resident Assessment Instrument (RAI), 105, 213
Resident Assessment Protocols (RAPs), 105
Resource-based relative value system (RBRVS),
    214
Resource intensity (RI), 169, 207–208
Resource utilization group (RUG), 212–213
Respite care, 109
Restoration, of lost information, 320
Restriction, 303
Retail care centers, 109
Retainer medicine, 202
Retention, 311–314, 342–347
  facility closure in, 311–312, 314
  patient rights and, 311–314
  policy, 311–312
Retrospective audit (review), 385–386
Retrospective consent, 306
Retrospective review, 272
Return on investment (ROI), 225–227
Revenue, 223
Revenue code, 211
Revenue cycle, 136, 385–386
Revenue cycle management (RCM), 148,
    215–222
RFP. See Request for proposal
RI. See Resource intensity
Right to complain, 304
Right to revoke, 304
Risk, assumption of, 196–198
Risk management, 316–320, 317f, 382
RN. See Registered nurse
ROI. See Release of information; Return on
    investment
Root cause analysis (RCA), 126–127
Rounding rule, 250
RUG. See Resource utilization group
Rule out, 75–76
RW. See Relative weight

S

Safety committee, 397
Same-day surgery records, 102
SAMHSA. See Substance Abuse and Mental
    Health Services Administration
Sample, of population, 245–246
Scanning, 130–131
Scope of work, 384
SCRUM, 407

SDLC. See System development life cycle
SDOs. See Standards-developing organizations
Secondary data, 239
  data collection and, 238, 240
  Quality Improvement Organization and, 384
Secondary payer, 67–68
Security, 299
  confidentiality and, 299
  destruction of information and, 310
  disaster planning and, 318–319
  restoration of lost information and, 320
  theft and tampering and, 319
Self-insurance, 201–203
Self-pay, 194
Semantic interoperability, 51
Semantic interpretability, 51
Sentinel event, 390
Severity of illness (SI), 91
Shared governance, in organizational structure,
    328–329
Short stay facility, 11
SI. See Severity of illness
Six Sigma, 395, 395f
Skewed, 256
Skilled nursing facility (SNF), 104t
Skilled Nursing Facility Prospective Payment
    System, 213–214
SNF. See Skilled nursing facility
SNOMED-CT. See Systemized Nomenclature of
    Medicine-Clinical Terms
Social determinants, of health, 30–31
Social media, 300
Social workers, 106
Socioeconomic data, 66–67
Span of control, 328
Special purpose classifications and code sets, 165
  Current Dental Terminology Codes, 169
  Diagnostic and Statistical Manual of Mental
      Disorders, Fifth Edition (DSM-5), 168
  ICD-O-3, 167–168, 168f
  National Drug Codes (NDCs), 168–169, 170t
  Systemized Nomenclature of Medicine-
      Clinical Terms (SNOMED CT)
    special purpose code sets and, 165–167,
        167f
  Systemized Nomenclature of Medicine-
      Clinical Terms (SNOMED-CT)
    ICD-10-CM codes and, 166
Special records
  autopsy reports as, 89
  clinical data and, 88
  intensive care unit records as, 88–89
  neonatal records as, 88
  operative records as, 88
  same-day surgery records as, 102
Specialized data collection systems, 272–274
Specialty care, 109
Sprinkler systems, fire damage and, 318
Staff model HMO, 201
Stakeholders, 58
Standard deviation, 256–258
Standardization, history and evolution of,
    381–382
Standards-developing organizations (SDOs), 54
Standards for code sets, 156–157
Standards of Ethical Coding, 157, 158f
Statistical process control, 392
Statistics, 237
  administration and, 148
  data reporting and, 271
  data retrieval and, 240
  health care formulas, 266

Statistics (Continued)
  institutional statistics, routine, 258–266
    admission and, 258–259
    average length of stay and, 260–262
    bed occupancy rate and, 264
    census and, 259, 262–263, 265f
    discharges and, 259
    hospital rates and percentages for,
        264–266
    length of stay and, 259–260
    transfers and, 262
  presentation and, 274–281
  registries, 272–273
Statute, 290, 314
Store-and-forward technology, 112
Strategic budget, 225
Strategic planning, 332, 334
  data and information governance, 333–334
  mission, vision, and values, 332–333
  rolling out the strategic plan, 334
Structural interoperability, 51
Structure, organizational, 326–332
  accountability in, 328
  HIM department organization, 329–330
  HIM department workflow in, 330–332
  management responsibilities in, 329
  shared governance in, 328–329
Subjective, 293
Subjective, objective, assessment, and plan
    (SOAP) format
  initial assessment and, 75, 77f
Subpoena, 293–295
Subpoena ad testificandum, 293–294
Subpoena duces tecum, 293–294
Substance Abuse and Mental Health
    Services Administration (SAMHSA),
    20, 106
Superbill, 217
Superuser, 59
Supportive standards, of Health level 7
    (HL7), 54
Surgeon, 88
Surplus, 17
Survey
  definition of, 401
  questions, 401t
  TJC accreditation and, 314–315
Swipe badge security feature, 319
Switchover implementation, in EHR migration
    and implementation, 59
Symptom, 68
Syntactic interoperability, 51
System development life cycle (SDLC), 57
Systemized Nomenclature of Medicine-Clinical
    Terms (SNOMED-CT)
  ICD-10-CM codes and, 166
  special purpose code sets and, 165–167, 167f

T

Tables, 274, 403
Tabular List of Diseases and Injuries, 161
Tampering, 319
Tax Equity and Fiscal Responsibility Act of 1982,
    205–206
Taxonomy, 159
Technical support hotline, 59–60
Telehealth, 110–114
Telemedicine, 110
Telephone orders (TOs), 82
The Joint Commission (TJC), 21–23, 382
  accreditation and, 314–315
  delinquent records and, 133–134

The Joint Commission (TJC) (Continued)
  H&P data collection and, 80
    operative report and, 88
    optimum data source and, 246
    timeliness and, 122
Theft, 319
Third-party payer, 18, 194, 255
Timekeeper, 363–364, 396
Timeliness, data quality and, 120t, 122–123
Timely processing, in coding quality, 179
Title II, of HIPAA, 301
TJC. See The Joint Commission
Topography axis, 168
Tort, 292
TOs. See Telephone orders
Tracer methodology, 318
Tracking records, 141
  batch by days processing and, 141
  efficiency and, 141
  for release, 310
Training, 367–373
  calendar of education, 369–370
  continuing education and, 371–373, 372f
  educating the public, 371
  in EHR migration and implementation, 59
  evaluation of, 370–371
  program, evaluating, 370–371
  session, planning for, 368–369
  technology, 369
Transaction code sets, 157
Transcription, postdischarge processing and, 141
Transfers, 262
Trauma registry, 273–274
Treatment
  clinical data and, 68
  physician's orders and, 81
Trend, 256
Triage, 99
TRICARE, 205
Trusted Exchange Framework and Common
    Agreement, 53
Tumor registry, 167–168, 273

**U**

UACDS. See Uniform Ambulatory Care Data Set
UB-04. See Uniform Bill

UCAOA. See Urgent Care Association of
    America
UCRs. See Usual, customary and reasonable fees
UHDDS. See Uniform Hospital Discharge Data
    Set
Unbilled list, 216
Uncompensated care, 204–205
Uniform Ambulatory Care Data Set (UACDS),
    98–99
Uniform Bill (UB-04), 218, 239–240
  defined data sets and, 39
  National Drug Codes and, 168–169
Uniform Hospital Discharge Data Set
    (UHDDS), 70f, 172, 184, 218,
    220f
  defined data sets and, 39
  discharge data set and, 92t–93t
Unity of command, 328
Upcoding, MS-DRG and, 176
UR. See Utilization review
Urgent, 71
Urgent Care Association of America (UCAOA), 95
Urgent care center, 95
U.S. Food and Drug Administration (FDA),
    National Drug Codes and, 168–169
U.S. Surgeon General, 148
Uses, of health information, 302–303
Usual, customary and reasonable fees (UCRs),
    206
Utilization review (UR), 90–91, 306
  data retrieval and, 244
  discharge and, 90–91

**V**

Validation, of record for release, 309–310
Validity, 179, 218
  data quality and, 120–121
Values statement, 333
Variable expenses, 227
Variance, 228–229
  measures of, 256–257
    definition of, 256–258
    normal curve and, 256
    population sampling and, 245–246
    skewedness and, 256
    standard deviation and, 256 258

Verbal orders (VOs), 82
Verification, 310
Veterans Health Administration (VHA),
    205
VHA. See Veterans Health Administration
Vicarious liability, 292
Vision, 333
Visit, 12, 94. See also Encounter
Vital records, 274
Vital signs, 86
Vital statistics, 34, 274
Vocational nurse, 5–6
Volume, in coding quality, 180
VOs. See Verbal orders

**W**

Water damage, 318–319
WHO. See World Health Organization
Workers' compensation, 307
Workflow, 330–332
  postdischarge processing and, 141–143
Workflow analysis, 330–331
Working DRG, 91
Working MS-DRG, 177
Workload, 348–349
World Health Organization (WHO), 159,
    167–168
Wraparound policies, 204
Wristband, 73–74, 75f
Written communication, 358–359

**X**

XML. See Extensible Markup Language
XP, 407

**Z**

Zero defects, 388

# Abbreviations

| | |
|---|---|
| **AAAHC** | Accreditation Association for Ambulatory Health Care |
| **AAPC** | American Academy of Professional Coders |
| **ABN** | Advance Beneficiary Notice |
| **ACA** | Affordable Care Act |
| **ACDIS** | Association of Clinical Documentation Improvement Specialists |
| **ACO** | Accountable Care Organization |
| **ACS** | American College of Surgeons |
| **ADA** | Americans With Disabilities Act |
| **ADLs** | activities of daily living |
| **AHA** | American Hospital Association |
| **AHIMA** | American Health Information Management Association |
| **AHRQ** | Agency for Healthcare Research and Quality |
| **AKA** | also known as |
| **ALOS** | average length of stay |
| **AMA** | against medical advice |
| **AMA** | American Medical Association |
| **AMRA** | American Medical Record Association |
| **ANA** | American Nursing Association |
| **AOA** | American Osteopathic Association |
| **APA** | American Psychiatric Association |
| **APC** | Ambulatory Payment Classification |
| **AP-DRG** | All Patient Diagnosis-Related Groups |
| **APR-DRG** | All Patient Refined Diagnosis-Related Groups |
| **APRN** | advanced practice registered nurse |
| **AR** | accounts receivable |
| **ARRA** | The American Recovery and Reinvestment Act |
| **ASC** | Ambulatory Surgery Center |
| **ATS** | American Trauma Society |
| **BCBSA** | Blue Cross and Blue Shield Association |
| **BCSW** | Board-Certified Social Worker |
| **BMI** | body mass index |
| **CABG** | coronary artery bypass graft |
| **CAC** | computer-assisted coding |
| **CAHIIM** | Commission on Accreditation of Health Informatics and Information Management |
| **CAP** | College of American Pathologists |
| **CARF** | Commission on Accreditation of Rehabilitation Facilities |
| **CBC** | complete blood count |
| **CC** | comorbidity or complication |
| **CCA** | certified coding associate |
| **CCC** | convenient care clinic |
| **CCHIIM** | Commission on Certification for Health Informatics and Information Management |
| **CCHIT** | Certification Commission for Health Information Technology |
| **CCI** | Correct Coding Initiative |
| **CCI** | Canadian Classification of Interventions |
| **CCS** | certified coding specialist |
| **CCS-P** | certified coding specialist–physician-based |
| **CCU** | coronary care unit |
| **CDC** | Centers for Disease Control and Prevention |
| **CDI** | clinical documentation improvement |
| **CDIP** | clinical documentation improvement professional |
| **CDM** | charge description master |
| **CDS** | clinical decision-making system |
| **CDT** | Current Dental Terminology |
| **CE** | continuing education |
| **CEO** | chief executive officer |
| **CEU** | continuing education unit |
| **CFO** | chief financial officer |
| **CFR** | Code of Federal Regulations |
| **CHAMPVA** | Civilian Health and Medical Program of the Veterans Administration |
| **CHAP** | Community Health Accreditation Program |
| **CHDA** | certified health data analyst |
| **CHF** | congestive heart failure |
| **CHIP** | Children's Health Insurance Program |
| **CHP** | certified in healthcare privacy |
| **CHPS** | certified in healthcare privacy and security |
| **CHS** | certified in healthcare security |
| **CIC** | certified hospital inpatient coder |
| **CIO** | chief information officer |
| **CLIA** | Clinical Laboratory Improvement Amendment |
| **CMAT** | case mix assessment tool |
| **CMG** | case mix group |
| **CMI** | case mix index |
| **CMS** | Centers for Medicare and Medicaid Services |
| **CNA** | certified nursing assistant |
| **CNO** | chief nursing officer |
| **COC** | certified hospital outpatient coder |
| **COO** | chief operating officer |
| **COP** | conditions of participation (Medicare) |
| **CPC** | certified professional coder |
| **CPOE** | computerized physician order entry |
| **CPT** | Current Procedural Terminology |
| **CQI** | continuous quality improvement |
| **CQM** | clinical quality measure |
| **CRNA** | certified registered nurse anesthetist |
| **CT** | computed tomography |
| **CTR** | certified tumor registrar |
| **CY** | calendar year |
| **DD** | date dictated |
| **DEEDS** | Data Elements for Emergency Department Systems |
| **DHHS** | Department of Health and Human Services |
| **DICOM** | Digital Imaging and Communications in Medicine |
| **DMADV** | definition, measurement, analysis, design, verification |
| **DMAIC** | definition, measurement, analysis, improvement, and control |
| **DME** | durable medical equipment |
| **DNFB** | discharged no final bill/discharged not final billed |
| **DNR** | do not resuscitate |
| **DNV** | Det Norske Veritas |
| **DO** | Doctor of Osteopathy |

| | |
|---|---|
| DOA | dead on arrival |
| DOB | date of birth |
| DRG | diagnosis-related group |
| DSM-5 | Diagnostic and Statistical Manual of Mental Disorders, 5th edition |
| DT | date transcribed |
| DTR | dietetic technician, registered |
| E/M | evaluation and management [code] |
| EBM | evidence-based medicine |
| ECG | electrocardiography |
| ED | emergency department |
| EDI | electronic data interchange |
| EDMS | electronic document management system |
| EEG | electroencephalography |
| EEOC | Equal Employment Opportunity Commission |
| EHR | electronic health record |
| EKG | electrocardiography |
| EMDS | emergency medical data set |
| EMPI | enterprise master patient index |
| EMTALA | Emergency Medical Treatment and Active Labor Act |
| ePHI | electronic protected health information |
| ESRD | end-stage renal disease |
| FAHIMA | Fellow of the American Health Information Management Association |
| FDA | Food and Drug Administration |
| FL | form locator |
| FLSA | Fair Labor Standards Act |
| FSMB | Federation of State Medical Boards |
| FTE | full-time equivalent |
| FY | fiscal year |
| GLOS | geometric length of stay |
| GMLOS | geometric mean length of stay |
| GUI | graphical user interface |
| H&P | History and Physical |
| HCA | home care aide |
| HCFA | Health Care Financing Administration (now CMS) |
| HCPCS | Healthcare Common Procedure Coding System |
| HFAP | Healthcare Facilities Accreditation Program |
| HFMA | Healthcare Financial Management Association |
| HH PPS | Home Health Prospective Payment System |
| HHRG | Home Health Resources Group |
| HHS | Department of Health and Human Services |
| HIAA | Health Insurance Association of America |
| HIE | health information exchange |
| HIM | health information management |
| HIMSS | Health Information Management Systems Society |
| HIPAA | Health Insurance Portability and Accountability Act |
| HIT | health information technology |
| HITECH | Health Information Technology for Economic and Clinical Health Act |
| HL7 | Health Level 7 |
| HMO | Health Maintenance Organization |
| HR | human resources |
| HRSA | Health Resources and Services Administration |
| ICD | International Classification of Diseases |
| ICD-0 | International Classification of Diseases for Oncology |
| ICD-0–3 | International Classification of Diseases for Oncology, Third Edition |
| ICD-9 | International Classification of Diseases, Ninth Revision |
| ICD-9-CM | International Classification of Diseases, Ninth Revision, Clinical Modification |
| ICD-10 | International Classification of Diseases, Tenth Revision |
| ICD-10-CM | International Classification of Diseases, Tenth Revision, Clinical Modification |
| ICD-10-PCS | International Classification of Diseases, Tenth Revision, Procedural Coding System |
| ICU | intensive care unit |
| IDS | integrated delivery system |
| IEEE | Institute of Electrical and Electronics Engineers |
| IHI | Institute for Healthcare Improvement |
| IHS | Indian Health Service |
| IHTSDO | International Health Terminology Standards Development Organisation |
| I-MAGIC | Interactive Map-Assisted Generation of ICD-10-CM Codes |
| IPA | Independent Practice Association |
| IPF PPS | Inpatient Psychiatric Facility Prospective Payment System |
| IPSD | inpatient service day |
| IRB | Institutional Review Board |
| IRF-PAI | Inpatient Rehabilitation Facility Patient Assessment Instrument |
| IS | intensity of service |
| ISO | International Standards Organization |
| IT | information technology |
| KPI | key performance indicator |
| LCD | local coverage determination |
| LOS | length of stay |
| LPN | licensed practical nurse |
| LTAC | long-term acute care |
| LTC | long-term care |
| LTCH-PPS | long-term care hospital prospective payment system |
| LVN | licensed vocational nurse |
| MAC | Medicare Administrative Contractor |
| MCC | major comorbidity or complication |
| MCE | Medicare Code Editor |
| MCO | managed care organization |
| MD | medical doctor |
| MDC | major diagnostic category |
| MDS | minimum data set |
| MEC | Medical Executive Committee |
| MI | myocardial infarction |
| MIC | Medicaid Integrity Contractor |
| MPI | master patient index |
| MRI | magnetic resonance imaging |
| MRN | medical record number |
| MS-DRG | Medicare Severity Diagnosis-related Group |
| NAM | National Academy of Medicine |
| NB | newborn |
| NCCI | National Correct Coding Initiative |
| NCD | National Coverage Determination |
| NCD | National Drug Code |
| NCHS | National Center for Health Statistics |
| NCI | National Cancer Institute |
| NCIPC | National Center for Injury Prevention and Control |
| NCQA | National Committee for Quality Assurance |
| NCVHS | National Committee on Vital and Health Statistics |
| NDC | National Drug Codes |
| NHIN | Nationwide Health Information Network |

| | |
|---|---|
| NHPCO | National Hospice and Palliative Care Organization |
| NHS | National Health Service |
| NIAHO | National Integrated Accreditation for Healthcare Organizations |
| NICU | neonatal intensive care unit |
| NIH | National Institutes of Health |
| NLM | National Library of Medicine |
| NLRA | National Labor Relations Act |
| NLRB | National Labor Relations Board |
| NMBE | National Board of Medical Examiners |
| NP | nurse practitioner |
| NPCR | National Program of Cancer Registries |
| NPI | National Provider Identifier |
| NUBC | National Uniform Billing Committee |
| OASIS | Outcome and Assessment Information Set |
| OB/GYN | obstetrics/gynecology |
| OCE | Outpatient Code Editor |
| OIG | Office of the Inspector General |
| ONC | Office of the National Coordinator of Health Information Technology |
| OPPS | outpatient prospective payment system |
| OR | operating room |
| OSHA | Occupational Safety and Health Administration |
| OT | occupational therapist |
| P&T | Pharmacy and Therapeutics |
| PA | physician assistant |
| PACS | picture archiving and communication system |
| PAI | patient assessment instrument |
| PCE | potentially compensable event |
| PCORI | Patient-Centered Outcomes Research Institute |
| PCP | primary care provider |
| PDCA | Plan, Do, Check, Act |
| PEPPER | Program for Evaluating Payment Patterns Electronic Reports |
| PERT | program evaluation and review technique |
| PET | positron emission tomography |
| PHI | protected health information |
| PHR | personal health record |
| PI | performance improvement |
| PIN | personal identification number |
| PIP | performance improvement plan |
| PKU | phenylketonuria |
| PPM | policy and procedure manual |
| PPO | preferred provider organization |
| PPS | prospective payment system |
| PT | physical therapist |
| QA | quality assurance |
| QI | quality improvement |
| QIO | Quality Improvement Organization |
| QM | quality management |
| RAC | Recovery Audit Contractor |
| RAI | Resident Assessment Instrument |

| | |
|---|---|
| RAID | redundant array of independent disks |
| RAP | resident assessment protocol |
| RBRVS | resource-based relative value system |
| RCM | revenue cycle management |
| RD | registered dietician |
| RFP | request for proposal |
| RHIA | registered health information administrator |
| RHIO | Regional Health Information Organization |
| RHIT | registered health information technician |
| RI | resource intensity |
| RM | risk management |
| RN | registered nurse |
| ROI | release of information |
| RPM | remote patient monitoring |
| RT | respiratory therapist |
| RUG | resource utilization group |
| RW | relative weight |
| SAMHSA | Substance Abuse and Mental Health Services Administration |
| SAN | storage area network |
| SDLC | system development life cycle |
| SDO | standards development organization |
| SEER | Surveillance, Epidemiology, and End Results |
| SI | severity of illness |
| SLP | speech/language therapist |
| SNF | skilled nursing facility |
| SNOMED CT | Systematized Nomenclature of Medicine Clinical Terms |
| SOAP | Subjective, Objective, Assessment, Plan |
| SOW | statement of work |
| SSN | Social Security Number |
| TD | terminal digit (filing) |
| TEFRA | Tax Equity and Fiscal Responsibility Act |
| TJC | The Joint Commission |
| TO | telephone order |
| UA | urinalysis |
| UACDS | Uniform Ambulatory Care Data Set |
| UB-04 | uniform bill |
| UCA | Urgent Care Association |
| UCR | usual, customary, and reasonable [fee] |
| UHDDS | Uniform Hospital Discharge Data Set |
| UM | utilization management |
| UPIN | unique personal/physician identification number |
| UR | utilization review |
| USMLE | United States Medical Licensing Examination |
| VA | Department of Veterans Affairs |
| VBP | value-based purchasing |
| VHA | Veterans Health Administration |
| VO | verbal order |
| VTE | venous thromboembolism |
| WBC | white blood cell |
| WHO | World Health Organization |
| YTD | year-to-date |